WG
148
OTT

A08775

D1585583

ECHOCARDIOGRAPHY
REVIEW GUIDE

MEDICAL LIBRARY
MORRISTON HOSPITAL

SECOND EDITION

ECHOCARDIOGRAPHY REVIEW GUIDE

Companion to the Textbook of Clinical Echocardiography

CATHERINE M. OTTO, MD

J. Ward Kennedy-Hamilton Endowed Professor of Cardiology
Director, Training Program in Cardiovascular Disease
University of Washington School of Medicine;
Associate Director, Echocardiography Laboratory
Co-Director, Adult Congenital Heart Disease Clinic
University of Washington Medical Center
Seattle, Washington

REBECCA GIBBONS SCHWAEGLER, BS, RDCS

Cardiac Sonographer
University of Washington Medical Center
Seattle, Washington

ROSARIO V. FREEMAN, MD

Associate Professor of Medicine
University of Washington School of Medicine;
Director, Echocardiography Laboratory
Medical Director, Coronary Care Unit
University of Washington Medical Center
Seattle, Washington

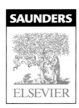

SAUNDERS

ELSEVIER

1600 John F. Kennedy Blvd.
Ste 1800
Philadelphia, PA 19103-2899

ECHOCARDIOGRAPHY REVIEW GUIDE: ISBN: 978-1-4377-2021-1
COMPANION TO THE TEXTBOOK OF CLINICAL
ECHOCARDIOGRAPHY, SECOND EDITION
Copyright © 2011, 2008 by Saunders, an imprint of Elsevier Inc. All rights reserved.

No part of this publication may be reproduced or transmitted in any form or by any means, electronic or
mechanical, including photocopying, recording, or any information storage and retrieval system, without
permission in writing from the publisher. Details on how to seek permission, further information about the
Publisher's permissions policies and our arrangements with organizations such as the Copyright Clearance
Center and the Copyright Licensing Agency, can be found at our website: www.elsevier.com/permissions.

This book and the individual contributions contained in it are protected under copyright by the Publisher
(other than as may be noted herein).

Notices

Knowledge and best practice in this field are constantly changing. As new research and experience
broaden our understanding, changes in research methods, professional practices, or medical treatment
may become necessary.

Practitioners and researchers must always rely on their own experience and knowledge in evaluating
and using any information, methods, compounds, or experiments described herein. In using such
information or methods they should be mindful of their own safety and the safety of others, including
parties for whom they have a professional responsibility.

With respect to any drug or pharmaceutical products identified, readers are advised to check the most
current information provided (i) on procedures featured or (ii) by the manufacturer of each product to be
administered, to verify the recommended dose or formula, the method and duration of administration,
and contraindications. It is the responsibility of practitioners, relying on their own experience and
knowledge of their patients, to make diagnoses, to determine dosages and the best treatment for each
individual patient, and to take all appropriate safety precautions.

To the fullest extent of the law, neither the Publisher nor the authors, contributors, or editors assume
any liability for any injury and/or damage to persons or property as a matter of products liability,
negligence or otherwise, or from any use or operation of any methods, products, instructions, or ideas
contained in the material herein.

International Standard Book Number: 978-1-4377-2021-1

Acquisitions Editor: Natasha Andjelkovic
Developmental Editor: Brad McIlwain
Publishing Services Manager: Anne Altepeter
Project Manager: Louise King
Designer: Louis Forgione

Printed in the United States of America

Last digit is the print number: 9 8 7 6 5 4 3 2 1

Working together to grow
libraries in developing countries

www.elsevier.com | www.bookaid.org | www.sabre.org

ELSEVIER   BOOK AID International   Sabre Foundation

INTRODUCTION

ECHOCARDIOGRAPHY REVIEW GUIDE, SECOND EDITION

A companion workbook for the fourth edition of the *Textbook of Clinical Echocardiography*

This *Echocardiography Review Guide* complements the *Textbook of Clinical Echocardiography*, fourth edition, providing a review of basic principles, additional details of data acquisition and interpretation, and a step-by-step approach to patient examination for each diagnosis. In addition, self-assessment questions allow the reader to be more actively involved in the learning process. All the self-assessment questions in the second edition are new and supplement the questions available in the first edition.

This book will be of interest to practicing cardiologists and sonographers as a quick update on echocardiography and will be of value to cardiology fellows and cardiac sonographer students who are mastering the material for the first time. Cardiac anesthesiologists will find helpful information about details of the examination and a chapter dedicated to intraoperative transesophageal echocardiography. In addition, primary care physicians using handheld echocardiography can use this book to get started and to improve their echocardiography skills. Multiple-choice questions provide a review and self-assessment for those preparing for echocardiography examinations and may be useful in echocardiography laboratories for continuous quality improvement processes.

The chapters are arranged in the same order as the *Textbook of Clinical Echocardiography*, and we recommend that these two books be used in parallel. As in the textbook, there are introductory chapters on basic principles of image acquisition, transthoracic and transesophageal echocardiography, other echocardiographic modalities, and clinical indications. Each of the subsequent chapters focuses on a specific clinical diagnosis, including ventricular systolic and diastolic function, ischemic cardiac disease, cardiomyopathies, valve stenosis and regurgitation, prosthetic valves, endocarditis, cardiac masses, aortic disease, adult congenital heart disease, and intraoperative transesophageal echocardiography.

A step-by-step approach to patient examination is detailed. Information is conveyed in bullet points, with each set of major principles followed by a list of key points. Potential pitfalls are identified, and approaches to avoiding errors are provided. Data measurements and calculations are explained with specific examples. Numerous illustrations with detailed figure legends demonstrate each major point and guide the reader through the teaching points. At the end of each chapter, the short Echo Review Guide from the *Textbook of Clinical Echocardiography* is included for quick reference. Self-assessment questions help the reader consolidate the information and identify areas where further study is needed. Along with the correct answer to each question, there is a brief discussion of how that answer was determined and why the other potential answers are not correct.

This review guide is intended as an adjunct to formal training programs in echocardiography; a book does not replace hands-on training or practical experience. The three of us fully endorse current standards for education and training of physicians and sonographers in clinical cardiac ultrasound as provided by the American Society of Echocardiography, American Heart Association, American College of Cardiology, and Society of Cardiovascular Anesthesiologists. We support training in accredited programs with formal certification of sonographers and evaluation of physician competency. The material in this book reflects the clinical practice of echocardiography at one point in time. Cardiac imaging is a rapidly changing field, and we encourage our readers to stay up to date by reading journals and other online sources, and by attending national meetings and continuing medical education courses.

ACKNOWLEDGMENTS

It is never possible to fully acknowledge all those who help make a book possible; however, we would like to thank some of those who helped us along the way. First, the cardiac sonographers at the University of Washington deserve our special appreciation for the excellence of their imaging skills and the time they dedicated to acquiring additional images for us and discussing the finer points of data acquisition: Pamela Clark, RDCS; Sarah Curtis, RDCS; Caryn D'Jang, RDCS; Michelle Fujioka, RDCS; Jennifer Gregov, RDCS; Yelena Kovalenko, RDCS; Carol Kraft, RDCS; Chris McKenzie, RDCS; Amy Owens, RDCS; Joannalyn Sangco, RDCS; and Todd Zwink, RDCS. Theresa Shugart and Joan Raney in the Cardiology Division also helped greatly in several aspects of book preparation. Special thanks are due to the many readers who provided comments and input on the text and questions. Our appreciation extends to Natasha Andjelkovic and Louise King at Elsevier and the production team who supported this project and helped us make it a reality.

Finally, we all want to sincerely thank our families: not only our husbands for their unwavering and continual encouragement, but even the younger members—Vea, Remy, Brendan, Sarah, Claire, Jack, and Anna—for their support and patience in the book-writing process. This book would not have been possible without their helping us find the time to complete it.

Rosario V. Freeman, MD
Catherine M. Otto, MD
Rebecca Gibbons Schwaegler, BS, RDCS

CONTENTS

GLOSSARY

2D = two-dimensional
3D = three-dimensional
A-long = apical long-axis
A-mode = amplitude mode (amplitude versus depth)
A = late diastolic ventricular filling velocity with atrial contraction
A′ = diastolic tissue Doppler velocity with atrial contraction
A2C = apical two-chamber
A4C = apical four-chamber
AcT = acceleration time
AF = atrial fibrillation
AMVL = anterior mitral valve leaflet
ant = anterior
Ao = aortic or aorta
AR = aortic regurgitation
AS = aortic stenosis
ASD = atrial septal defect
ATVL = anterior tricuspid valve leaflet
AV = atrioventricular
AVA = aortic valve area
AVR = aortic valve replacement
BAV = bicuspid aortic valve
BP = blood pressure
BSA = body surface area
c = propagation velocity of sound in tissue
CAD = coronary artery disease
cath = cardiac catheterization
cm/s = centimeters per second
cm = centimeters
CMR = cardiac magnetic resonance imaging
CO = cardiac output
cos = cosine
CS = coronary sinus
CSA = cross-sectional area
CT = computed tomography
CW = continuous wave
Cx = circumflex coronary artery
D = diameter
DA = descending aorta
dB = decibels
dP/dt = rate of change in pressure over time
dT/dt = rate of increase in temperature
dyne $\cdot$ s $\cdot$ cm^{-5} = units of resistance
E = early diastolic peak velocity
E′ = early diastolic tissue Doppler velocity
ECG = electrocardiogram

echo = echocardiography
ED = end-diastole
EDD = end-diastolic dimension
EDV = end-diastolic volume
EF = ejection fraction
endo = endocardium
epi = epicardium
EPSS = E-point septal separation
EROA = effective regurgitant orifice area
ES = end-systole
ESD = end-systolic dimension
ESV = end-systolic volume
ETT = exercise treadmill test
Δf = frequency shift
f = frequency
FL = false lumen
F_n = near field frequency
F_o = resonance frequency
F_s = scattered frequency
FSV = forward stroke volume
F_t = transmitted frequency
HCM = hypertrophic cardiomyopathy
HPRF = high pulse repetition frequency
HR = heart rate
HV = hepatic vein
Hz = Hertz (cycles per second)
I = intensity of ultrasound exposure
IAS = interatrial septum
inf = inferior
IV = intravenous
IVC = inferior vena cava
IVCT = isovolumic contraction time
IVRT = isovolumic relaxation time
kHz = kilohertz
L = length
LA = left atrium
LAA = left atrial appendage
LAD = left anterior descending coronary artery
LAE = left atrial enlargement
lat = lateral
LCC = left coronary cusp
LMCA = left main coronary artery
LPA = left pulmonary artery
LSPV = left superior pulmonary vein
L-TGA = congenitally corrected transposition of the great arteries
LV = left ventricle

LV-EDP = left ventricular end-diastolic pressure
LVH = left ventricular hypertrophy
LVID = left ventricular internal dimension
LVOT = left ventricular outflow tract
M-mode = motion display (depth versus time)
MAC = mitral annular calcification
MI = myocardial infarction
MR = mitral regurgitation
MS = mitral stenosis
MVA = mitral valve area
MVL = mitral valve leaflet
MVR = mitral valve replacement
n = number of subjects
NBTE = nonbacterial thrombotic endocarditis
NCC = noncoronary cusp
ΔP = pressure gradient
P = pressure
PA = pulmonary artery
PAP = pulmonary artery pressure
PDA = patent ductus arteriosus or posterior descending artery (depends on context)
PE = pericardial effusion
PEP = preejection period
PET = positron-emission tomography
PISA = proximal isovelocity surface area
PLAX = parasternal long-axis
PM = papillary muscle
PMVL = posterior mitral valve leaflet
post = posterior (or inferior-lateral) ventricular wall
PR = pulmonic regurgitation
PRF = pulse repetition frequency
PRFR = peak rapid filling rate
PS = pulmonic stenosis
PSAX = parasternal short-axis
PCI = percutaneous coronary intervention
PV = pulmonary vein
PVC = premature ventricular contraction
PVR = pulmonary vascular resistance
PWT = posterior wall thickness
Q = volume flow rate
Q_p = pulmonic volume flow rate
Q_s = systemic volume flow rate
r = correlation coefficient
R = ventricular radius
R_{FR} = regurgitant instantaneous flow rate
RA = right atrium
RAE = right atrial enlargement
RAO = right anterior oblique
RAP = right atrial pressure
RCA = right coronary artery
RCC = right coronary cusp

Re = Reynolds number
RF = regurgitant fraction
RJ = regurgitant jet
R_o = radius of microbubble
ROA = regurgitant orifice area
RPA = right pulmonary artery
RSPV = right superior pulmonary vein
RSV = regurgitant stroke volume
RV = right ventricle or regurgitant volume, depending on context
RVE = right ventricular enlargement
RVH = right ventricular hypertrophy
RVOT = right ventricular outflow tract
s = second
SAM = systolic anterior motion
SC = subcostal
SEE = standard error of the estimate
SPPA = spatial peak pulse average
SPTA = spatial peak temporal average
SSN = suprasternal notch
ST = septal thickness
STJ = sinotubular junction
STVL = septal tricuspid valve leaflet
SV = stroke volume or sample volume (depends on context)
SVC = superior vena cava
T 1/2 = pressure half-time
TD = thermodilution
TEE = transesophageal echocardiography
TGA = transposition of the great arteries
TGC = time gain compensation
Th = wall thickness
TL = true lumen
TN = true negatives
TOF = tetralogy of Fallot
TP = true positives
TPV = time to peak velocity
TR = tricuspid regurgitation
TS = tricuspid stenosis
TSV = total stroke volume
TTE = transthoracic echocardiography
TV = tricuspid valve
v = velocity
V = volume or velocity (depends on context)
VAS = ventriculo-atrial septum
Veg = vegetation
V_{max} = maximum velocity
VSD = ventricular septal defect
VTI = velocity-time integral
WPW = Wolff-Parkinson-White syndrome
Z = acoustic impedance

Symbols	Greek Name	Used for
α	alpha	frequency
γ	gamma	viscosity
Δ	delta	difference
θ	theta	angle
λ	lambda	wavelength
μ	mu	micro-
π	pi	mathematical constant (approx. 3.14)
ρ	rho	tissue density
σ	sigma	wall stress
τ	tau	time constant of ventricular relaxation

UNITS OF MEASURE

Variable	Unit	Definition
Amplitude	dB	Decibels = a logarithmic scale describing the amplitude ("loudness") of the sound wave
Angle	degrees	Degree = $(\pi/180)$rad. Example: intercept angle
Area	cm^2	Square centimeters. A two-dimensional measurement (e.g., end-systolic area) or a calculated value (e.g., continuity equation valve area)
Frequency (f)	Hz kHz MHz	Hertz (cycles per second) Kilohertz = 1000 Hz Megahertz = 1 million Hz
Length	cm mm	Centimeter (1/100 m) Millimeter (1/1000 m or 1/10 cm)
Mass	g	Grams. Example: LV mass
Pressure	mm Hg	Millimeters of mercury, 1 mm Hg = 1333.2 dyne/cm^2, where dyne measures force in $cm \cdot g \cdot s^{-2}$
Resistance	$dyne \cdot s \cdot cm^{-5}$	Measure of vascular resistance
Time	s ms μs	Second Millisecond (1/1000 s) Microsecond
Ultrasound intensity	W/cm^2 mW/cm^2	Where watt (W) = joule per second and joule = $m^2 \cdot kg \cdot s^{-2}$ (unit of energy)
Velocity (v)	m/s cm/s	Meters per second Centimeters per second
Velocity-time integral (VTI)	cm	Integral of the Doppler velocity curve (cm/s) over time (s), in units of cm

Variable	Unit	Definition
Volume	cm^3	Cubic centimeters
	mL	Milliliter, 1 mL = 1 cm^3
	L	Liter = 1000 mL
Volume flow rate (Q)	L/min	Rate of volume flow across a valve or in cardiac output
	mL/s	L/min = liters per minute
		mL/s = milliliters per second
Wall stress unit	$dyne/cm^2$	Units of meridional or circumferential wall stress
	$kdyn/cm^2$	Kilodynes per cm^2
	kPa	Kilopascals, where 1 kPa = 10 $kdyn/cm^2$

KEY EQUATIONS

Ultrasound physics

Frequency	f = cycles/s = Hz
Wavelength	$\lambda = c/f = 1.54/f$ (MHz)
Doppler equation	$v = c \times \Delta F/[2\ F_T(\cos\theta)]$
Bernoulli equation	$\Delta P = 4V^2$

LV imaging

Stroke volume	SV = EDV − ESV
Ejection fraction	EF (%) = (SV/EDV) × 100%
Wall stress	$\sigma = PR/2Th$

Doppler ventricular function

Stroke volume	SV = CSA × VTI
Rate of pressure rise	dP/dt = 32 mm Hg/time from 1 to 3 m/s of MR CW jet (sec)

Pulmonary pressures and resistance

Pulmonary systolic pressure $\quad PAP_{systolic} = 4(V_{TR})^2 + RAP$

PAP (when PS is present)
$PAP_{systolic} = [4(V_{TR})^2 + RAP] - \Delta P_{RV-PA}$

Pulmonary vascular resistance $\quad PVR \cong 10(V_{TR})/VTI_{RVOT}$

Aortic stenosis

Maximum pressure gradient $\quad \Delta P_{max} = 4(V_{max})^2$ (integrate over ejection period for mean gradient)

Continuity equation valve area
$AVA\ (cm^2) = [\pi(LVOT_D/2)^2 \times VTI_{LVOT}]/VTI_{AS-Jet}$

Simplified continuity equation
$AVA\ (cm^2) = [\pi(LVOT_D/2)^2 \times V_{LVOT}]/V_{AS-Jet}$

Velocity ratio $\quad$ Velocity ratio = V_{LVOT}/V_{AS-Jet}

Mitral stenosis

Pressure half-time valve area $\quad MVA_{Doppler} = 220/T\ ½$

Aortic regurgitation

Total stroke volume
$TSV = SV_{LVOT} = (CSA_{LVOT} \times VTI_{LVOT})$

Forward stroke volume
$FSV = SV_{MA} = (CSA_{MA} \times VTI_{MA})$

Regurgitant volume $\quad$ RV = TSV − FSV

Regurgitant orifice area $\quad ROA = RSV/VTI_{AR}$

Mitral regurgitation

Total stroke volume
$TSV = SV_{MA} = (CSA_{MA} \times VTI_{MA})$ *or 2D LV stroke volume*

Forward stroke volume
$FSV = SV_{LVOT} = (CSA_{LVOT} \times VTI_{LVOT})$

Regurgitant volume $\quad$ RV = TSV − FSV

Regurgitant orifice area $\quad ROA = RV/VTI_{MR}$

PISA method Regurgitant flow rate $\quad R_{FR} = 2\pi r^2 \times V_{aliasing}$

Orifice area (maximum) $\quad ROA_{max} = R_{FR}/V_{MR}$

Regurgitant volume $\quad$ RV = ROA × VTI_{MR}

Aortic dilation

Predicted sinus diameter
  Children (<18 years): predicted sinus dimension = 1.02 + (0.98 BSA)
  Adults (age 18–40 years): predicted sinus dimension = 0.97 + (1.12 BSA)
  Adults (>40 years): predicted sinus dimension = 1.92 + (0.74 BSA)
Ratio = measured maximum diameter/predicted maximum diameter

Pulmonary (Q_p) to Systemic (Q_s) Shunt Ratio

$$Qp{:}Qs = [CSA_{PA} \times VTI_{PA}]/[CSA_{LVOT} \times VTI_{LVOT}]$$

1 Principles of Echocardiographic Image Acquisition and Doppler Analysis

BASIC PRINCIPLES	Color Doppler
Ultrasound Waves	Continuous Wave (CW) Doppler
Transducers	Doppler Artifacts
Ultrasound Imaging	Bioeffects and Safety
Principles	THE ECHO EXAM
Imaging Artifacts	SELF-ASSESSMENT QUESTIONS
Doppler	
Pulsed Doppler	

BASIC PRINCIPLES

- Knowledge of basic ultrasound principles is needed for interpretation of images and Doppler data.
- Appropriate adjustment of instrument parameters is needed to obtain diagnostic information.

Key points:

- ❏ The appropriate ultrasound modality (two-dimensional [2D] imaging, pulsed Doppler color Doppler, etc.) is chosen for each type of needed clinical information.
- ❏ Current instrumentation allows modification of many parameters during data acquisition, such as depth, gain, harmonic imaging, wall filters, and so on.
- ❏ Artifacts must be distinguished from anatomic findings on ultrasound images.
- ❏ Accurate Doppler measurements depend on details of both blood flow interrogation and instrument acquisition parameters.

Ultrasound waves

- Ultrasound waves (Table 1-1) are mechanical vibrations with basic descriptors including:
  - Frequency (cycles per second = Hz, 1000 cycles/second = MHz)
  - Propagation velocity (about 1540 m/s in blood)
  - Wavelength (equal to the propagation velocity divided by frequency)
  - Amplitude (decibels or dB)

- Ultrasound waves interact with tissues (Table 1-2) in four different ways:
  - Reflection (used to create ultrasound images)
  - Scattering (the basis of Doppler ultrasound)
  - Refraction (used to focus the ultrasound beam)
  - Attenuation (loss of signal strength in the tissue)

Key points:

- ❏ Tissue penetration is greatest with a lower frequency transducer (e.g., 2-3 MHz)
- ❏ Image resolution is greatest (about 1 mm) with a higher frequency transducer (e.g., 5-7.5 MHz) (Figure 1–1)
- ❏ Amplitude ("loudness") is described using the logarithmic decibel (dB) scale; a 6 dB change represents a doubling or halving of signal amplitude.
- ❏ Acoustic impedance depends on tissue density and the propagation velocity of ultrasound in that tissue.
- ❏ Ultrasound reflection occurs at smooth tissue boundaries with different acoustic impedances (such as between blood and myocardium). Reflection is greatest when the ultrasounds beam is *perpendicular* to the tissue interface.
- ❏ Ultrasound scattering that occurs with small structures (such as red blood cells) is used to generate Doppler signals. Doppler velocity recordings are most accurate when the ultrasound beam is *parallel* to the blood flow direction.

1

TABLE 1-1 Ultrasound Waves

	Definition	Examples	Clinical Implications
Frequency (f)	The number of cycles per second in an ultrasound wave f = cycles/s = Hz	Transducer frequencies are measured in MHz (1,000,000 cycles/s). Doppler signal frequencies are measured in KHz (1000 cycles/s).	Different transducer frequencies are used for specific clinical applications because the transmitted frequency affects ultrasound tissue penetration, image resolution and the Doppler signal.
Velocity of propagation (c)	The speed that ultrasound travels through tissue	The average velocity of ultrasound in soft tissue about 1540 m/s.	The velocity of propagation is similar in different soft tissues (blood, myocardium, liver, fat, etc.) but is much lower in lung and much higher in bone.
Wavelength (λ)	The distance between ultrasound waves: $\lambda = c/f = 1.54/f$ (MHz)	Wavelength is shorter with a higher frequency transducer and longer with a lower frequency transducer.	Image resolution is greatest (about 1 mm) with a shorter wavelength (higher frequency). Depth of tissue penetration is greatest with a longer wavelength (lower frequency).
Amplitude (dB)	Height of the ultrasound wave or "loudness" measured in decibels (dB)	A log scale is used for dB On the dB scale, 80 dB represents a 10,000-fold and 40 dB indicates a 100-fold increase in amplitude.	A very wide range of amplitudes can be displayed using a gray scale display for both imaging and spectral Doppler.

TABLE 1-2 Ultrasound Tissue Interaction

	Definition	Examples	Clinical Implications
Acoustic impedance (Z)	A characteristic of each tissue defined by tissue density (ρ) and propagation of velocity (c) as: $Z = \rho \times c$	Lung has a low density and slow propagation velocity, whereas bone has a high density and fast propagation velocity. Soft tissues have smaller differences in tissue density and acoustic impedance.	Ultrasound is reflected from boundaries between tissues with differences in acoustic impedance (e.g., blood versus myocardium).
Reflection	Return of ultrasound signal to the transducer from a smooth tissue boundary	Reflection is used to generate 2D cardiac images.	Reflection is greatest when the ultrasound beam is perpendicular to the tissue interface.
Scattering	Radiation of ultrasound in multiple directions from a small structure, such as blood cells	The change in frequency of signals scattered from moving blood cells is the basis of Doppler ultrasound.	The amplitude of scattered signals is 100 to 1000 times less than reflected signals.
Refraction	Deflection of ultrasound waves from a straight path due to differences in acoustic impedance	Refraction is used in transducer design to focus the ultrasound beam.	Refraction in tissues results in double image artifacts.
Attenuation	Loss in signal strength due to absorption of ultrasound energy by tissues	Attenuation is frequency dependent with greater attenuation (less penetration) at higher frequencies.	A lower frequency transducer may be needed for apical views or in larger patients on transthoracic imaging.
Resolution	The smallest resolvable distance between two specular reflectors on an ultrasound image	Resolution has three dimensions—along the length of the beam (axial), lateral across the image (azimuthal), and in the elevational plane.	Axial resolution is most precise (as small as 1 mm), so imaging measurements are best made along the length of the ultrasound beam.

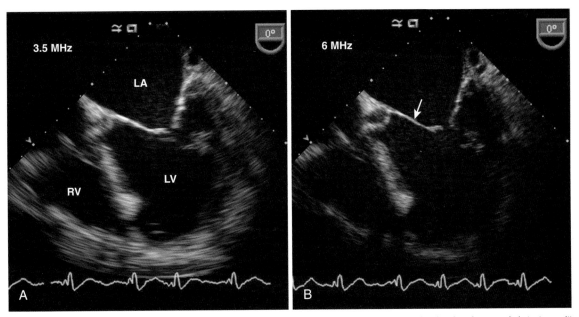

Figure 1–1. The effect of transducer frequency on penetration and resolution is shown by this transesophageal 4-chamber view recorded at a transmitted frequency of (*A*) 3.5 MHz and (*B*) 6 MHz. The higher frequency transducer provides better resolution—for example, the mitral leaflets (*arrow*) look thin, but the depth of penetration of the signal is very poor so the apical half of the LV is not seen. With the lower frequency transducer, improved tissue penetration provides a better image of the LV apex but image resolution is poorer, with the mitral leaflets looking thicker and less well defined.

❏ Refraction of ultrasound can result in imaging artifacts due to deflection of the ultrasound beam from a straight path.

Transducers

■ Ultrasound transducers use a piezoelectric crystal to alternately transmit and receive ultrasound signals (Figure 1–2).
■ Transducers are configured for specific imaging approaches—transthoracic, transesophageal, intracardiac, and intravascular (Table 1-3).
■ The basic characteristics of a transducer are:
  • Transmission frequency (from 2.5 MHz for transthoracic to 20 MHz for intravascular ultrasound)
  • Bandwidth (range of frequencies in the transmitted ultrasound pulse)
  • Pulse repetition frequency (the number of transmission-receive cycles per second)
  • Focal depth (depends on beam shape and focusing)
  • Aperture (size of the transducer face or "footprint")
  • Power output

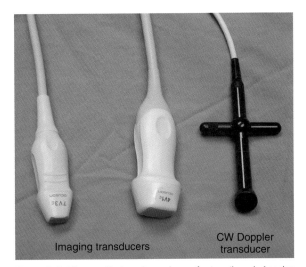

Imaging transducers

CW Doppler transducer

Figure 1–2. The specific transducer chosen for transthoracic imaging depends on the transmitted frequency, transducer size, and the specific application. A small phased array imaging transducer used in children and to view the apex in adults; a larger lower frequency phased array imaging transducer for better ultrasound penetration; and a non-imaging dedicated dual-crystal continuous wave Doppler transducer are shown here. Typically, multiple transducers are used during the examination.

Key points:

❏ The time delay between transmission of an ultrasound burst and detection of the reflected wave indicates the depth of the tissue reflector.
❏ The pulse repetition frequency is an important factor in image resolution and frame rate.

❏ A shorter transmitted pulse length results in improved depth (or axial) resolution.
❏ A wider bandwidth provides better resolution of structures distant from the transducer.
❏ The shape of the ultrasound beam depends on several complex factors. Each type of

TABLE 1-3 Ultrasound Transducers

	Definition	Examples	Clinical Implications
Type	Transducer characteristics and configuration Most cardiac transducers use phased array of piezoelectric crystals	Transthoracic (adult and pediatric) Non-imaging CW Doppler 3D echocardiography TEE Intracardiac	Each transducer type is optimized for a specific clinical application. More than one transducer may be needed for a full examination.
Transmission frequency	The central frequency emitted by the transducer	Transducer frequencies vary from 2.5 MHz for transthoracic echo to 20 MHz for intravascular imaging.	A higher frequency transducer provides improved resolution but less penetration. Doppler signals are optimal at a lower transducer frequency than used for imaging.
Power output	The amount of ultrasound energy emitted by the transducer	An increase in transmitted power increases the amplitude of the reflected ultrasound signals.	Excessive power output may result in bioeffects measured by the mechanical and thermal indexes.
Bandwidth	The range of frequencies in the ultrasound pulse	Bandwidth is determined by transducer design.	A wider bandwidth allows improved axial resolution for structures distant from the transducer.
Pulse (or burst) length	The length of the transmitted ultrasound signal	A higher frequency signal can be transmitted in a shorted pulse length compared with a lower frequency signal.	A shorter pulse length improves axial resolution.
Pulse repetition frequency (PRF)	The number of transmission-receive cycles per second	The PRF decreases as imaging (or Doppler) depth increases because of the time needed for the signal to travel from and to the transducer.	Pulse repetition frequency affects image resolution and frame rate (particularly with color Doppler)
Focal depth	Beam shape and focusing are used to optimize ultrasound resolution at a specific distance from the transducer	Structures close to the transducer are best visualized with a short focal depth, distant structures with a long focal depth.	The length and site of a transducer's focal zone is primarily determined by transducer design but adjustment during the exam may be possible.
Aperture	The surface of the transducer face where ultrasound is transmitted and received	A small non-imaging CW Doppler transducer allows optimal positioning and angulation of the ultrasound beam.	A larger aperture allows a more focused beam. A smaller aperture allows improved transducer angulation on TTE imaging.

transducer focuses the beam at a depth appropriate for the clinical application. Some transducers allow adjustment of focal depth.

❑ A smaller aperture is associated with a wider beam width; however, the smaller "footprint" may allow improved angulation of the beam in the intercostal spaces. This is most evident clinically with a dedicated non-imaging continuous wave (CW) Doppler transducer.

Ultrasound imaging

Principles

■ The basic ultrasound imaging modalities are:
  • M-mode—a graph of depth versus time
  • Two-dimensional—a sector scan in a tomographic image plane with real-time motion
  • Three-dimensional (3D)—a selected cutaway real-time image in a 3D display format (see Chapter 4)

- System controls for 2D imaging typically include:
  - Power output (transmitted ultrasound energy)
  - Gain (amplitude of the received signal)
  - Time gain compensation (differential gain along the ultrasound beam)
  - Depth of the image (affects pulse repetition frequency and frame rate)
  - Gray scale/dynamic range (degree of contrast in the images)

Key points:

❏ M-mode recordings allow identification of very rapid intracardiac motion because the sampling rate is about 1800 times per second compared to a 2D frame rate of 30 frames per second (Figure 1–3)

❏ Ultrasound imaging resolution is more precise along the length of the ultrasound beam (axial resolution) compared with lateral (side to side) or elevational ("thickness" of the image plane) resolution.

❏ Lateral resolution decreases with increasing distance from the transducer (Figure 1–4).

❏ Harmonic imaging improves endocardial definition and reduces near-field and side-lobe artifacts (Figure 1–5).

Imaging artifacts

- Common imaging artifacts result from:
  - A low signal-to-noise ratio
  - Acoustic shadowing
  - Reverberations
  - Beam width
  - Lateral resolution
  - Refraction
  - Range ambiguity
  - Electronic processing

Key points:

❏ A shadow occurs distal to a strong ultrasound reflector because the ultrasound wave does not penetrate past the reflector (Figure 1–6).

❏ Signals originating from the edges of the ultrasound beam or from side lobes can result in imaging or Doppler artifacts.

❏ Deviation of the ultrasound beam from a straight pathway due to refraction in the tissue results in the structure appearing in the incorrect location across the sector scan (Figure 1–7).

❏ Ultrasound reflected back and forth between two strong reflectors creates a reverberation artifact.

❏ Reflected ultrasound signals received at the transducer are assumed to originate from the preceding transmitted pulse. Signals from very deep structures or signals that have been re-reflected will be displayed at $\frac{1}{2}$ or twice the actual depth of origin.

Doppler

- Doppler ultrasound is based on the principle that ultrasound backscattered (F_s) from moving red blood cells will appear higher or lower in frequency than the transmitted frequency (F_T) depending on the speed and direction of blood flow (v) (Table 1-4).
- The Doppler equation is:

$$v = c(F_s - F_T)/[2\,F_T(\cos\theta)]$$

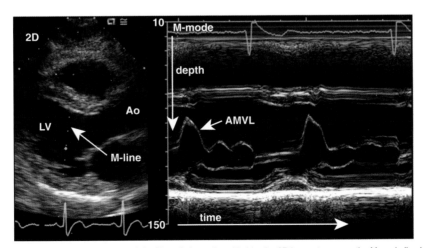

Figure 1–3. M-mode echocardiography. The location of the M-mode beam is guided by the 2D image to ensure the M-mode line is perpendicular to the long axis of the ventricle and centered in the chamber. This M-mode (*M* for motion) tracing of time (on the horizontal axis) versus depth (on the vertical axis) shows the rapid diastolic motion of the anterior mitral valve leaflet (*AMVL*) in a patient in atrial flutter.

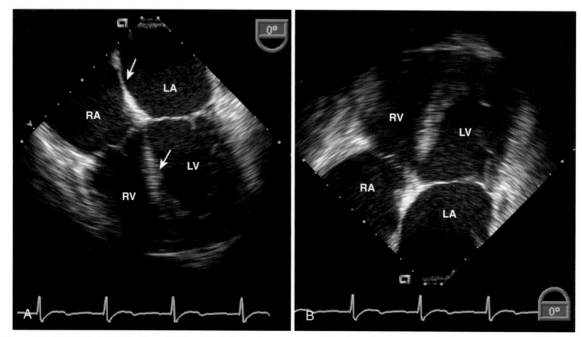

Figure 1–4. Lateral resolution with ultrasound decreases with the distance of the reflector from the transducer. In this TEE image oriented with the origin of the ultrasound signal at the top of the image (*A*), thin structures close to the transducer, such as the atrial septum (*small arrow*), appear as a dot because lateral resolution is optimal at this depth. Reflections from more distant structures, such as the ventricular septum (*large arrow*), appear as a broad line due to poor lateral resolution. When the image is oriented with the transducer at the bottom of the image (*B*), the effects of depth on lateral resolution are more visually apparent. The standard orientation for echocardiography with the transducer as the top of the image is based on considerations of ultrasound physics, not on cardiac anatomy.

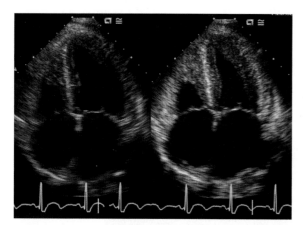

Figure 1–5. Harmonic imaging improves identification of the LV endocardial border, as seen in this apical 4-chamber view recorded with a 4-MHz transducer using (*A*) fundamental frequency imaging and (*B*) harmonic imaging.

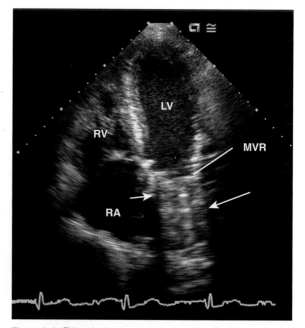

Figure 1–6. This apical 4-chamber view in a patient with a mechanical mitral valve prosthesis illustrates the shadowing (dark area, *small arrow*) and reverberations (white band of echoes, *large arrow*) that obscure structures (in this case the left atrium) distal to the valve.

- Accurate blood flow measurements depend on a parallel intercept angle (θ) between the ultrasound beam and direction of blood flow.
- There are three basic Doppler modalities: pulsed Doppler, color flow imaging, and continuous wave Doppler ultrasound.

TABLE 1-4   Doppler Physics

	Definition	Examples	Clinical Implications
Doppler effect	The change in frequency of ultrasound scattered from a moving target $$v = c \times \Delta F/[2\,F_T(\cos\theta)]$$	A higher velocity corresponds to a higher Doppler frequency shift, ranging from 1 to 20 kHz for intracardiac flow velocities.	Ultrasound systems display velocity, which is calculated using the Doppler equation, based on transducer frequency and the Doppler shift, assuming $\cos\theta$ equals 1.
Intercept angle	The angle (θ) between the direction of blood flow and the ultrasound beam	When the ultrasound beam is parallel to the direction of blood flow (0° or 180°), $\cos\theta$ is 1 and can be ignored in the Doppler equation.	Velocity is underestimated when the intercept angle is not parallel. This can lead to errors in hemodynamic measurements.
CW Doppler	Continuous ultrasound transmission with reception of Doppler signals from the entire length of the ultrasound beam	CW Doppler allows measurements of high velocity signals but does not localize the depth of origin of the signal.	CW Doppler is used to measure high velocities in valve stenosis and regurgitation.
Pulsed Doppler	Pulsed ultrasound transmission with timing of reception determining depth of the backscattered signal	Pulsed Doppler samples velocities from a specific site but can only measure velocity over a limited range.	Pulsed Doppler is used to record low velocity signals at a specific site, such as LV outflow velocity or LV inflow velocity.
Pulse repetition frequency (PRF)	The number of pulsed transmitted per second	The PRF is limited by the time needed for ultrasound to reach and return from the depth of interest. PRF determines thxe maximum velocity that can be unambiguously measured.	The maximum velocity measurable with pulsed Doppler is about 1 m/s at 6 cm depth.
Nyquist limit	The maximum frequency shift (or velocity) measurable with pulsed Doppler equal to ½ PRF	The Nyquist limit is displayed as the top and bottom of the velocity range with the baseline centered.	The greater the depth, the lower the maximum velocity measurable with pulsed Doppler.
Signal aliasing	The phenomenon that the direction of flow for frequency shifts greater than the Nyquist limit cannot be determined	With aliasing of the LV outflow signal, the peak of the velocity curve is "cut off" and appears as flow in the opposite direction.	Aliasing can result in inaccurate velocity measurements if not recognized.
Sample Volume	The intracardiac location where the pulsed Doppler signal originated	Sample volume depth is determined by the time interval between transmission and reception. Sample volume length is determined by the duration of the receive cycle.	Sample volume depth and length are adjusted to record the flow of interest.
Spectral analysis	Method used to display Doppler velocity data versus time, with gray scale indicating amplitude	Spectral analysis is used for both pulsed and CWD.	The velocity scale, baseline position, and time scale of the spectral display are adjusted for each Doppler velocity signal.

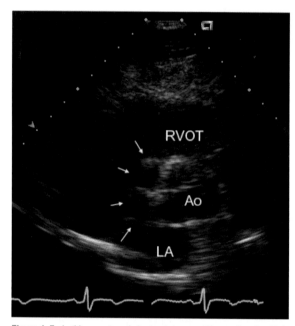

Figure 1–7. In this parasternal short axis image of the aortic valve (*Ao*), a refraction artifact results in the appearance of a "second" aortic valve (*arrows*), partly overlapping with the actual position of the aortic valve. *LA*, left atrium. *RVOT*, right ventricular outflow tract.

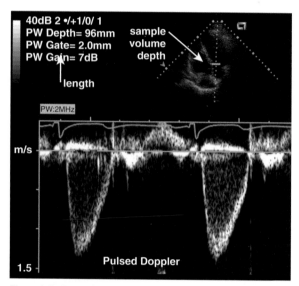

Figure 1–8. Doppler spectral tracing of LV outflow recorded with pulsed Doppler ultrasound from the apex. The sample volume depth (time for transmission and reception of the signal) is shown on a small 2D image with the length (sampling duration) indicated by the pulsed wave (*PW*) gate size. The spectral tracing shows time (horizontal axis), velocity (vertical axis) and signal strength (gray scale). The baseline has been shifted upward to show the entire velocity curve directed away from the transducer. Some diastolic LV inflow is seen above the baseline, directed toward the transducer.

Key points:

❑ The speed (c) of ultrasound in blood is about 1540 m/s
❑ Blood flow velocity will be underestimated with a non-parallel intercept angle; the error is only 6% with an angle of 20 degrees but increases to 50% at a 60-degree angle.
❑ When the ultrasound beam is perpendicular to flow, there is no Doppler shift and blood flow is not detected, even when present.
❑ The standard Doppler velocity display (or spectral recording) shows time on the horizontal axis and velocity on the vertical axis with signal amplitude displayed using a decibel gray scale (Figure 1–8).
❑ Standard Doppler instrument controls are:
  • Power output
  • Receiver gain (Figure 1–9)
  • High-pass ("wall") filters (Figure 1–10)
  • Velocity range and baseline shift
  • Post-processing options

Pulsed Doppler

■ Pulsed Doppler allows measurement of blood flow velocity at a specific intracardiac site.
■ The depth of interrogation (or sample volume) is determined by the time interval between transmission and sampling of the backscattered signal.
■ Signal aliasing limits the maximum velocity measurable with pulsed Doppler.

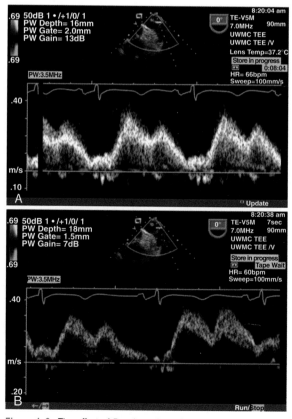

Figure 1–9. The effect of Doppler gain settings are shown for a TEE recording of pulmonary vein inflow. Excess noise is eliminated; then the gain is decreased from 13 dB (*A*) to 7 dB (*B*).

Key points:

- ❑ A pulse of ultrasound is transmitted and then the backscattered signal is analyzed at a time interval corresponding to the transit time from the depth of interest.
- ❑ The pulsed Doppler interrogation line and sample volume are displayed on the 2D image, with the transducer switched to Doppler only during data recording.
- ❑ Pulse repetition frequency is the number of transmission/receive cycles per second, which is determined by the depth of the sample volume.
- ❑ The maximum frequency detectable with intermittent sampling is one half the pulse repetition frequency (or Nyquist limit).
- ❑ The direction of blood flow for frequencies in excess of the Nyquist limit is ambiguous, a phenomenon called signal aliasing (Figure 1–11)
- ❑ The effective velocity range for pulsed Doppler can be doubled by moving the baseline to the edge of the spectral display.
- ❑ The sample volume length can be adjusted to localize the signal (short length) or improve signal strength (long length).
- ❑ Pulsed Doppler is used to measure normal intracardiac transvalvular flow velocities.
- ❑ Variations of the pulsed Doppler principle are used to generate color Doppler flow images and tissue Doppler recordings.

Color Doppler

- ■ Color Doppler uses the pulsed Doppler principle to generate a 2D image or "map" of blood flow velocity superimposed on the 2D real-time image (Table 1-5).
- ■ Color Doppler signals, like all pulsed Doppler velocity data, are angle dependent and are subject to signal aliasing.
- ■ The frame rate for color Doppler imaging depends on:
  - • Pulse repetition frequency (depth of color sector)
  - • Number of scan lines (width of color sector and scan line density)
  - • Number of pulses per scan line (affects accuracy of mean velocity calculation)

Key points:

- ❑ Color Doppler is recorded in real-time simultaneous with 2D imaging.
- ❑ Flow toward the transducer typically is shown in red with flow directed away from the transducer in blue (Figure 1–12).
- ❑ When velocity exceeds the Nyquist limit, signal aliasing occurs so that faster flows toward the transducer alias from red to blue and vice versa for flow away from the transducer.
- ❑ The amount of variation in the velocity signal from each site can be coded on the color scale as variance.
- ❑ Variance reflects either signal aliasing (high velocity flow) or the presence of multiple flow velocities or directions (flow disturbance).

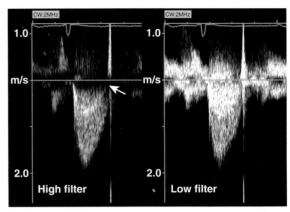

Figure 1–10. Continuous wave Doppler recording of an aortic outflow signal with the high pass ("wall") filter set at a high and low level. With the higher filter, low velocity signal are eliminated reflected in the blank space adjacent to the baseline. This tracing enhances identification of the maximum velocity and recognition of the valve closing click. At the lower filter setting, the velocity signals extend to the baseline, making measurement of time intervals more accurate, but there also is more low velocity noise in the signal, related to motion of cardiac structures.

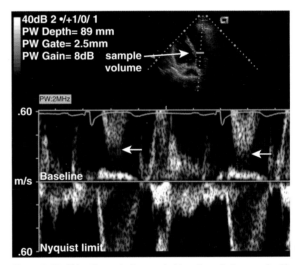

Figure 1–11. LV outflow velocity recorded from the apical approach with the sample volume on the LV side of the aortic valve. The spectral tracing is shown in the standard format with the baseline in the center of the scale and the Nyquist limit at the top and bottom of the scale. Signal aliasing is present with the top of the LV outflow signal seen in the reverse channel (*arrows*). This degree of aliasing is easily resolved by shifting the baseline, as seen in Figure 1–7. Aliasing with higher velocity flow is best resolved using continuous wave Doppler ultrasound.

TABLE 1-5 Color Doppler Flow Imaging

	Definition	Examples	Clinical Implications
Sampling line	Doppler data is displayed from multiple sampling lines across the 2D image	Instead of sampling backscattered signals from one depth (as in pulsed Doppler), signals from multiple depths along the beam are analyzed.	A greater number of sampling lines results in denser Doppler data but a slower frame rate.
Burst length	The number of ultrasound bursts along each sampling line	Mean velocity is estimated from the average of the backscattered signals from each burst.	A greater number of bursts results in more accurate mean velocity estimates but a slower frame rate.
Sector scan width	The width of the displayed 2D and color image	A greater sector width requires more sampling lines or less dense velocity data.	A narrower sector scan allows a greater sampling line density and faster frame rate.
Sector scan depth	The depth of the displayed color Doppler image	The maximum depth of the sector scan determines PRF (as with pulsed Doppler) and the Nyquist limit.	The minimum depth needed to display the flow of interest provides the optimal color display.
Color scale	Color display of Doppler velocity and flow direction	Most systems use shades of red for flow toward the transducer and blue for flow away from the transducer.	The color scale can be adjusted by shifting the baseline and adjusted the maximum velocity displayed (within the Nyquist limit).
Variance	The degree of variability in the mean velocity estimate at each depth along a sampling line	Variance typically is displayed as a green scale superimposed on the red–blue velocity scale. Variance can be turned on or off.	A variance display highlights flow disturbances and high velocity flow, but even normal flows will be displayed as showing variance if velocity exceeds the Nyquist limit.

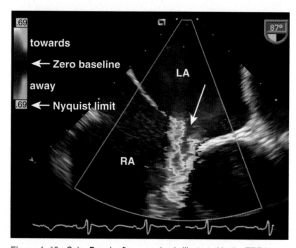

Figure 1–12. Color Doppler flow mapping is illustrated in the TEE image of an atrial septal defect. The Doppler signal is superimposed on the 2D image using a color scale for flow toward the transducer in red and flow away from the transducer in blue. The color density indicates velocity as shown by the scale. This scale includes variance as the addition of green to the color scale. The flow (*arrow*) from the left atrium (*LA*) to the right atrium (*RA*) across the septal defect should be blue (away from the transducer) but has aliased to red because the velocity exceeds the Nyquist limit of 60 cm/s.

❏ Color Doppler is most useful for visualization of spatial flow patterns; for this purpose, examiner preference determines the most appropriate color scale.

❏ For color Doppler measurements, such as vena contracta width or proximal isovelocity surface area (PISA) measurements, a color scale without variance is optimal.

❏ The maximum velocity measurable with color Doppler is determined by the Nyquist limit but the baseline can be shifted or the velocity scale can be reduced.

Continuous Wave (CW) Doppler

■ CW Doppler uses two ultrasound crystals to continuously transmit and receive ultrasound signals.

■ CW Doppler allows accurate measurement of high flow velocities without signal aliasing.

■ Signals from the entire length of the ultrasound beam are included in the spectral CW Doppler recording.

Key points:

❐ CW Doppler is used to measure high velocity flows, for example, across stenotic and regurgitant valves (Figure 1–13).

❐ The CW Doppler signal is recorded as a spectral tracing with the scale and baseline adjusted as needed to display the signal of interest.

❐ CW Doppler can be recorded with a standard transducer with the CW interrogation line shown on the 2D image; however, a dedicated non-imaging CW transducer is optimal due to a higher signal-to-noise ratio and better angulation with a smaller transducer.

❐ The lack of range resolution means that the origin of the CW signal must be inferred from:

• Characteristics of the signal itself (timing, shape, and associated flow signals)

• Associated 2D imaging and pulsed or color Doppler findings

❐ Underestimation of blood flow velocity occurs when the CW Doppler beam is not parallel to the flow of interest.

Doppler artifacts

■ Artifacts with pulsed or CW Doppler spectral recordings include:

• Underestimation of velocity because of a non-parallel intercept angle
• Signal aliasing (with pulsed Doppler)
• Range ambiguity
• Beam width artifacts with superimposition of multiple flow signals
• Mirror image artifact (Figure 1–14)
• Transit time effect
• Electronic interference

■ Artifacts with color Doppler flow imaging (Table 1-6) include:

• Shadowing resulting in inability to detect flow abnormalities
• Ghosting from strong reflectors leading to flashes of color across the image plane
• Gain too low (loss of true signal) or gain too high (speckle pattern across the image)
• Intercept angle with absence of detectable flow at 90-degree angle
• Signal aliasing (Figure 1–15)
• Electronic interference

Key points:

❐ The potential for underestimation of velocity is the most important clinical limitation of Doppler ultrasound.

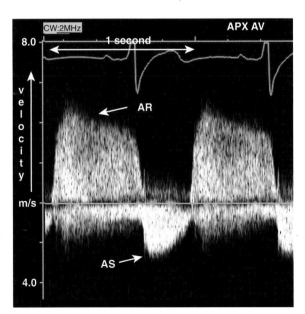

Figure 1–13. Continuous wave (*CW*) Doppler recording of the antegrade (aortic stenosis, *AS*) and retrograde flow (aortic regurgitation, *AR*) across the aortic valve. The spectral recording shows time (horizontal axis in seconds), velocity (vertical axis in m/s) and signal strength (gray scale). High velocity flow can be measured without aliasing using continuous wave Doppler as shown in the aortic regurgitant velocity over 4 m/s in this example.

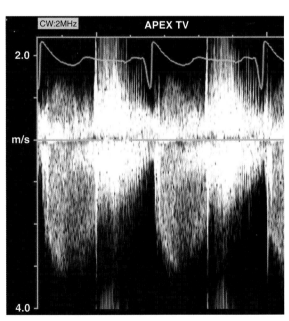

Figure 1–14. Appropriate use of instrumentation allows minimization of many ultrasound artifacts. This recording of the tricuspid regurgitant jet velocity shows marked channel cross-talk (signal below the baseline that does not correlate with an actual intracardiac flow) from the diastolic signal across the tricuspid valve. This recording would be improved by a higher wall filter and lower gain setting.

TABLE 1-6 Ultrasound Terminology: Ultrasound Safety

	Definition	Examples	Clinical implications
Exposure Intensity (I)	Ultrasound exposure depends on power and area: $I = power/area = watt/cm^2$	Common measures of intensity are the spatial peak temporal average (SPTA) or the spatial peak pulse average (SPPA).	Transducer output and tissue exposure affect the total ultrasound exposure of the patient.
Thermal bioeffects	Heating of tissue due to absorption of ultrasound energy described by the thermal index (TI)	The degree of tissue heating is affected by tissue density and blood flow. TI is the ratio of transmitted acoustic power to the power needed to increase temperature by $1°C$. TI is most important with Doppler and color flow imaging.	Total ultrasound exposure depends on transducer frequency, power output, focus, depth, and exam duration. When the TI exceeds 1, the benefits of the study should be balanced against potential biologic effects.
Cavitation	Creation or vibration of small gas-filled bodies by the ultrasound wave	Mechanical index (MI) is the ratio of peak rarefactional pressure to the square root of the transducer frequency. MI is most important with 2D imaging.	Cavitation or vibration of microbubbles occurs with higher intensity exposure. Power output and exposure time should be monitored.

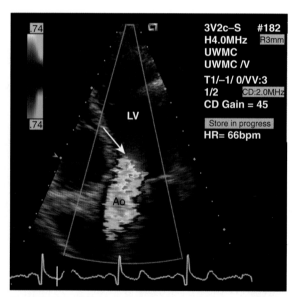

Figure 1–15. In this apical view angulated anteriorly to visualize the aorta, the antegrade flow in the LV outflow tract aliased from blue to orange because the velocity exceeds the Nyquist limit of 74 cm/s. Variance is seen because of signal aliasing.

❏ Signal aliasing limits measurement of high velocities with pulsed Doppler and may confuse interpretation of color Doppler images.
❏ Range ambiguity with CW Doppler is obvious. With pulsed Doppler, range ambiguity occurs when signals from 2x, 3x, or more of the depth of the sample volume return to the transducer during a receive cycle.

❏ A mirror image artifact is common on spectral tracings and may be reduced by lowering power output and gain.
❏ As ultrasound propagates through moving blood, there is a slight change in ultrasound frequency, called the transit time effect. The transit time effect results is slight blurring of the edge of the CW Doppler signal, particularly for high velocity flows.
❏ Acoustic shadowing can be avoided by using an alternate transducer position; for example, transesophageal imaging of a mitral prosthetic valve.
❏ Color ghosting is seen in only one or two frames of the cardiac cycle, whereas blood flow signals demonstrate physiologic timing.

Bioeffects and safety

■ Two types of ultrasound bioeffects are important with diagnostic imaging:
  • Thermal (heating of tissue due to the interaction of ultrasound energy with tissue)
  • Cavitation (the creation or vibration of small gas-filled bodies)
■ Ultrasound exposure is measured by the:
  • Thermal index (TI, the ratio of transmitted acoustic power to the power needed to increase temperature by $1°C$)
  • Mechanical index (MI, the ratio of peak rarefactional pressure to the square root of transducer frequency)

Key points:

❐ The degree of tissue heating depends on the ultrasound energy imparted to the tissue and on characteristics of the tissue, including tissue density and blood flow.

❐ The total ultrasound exposure depends on transducer frequency, focus, power output, and depth, as well as the duration of the examination.

❐ Cavitation or vibration of microbubbles occurs with higher intensity ultrasound exposure.

❐ When the TI or MI exceeds 1, the benefit of the ultrasound examination should be balanced against potential biologic effects.

❐ Power output and exposure time should be monitored during the echocardiographic examination.

THE ECHO EXAM

Basic Principles
Optimization of Echocardiographic Images

Instrument Control	Data Optimization	Clinical Issues
Transducer	• Different transducer types and transmission frequencies are needed for specific clinical applications. • Transmission frequency is adjusted for tissue penetration in each patient and for ultrasound modality (Doppler vs. imaging).	• A higher transducer frequency provides improved resolution but less penetration. • A larger aperture provides a more focused beam.
Power output	• Power output reflects the amount of ultrasound energy transmitted to the tissue. • Higher power output results in greater tissue penetration.	• Potential bioeffects must be considered. • Exam time and mechanical and thermal indexes should be monitored.
Imaging mode	• 2D imaging is the clinical standard for most indications. • M-mode provides high time resolution along a single scan line. • 3D imaging provides appreciation of spatial relationships.	• Optimal measurement of cardiac chambers and vessels may require a combination of imaging modes.
Transducer position	• Acoustic windows allow ultrasound tissue penetration without intervening lung or bone tissue. • Transthoracic acoustic windows include parasternal, apical, subcostal, and suprasternal. • TEE acoustic windows include high esophageal and transgastric.	• Optimal patient positioning is essential for acoustic access to the heart. • Imaging resolution is optimal when the ultrasound beam is reflected perpendicular to the tissue interface. • Doppler signals are optimal with the ultrasound beam is aligned parallel to flow.
Depth	• Depth is adjusted to show the structure of interest. • Pulse repetition frequency (PRF) depends on maximum image depth.	• PRF is higher at shallow depths, which contributes to improved image resolution. • Axial resolution is the same along the entire length of the ultrasound beam. • Lateral and elevational resolution depends on the 3D shape of the ultrasound beam at each depth.
Sector width	• Standard sector width is 60 degrees, but a narrower sector allows a higher scan line density and faster frame rate.	• Sector width should be adjusted as needed to optimize the image. • Too narrow a sector may miss important anatomic or Doppler findings.
Gain	• Overall gain affects the display of the reflected ultrasound signals.	• Excessive gain obscures border identification. • Inadequate gain results in failure to display reflections from tissue interfaces.
TGC	• Time gain compensation adjusts gain differentially along the length of the ultrasound bean to compensate for the effects of attenuation.	• An appropriate TGC curve results in an image with similar brightness proximally and distally in the sector image.
Gray scale/dynamic range	• Ultrasound amplitude is displayed using a decibel scale in shades of gray.	• The range of displayed amplitudes is adjusted to optimize the image using the dynamic range or compression controls.
Harmonic imaging	• Harmonic frequencies are proportional to the strength of the fundament frequency but increase with depth of propagation.	• Harmonic imaging improves endocardial definition and decreases near field and side lobe artifacts. • Flat structures, such as valves, appear thicker with harmonic than with fundamental imaging. • Axial resolution is reduced.

Basic Principles—cont'd

Instrument Control	Data Optimization	Clinical Issues
Focal depth	• Transducer design parameters that affect focal depth include array pattern, aperture size, and acoustic focusing.	• The ultrasound beam is most focused at the junction between the near zone and far field of the beam pattern. • Transducer design allows a longer focal zone. In some cases, focal zone can be adjusted during the examination.
Zoom mode	• The ultrasound image can be restricted to a smaller depth range and narrow section. The maximum depth still determines PRF, but scan line density and frame rate can be optimized in the region of interest.	• Zoom mode is used to examine areas on interest identified on standard views.
ECG	• The ECG signal is essential for triggering digital cine loop acquisition.	• A noisy signal or low amplitude QRS results in incorrect triggering or inadvertent recording of an incomplete cardiac cycle.

2D, two-dimensional; 3D, three-dimensional; ECG, electrocardiogram; PRF, pulse repetition frequency; TEE, transesophageal echocardiography; TGC, time gain compensation.

Optimization of Doppler Recordings

Modality	Data Optimization	Common Artifacts
Pulsed	• 2D guided with "frozen" image • Parallel to flow • Small sample volume • Velocity scale at Nyquist limit • Adjust baseline for aliasing • Use low wall filters • Adjust gain and dynamic range	• Non-parallel angle with underestimation of velocity • Signal aliasing; Nyquist limit = $\frac{1}{2}$ PRF • Signal strength/noise
Continuous wave (CW)	• Dedicated non-imaging transducer • Parallel to flow • Adjust velocity scale so flow fits and fills displayed range • Use high wall filters • Adjust gain and dynamic range	• Non-parallel angle with underestimation of velocity • Range ambiguity • Beam width • Transit time effect
Color flow	• Use minimal depth and sector width for flow of interest (best frame rate) • Adjust gain just below random noise • Color scale at Nyquist limit • Decrease 2D gain to optimize Doppler signal	• Shadowing • Ghosting • Electronic interference

SELF-ASSESSMENT QUESTIONS

QUESTION 1

Compared to fundamental imaging, use of tissue harmonic imaging has the most benefical effect on:

A. Temporal resolution
B. Lateral resolution
C. Axial resolution

QUESTION 2

The width of the 2D sector scan has the greatest adverse effect on:

A. Temporal resolution
B. Lateral resolution
C. Axial resolution

QUESTION 3

M-mode imaging has the greatest beneficial effect on:

A. Temporal resolution
B. Lateral resolution
C. Axial resolution

QUESTION 4

A patient is referred for a transthoracic echocardiogram (Figure 1–16). A parasternal long-axis view is shown.

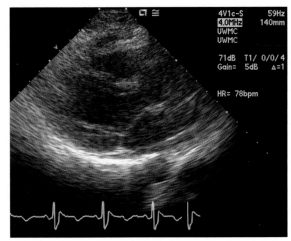

Figure 1–16.

The next best step to improve image quality would be:

A. Narrow 2D sector scan
B. Decrease image depth
C. Use tissue harmonic imaging
D. Increase transducer frequency
E. Increase overall gain

QUESTION 5

In this color Doppler image of the aortic arch (Figure 1–17), the interposed "black" region between the red and blue color Doppler shift is the result of:

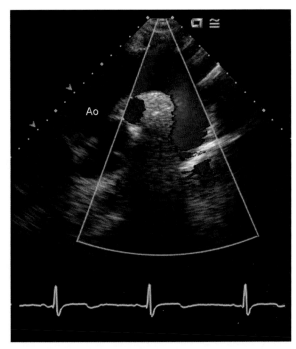

Figure 1–17.

A. Acoustic shadowing
B. Intercept angle
C. Electronic interference
D. Signal aliasing
E. Flow disruption

QUESTION 6

For the following ultrasound artifacts, circle the position of the artifact on the two-dimensional image relative to the actual anatomic structure.

1. Reverberation same distance more distant
2. Side lobe same distance more distant
3. Refraction same distance more distant

QUESTION 7

The black signal seen on the parasternal long-axis view (Figure 1–18, *arrow*) is best explained by:

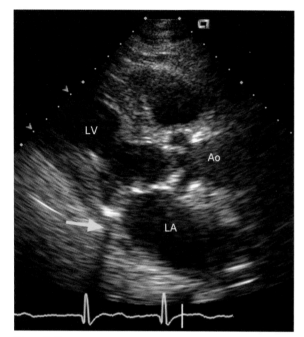

Figure 1–18.

A.   Acoustic shadowing
B.   Intercept angle
C.   Electronic interference
D.   Reverberations
E.   Refraction of the ultrasound beam

QUESTION 8

For each of these clinical situations, select the Doppler modality that offers the best diagnostic data:

    I.   Velocity of the aortic jet in a patient with severe aortic stenosis
    II.   Width of the mitral regurgitant jet in a patient with mitral valve prolapse and eccentric regurgitation.
    III.   LV outflow velocity in a patient with severe aortic stenosis
    IV.   Tricuspid regurgitation velocity in a patient with pulmonary hypertension.

Use one of the following choices:

A.   Color Doppler imaging
B.   Pulsed Doppler imaging
C.   Continuous wave Doppler imaging

ANSWERS

ANSWER 1: B

Tissue harmonic imaging improves both axial and lateral resolution. Axial resolution is improved by reducing near-field clutter and improving image quality in the far field. Fundamental frequencies produce large signals from strong specular reflectors and can result in near-field artifact, or "clutter." Tissue harmonic imaging utilizes the harmonic frequency energy rather than the fundamental transmitted frequency, reducing near-field clutter. With fundamental imaging, ultrasound reflection from planar structures perpendicular to the ultrasound beam produces the strongest signal. Structures that are parallel to the ultrasound beam, such as the endocardial walls of the LV, are poorly seen with fundamental imaging. Harmonic imaging allows for improved imaging of more parallel structures. However, strong planar reflectors, such as valve leaflets appear thicker than the actual structure, adversely affecting axial resolution for these structures. Additionally, the strength of the harmonic signal increases with increased depth of ultrasound propagation. Thus, tissue harmonic imaging improves lateral resolution, and is particularly helpful in delineating the LV endocardial border. Harmonic imaging does not affect temporal resolution.

ANSWER 2: A

With scanned (2D) imaging, the image sector is formed by multiple adjacent scan lines where the transducer sweeps the ultrasound beam across the imaging field. Rapid image processing allows for real-time imaging with improved spatial resolution across the imaging field. However, because time is incurred sweeping the ultrasound beam across the imaging field, temporal resolution is not optimal to M-mode, which images along a single scan line. A narrower 2D sector allows a higher frame rate.

ANSWER 3: A

With M-mode imaging, the transducer sends and receives an ultrasound signal along a single scan line, and the time to sweep the ultrasound beam across a sector is not incurred. Thus, the time transmit/receive cycle is very rapid (about 1800 times per second), which improves the temporal resolution of the image, allowing evaluation of rapidly moving structures, such as valve leaflets, dissection flaps, and valve vegetations.

ANSWER 4: C

Tissue harmonic imaging improves overall image quality. With harmonic imaging, parallel dropout of specular reflectors is decreased, improving endocardial border definition. With increased depth of ultrasound propagation, the strength of the harmonic signal increases, improving image quality in the far field. Additionally, harmonic imaging reduces near-field clutter and side-lobe artifacts (Figure 1–19).

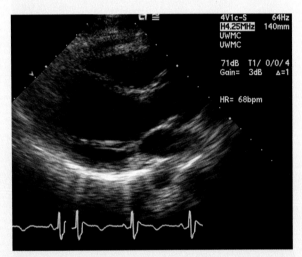

Figure 1–19.

A narrow 2D sector might increase sample line density and frame rate but would not improve image quality as much as harmonic imaging. Decreased depth might slightly improve near-field image quality, but the structures of interest would no longer be seen. Although increasing the transducer frequency will improve image quality in the near field, ultrasound tissue penetration would decrease, resulting in poor image quality in the far field. Increasing gain would increase signal strength across the image plane but would also increase noise with no improvement in resolution of anatomic structures. Another approach would be to alter the transducer position (for example, move up an interspace or move closer to the sternum) in order to gain better acoustic access.

ANSWER 5: B

Color Doppler imaging samples blood velocity moving toward (displayed as red) or away (displayed as blue) from the transducer. In this image, flow up toward the ascending aorta and through the aortic arch is shown. Maximal velocities are obtained when flow is parallel with the transducer. Flow perpendicular to the transducer, in this case the interposed "black" region, is recorded as an absent signal. Thus, this black region is due to a perpendicular intercept angle in this image. Acoustic shadowing occurs when a strong specular reflector, such as prosthetic valves or calcium, blocks ultrasound penetration distal to the reflector. Electronic interference is displayed as an overlaying artifact that is not associated with the image and may extend beyond tissue borders. Signal aliasing results in flow being displayed as if it were due to flow opposite in direction to actual flow. So flow toward the transducer, by convention shown in red, would be displayed as blue, and vice versa. Signal aliasing often is seen on subcostal images of the proximal abdominal aorta. However, in this image flow in the ascending aorta is correctly shown toward the transducer in red and flow down the descending aorta away from the transducer in blue. (Notice the right pulmonary artery seen as a blue circle under the arch.) Disruption of flow would be accompanied by turbulent and disarrayed flow with aliasing of the color Doppler signal at the point of disruption, which is not seen on this image of a normal aortic arch.

ANSWER 6:

Reverberation artifacts occur distant to the actual anatomic structure, whereas side lobe and refraction artifacts occur at the same distance.

An ultrasound image is produced based on the time delay between the initial ultrasound burst from the transducer and the time that signal is reflected by an anatomic structure and received back by the transducer. Because more distal anatomic structures are associated with a longer time delay back to the transducer, they are placed further from the transducer on the generated image. With reverberations, a portion of the ultrasound wave is reflected back and forth between cardiac structures that are strong specular reflectors, such as the pericardium or mitral valve leaflets. This additional time delay will result in display of the structure as an artifact distal to the primary image source. Refraction occurs when a portion of the ultrasound beam is transmitted and deflected through tissue, resulting in an artifact that is displayed equidistant but lateral to the actual anatomic structure. Side-lobe artifacts are also equidistant to the actual anatomic structure. For this artifact, in the far zone of the ultrasound beam, strong reflectors at the edges of the beam are superimposed on central structures in the generated image.

ANSWER 7: A

This two-dimensional image from the parasternal long-axis view shows moderate mitral annular calcification at the posterior mitral valve annulus, just at the base of the posterior mitral valve leaflet. Calcium is a strong specular reflector that blocks ultrasound penetration distally. Most of the transmitted ultrasound beam reflects from the calcium back to the transducer. This is shown on the generated image as a bright echodensity at the site of calcium with shadowing of the signal in the distal field. On 2D imaging, a parallel intercept angle between the structure of interest and the ultrasound beam results in image "dropout" as few signals are reflected from the anatomic structure. Electronic interference typically has a geometric pattern and affects the entire 2D image. Reverberations appear as multiple bright echodensities distal to the anatomic structure, whereas refraction results in the structure of interest appearing lateral to the actual location.

ANSWER 8: I, C; II, A; III, B; IV, C

Continuous wave Doppler imaging allows accurate measurement of high velocity flow without aliasing of the signal. Clinically, CW Doppler is used whenever a high velocity signal is present, for example, with aortic stenosis, tricuspid regurgitation, mitral regurgitation, or a ventricular septal defect. However, with CW Doppler, sampling occurs along the line of interrogation without localization of the point of maximum velocity along that line (lack of range resolution). The origin of the high velocity signal is inferred from imaging data or localized using pulsed Doppler or color flow imaging.

Color Doppler imaging is useful for evaluating the spatial distribution of flow, which is especially helpful in determining the severity and mechanism of regurgitant flow. The width of the color Doppler regurgitant jet, the vena contracta, is a reliable measure of regurgitation severity.

Pulsed wave Doppler imaging allows spatial localization of a velocity signal but is best used for low velocity signals with a maximum velocity that is below the Nyquist level. Clinical examples of the use of pulsed Doppler include LV inflow across the mitral valve, pulmonary venous flow, and LV outflow velocity proximal to the aortic valve (even when aortic stenosis is present). With velocities that exceed the Nyquist limit, aliasing of the pulsed wave Doppler signal occurs, which precludes accurate velocity measurements.

2 The Transthoracic Echocardiogram

Step 1: Clinical Data

- The indication for the study determines the focus of the examination.
- Key clinical history and physical examination findings and results of any previous cardiac imaging studies are noted.

Key points:

- ❑ The goal of the echo study is to answer the specific question asked by the referring provider.
- ❑ Blood pressure is recorded at the time of the echo because many measurements vary with loading conditions.
- ❑ Knowledge of clinical data ensures that the echo study includes all the pertinent images and Doppler data. For example, when a systolic murmur is present, the echo study includes data addressing all the possible causes for this finding.
- ❑ Data from previous imaging studies may identify specific areas of concern, such as a pericardial effusion noted on chest computed tomography (CT) imaging.
- ❑ Detailed information about previous cardiac procedures assists in interpretation of postoperative findings, evaluation of implanted devices (such as prosthetic valves or percutaneous closure devices), and detection of complications.
- ❑ Use of precise anatomic terminology facilitates accurate communication of imaging results (Table 2-1).

Step 2: Patient Positioning (Figure 2–1)

- A steep left lateral position provides acoustic access for parasternal and apical views.
- The subcostal views are obtained when the patient is supine; if needed, the legs are bent to relax the abdominal wall.
- Suprasternal notch views are obtained when the patient is supine with the head turned toward either side.

Key points:

- ❑ Images may be improved with suspended respiration, typically at end-expiration but sometimes at other phases of the respiratory cycle.
- ❑ An examination bed with an apical cutout allows a steeper left lateral position, often providing improved acoustic access for apical views.

❏ Imaging can be performed with either hand holding the transducer and with the examiner on either side of the patient. However, imaging from the patient's left side avoids reaching over the patient and is essential for apical views when the patient's girth is larger than the arm span of the examiner.

❏ Prolonged or repetitive imaging requires the examiner to learn ergonomic approaches to minimize mechanical stress and avoid injury.

TABLE 2-1 Terminology for Normal Echocardiographic Anatomy

Aorta*	Sinuses of Valsalva
	Sinotubular junction
	Coronary ostia
	Ascending aorta
	Descending thoracic aorta
	Proximal abdominal aorta
Aortic valve	Right, left, and non-coronary cusps
	Nodules of Arantius
	Lambl's excrescence
Mitral valve	Anterior and posterior leaflets
	Posterior leaflet scallops (lateral, central, medial)
	Chordae (primary, secondary, tertiary; basal, and marginal)
	Commissures (medial and lateral)
Left ventricle	Wall segments (see Chapter 8)
	Septum, free wall
	Base, apex
	Medial and lateral papillary muscles
Right ventricle	Inflow segment
	Moderator band
	Outflow tract (conus)
	Supraventricular crest
	Anterior, posterior, and conus papillary muscles
Tricuspid value	Anterior, septal, and posterior leaflets
	Chordae
	Commissures
Right atrium	RA appendage
	SVC and IVC junctions
	Valve of IVC (Chiari network)
	Coronary sinus ostium
	Crista terminalis
	Fossa ovalis
	Patent foramen ovale
Left atrium	LA appendage
	Superior and inferior left pulmonary veins
	Superior and inferior right pulmonary veins
	Ridge at junction of LA appendage and left superior pulmonary vein
Pericardium	Oblique sinus
	Transverse sinus

*The term aortic root is used inconsistently, sometimes meaning the aortic sinuses and sometimes meaning the entire segment of the aorta from the annulus to the arch (including sinuses and ascending aorta).
SVC, superior vena cava; IVC, inferior vena cava.

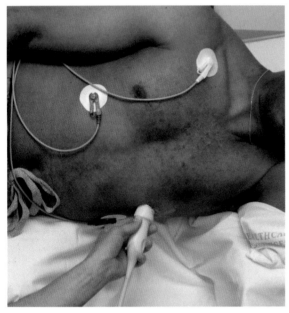

Figure 2–1. The patient is positioned in a steep left lateral decubitus position on an examination bed with a removable section cut out of the mattress to allow placement of the transducer on the apex by the sonographer as shown. Ultrasound gel is used to enhance coupling between the transducer face and the patient's skin. The sonographer sits on an adjustable chair and uses the left hand for scanning and the right hand to adjust the instrument panel. The room is darkened to improve visualization on the ultrasound instrument display screen.

Step 3: Instrumentation Principles (Figure 2–2)

- A higher transducer frequency provides improved resolution but less penetration of the ultrasound signal.
- Harmonic imaging is frequently used to improve image quality, particularly recognition of endothelial borders.
- Depth, zoom mode, and sector width are adjusted to optimize the image and frame rate, depending on the structure or flow of interest.
- Gain settings are adjusted to optimize the data recording while avoiding artifacts.

Key points:

- Although the control panel varies for each instrument, the basic functions are similar for all ultrasound systems.
- The highest frequency that penetrates adequately to the depth of interest is used for optimal imaging.
- With harmonic imaging, flat structures, such as valve leaflets, appear thicker than with fundamental imaging.
- Frame rate is higher for a shorter depth or a narrower sector; a fast frame rate is especially important with Doppler color flow imaging.

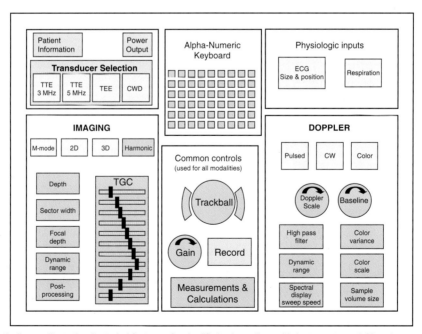

Figure 2–2. Schematic diagram illustrating the typical features of a simplified echocardiographic instrument panel. Many instrument controls affect different parameters depending on the imaging modality. For example, the trackball is used to adjust the position of the M-mode and Doppler beams, sample volume depth, and the size and position of the color Doppler box. The trackball also may be used to adjust two-dimensional image depth and sector width and the position of the zoom box. The gain control adjusts gain for each modality, imaging, pulsed, or continuous wave Doppler. Only a simplified model of an instrument panel is shown. The transducer choices are examples; other transducers are available depending on the system. In addition to the time gain compensation (TCG) controls, a lateral control scale may also be present.

- Too narrow a sector may miss important anatomic or physiologic findings.
- Excessive gain results in artifacts with both imaging and Doppler, whereas inadequate gain results in data loss.

Step 4: Data Recording

- Representative images from the echo study are recorded, usually digitally, to document the findings and for later review and measurement.

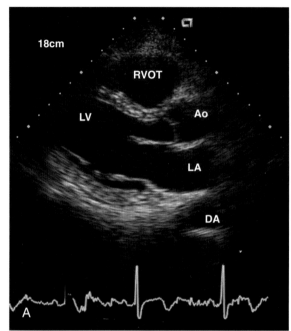

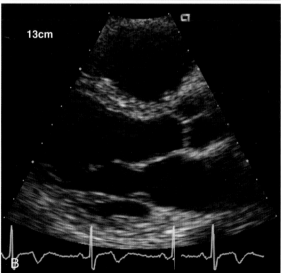

Figure 2–3. Parasternal long axis view recorded at a depth of 18 cm to show the structures posterior to the heart (*top*) and then with the depth decreased to 13 cm and the resolution mode used (note that the top of the displayed image now is 2 cm from the skin) to focus on the aortic and mitral valves.

- Echo images typically include an electrocardiogram (ECG) tracing for timing purposes.

Key points:

- Echo images in each view are recorded first with a depth and sector width that encompasses all the structures in the image plane and then at a depth and sector width optimized for the structures of interest (Figure 2–3).
- Additional zoom mode images of normal and abnormal findings are recorded as needed.
- Spectral pulsed and continuous wave (CW) Doppler data are recorded with the baseline and velocity range adjusted so the flow signal fits but fills the vertical axis. The time scale is adjusted to maximize the accuracy of measurements (usually an x-axis of 100 mm/s) (Figure 2–4).
- Color Doppler is recorded after sector width and depth are adjusted to optimize frame rate and gain is set just below the level that results in background speckle.
- The variance mode on the color scale is preferred by many examiners (including the authors) to enhance recognition of abnormal flows.
- Some normal flows result in a variance display—for example, when left ventricular outflow velocity exceeds the Nyquist limit and signal aliasing occurs (Figure 2–5).
- Conversely, when variance is not used, it is more difficult to distinguish abnormal flows (such as mitral regurgitation) from normal flows (such as pulmonary vein flow) when both occur in the same anatomic region.

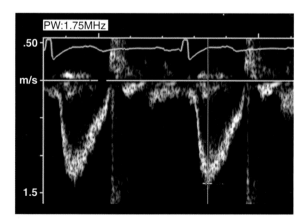

Figure 2–4. The spectral display of the pulsed Doppler signal is shown with the baseline shifted and velocity scale adjusted to avoid aliasing and to use the full vertical axis to improve measurement accuracy; for example, the signal "fits but fills" the graphical display. The horizontal time scale is 100 mm/s, which is standard for most Doppler recordings.

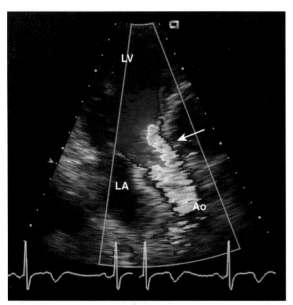

Figure 2–5. This color Doppler image of LV outflow in an apical long axis view shows signal aliasing adjacent to the septum in the subaortic region. Although this appearance may be due to an asymmetric flow profile, the effects of intercept angle also may be important. Even if the velocity is identical across the outflow tract, compared with the region along the anterior mitral valve leaflet, in the region adjacent to the septum the Doppler beam is more parallel to the flow direction. The higher Doppler shift results in signal aliasing. Aliasing at the aortic valve level is expected because the aortic velocity typically exceeds the Nyquist limit at this depth (0.74 m/s in this example).

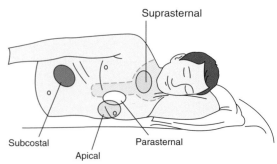

Figure 2–6. The standard acoustic "windows" where ultrasound can reach the cardiac structures without intervening lung or bone include the parasternal, apical, subcostal, and suprasternal notch windows. The parasternal and apical windows typically are optimal with the patient in a steep left lateral position. For the subcostal window, the patient is supine with the knees flexed to relax the abdominal vasculature. For the suprasternal notch window, the patient is supine with the head tilted back and to one side.

Step 5: Examination Sequence

■ In subsequent chapters, the elements of the examination for each clinical condition are presented in the order needed for a final diagnosis.
■ Typically, these examination elements are incorporated into a systemic examination sequence.

Key points:

❑ There are several approaches to an examination sequence; any of these are appropriate if a complete systemic examination is performed.
❑ In some clinical situations, a limited examination may be appropriate, with the study components selected by the referring or performing physician.
❑ The approach suggested here is based on obtaining all data (imaging and Doppler) for each acoustic window (parasternal, apical, subcostal, and suprasternal) before moving to the next acoustic window; this approach minimizes the time needed to reposition the patient between acoustic windows (Figure 2–6).
❑ Some examiners prefer to obtain all the imaging data and then obtain all the Doppler data; this approach allows the Doppler data recording to be tailored to the imaging findings.
❑ With any approach, the examiner may need to go back to previous acoustic windows at the end of the examination if additional views or measurements are needed based on abnormal findings.
❑ The examination sequence also may need to be modified depending on patient factors (inability to move, bandages, etc.) or the urgency of the examination.
❑ Basic measurements are made as the examination is performed (Table 2-2) or during review of images at completion of the study. Normal values for chamber sizes are provided in Chapter 6 (Tables 6-2 and 6-3) and for the aorta in Chapter 16 (Tables 16-1 and 16-2).

Step 6: Parasternal Window

Step 6A: Long axis view

■ Many echocardiographers start with the parasternal long axis view with:
  • Imaging to show the aortic and mitral valves, left atrium and aortic root, the LV base, and the RV outflow tract
  • Color Doppler to screen for aortic and mitral regurgitation
■ Standard measurements include:
  • LV end-diastolic and end-systolic diameters; diastolic thickness of the septum and LV inferior-lateral wall just apical from the mitral leaflet tips (Figure 2–7)
  • Aortic diameter at end-diastole (Figure 2–8)
  • Left atrial anterior-posterior dimension
  • Vena contracta width for aortic, mitral, and tricuspid regurgitation

TABLE 2-2   Basic Echo Imaging Measurements

Cardiac Structure	Basic Measurements	Additional Measurements	Technical Details
Left ventricle	• ED dimension • ES dimension • Wall thickness	• ED volume • ES volume • 2D stroke volume • Ejection fraction • LV mass	• 2D imaging is used to ensure measurements are centered and perpendicular to the long axis of the LV. • M-mode provides superior time resolution and more accurate identification of endocardial borders.
Left atrium	• AP diameter	• LA area • LA volume	• Left atrial anterior-posterior dimension provides a quick screen but may underestimate LA size. • When LA size is important for clinical decision making, measurement of LA volume is helpful.
Right ventricle	• Visual estimate of size	• ED RV outflow tract diameter • ED RV length and diameter	• Quantitation of RV size by echo is challenging due to the complex 3D shape of the chamber. • Tricuspid annular plane systolic excursion via M-mode is a quantitative measure of RV systolic function.
Right atrium	• Visual estimate of size		• RA size is usually compared to the LA in the apical 4-chamber view.
Aorta	• ED diameter at sinuses	• Maximum diameter indexed to expected dimension • Diameter at multiple sites in aorta	• With 2D echo, inner edge to inner edge measurements are more reproducible. • Measurements are made at end-diastole by convention, but end-systolic measurements also may be helpful.
Pulmonary artery		• Diameter	

3D, three-dimensional; AP, anterior-posterior; ED, end-diastole (onset of the QRS); ES, end-systole (minimum LV volume).

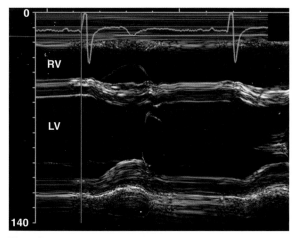

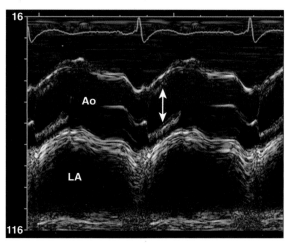

Figure 2–7. Two-dimensional guided M-mode recording of the LV at the mitral chordal level. End-diastolic measurements of wall thickness and cavity dimension are made at the onset of the QRS, as shown. End-systolic measurements are made at the maximum posterior motion of the septum (when septal motion is normal) or at minimal LV size. The rapid sampling rate with M-mode allows more accurate identification of the endocardial border, which is distinguished from chordae or trabeculations as being a continuous line in diastole, with the steepest slope during systole.

Figure 2–8. Two-dimensional guided M-mode recording of the aortic valve (Ao) and left atrium (LA) allows measurement of aortic root dimension at end-diastole using a leading edge to leading edge approach; the aortic leaflet separation (arrows); and the left atrial maximum anterior-posterior dimension in early diastole. The fine fluttering of the aortic valve leaflets is normal.

Key points:

❑ Images are initially recorded at a depth that includes the descending thoracic aorta to detect pleural and pericardial effusions.

❑ Depth then is reduced to the level of the posterior wall for assessment of the size and function of the base of the LV and the RV outflow tract.

❑ The aortic and mitral valves are examined with zoom mode sweeping through the valve planes from medial to lateral to assess valve anatomy and motion (Figure 2–9).

❑ M-mode tracings of the mitral valve can aid in timing of leaflet motion, such as systolic anterior motion in hypertrophic cardiomyopathy or posterior buckling in mitral valve prolapse.

❑ LA anterior-posterior dimension may underestimate LA enlargement; when clinically indicated, additional measurements are made from apical views.

❑ The aortic root (sinuses of Valsalva and sinotubular junction) is visualized first from the standard window and then with the transducer moved up one or more interspaces to visualize the ascending aorta (Figure 2–10).

❑ Color Doppler of aortic and mitral valves is used to screen for valve regurgitation. If more than physiologic regurgitation is present, further evaluation is needed as discussed in Chapter 12.

Step 6B: Right ventricular inflow view

■ From the long axis view, the image plane is angled medially to show the right ventricular inflow view (Figure 2–11) with:
  • Imaging of the right atrium, tricuspid valve, and right ventricle
  • Color Doppler evaluation of tricuspid regurgitation
  • CW Doppler recording of tricuspid regurgitant jet velocity
■ Standard measurements include:
  • Maximum tricuspid regurgitant velocity (Figure 2–12)

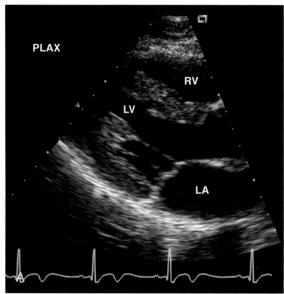

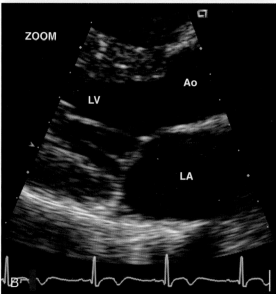

Figure 2–9. First the mitral valve is examined at a standard depth (*PLAX*), then zoom mode (*ZOOM*) is used to optimize visualization of the aortic and mitral valves. The image plane is angled slightly medial and lateral to encompass the medial and lateral aspects of the valve. Some normal thin mitral chords are well seen in this slightly laterally angulated view, extending from the mitral closure plane to the papillary muscle.

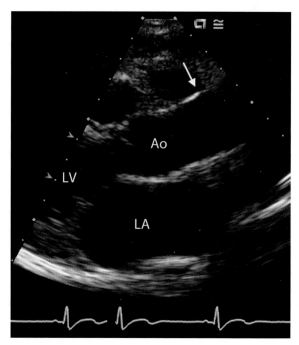

Figure 2–10. The ascending aorta is visualized by moving the transducer up an interspace from the parasternal long axis view.

Key points:

- ❏ Slide apically one interspace if views are not obtained from the standard window.
- ❏ Adjust depth to include the RA, RV, and tricuspid valve.
- ❏ The entrance of the coronary sinus and the inferior vena cava into the RA are seen in this view.

- ❏ A small amount of tricuspid regurgitation on color Doppler is seen in most (>80%) normal individuals and sometimes is referred to as "physiologic."
- ❏ The CW Doppler tricuspid regurgitant jet is recorded from multiple views; the highest velocity represents the most parallel intercept angle with flow and is used to estimate pulmonary pressure; the lower velocity recordings are ignored.

Step 6C: Right ventricular outflow view

- ■ From the long axis view, the image plane is angled laterally to show the right ventricular outflow view (Figure 2–13) with:
  - Imaging of the RV outflow tract, pulmonic valve, and main pulmonary artery
  - Color Doppler evaluation of pulmonic regurgitation (Figure 2–14)
  - Pulsed Doppler recording of pulmonary artery flow (Figure 2–15)
- ■ Standard measurements include:
  - Antegrade velocity in the pulmonary artery

Key points:

- ❏ Slide cephalad one interspace if views are not obtained from the standard window.
- ❏ Adjust depth to include the RV outflow tract, main pulmonary artery, and pulmonary artery bifurcation.

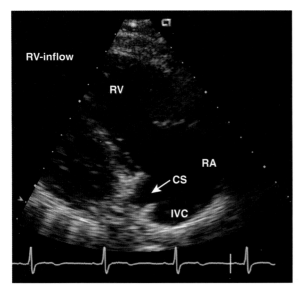

Figure 2–11. From the parasternal long axis view, the image plane is angulated medially to visualize the right ventricular inflow view with the right ventricle (*RV*), right atrium (*RA*), coronary sinus (*CS*), inferior vena cava (*IVC*) and tricuspid valve.

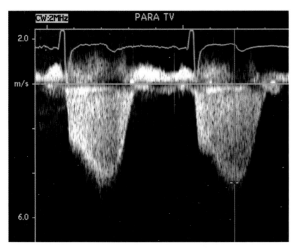

Figure 2–12. The tricuspid regurgitation jet is recorded with CW Doppler from both the parasternal RV inflow view and from the LV apex. Only the highest velocity is reported, in normal sinus rhythm, because the apparent lower velocity signal is due to a non-parallel intercept angle between the ultrasound beam and regurgitant jet. This example shows a high velocity jet consistent with severe pulmonary hypertension. The maximum velocity is measured at the edge of the dense "envelope" of flow, avoiding the faint signals due to gain and transit time effects.

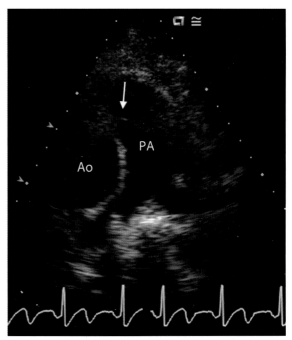

Figure 2–13. Right ventricular outflow tract view, obtained by angulating the transducer laterally from the parasternal long axis view, shows the RV outflow tract, pulmonic valve (arrow) and main pulmonary artery.

- The pulmonic valve often is difficult to visualize in adults, but a small amount of pulmonic regurgitation typically is present with a normally functioning valve.
- The pulsed Doppler recording of flow in the main pulmonary artery is helpful for assessment of pulmonary pressures and to exclude pulmonic stenosis or a patent ductus arteriosus.

Step 6D: Short axis view

- From the long axis view, the image plane is rotated 90 degrees to show the short axis plane with:
  - Imaging and color Doppler at the level of the aortic valve to evaluate the aortic, tricuspid, and pulmonic valves (Figure 2–16)
  - Imaging at the level of the mitral valve for evaluation of mitral leaflet anatomy and motion and LV size and function (Figure 2–17)
  - Imaging at the mid-papillary muscle level to evaluate global and regional LV size and function (Figure 2–18)

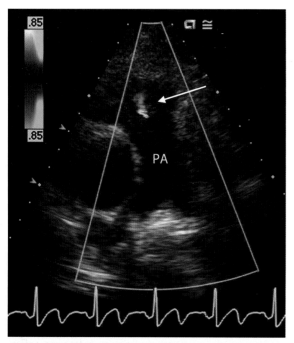

Figure 2–14. Color Doppler in a right ventricular outflow view showing a narrow jet of pulmonic regurgitation (*arrow*) in diastole. Mild pulmonic regurgitation is seen in about 80% of normal adults.

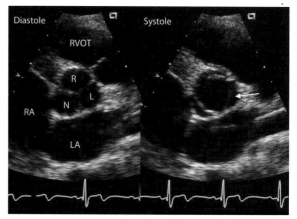

Figure 2–16. Parasternal short axis view of a normal trileaflet aortic valve in diastole (*left*) and in systole (*right*). The normal positions of the right (*R*), left (*L*) and non-coronary (*N*) cusps are seen in diastole. In systole, the open left coronary cusp often is difficult to see (*arrow*) because the leaflet edge is parallel to the ultrasound beam. However, the three commissures of the open valve are clearly visualized.

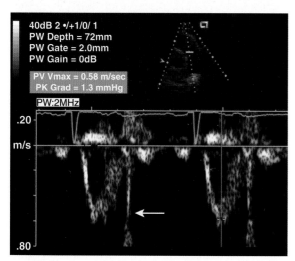

Figure 2–15. Pulsed Doppler recording of normal flow in the right ventricular outflow tract (notice the pulmonic valve closure click indicated the sample volume is on the RV side of the valve) shows a smooth velocity curve that peaks in mid-systole with a velocity less than 1 m/s.

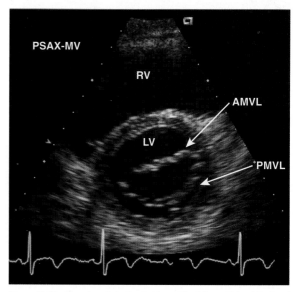

Figure 2–17. Parasternal short axis view of the left ventricle at the level of the mitral valve showing both anterior and posterior valve leaflets.

- Standard measurements include:
  - M-mode or 2D measurements of the aorta, LA, and LV using the combination of long and short axis view to ensure the dimensions are measured in the minor axis of each chamber or vessel (see Table 2-1)

Key points:

- ❒ The aortic and pulmonic valves normally are perpendicular to each other (when the aortic valve is seen in short axis, the pulmonic valve is seen in long axis).
- ❒ Zoom mode is used to identify the number of aortic valve leaflets, taking care to visualize the leaflets in systole.
- ❒ A bicuspid aortic valve is a common abnormality with a prevalence of about 1% of the total population and often is diagnosed on echocardiography requested for other indications.
- ❒ The coronary artery os may be seen originating in expected positions from the right and left coronary sinuses.
- ❒ The atrial septum is seen in the short axis view at the aortic valve level. Color flow imaging may help detect a patent foramen ovale but must be distinguished from normal flow in the right atrium (inflow from the superior and inferior vena cava and regurgitation across the tricuspid valve), all of which are adjacent to the atrial septum.

- ❒ Parasternal views of the LV at the papillary muscle level provide optimal endocardial definition and are used in conjunction with apical views for detection of regional wall motion abnormalities.

Step 7: Apical Window

Step 7A: Imaging four-chamber, two-chamber, and long axis views

- The apical window usually corresponds to the point of maximal impulse and is optimized with the patient in a steep left lateral position.
- Images are obtained in 4-chamber (Figure 2–19), 2-chamber (Figure 2–20), and long axis (Figure 2–21) views to evaluate:
  - LV size, wall thickness, and global and regional systolic function
  - RV size, wall thickness, and systolic function
  - Anatomy and motion of the mitral and tricuspid valves
  - Left and right atrial size and coronary sinus anatomy
  - The amount of pericardial fluid, if present
- Standard measurements include:
  - Visual estimate of LV ejection fraction
  - Quantitative apical biplane ejection fraction when clinically indicated (see Chapter 5)

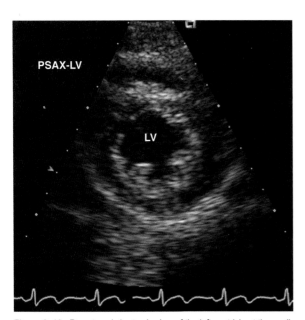

Figure 2–18. Parasternal short axis view of the left ventricle at the papillary muscle level. The LV cavity should appear circular in this view, an elliptical shape suggest an oblique intercept angle. This view sometimes requires the transducer be moved slightly apically from the short axis view of the aortic valve, instead of just tilting the transducer towards the apex from a fixed position on the chest wall.

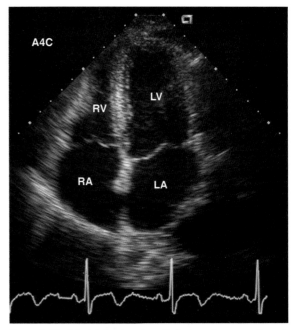

Figure 2–19. Apical 4-chamber view with the transducer correctly positioned over the LV apex. Foreshortening of this view results in a more spherical appearance of the left ventricle. This older adult has enlargement of both atrium and some benign thickening (lipomatous hypertrophy) of the atrial septum. The loss of signal in the mid segment of the atrial septum is an artifact because the thin fossa ovalis is parallel to the ultrasound beam at this point resulting in echo "dropout."

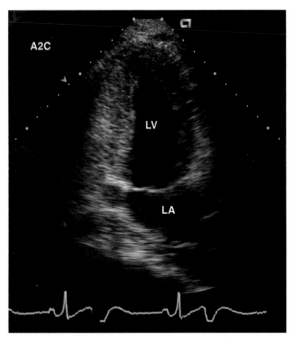

Figure 2–20. Apical 2-chamber view obtained by rotating the transducer about 60 degrees counterclockwise from the 4-chamber view.

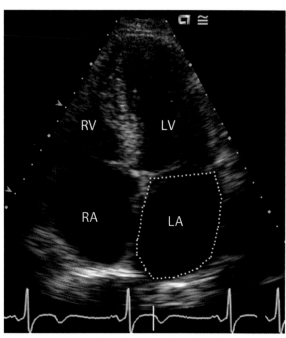

Figure 2–22. Left atrial volume is measured in the apical 4-chamber view by tracing the inner edge of the atrial border at end-systole. At the mitral annulus, a straight line from leaflet insertion to leaflet insertion is used for this calculation.

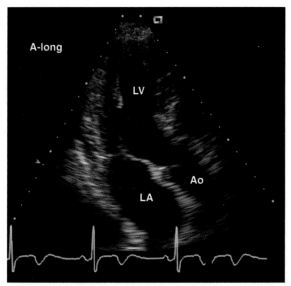

Figure 2–21. Apical long axis view is obtained by rotating an additional 60 degrees counterclockwise to obtain an image similar to the parasternal long axis view.

- Measurement of LA area or volume when clinically indicated (Figure 2–22)
- Visual estimate of RV size and systolic function
- Tricuspid annular plane systolic excursion via M-mode is a quantitative measure of RV systolic function

Key points:

☐ The three apical views are at approximately 60 degrees of rotation from each other; however, image planes are based on cardiac anatomy, not external reference points, so that slight adjustment of transducer position and angulation often is needed to optimize the image.

☐ Initial views are recorded at the maximum depth to see all the cardiac chambers and surrounding pericardium.

☐ Evaluation of the LV and RV are based on images with the depth adjusted to just beyond the valve annular plane. The RV is best visualized using zoom mode (Figure 2–23).

☐ From the 4-chamber view, the image plane is angled anteriorly to visualize the aortic valve (sometimes called the 5-chamber view); this view is useful for Doppler recordings, but image quality is suboptimal at the depth of the aortic valve from the apical window (Figure 2–24).

☐ The image plane is angled posteriorly to visualize the length of the coronary sinus and its entrance into the right atrium (Figure 2–25).

☐ The LA appendage is not well visualized on transthoracic imaging, and the sensitivity for detection of LA thrombus is low. Transesophageal imaging is needed when atrial thrombus is suspected.

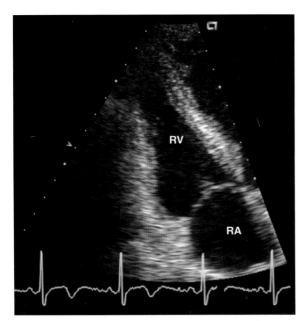

Figure 2–23. Right ventricular size and function are best estimated by centering the RV in the image plane and adjusting depth and zoom appropriately.

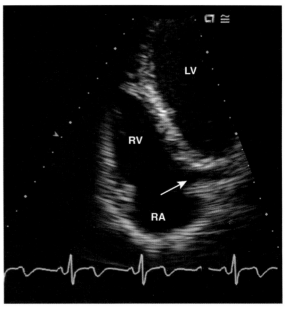

Figure 2–25. The entrance of the coronary sinus (*arrow*) into the right atrium is visualized by posterior angulation from the apical 4-chamber view.

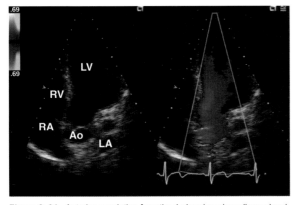

Figure 2–24. Anterior angulation from the 4-chamber view allows visualization of the LV outflow tract and an oblique view of the aortic valve. Laminar flow in the LV outflow tract is demonstrated with color Doppler. This view sometimes is colloquially called the 5-chamber view.

□ The descending thoracic aorta is seen in cross section behind the left atrium in the long axis view and in a longitudinal plane from the 2-chamber view with lateral angulation.

Step 7B: Doppler Data

■ The apical window provides an intercept angle that is relatively parallel to flow for the aortic, mitral, and tricuspid valves. Standard data recording includes:
  • Pulsed Doppler recordings of transmitral flow, pulmonary vein inflow, and LV outflow (Figure 2–26)
  • Color Doppler evaluation of mitral and tricuspid regurgitation

  • CW Doppler recordings of mitral, tricuspid, and aortic antegrade flow and regurgitation (Figure 2–27)
■ Standard measurements include:
  • Pulsed Doppler antegrade mitral early diastolic filling (E) and atrial filling (A) velocities
  • Pulsed Doppler LV outflow and CW Doppler aortic flow velocities
  • Maximum velocity of the tricuspid regurgitant jet
  • Additional measurements as clinically indicated (see specific chapters for each clinical condition)

Key points:

□ Transmitral and pulmonary venous inflow velocities are helpful for evaluation of LV diastolic dysfunction (see Chapter 7). Pulsed Doppler tissue velocities of the myocardial septal or lateral wall also are helpful for evaluation of diastolic function.
□ There is only a small increase in velocity from the LV outflow tract to the ascending aorta in normal individuals (see Chapter 11).
□ The CW Doppler recordings of aortic, mitral, and tricuspid regurgitation provide data on the severity of regurgitation (based on the density of the signal) and the transvalvular hemodynamics (based on the shape and density of the time velocity curve).
□ Color flow Doppler from the apical approach is helpful for evaluation of jet direction and for visualization of proximal jet geometry (vena

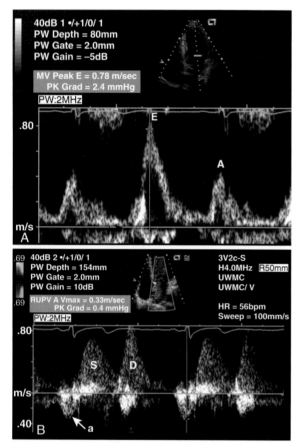

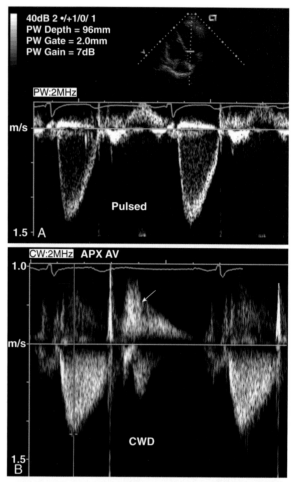

Figure 2–26. *A,* Left ventricular inflow is recorded using pulsed Doppler with the sample volume positioned at the mitral leaflet tips in diastole. The typical early (*E*) diastolic filling velocity and atrial (*A*) velocity are seen. *B,* Left atrial inflow is recorded with the pulsed Doppler sample volume in the right superior pulmonary vein in an apical 4-chamber view. The normal pattern of systolic (*S*) and diastolic (*D*) inflow with a small atrial (*a*) flow reversal are seen.

Figure 2–27. *A,* Left ventricular outflow is recorded with the Doppler sample volume on the left ventricular side of the aortic valve either in an anteriorly angulated 4-chamber view or in an apical long axis view. The normal smooth "envelope" of flow with dense signals along the outer edge and few velocity signals within the curve are seen. Again, the baseline and scale are adjusted to prevent aliasing and allow accurate measurements. *B,* Aortic flow velocity is recorded from an apical approach using CW Doppler. This velocity tracing includes signals from the entire length of the ultrasound beam so that the velocity curve is filled in by lower velocities proximal to the valve. The aortic closing click is seen. In diastole, the relatively broad CW beam intersects the left ventricular inflow curve (*arrow*).

contracta) and proximal isovelocity surface area (PISA) for mitral regurgitation

❏ Apical color Doppler is less helpful for aortic regurgitation because beam width is greater at the depth of the aortic valve than at the mitral valve.

Step 8: Subcostal Window

■ The subcostal window provides:
- An alternate acoustic window for evaluation of LV and RV systolic function (Figure 2–28)
- An optimal angle to evaluate the interatrial septum
- Estimation of RA pressure based on the size and respiratory variation in the inferior vena cava (Figure 2–29)
- Pulsed Doppler evaluation of hepatic vein flow (right atrial inflow) and proximal abdominal aortic flow, when clinically indicated (Figure 2–30)

Key points:

❏ Estimation of RA pressure is a standard part of the examination used to calculate pulmonary systolic pressure.
❏ Atrial septal defects often are best visualized on imaging and with color Doppler using a low Nyquist setting from the subcostal window.
❏ Hepatic vein flow patterns are helpful for detection of severe tricuspid regurgitation and for evaluation of pericardial disease.

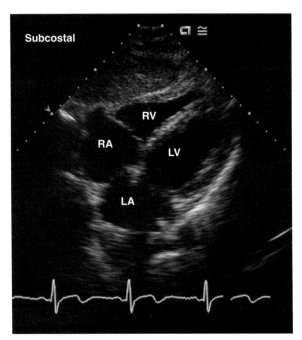

Figure 2–28. The subcostal 4-chamber view provides a useful view for evaluation of RV and LV function. This view also is best for evaluation of the atrial septum because the ultrasound beam is perpendicular to the septum from this transducer position.

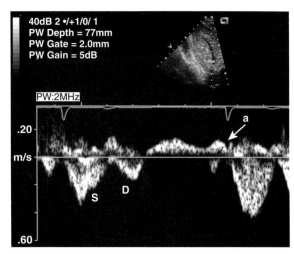

Figure 2–30. Hepatic vein flow can be recorded from the subcostal view to evaluate right atrial filling when tricuspid regurgitation or pericardial disease is of concern.

☐ Descending aortic holodiastolic flow reversal is seen with severe aortic regurgitation; persistent holodiastolic antegrade flow is seen with aortic coarctation.

Step 9: Suprasternal Window

■ The suprasternal window is a standard part of the examination of patients with diseases of the aortic valve or aorta.
■ The suprasternal window provides:
  • Images of the aortic arch and proximal descending thoracic aorta (Figure 2–31)
  • Pulsed and CW Doppler evaluation of descending aortic flow, when clinically indicated (Figure 2–32)
  • A parallel intercept angle with the aortic velocity in some patients with native or prosthetic aortic valve disease

Key points:

☐ Aortic disease, such as aortic dissection, may be visualized from this window.
☐ An increased systolic velocity with persistent antegrade flow ("runoff") in diastole is seen with an aortic coarctation.
☐ Holodiastolic flow reversal in the descending aorta suggests significant aortic valve regurgitation.

Step 10: The Echo Report

■ The echo report consists of four sections:
  • Clinical data
  • Measurements
  • Echo findings
  • Conclusions (with recommendations)

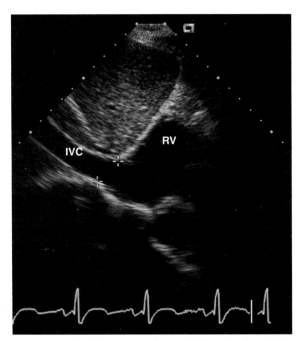

Figure 2–29. The inferior vena cava is examined from the subcostal view with the size and respiratory variation used to estimate right atrial pressure, as discussed in Chapter 6.

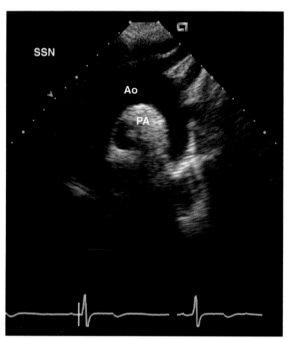

Figure 2–31. The suprasternal notch view showing the ascending aorta (*Ao*), arch, and descending thoracic aorta. A small segment of the right pulmonary artery (*PA*) is seen in cross section.

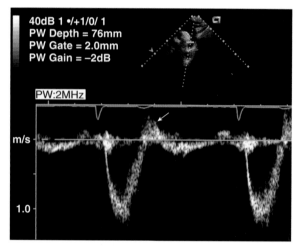

Figure 2–32. Normal pattern of flow in the descending thoracic aorta with antegrade flow in systole, brief diastolic flow reversal as a result of aortic recoil and coronary blood flow, a small amount of antegrade flow in mid-diastole, and slight reversal just before the next cardiac cycle.

Key points:

❏ The clinical data section includes the reason for the study, pertinent history and physical examination findings, cardiac medications, and blood pressure.

❏ Standard measurements are indicated in the example (Table 2-3) with additional measurements as clinically indicated.

❏ The findings section documents what views and flow were recorded and describes any abnormal and key normal findings.

❏ The conclusions indicate the major diagnosis, associated findings, and pertinent negative findings (depending on the indication for the study).

❏ When clinically appropriate, specific recommendations are made. These include:

• The clinical significance of the findings

• Recommendations for cardiology evaluation and periodic follow-up

❏ Serious unexpected findings are communicated promptly directly to the referring physician.

❏ When data are not definitive, the findings are described along with a differential diagnosis to explain these findings.

❏ Additional diagnostic approaches are recommended as appropriate.

TABLE 2-3 Sample Echo Report

Name_____ Date of Study_____

Age: 45 years Sex: M

Indication: Systolic murmur on auscultation

Cardiac medications: None

Clinical history: Chest pain on exertion, systolic murmur, no prior cardiac procedures

Blood pressure: 118/68 mm Hg Heart rate: 60 bpm Rhythm: NSR

Sonographer: BKS Image quality: Excellent

MEASUREMENTS

	Dimensions (cm)	Normal Values (men)
LV Chamber		
End-systole	3.2	2.1-4.0 cm
End-diastole	5.4	4.2-5.9 cm
Wall thickness (diastole)	0.8	0.6-1.0 cm
2D Ejection fraction	65% (estimate)	≥55 %
Left atrium	3.6	3.0-4.0 cm
Aortic sinus	2.9	<4.0 (<2.1 cm/m^2)

DOPPLER FLOWS

	Regurgitation	Velocity (m/s)	
Aortic valve	None	LVOT	1.0
		Ao	1.4
Mitral valve	Trace	E	1.0
		A	0.4
Pulmonary valve	Trace		
Tricuspid valve	Mild	TR-Jet	2.3

		Normal Values
RA pressure estimate (mm Hg)	5	0-5
PA pressure estimate (mm Hg)	26	20-30

FINDINGS

Left ventricle	Wall thickness, internal dimension and systolic function are normal with an estimated ejection fraction of 65%. There are no resting regional wall motion abnormalities.
Left atrium	Size is normal.
Aortic valve	Trileaflet with normal systolic opening and no regurgitation.
Aortic root	Normal dimensions with normal contours of the sinuses of Valsalva.
Mitral valve	Normal anatomy and motion with no stenosis and only physiologic regurgitation.
PA pressures	Estimated pulmonary systolic pressure is normal at 21-16 mm Hg, based on the velocity in the TR jet and the size and respiratory variation of the inferior vena cava.
Right heart	Right ventricular size and systolic function are normal. Tricuspid and pulmonic valves show normal anatomy and Doppler flows. Right atrial size is normal.
Pericardium	No effusion.

CONCLUSIONS

1. Normal valve anatomy and function.
2. Normal left ventricle with an estimated ejection fraction of 65%.
3. Normal pulmonary pressures and right heart.

Given these findings, the murmur appreciated on physical examination most likely is a benign flow murmur. Although resting left ventricular regional function is normal, coronary disease cannot be excluded on a resting study. If there is concern that chest pain may be due to coronary disease, a stress study should be considered.

Signed: _____MD

MEDICAL LIBRARY
RRISTON HOSPITAL

THE ECHO EXAM

Core Elements
A Complete Echo Exam Consists of Core Elements Plus Additional Components

Modality	Window	View/Signal	Measurements
Clinical data		Indication for echo Key history and physical findings Previous cardiac imaging data	Blood pressure at time of echo exam
2D imaging	*Parasternal*	Long axis Short axis aortic valve Short axis mitral valve Short axis LV (papillary muscle level) Right ventricular inflow	LV ED and ES dimensions LV ED wall thickness Aortic sinus ED dimension LA dimension
	Apical	4-chamber Anteriorly angulated 4-chamber 2-chamber Long axis	Visual estimate or biplane ejection fraction
	Subcostal	4-chamber IVC with respiration Proximal abdominal aorta	
	Suprasternal	Aortic arch	
Pulsed Doppler	*Parasternal* *Apical*	Pulmonary artery flow LV inflow at leaflet tips LV outflow	PA velocity E velocity A velocity LV outflow velocity
Color flow	*Parasternal*	Long axis: aortic and mitral valves Short axis: aortic and pulmonic valves RV inflow: tricuspid valve	Color flow to identify regurgitation of all four valves; if more than mild, measure vena contracta
	Apical	4-chamber: mitral and tricuspid valves Long axis: aortic and mitral valves	
CW Doppler	*Parasternal*	Tricuspid valve Pulmonic valve	TR-jet velocity
	Apical	Aortic valve Mitral valve Tricuspid valve	Aortic velocity TR-jet (PAP)

2D, Two-dimensional; A, atrial filling; E, early diastolic filling; ED, end-diastole; ES, end-systole; IVC, inferior vena cava; LV, left ventricle; PAP, pulmonary artery pressure; TR, tricuspid regurgitation.

Additional Components*

Abnormality on Core Elements	Additional Echo Exam Components (Chapter)
REASON FOR ECHO	Additional components to address specific clinical question*
LEFT VENTRICLE	
Decreased ejection fraction	See Systolic Function (6)
Abnormal LV filling velocities	See Diastolic Function (7)
Regional wall motion abnormality	See Ischemic Heart Disease (8)

Additional Components—cont'd

Abnormality on Core Elements	Additional Echo Exam Components (Chapter)
Increased wall thickness	See Hypertrophic Cardiomyopathy, Restrictive Cardiomyopathy, and Hypertensive Heart Disease (9)
VALVES	
Imaging evidence for stenosis or an increased antegrade transvalvular velocity	See Valve Stenosis (11)
Regurgitation greater than mild on color flow imaging or CW Doppler	See Valve Regurgitation (12)
Prosthetic valve	See Prosthetic Valves (13)
Valve mass or suspected endocarditis	See Endocarditis and Masses (14,15)
RIGHT HEART	
Enlarged RV	See Pulmonary Heart Disease and Congenital Heart Disease (9,17)
Elevated TR-jet velocity	See Pulmonary Pressures (6)
PERICARDIUM	
Pericardial effusion	See Pericardial Effusion (10)
Pericardial thickening	See Constrictive Pericarditis (10)
GREAT VESSELS	
Enlarged aorta	See Aortic Disease (16)

*The echo exam should always include additional components to address the clinical indication. For example, if the indication is "heart failure," additional components to evaluate systolic and diastolic function are needed even if the core elements do not show obvious abnormalities. If the indication is "cardiac source of embolus," the additional components for that diagnosis are needed.

CW, continuous wave; TR, tricuspid regurgitation.

Principles of Doppler Quantitation

Method	Assumptions/Characteristics	Examples of Clinical Applications
Volume flow $SV = CSA \times VTI$	Laminar flow Flat flow profile Cross-sectional area (CSA) and velocity time integral (VTI) measured at same site	Cardiac output Continuity equation for valve area Regurgitant volume calculations Intracardiac shunts, pulmonary to systemic flow ratio
Velocity-pressure relationship $\Delta P = 4v^2$	Flow limiting orifice CW Doppler signal recorded parallel to flow	Stenotic valve gradients Calculation of pulmonary pressures LV dP/dt
Spatial flow patterns	Proximal flow convergence region Narrow flow stream in orifice (vena contracta) Downstream flow disturbance	Detection of valve regurgitation and intracardiac shunts Level of obstruction Quantitation of regurgitant severity

CW, continuous wave; dP/dt, rate of change over time; LV, left ventricle.

SELF-ASSESSMENT QUESTIONS

QUESTION 1

Identify the numbered "spaces" shown in Figure 2–33.

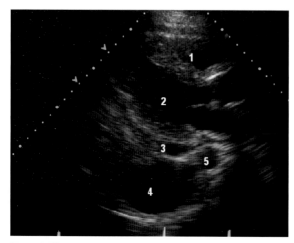

Figure 2–33.

1. _____
2. _____
3. _____
4. _____
5. _____

QUESTION 2

The aortic valve in Figure 2–34 is shown from the parasternal short axis view. Identify the aortic valve cusps.

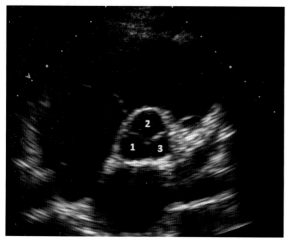

Figure 2–34.

1. _____
2. _____
3. _____

QUESTION 3

The atrial border tracing for left atrial volume measurement should be traced:

    A. In the parasternal long axis view
    B. To include the atrial appendage
    C. From the mitral annular plane
    D. At end-diastole

QUESTION 4

You are asked to review an echocardiogram of a patient who is a cardiac transplant recipient. Serial echocardiograms in the past documented an LV end-diastolic dimension of 4.5 cm (Figure 2–35).

The LV dimension from today's study is shown. The most likely explanation for the change between studies is:

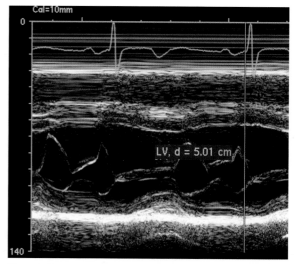

Figure 2–35.

    A. Measurement error
    B. Interval LV enlargement
    C. Measurement variability
    D. Misaligned ultrasound

QUESTION 5

The structure indicated by the arrow in the right ventricular inflow view shown in Figure 2–36 is:

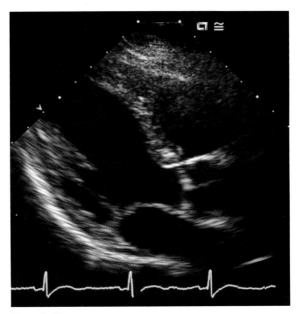

Figure 2–37.

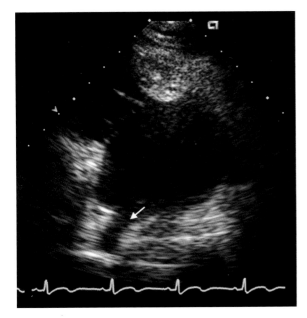

Figure 2–36.

A. Inferior vena cava
B. Right atrial appendage
C. Superior vena cava
D. Coronary sinus

QUESTION 6

The best view for visualization of an atrial septal defect is:

A. Parasternal short axis
B. Subcostal 4-chamber
C. Parasternal long axis
D. Anteriorly angled apical 4-chamber

QUESTION 7

The parasternal long axis view in Figure 2–37 is obtained. What is the next best step in improving this image?

A. Decrease the transducer frequency
B. Turn the harmonic imaging off
C. Move the transducer up an interspace
D. Position the patient in a steep left lateral decubitus position
E. Rotate the transducer slightly counter-clockwise

QUESTION 8

The Doppler flow signal shown in Figure 2–38 is most consistent with:

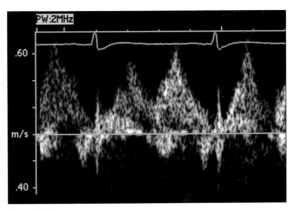

Figure 2–38.

A. Left ventricular inflow
B. Left ventricular outflow
C. Pulmonary vein flow
D. Pulmonary artery flow
E. Descending aorta flow

A. Aortic stenosis
B. Aortic regurgitation
C. Mitral stenosis
D. Mitral regurgitation
E. Tricuspid regurgitation

QUESTION 9

The Doppler tracing shown in Figure 2–39 is most consistent with:

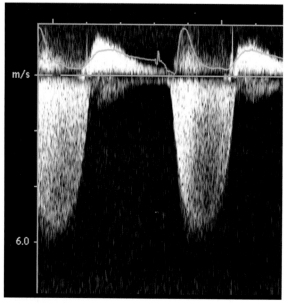

Figure 2–39.

QUESTION 10

Which of the following would improve the signal quality of the CW Doppler LV outflow recording shown in Figure 2–40?

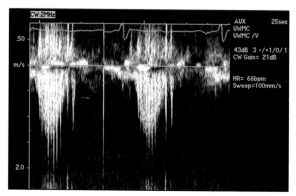

Figure 2–40.

A. Increase transducer frequency
B. Increase wall (high pass) filters
C. Increase gain
D. Increase velocity range
E. Use a different electrical outlet

ANSWERS

ANSWER 1

1. Right ventricle
2. Left ventricle
3. Pericardial effusion
4. Pleural effusion
5. Descending thoracic aorta

This is a parasternal long axis view of the heart, set to A depth of more than 18 cm. The numbered echolucent space closest to the transducer (*1*) is the right ventricle and the adjacent chamber (*2*) is the left ventricle. This patient has a small pericardial effusion that is circumferential, but more prominent posterior to the heart (*3*). The pericardial effusion is easily seen tracking anteriorly to the descending thoracic aorta (*5*), which is imaged in cross-section. A small strip of pericardial fluid is seen anterior to the right ventricle as well. Posterior to the heart is a large left-sided pleural effusion (*4*), which is seen tracking posterior to the descending thoracic aorta.

ANSWER 2

1. Non-coronary cusp
2. Right coronary cusp
3. Left coronary cusp

The normal aortic valve has three valve cusps. The non-coronary cusp (*1*) is adjacent to the interatrial septum. The right and left coronary artery cusps are named based on the origins of the coronary artery ostia from the respective cusp. The right coronary cusp (*2*) is adjacent to the right ventricle, and the left coronary cusp (*3*) is adjacent to the left atrium. Recognition of the relevant anatomic landmarks is important because variations in imaging modality may change image aspect. For example, with TEE, the aortic valve is imaged from a transducer placed posterior to the heart, which produces a "mirrored" image of the aortic valve compared with transthoracic imaging.

ANSWER 3: C

The left atrial border tracing for volume measurement should be performed from an apical window when the atria are maximally filled, which occurs at end-systole. Measurements should be taken from both the apical 2-chamber and apical 4-chamber views (Figures 2–41 and 2–42).

Care should be taken that images are optimized and not foreshortened, so volumes are not underestimated. The border tracing should follow the blood-tissue border of the LA and a horizontal line across the mitral annulus. The atrial area between the mitral

annular plane and the mitral leaflet coaptation point should be excluded. The left atrial appendage and the pulmonary vein ostia should also be excluded from the atrial area measurement. If either the 2-chamber or 4-chamber view is suboptimal, then a single apical view measurement can be used twice in the left atrial volume calculation. The parasternal long axis view is useful to provide an anterior-posterior LA dimension but, because it is a single linear measurement of the atria, may underestimate overall LA size. Border tracings from the parasternal long axis view would be inaccurate because this view does not allow for full visualization of the atria.

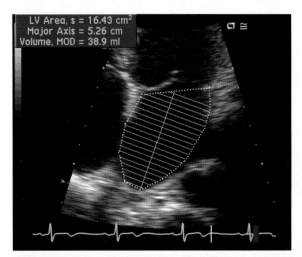

Figure 2–41.

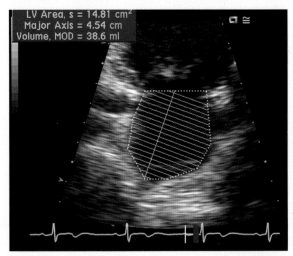

Figure 2–42.

ANSWER 4: D

The LV end-diastolic dimension is measured at 5.0 cm by the provided M-mode tracing. This is 0.5 cm larger than previous measurements. Interval change from the prior study or measurement variability should be considered, but only once proper alignment of the M-mode ultrasound beam is ensured. Two-dimensional guided M-mode allows for spatial alignment of the M-mode ultrasound beam to ensure cardiac dimension measurements are perpendicular to the endocardial border. Misaligned M-mode tracings lead to oblique images of the LV and overestimation of cardiac dimensions. The dimension was measured correctly from the M-mode image, but the beam itself is misaligned. A 2D image (Figure 2–43) from the same patient shows misalignment of the M-mode beam (*dashed line*), compared with the minor axis dimension perpendicular to the left ventricular long axis (*marked points*). In fact, the end-diastolic dimension is unchanged from previous, at 4.49 cm (Figure 2–43).

Although 2D imaging improves spatial resolution, M-mode has significantly improved temporal resolution, which may allow for better visualization of the blood-tissue border if image quality is suboptimal.

ANSWER 5: A

This image shows the inferior vena cava draining into the right atrium. In some patients there is an adjacent Eustachian valve at the ostium of the inferior vena cava. The coronary sinus also drains into the right

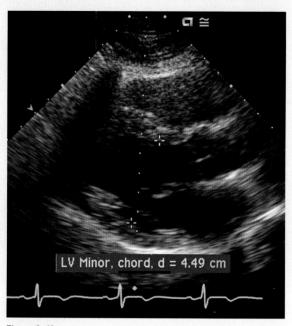

Figure 2–43.

atrium but inserts closer to the posterior leaflet of the tricuspid valve. The right atrial appendage is situated more anteriorly and is not optimally seen in this view. The superior vena cava also is more superiorly located and not seen in this view.

ANSWER 6: B

If image quality is adequate, the subcostal 4-chamber view allows 2D visualization of the entire atrial septum. Additionally, the atrial septum is perpendicular to the ultrasound beam and any flow across the septum would be directed toward the transducer, detectable by color Doppler imaging. Although the parasternal short axis view also allows for visualization of the atrial septum, the ultrasound beam is parallel to the atrial septum. Lack of reflection from the thin atrial septum at a parallel intercept angle often results in "dropout" of ultrasound signals and an apparent defect even when the atrial septum is normal. In the parasternal long axis view, the interatrial septum is not seen because it is medial to the standard image plane. Anterior angulation of the transducer in the apical 4-chamber view brings the aortic valve and aortic root into view and the interatrial septum is no longer in the imaging plane. In a standard apical 4-chamber view, the atrial septum is parallel to the ultrasound beam direction, resulting in signal dropout and an apparent defect even when the atrial septum is normal. However, color Doppler flow imaging in the apical 4-chamber and parasternal short axis views may be helpful if a flow stream from left to right across the septum is demonstrated.

ANSWER 7: C

This parasternal long axis image is recorded from a low interspace so that the septum appears relatively vertical on the image and the aortic valve not centered. This image plane results in inaccurate LV measurements by M-mode (oblique angle to LV minor axis dimension) and on 2D imaging (poorer axial resolution for endocardial edges than with correct alignment).

When the transducer is moved up an interspace (Figure 2–44), the ultrasound beam is now perpendicular to endocardial borders, the aortic valve is centered and closer to the transducer, and more of the ascending aorta is visualized. When tissue penetration is poor, a decrease in transducer frequency may be helpful, but this image has adequate image quality at every depth. Turning off tissue harmonic imaging would result in poor lateral resolution and poorer endocardial definition. When an adequate image cannot be obtained, positioning the patient in a steep left lateral position brings the cardiac structures closer to the chest wall; this image has adequate

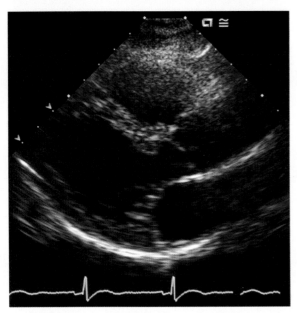

Figure 2–44.

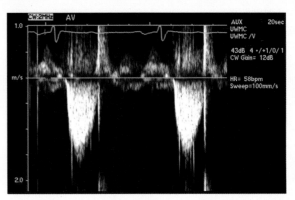

Figure 2–45.

quality, but does not have correct image position. Rotation of the transducer is not needed because the image plane is correctly aligned along the long axis of the aorta, aortic valve, mitral valve, and LV. The linear and symmetric closure of the aortic leaflets help confirm the correct image plane.

ANSWER 8: C

This pulsed Doppler recording shows pulmonary vein flow with the typical inflow curves in systole and diastole and slight reversal of flow after atrial contraction. This biphasic systolic-diastolic flow pattern is characteristic of venous flow, and a similar pattern is seen in the hepatic veins (or inferior vena cava) and in the superior vena cava. Aortic and pulmonary outflow occur in systole with an ejection curve shape, with a mid-systolic peak for the pulmonary artery and an early systolic peak for aortic flow. Descending aortic flow also occurs in systole, directed away from the transducer. LV inflow in diastole consists of an early (*E*) diastolic peak with a second peak occurring with atrial (*A*) contraction.

ANSWER 9: D

This is a CW Doppler recording (note velocity scale) showing a systolic flow signal, directed away from the transducer, with a maximum velocity of more than

5 m/s. This is most consistent with mitral regurgitation recorded from an apical window, reflecting the more than 100 mm Hg pressure difference between the LV and LA in systole. The diastolic flow signal is consistent with normal LV inflow; if mitral stenosis were present, the diastolic velocity would be higher and the slope of the deceleration slope would be flatter. The Doppler signal also indicates that the patient is in atrial fibrillation because there is no A-velocity seen on the diastolic signal. Aortic stenosis also occurs in systole and may be high velocity, but flow would end before mitral valve opening (reflecting isovolumic relaxation). Aortic regurgitation results in a high velocity diastolic flow signal as a result of the diastolic pressure difference between the aorta and LV. Tricuspid regurgitation typically is longer in duration than mitral regurgitation and the diastolic inflow signal across the tricuspid valve is lower in velocity. However, it may be difficult to distinguish mitral from tricuspid regurgitation unless both signals are recorded so that timing can be compared. If this were tricuspid regurgitation, the velocity would indicate very severe pulmonary hypertension.

ANSWER 10: C

This Doppler signal has excessive noise from high gain and low wall filters. With gain decreased and wall filters increased, the signal to noise ratio is improved as shown here (Figure 2–45).

Increasing the transducer frequency would decrease signal strength but not affect the signal to noise ratio, and is not usually an option with CW Doppler. Changing the velocity range would not affect signal to noise ratio. If electronic interference is a concern, using a different electrical outlet may be helpful.

3 The Transesophageal Echocardiogram

STEP-BY-STEP APPROACH

Step 1: Clinical Data

- In addition to the indication for the study and the cardiac history, clinical data establishing the safety of the TEE procedure are needed.
- The risk of the TEE procedure is related to both conscious sedation and esophageal intubation.
- Informed consent is obtained before the procedure.

Key points:

- ❏ Informed consent includes a description of the procedure with explanation of the expected benefits and potential risks.
- ❏ Complications serious enough to interrupt the procedure occur in less than 1% of cases, and the reported mortality rate is less than 1 in 10,000.
- ❏ Significant esophageal disease, excessive bleeding risk, and tenuous respiratory status are contraindications to TEE.
- ❏ The risk of hemodynamic compromise and respiratory depression are assessed using standard pre-anesthesia protocols and risk levels.
- ❏ Risk is higher in patients with impaired respiratory status or a history of sleep apnea.

- ❏ Patients typically have no oral intake for at least 6 hours before the procedure, except in emergencies.
- ❏ In anticoagulated patients, the level of anticoagulation is checked before the TEE to ensure it is in the therapeutic range.

Step 2: TEE Protocol

- The conscious sedation standards at each institution apply to TEE procedures.
- Typically these include having a skilled health care provider monitor level of consciousness, blood pressure, electrocardiogram (ECG), and arterial oxygen saturation.
- Oral suction is used to clear secretions and maintain an open airway.
- The study is optimally performed with a physician to manipulate the probe and direct the examination, a cardiac sonographer to optimize image quality and record data, and a nurse to monitor the patient.

Key points:

- ❏ Endocarditis prophylaxis is not routinely recommended for TEE.
- ❏ Adequate local anesthesia of the pharynx improves patient comfort and tolerance.

- ❏ The specific choice and dose of pharmacologic agents for sedation are based on institutional protocols.
- ❏ The TEE probe is inserted via a bite block using ultrasound gel for lubrication and to provide acoustic coupling between the ultrasound transducer on the probe and the wall of the esophagus.
- ❏ The TEE is advanced and angulated, with rotation of the image plane, to obtain diagnostic images in standard tomographic views.
- ❏ All health care providers involved in the procedure use universal precautions to prevent exposure to body fluids.

Step 3: Basic Examination Principles

- ▪ Although the TEE study is directed toward answering the clinical question, a complete systemic examination is recorded unless precluded by the clinical situation.
- ▪ Standard tomographic planes are used to evaluate cardiac chambers and valves.

Key points:

- ❏ In unstable patients, the examination should focus on the key diagnostic issues first, with additional recordings as tolerance and time allow.
- ❏ Each cardiac structures is evaluated in at least two orthogonal views or, ideally, using a rotational scan of the structure.
- ❏ Transducer frequency, depth, and zoom are adjusted to optimize visualization of each structure.
- ❏ With color Doppler, frame rate is optimized by decreasing depth and sector width to focus on the flow of interest.
- ❏ Only 1 to 2 beats of each view are recorded so the examiner can move quickly through the examination sequence. The total intubation time for a complete TEE ranges from less than 10 minutes for a relatively normal study to up to 30 minutes for complex examinations.

Step 4: Imaging Sequence

- ▪ The basic imaging sequence suggested in the Echo Exam: Basic Transesophageal Exam table at the end of this chapter is organized by probe position because this is the most efficient approach to examination in most cases.
- ▪ The imaging sequence is adjusted to focus on the key issues in unstable patients.
- ▪ This step-by-step approach describes the evaluation of each anatomic structure. This evaluation often is incorporated into the standard exam sequence shown in the Echo Exam table.

Key points:

- ❏ The probe position is constrained by the position of the esophagus so that optimal views are not always possible.
- ❏ The terms *advance* and *withdraw* refer to the vertical motion of the probe in the esophagus and stomach (Figure 3–1).
- ❏ The term *turn* refers to manual rotation of the entire probe toward the patient's right or left side (Figure 3–1).
- ❏ The terms *bending* and *extension* refer to motion of the tip of the probe in a plane parallel to the long axis of the probe, controlled by a large dial at the base of the probe (Figure 3–2).
- ❏ The term *rotation* refers to the electronic movement of the image plane in a circular fashion,

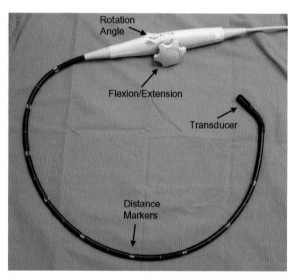

Figure 3–1. The transesophageal multiplane transducer is at the tip of a steerable probe. The probe motion is controlled by the dials, with the rotational angle of the image plane adjusted with a button.

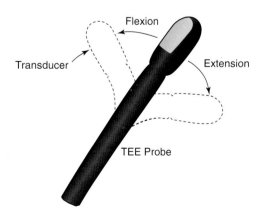

Figure 3–2. The tip of the probe can be extended or flexed to obtain standard image planes.

controlled by a button on the probe and displayed as an angle on the image (Figure 3–3).

❏ The exact degree of rotation needed for a specific view varies from patient to patient depending on the relationship between the heart and esophagus. The values given here are a starting point; image planes are adjusted based on cardiac anatomy, not specific rotation angles.

❏ If a specific view or flow is difficult to obtain, continue with the examination and return to this view later in the study.

❏ The specific views and flows recorded depend on the clinical indication and the findings of the study.

❏ Although modification of the exam sequence often is necessary, the examiner should quickly review a checklist of the recorded data before removing the probe to ensure a complete exam.

Step 5: Left Ventricle

■ The LV is evaluated in the high esophageal 4-chamber, 2-chamber, and long axis views.

■ Additional views of the LV include the transgastric short axis view and the transgastric apical view.

Key points:

❏ The starting point for a TEE is a 4-chamber view recorded from a high esophageal position (0 degree rotation) at maximum depth to show the entire LV. Typically the probe is extended to include as much of the apex as possible (Figure 3–4).

❏ With the probe centered behind the LA and the LV apex in the center of the image, the image plane is rotated to about 60 degrees to obtain a 2-chamber view and then rotated further to about 120 degrees for a long axis view (Figures 3–5 and 3–6).

❏ The transducer position, angulation, and exact degree of rotation are adjusted to optimize each view.

❏ Regional ventricular function is evaluated as follows:
  • Lateral and septal (inferior) walls in the 4-chamber view
  • Anterior and inferior walls in the 2-chamber view
  • Anterior septum and the inferior-lateral (or posterior) wall in the long axis view

❏ Ejection fraction is estimated from these three views. If a quantitative ejection fraction is needed, the biplane approach is used tracing endocardial borders at end-diastole and end-systole in 4-chamber and 2-chamber views.

❏ The LV apex often is foreshortened on TEE, even with careful positioning, which may result in underestimation of LV volumes.

❏ An apical LV thrombus may be missed because the apex is in the far field of the TEE image; transthoracic imaging is more sensitive for detection of apical thrombus.

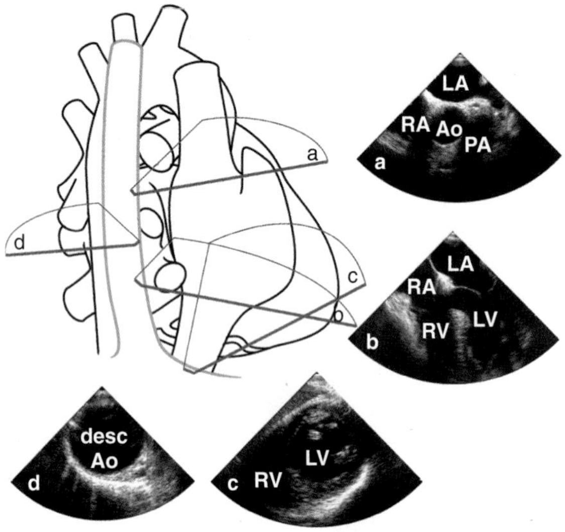

Figure 3–3. Diagram showing the TEE transducer locations for the four standard imaging views: basal (a), 4-chamber (b), transgastric (c), and aortic (d). Ao, aorta; desc Ao, descending aorta; LA, left atrium; LV, left ventricle; PA, pulmonary artery; RA, right atrium; RV, right ventricle. *From Burwash IG, Chan KL: Transesophageal Echocardiography. In Otto CM (ed): The Practice of Clinical Echocardiography, 3rd ed. Philadelphia, Elsevier, 2007.*

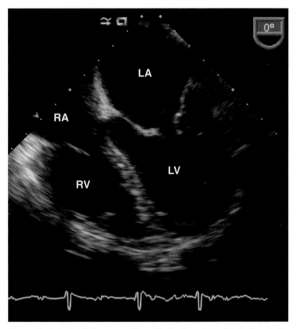

Figure 3–4. In the 0 degree position with the transducer located posterior to the LA, the probe tip is flexed or extended to obtain a 4-chamber view. The apparent apex in this view often is part of the anterior wall because it may not be possible to adjust the image plane to intersect the true apex.

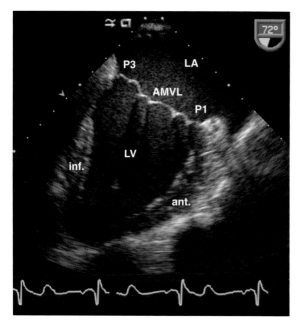

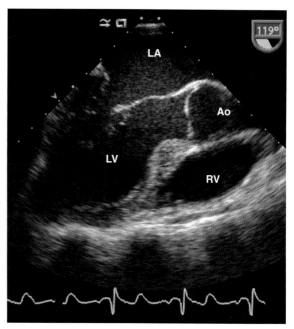

Figure 3–5. With the LV apex centered in the image plane at 0 degrees, the angle is adjusted to about 60 degrees to obtain a 2-chamber view, with the anterior and inferior LV walls. The lateral (*P1*) and medial (*P3*) scallops of the posterior mitral leaflet and the central segment of the anterior leaflet (*AMVL*) are typically seen in this view.

Figure 3–6. With further rotation of the image plane to about 120 degrees, a long axis view is obtained with the aortic valve and ascending aorta (*Ao*) and the inferior-lateral (posterior) and anterior septal walls of the LV.

Step 6: Left Atrium and Atrial Septum

- The body of the LA is evaluated in the high esophageal 4-chamber, 2-chamber, and long axis views.
- The LA appendage is imaged in at least two orthogonal planes at 0 and 90 degrees.
- The pulmonary veins are identified using two-dimensional (2D) and color Doppler imaging most easily in the 0 degree image plane, although views at 90 degrees also may be helpful.

Key points:

- ❐ Images of the LA are recorded at a shallow depth to focus on the structure of interest.
- ❐ The atrial septum is best examined by centering the septum in the image plane in the 4-chamber view and then slowly rotating the image plane, keeping the septum centered, from 0 to 120 degrees (Figure 3–7).
- ❐ The atrial appendage is imaged using a high frequency transducer, zoom mode, and a narrow sector to improve image resolution (Figure 3–8).
- ❐ Flow in the atrial appendage is recorded with a pulsed Doppler sample volume about 1 cm from the mouth of the appendage (Figures 3–9 and 3–10).
- ❐ The pulmonary veins are most easily identified using color Doppler with the aliasing velocity decreased to about 20 to 30 cm/s.

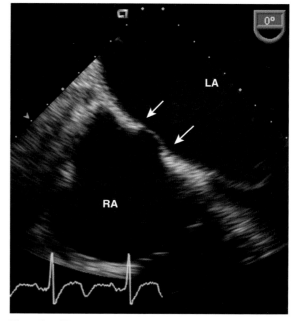

Figure 3–7. The atrial septum is examined by centering the septum in the image plane at 0 degrees rotation and then slowly rotating the image plane to 120 degrees. The thin fossa ovalis (between *arrows*) is well seen on this image.

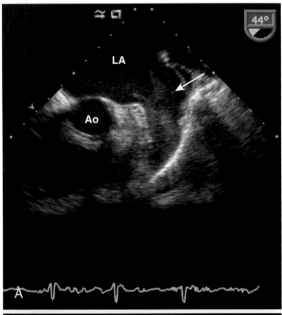

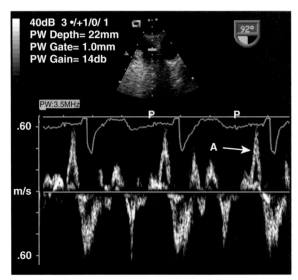

Figure 3–9. Doppler flow patterns in the atrial appendage are recorded with the sample volume in the appendage about 1 cm from the entrance into the LA. In this patient in sinus rhythm, the normal antegrade flow, with a velocity greater than 0.4 m/s after the p-wave, is seen (arrow).

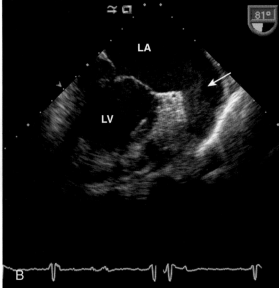

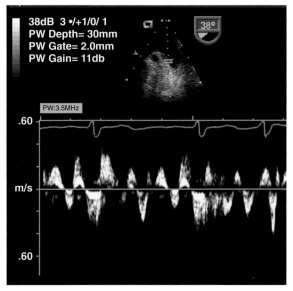

Figure 3–10. Atrial appendage flow in a patient in atrial fibrillation shows a rapid, irregular low velocity flow pattern.

Figure 3–8. Two views of the LA appendage at about 40 (A) and 80 (B) degrees rotation. The typical crescent shape of the appendage is seen, and the normal ridge (arrow) is seen between the LA appendage and left superior pulmonary view. In this patient with a dilated cardiomyopathy and atrial fibrillation, spontaneous contrast (arrows) is seen in the appendage, consistent with a low flow state.

❐ The left superior pulmonary vein is located adjacent to the atrial appendage and enters the atrium in an oblique anterior to posterior direction. The left inferior pulmonary vein, seen by advancing the probe a few centimeters, enters the atrium in a left lateral to medial direction (Figure 3–11).

❐ The right pulmonary veins are imaged in the 0 degree plane by turning the probe toward the patient's right side. Again the superior vein enters the atrium in an anterior-posterior direction; the inferior vein is seen by advancing the probe and enters in a right lateral to medial direction (Figure 3–12).

❐ Pulmonary vein flow is recorded with pulsed Doppler in one or more pulmonary veins, depending on the clinical indication for the study (Figure 3–13).

❐ An orthogonal view at 90 degrees also may be helpful, turning the probe rightward for the

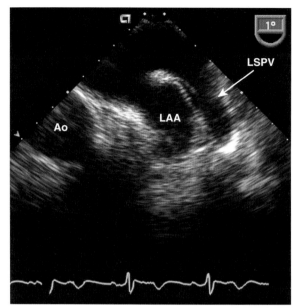

Figure 3–11. From the standard 4-chamber view at 0 degrees, the LA appendage (*LAA*) and left superior pulmonary vein (*LSPV*) are visualized by moving the transducer up in the esophagus and flexing the probe tip. There often is a normal prominent ridge, seen as a rounded mass in this view, between the atrial appendage and pulmonary vein.

right pulmonary veins and leftward for the left pulmonary veins (Figure 3–14).

Step 7: Mitral Valve

- The mitral valve is evaluated starting in the 4-chamber view and then rotating the image plane slowly to 120 degrees (long axis view), keeping the valve centered in the image.
- Additional views of the mitral valve include the transgastric short axis and 2-chamber view.
- TEE provides optimal evaluation of mitral regurgitant severity, allowing a parallel angle between the flow direction and ultrasound beam for CW Doppler, excellent visualization of the jet origin and direction, and accurate measurement of vena contracta width and proximal isovelocity surface area (PISA) radius.

Key points:

- ❏ The image depth is adjusted to just fit the mitral valve on the image. Transducer frequency, harmonic imaging, and gain are adjusted to improve the image (Figure 3–15).
- ❏ The mitral valve is first evaluated with 2D imaging alone to focus on the details of valve anatomy.
- ❏ A second rotational scan is performed using color Doppler to evaluate for mitral

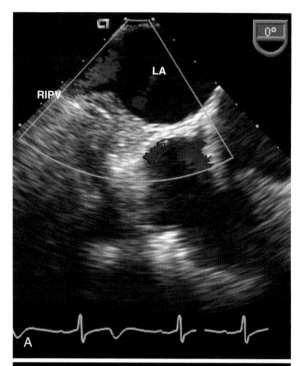

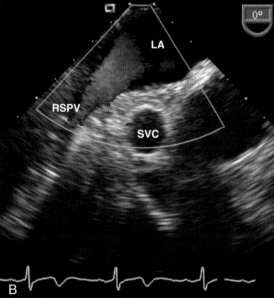

Figure 3–12. The right pulmonary veins are identified in the 0 degree image plane by turning the transducer toward the patient's right side. The right inferior pulmonary view (*A*) is seen with color Doppler entering the LA at a relatively perpendicular angle to the ultrasound beam. The probe is withdrawn 1 to 2 cm to visualize the right superior pulmonary vein (*B*), which enters the atrium relatively parallel to the ultrasound beam direction.

regurgitation. Regurgitation is evaluated based on measurement of the vena contracta, evaluation of pulmonary venous flow pattern, the CW Doppler signal, and quantitative parameters as discussed in Chapter 12 (Figure 3–16).

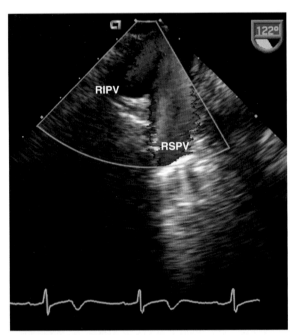

Figure 3–13. The right pulmonary veins also can be imaged in the orthogonal plane by rotating the image plane to a longitudinal view, with the right superior pulmonary vein on the right and the inferior pulmonary vein on the left.

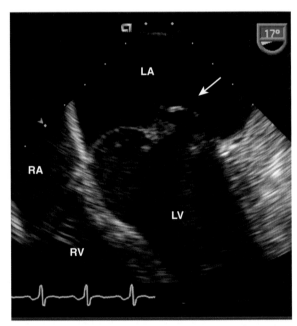

Figure 3–15. The mitral valve is imaged starting at 0 degrees rotation with the valve centered in the image plane and the depth adjusted to focus on the valve. The image plane is then slowly rotated, keeping the mitral valve centered, to examine the entire valve apparatus. In this patient, prolapse of the central (*P2*) segment of the posterior leaflet (arrow) is best seen at 17 degrees rotation.

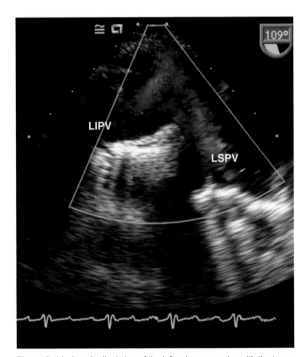

Figure 3–14. Longitudinal view of the left pulmonary veins with the transducer turned toward the patient's left side. In this image, superior structures are to the right of the image and inferior structures to the left. As for the right pulmonary veins, the left inferior pulmonary vein (*LIPV*) enters the atrium at a perpendicular angle to the ultrasound beam, whereas the left superior pulmonary vein (*LSPV*) enters with the flow direction parallel to the ultrasound beam.

□ The transgastric view of the mitral valve offers improved visualization of the subvalvular apparatus, although concurrent evaluation by transthoracic imaging also may be needed (Figure 3–17).

□ Regurgitation is evaluated based on vena contracta width, and calculation of regurgitant volume and orifice areas using the PISA method, and CW Doppler recording of regurgitant flow (see Chapter 12).

Step 8: Aortic Valve and Ascending Aorta

■ The aortic valve and proximal ascending aorta are evaluated in standard long and short axis views.

■ Aortic regurgitation is evaluated by color Doppler in high esophageal views.

Key points:

□ The aortic valve is best seen in the long axis view (at about 120 degrees) and in a short axis view of the valve (at about 30 to 50 degrees rotation), using a shallow depth, high frequency transducer, zoom mode, and narrow 2D sector (Figures 3–18 and 3–19).

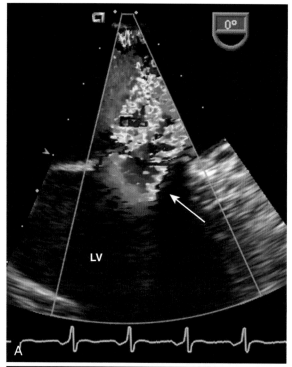

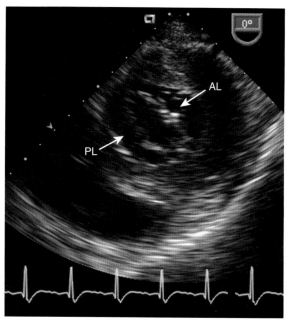

Figure 3–17. From the transgastric short axis view of the LV, the transducer is withdrawn about 1 cm to obtain a short axis view of the mitral valve with the anterior leaflet (*AL*) and posterior leaflet (*PL*) seen.

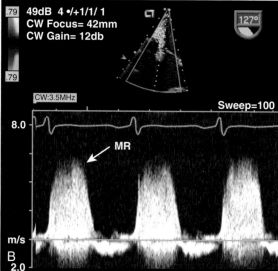

Figure 3–16. *A,* Color Doppler is used to identify the presence of mitral regurgitation and to evaluate severity based on vena contracta width (*arrow*) and by the proximal isovelocity surface area (*PISA*) approach (see Chapter 12). *B,* The continuous wave Doppler velocity curve also is useful for confirming the identify and evaluating severity of regurgitation.

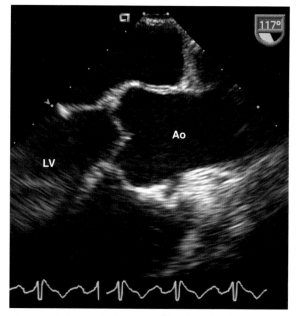

Figure 3–18. A long axis view of the aortic valve and aortic root typically is obtained at about 120 degrees rotation. The exact rotation angle needed varies between patients; the image plane is adjusted to the standard image plane based on anatomy, not a specific rotation angle. Note that the right coronary ostium is seen in this view.

❏ From the standard long axis view, the TEE probe is turned rightward and leftward to see the medial and lateral aspects of the valve. The probe also is withdrawn higher in the esophagus to see as much of the ascending aorta as possible.

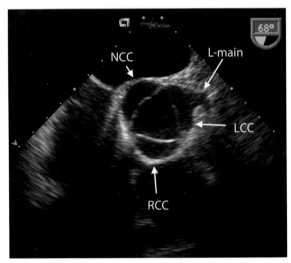

Figure 3–19. The short axis view of the aortic valve is obtained by centering the valve in the image in the long axis image and then rotating the image plane to about 45 degrees. This zoomed image shows the right coronary cusp (RCC), left coronary cusp (LCC), and non-coronary cusp (NCC) in systole. The left main coronary artery is also seen.

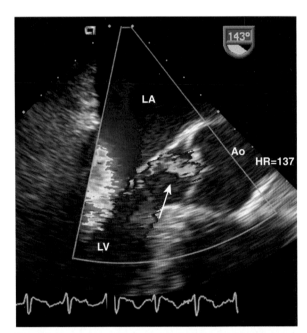

Figure 3–20. Aortic regurgitation is evaluated using color Doppler in long and short axis images. Regurgitant severity is evaluated by measurement of vena contracta width in the long axis view. This example shows a narrow jet, consistent with mild regurgitation.

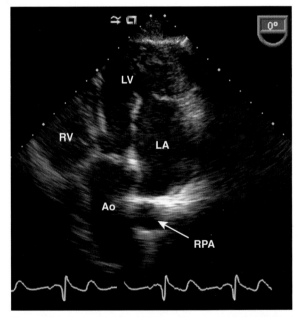

Figure 3–21. From a deep transgastric position, an anteriorly angulated 4-chamber view is obtained by flexion of the probe tip. This image plane does not pass through the true LV apex, with obvious foreshortening of the LV in this image. The ascending aorta (Ao) and right pulmonary artery (RPA) are seen.

- ❏ From the short axis view, the probe is slowly advanced and withdrawn to visualize the areas immediately inferior and superior to the valve plane.
- ❏ Aortic regurgitation can be evaluated by color Doppler, with measurement of vena contracta, although precise quantitation of regurgitant severity may be difficult on TEE because the Doppler beam cannot be aligned parallel to flow (Figure 3–20).
- ❏ CW Doppler of the aortic regurgitant jet sometimes can be recorded from a transgastric apical view, but underestimation of velocity is likely because of a non-parallel intercept angle between the ultrasound beam and regurgitant jet (Figure 3–21).
- ❏ Transthoracic imaging often provides more precise quantitation of regurgitant severity.

Step 9: Coronary Arteries

- The left main coronary artery is easily seen in the short axis view of the aorta valve (Figure 3–22).
- The right coronary artery may be seen in a long axis view of the ascending aorta or in the short axis view of the aortic valve, but can be identified in only about 20% of cases (see Figure 3–18).

Key points:

- ❏ The left main coronary is slightly superior to the aortic valve plane.

- ❏ Visualization of the coronary ostium is enhanced by using a high frequency transducer and zoom mode.
- ❏ The bifurcation of the left main into the left anterior descending and circumflex coronaries

is frequently visualized, but the more distal vessels are not seen in most patients.

❏ Identification of the coronary ostium is most important in adolescents and young adults with exertional symptoms and in patients with prior aortic root surgery with coronary reimplantation.

Step 10: Right Ventricle and Tricuspid Valve

■ The RV and tricuspid valve are evaluated in the high esophageal 4-chamber and RV inflow views (Figure 3–23).

■ Additional views of the RV and tricuspid valve include the transgastric short axis view and RV inflow views.

Key points:

❏ In the initial TEE 4-chamber images, RV size and systolic function are evaluated.

❏ The RV also is seen in the short axis view starting at the aortic valve level and slowly advancing the transducer to see the tricuspid valve and RV.

❏ From the transgastric short axis view, the image plane is rotated to 90 degrees and the probe is turned rightward to obtain a view of the RA,

tricuspid valve, and RV, similar to a transthoracic RV inflow view (Figure 3–24).

❏ Tricuspid valve anatomy and motion and color Doppler tricuspid regurgitation are evaluated in each of these views.

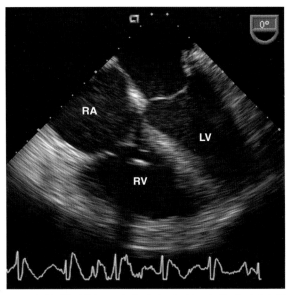

Figure 3–23. The RV is seen in the 4-chamber view, but it often is helpful to turn the transducer toward the RV to focus on RV size and systolic function. This patient has moderate RV dilation and systolic dysfunction. Rotation of the image plane allows evaluation of the RV outflow tract in the short axis view at the aortic valve level.

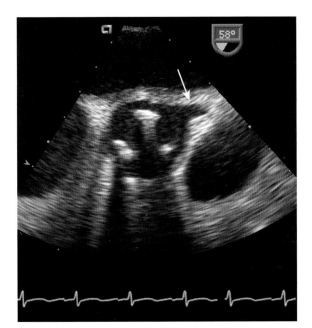

Figure 3–22. The left coronary artery is seen by moving the image plane slightly superior to the aortic valve short axis image plane. In this patient, the three stents of a tissue aortic valve prosthesis are seen at the same level as the left main coronary artery (arrow) ostium.

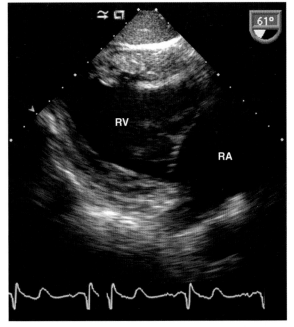

Figure 3–24. From the transgastric short axis view, the image plane is rotated to between 60 and 90 degrees. From the 2-chamber view of the LV, the probe is turned toward the patient's right side to obtain this view of the right atrium (RA), tricuspid valve, and right ventricle (RV).

❑ A CW Doppler recording of tricuspid regurgitant jet velocity may be obtained from the esophageal 4-chamber or short axis view, although underestimation of velocity because of a poor intercept angle is possible.

Step 11: Right Atrium

■ The RA is evaluated in the high esophageal 4-chamber view and in the 90-degree view of the RA (Figure 3–25).
■ Additional views of the RA include a low atrial view, at the level of the coronary sinus, and the transgastric 2-chamber view of the right side of the heart.

Key points:

❑ The RA is visualized by rotating the image plane to 90 degrees and turning the probe rightward to obtain a longitudinal view of the RA, including the entrances of the superior and inferior vena cava.
❑ The trabeculated RA appendage may be seen adjacent to the entry of the superior vena cava into the atrium.
❑ The inferior vena cava (IVC) can be evaluated by advancing the probe slowly toward the gastroesophageal junction.

❑ The central hepatic vein enters the IVC at a perpendicular angle, allowing Doppler recording of hepatic vein flow when indicated.
❑ From the standard 4-chamber plane at 0 degrees, the probe is advanced to obtain a low atrial view and the junction of the coronary sinus with the RA. The size and flow characteristics of the coronary sinus can be evaluated in this view when needed.

Step 12: Pulmonary Valve and Pulmonary Artery

■ The pulmonary valve and pulmonary artery are visualized in a very high esophageal view in the 0 degree image plane or in a 90 degree image plane with the transducer turned toward the left (RV outflow view) (Figure 3–26).
■ Images of the pulmonic valve may be suboptimal because the valve is in the far field of the image and it may be obscured by the air-filled bronchus at this level of the esophagus.

Key points:

❑ The pulmonic valve also may be visualized in the transgastric short axis view.
❑ Doppler flow in the pulmonary artery can be recorded from the high esophageal position.

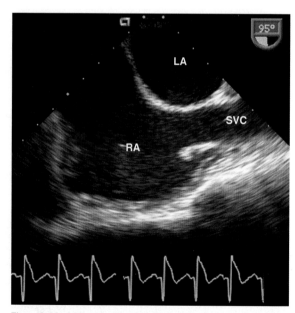

Figure 3–25. A long axis view of the RA is obtained with the image plane rotated to 90 degrees and the transducer turned toward the patient's right side. The superior vena cava (*SVC*) enters the atrium near the trabeculated atrial appendage. When the transducer is advanced in the esophagus, the entrance of the inferior vena cava into the atrium also may be seen in this view.

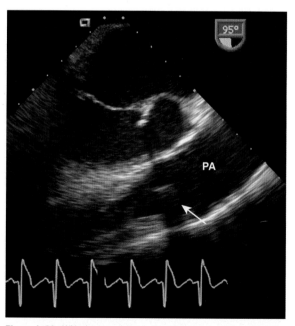

Figure 3–26. With the transducer in the high esophageal position, the pulmonary artery (*PA*) is seen with the image plane rotated to 90 degrees and the transducer turned slightly toward the patient's left side. The anteriorly located pulmonic valve (*arrow*) is relatively distant from the transducer, so image quality often is suboptimal.

- Evaluation of pulmonic regurgitation with color Doppler is performed in the RV outflow view. However, transthoracic imaging of the pulmonic valve often provides more accurate data.
- The pulmonary artery bifurcation and proximal right and left pulmonary arteries may be seen in a high esophageal view, but visualization of more distal pulmonary arteries is rarely possible (Figure 3–27).
- Cardiac magnetic resonance imaging provides an alternate approach to evaluation of the pulmonic valve and pulmonary artery.

Step 13: Descending Aorta and Aortic Arch

- The descending aorta is evaluated in a short axis view, starting at the transgastric level, by turning the probe leftward to identify the vessel and then slowly withdrawing the probe to visualize each segment of the descending thoracic aorta (Figure 3–28).
- Once the probe reaches the level of the aortic arch, the image plane is turned rightward and the probe extended to visualize the arch and ascending aorta.

Key points:

- Between the segment of the ascending aorta visualized in the high esophageal long axis view

and the aortic arch, there is a segment of the ascending aorta that may be missed on TEE imaging.
- In addition to short axis images of the descending aorta, the image plane may be rotated to 90 degrees to provide a longitudinal view of the extent of disease. However, the short axis view should always be used to ensure that the medial and lateral aspects of the aorta are examined, which would be missed in a single longitudinal image plane.
- Normal structures adjacent to the aorta (connective tissue, lymph nodes) should not be mistaken for pathologic aortic conditions.

Step 14: The TEE Report

- The TEE report provides a systematic summary of the findings arranged by anatomic structure.
- The study includes the diagnostic implications of the findings, notes any limitations of the study, and suggests further evaluation as appropriate.

Key points:

- The TEE report includes evaluation of:
  - LV size and function
  - RV size and function
  - LA and atrial appendage anatomy and evidence for thrombus

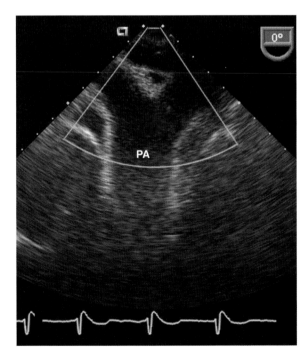

Figure 3–27. The main pulmonary artery and pulmonary artery bifurcation seen in a very high transesophageal view. This probe position may not be well tolerated in some patients, and this image cannot be obtained in all patients.

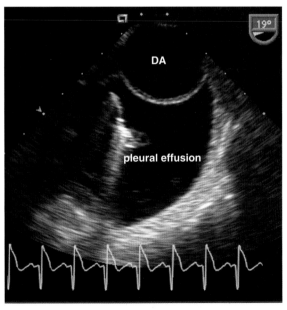

Figure 3–28. With the transducer turned toward the patient's left side, the descending thoracic aorta (*DA*) is imaged in cross section. This patient also has a pleural effusion.

- Anatomy of the interatrial septum and location of the four pulmonary veins
- Aortic, mitral, tricuspid, and pulmonic valve anatomy and function
- Abnormalities of the ascending aorta, descending aorta, or aortic arch

❐ Integration of the data to provide a specific diagnosis (such as "these findings are diagnostic for endocarditis") is provided whenever possible.

❐ Any unresolved clinical issues and areas of uncertainty are identified, and specific approaches to resolving these issues are recommended.

❐ The TEE report also includes the details of the procedure, including informed consent, patient monitoring, medications, and any procedural complications.

THE ECHO EXAM

Basic Transesophageal Exam

Probe Position	Rotation Angle	Views	Focus On
High esophageal *Set depth to include LV apex*	0° 60° 120°	4-chamber 2-chamber Long axis	• LV size, global, and regional function • RV size and systolic function • LA and RA size
High esophageal *↓ depth to optimize valves*	120° 120° → 0°	Long axis 2-chamber 4-chamber	• Mitral valve
	120° 30-50°	Long axis Short axis	• Aortic valve • Aorta
	0° 60° 90°	Depth	• LA appendage (resolution mode, 7 MHz) • Pulmonary veins
	0° → 90°	Rotational scan	• Atrial septum
	0° 90°	4-chamber SVC/IVC view	• RV • RA • Superior and inferior vena cava
	0° 60° 90°	4-chamber Short axis RV outflow	• Tricuspid valve • Pulmonic valve and pulmonary artery
Transgastric	0°	Short-axis	• LV wall motion , wall thickness, chamber dimensions • RV size and function
	90°	Long-axis	• LV and mitral valve • Turn medially to image RV and tricuspid valve
Transgastric apical	0°	4-chamber	• Useful for antegrade aortic flow but may still be non-parallel intercept angle
Transgastric to high esophageal	0°	Short axis descending aorta	• Image aorta from the diaphragm to aortic arch

IVC, inferior vena cava; LV, left ventricular; RV, right ventricular; LA, left atrial; RA, right atrial; SVC, superior vena cava.

SELF-ASSESSMENT QUESTIONS

QUESTION 1

A transesophageal echocardiogram is performed on a critically ill patient who has intermittent hypoxia despite mechanical ventilator support (Figure 3–29). The image provided is most consistent with:

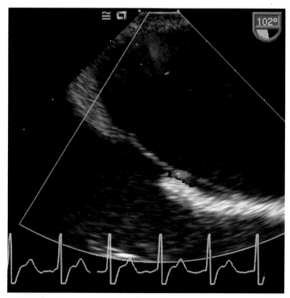

Figure 3–29.

A. Anomalous pulmonary vein
B. Sinus venosus septal defect
C. Patent foramen ovale
D. Thrombus in transit

QUESTION 2

A 50-year-old man with a history of dilated cardiomyopathy presents with fever and *Staphylococcus* bacteremia. TEE is performed. An image of the mitral valve is shown in Figure 3–30. This is most consistent with:

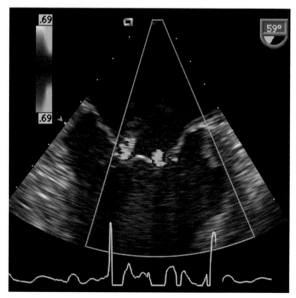

Figure 3–30.

A. Paravalvular abscess
B. Mitral leaflet perforation
C. Mitral valve prolapse
D. Functional mitral regurgitation

QUESTION 3

An 86-year-old woman presents with dyspnea. Electrocardiography demonstrates newly diagnosed atrial fibrillation, and a transesophageal echocardiogram is ordered to evaluate for LA appendage thrombus before direct current cardioversion. An image of the LA appendage is shown in Figure 3–31. It is consistent with:

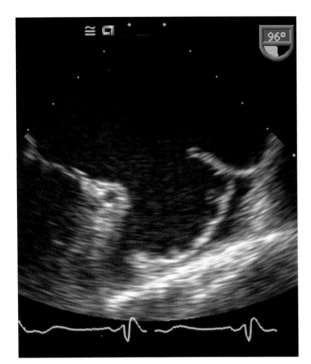

Figure 3–31.

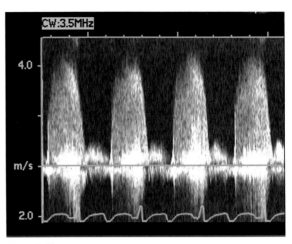

Figure 3–32.

A. Aortic stenosis
B. Aortic regurgitation
C. Mitral stenosis
D. Mitral regurgitation
E. Tricuspid regurgitation

QUESTION 6

TEE was requested for evaluation of mitral regurgitation in a 64-year-old man with dyspnea, and the images shown in Figure 3–33, A and B, were obtained. Why does the mitral regurgitation jet look larger in image B compared with image A?

A. Different image plane
B. Later in cardiac cycle
C. Higher transducer frequency
D. Lower Nyquist limit
E. Faster frame rate

A. Reverberation artifact
B. LA appendage thrombus
C. Atrial trabeculation
D. Spontaneous echo contrast

QUESTION 4

A 55-year-old man with recent history of an ST elevation anterior myocardial infarction presents with acute ischemia of the right lower extremity. Transthoracic echocardiogram images done at the time of his infarction demonstrated poor image quality. The best option for further diagnostic evaluation to evaluate the source of limb ischemia in this patient is:

A. Microbubble transpulmonary contrast
B. Transesophageal echocardiogram
C. Abdominal vascular ultrasound
D. Lower extremity venous Doppler

QUESTION 5

The Doppler tracing shown in Figure 3–32 was acquired on TEE imaging. This signal is most consistent with:

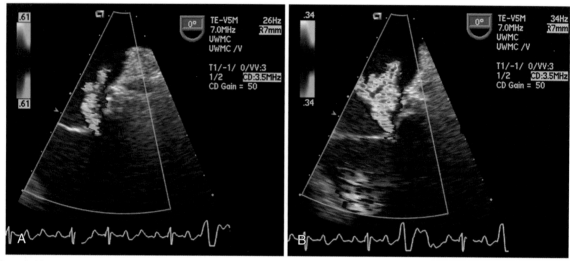

Figure 3–33.

QUESTION 7

The structure indicated by the question mark in Figure 3–34 is:

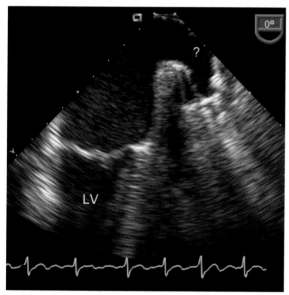

Figure 3–34.

A. Left atrial appendage
B. Pulmonary vein
C. Coronary sinus ostium
D. Right lower pulmonary vein

QUESTION 8

A transesophageal echocardiogram is performed to evaluate for endocarditis. The procedure is completed and all views are obtained. After recording the transgastric view, the probe is withdrawn back into the esophagus. In this position, there is resistance to further withdrawal of the probe. The next best step is to:

A. Withdraw the probe
B. Retroflex the probe
C. Rotate the probe
D. Advance the probe

QUESTION 9

Identify the structure indicated by the asterisk or arrow on each of the TEE images shown in Figure 3–35:

A. _____
B. _____
C. _____
D. _____

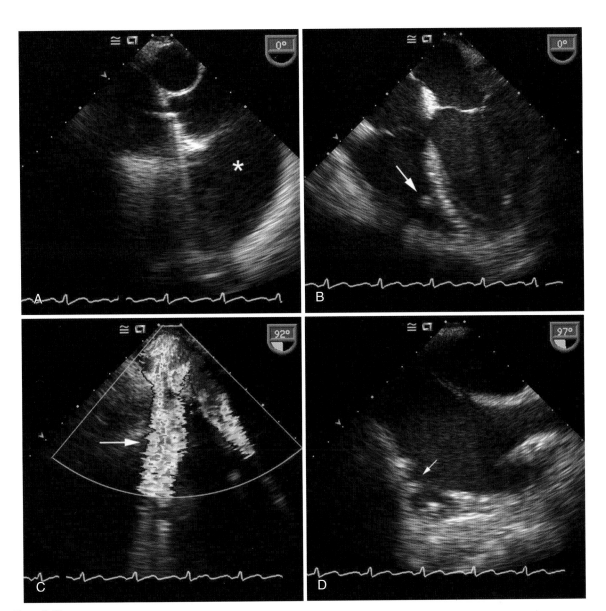

Figure 3-35.

ANSWERS

ANSWER 1: C

This image is taken from a bicaval view (100 degree mid-esophageal view) where the SVC and IVC are seen at their entry into the RA. In this case, color Doppler flow is shown in the mid-portion of the intraatrial septum, adjacent to the thin tissue layer that overlays the fossa ovalis, consistent with a patent foramen ovale (PFO). If RA pressure transiently increases over LA pressure, intra-atrial right to left shunting may occur across the PFO, leading to systemic hypoxia. A sinus venosus septal defect is a shunt at the base of the atrial septum, near either the inferior or superior vena cava, and is also best seen from the bicaval view with the probe slightly withdrawn. An anomalous pulmonary vein would not cause hypoxia because the pulmonary vein enters into the RA (left to right shunt only), with no channel that would allow right to left intra-cardiac flow. An anomalous pulmonary vein is identified by showing the absence of one view entering the LA and then identifying the location of the vein entry into the RA, SVC, or IVC. This patient is also incidentally noted to have mild lipomatous hypertrophy of the base of the interatrial septum (adjacent to the SVC), a benign finding that is not consistent with intracardiac thrombus.

ANSWER 2: D

In the normal mitral valve, leaflet size is asymmetric. The anterior mitral valve leaflet occupies less of the mitral annular circumference than the posterior mitral valve leaflet and "sits within" the posterior leaflet during leaflet coaptation. This normal anatomy is seen in Figure 3–36, a parasternal short axis view of the mitral valve taken during diastole.

In the transesophageal 60-degree view of an anatomically normal mitral valve, the image plane cuts horizontally through the tip of the anterior mitral valve leaflet. The two commissures are seen on either side of the valve, producing the two regurgitant jets. The tip of the anterior mitral valve leaflet is seen in the center of the two regurgitant jets. In this case, the dilated LV leads to leaflet tethering and mild, functional mitral regurgitation. There is no prolapse or flattening of the valve leaflets in systole. TEE is reasonable to evaluate for endocarditis in this patient who presents with fever and bacteremia. Leaflet perforation is usually the result of endocarditis or iatrogenic leaflet trauma (as would occur during cardiac surgery or cardiac catheterization) and would appear as regurgitation distant from expected commissures, within the body of the leaflet. Paravalvular abscess is another potential complication of endocarditis. This is usually seen along the aortic mitral intervalvular fibrosa, appearing as an echolucent space at the base of the anterior mitral valve leaflet adjacent to the aortic valve annulus, and is not seen in this case.

ANSWER 3: C

In patients with atrial fibrillation undergoing evaluation for direct current cardioversion who have not been on chronic anticoagulation, TEE is needed to visualize the LA appendage. The appendage should be visualized from several views. In this image, atrial trabeculations, atrial muscle seen in cross section, are seen protruding along the lateral wall of the appendage. Because trabeculations are contiguous with the atrial wall, contractile motion of the trabeculations should be seen with atrial activity and make thrombus less likely. A thrombus, if present, should be seen from multiple views to confirm its presence. A second view in this patient (Figure 3–37) shows no evidence of thrombus.

The normal ridge (*arrow*) between the LA appendage and left superior pulmonary vein is seen in both views. Spontaneous echo contrast appears as swirling echodensities within the body of the appendage and is consistent with low velocity flow. Often, spontaneous echo contrast coexists with a true appendage thrombus. A reverberation artifact from the ridge between the appendage and the left upper pulmonary vein is common and often difficult to differentiate from a thrombus. Artifact is more likely if the abnormality cannot be demonstrated from multiple image planes.

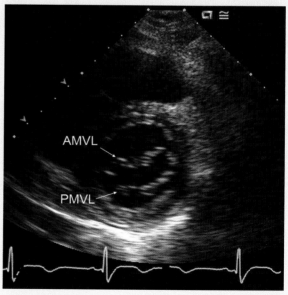

Figure 3–36.

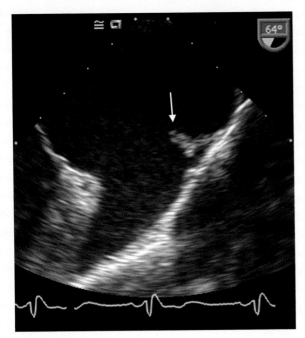

Figure 3–37.

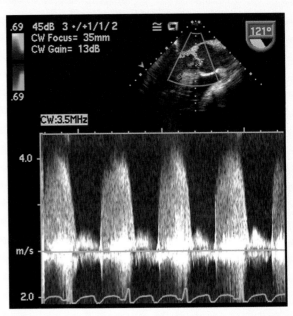

Figure 3–38.

ANSWER 4: A

This patient is presenting with acute limb ischemia, concerning for peripheral embolism. In the setting of a recent anterior wall myocardial infarction, an embolic source from apical thrombus should be considered. The cardiac apex is usually anteriorly situated and is generally well seen by transthoracic imaging. However, recent transthoracic images in this patient documented poor image quality. Microbubble transpulmonary contrast enhances endocardial border definition, allowing for improved visualization of the LV apex. An apical thrombus, if present, may displace microbubble contrast, creating a negative filling effect. Image planes for TEE imaging are constrained by esophageal anatomy. With TEE, the LV is foreshortened and the apex is not optimally seen to exclude thrombus. In a patient with limb ischemia, complications of the cardiac catheterization should be considered; however, any complication identified at the abdominal aorta level would cause bilateral limb ischemia, not unilateral limb ischemia as seen in this case. Lower extremity Doppler would diagnose a venous thrombus and might document the arterial blockage but would not aid in evaluation of the source of the arterial occlusion.

ANSWER 5: B

This is a CW Doppler tracing (note velocity scale) with a maximum velocity of about 4 m/s and with flow occurring in diastole, directed toward the transducer, consistent with aortic regurgitation. Aortic stenosis, mitral regurgitation, and tricuspid regurgitation might have a similar velocity, but all occur in systole. Mitral stenosis would be a lower velocity diastolic signal, usually directed away from the transducer from a high TEE 4-chamber view. The tracing was obtained in a patient with a bicuspid aortic valve in whom the aortic regurgitant jet was directly posteriorly (Figure 3–38).

ANSWER 6: D

These two images are in the same image plane (0 degrees) with an enlarged image of mitral valve closure in a TEE 4-chamber view. The Nyquist limit in *A* is 0.61 m/s, compared with 0.34 m/s in *B*, so that the mitral regurgitant jet appears larger as a result of lower velocities in the regurgitant jet coded as color flow at the lower aliasing velocity. Although mitral regurgitant severity may vary from frame to frame during the cardiac cycle, particularly with late systolic prolapse in mitral prolapse, both these frames were recorded in early systole, as seen by the break in the ECG signal at the bottom of the image. The transducer frequency is the same on both images (7 MHz); a higher transducer frequency would result in a smaller regurgitant jet color area. The frame rate is slightly faster (34 vs. 24 Hz) on the second image, but this is unlikely to affect the color jet size because both frame rates are adequate for diagnosis. Notice that the size of the jet as it crosses the mitral valve, the vena contracta, is similar on both images. Vena contracta size is a better measure of regurgitant severity than jet area because it is less dependent on imaging parameters, as shown in this example.

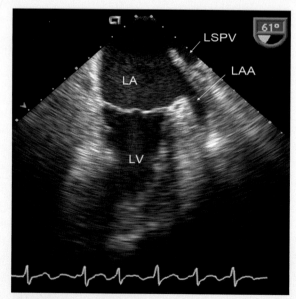

Figure 3–39.

ANSWER 7: B

The entrance of the pulmonary veins to the LA is easily seen by TEE. This is the left upper pulmonary vein which is typically the easiest to image and enters the LA superior to the LA appendage. This is not the LA appendage because a ridge of tissue separates the left upper pulmonary vein and the atrial appendage and would be seen adjacent to the transducer. The LA appendage lies just superior to the posterior mitral valve leaflet long the atrial wall, as seen in the image shown in Figure 3–39, taken from the same patient. The left lower pulmonary vein is best seen with the probe at 0 degrees and slightly advanced, where it enters the LA at a horizontal angle from the transducer. The right pulmonary veins are also seen best with the probe at 0 degrees and turned toward the patient's right side. The coronary sinus drains into the RA, adjacent to the inferior vena cava, and is best seen in the 0 degree view with the probe advanced to the gastroesophageal junction.

ANSWER 8: D

In the transgastric view, optimization of the short axis view of the LV typically involves flexion of the transducer for superior angulation of the probe tip. Once completed, flexion of the probe tip should be relaxed before withdrawal back into the esophagus; otherwise, the tip may be withdrawn in the fully flexed/folded position. In this probe position, withdrawing, retroflexing, or rotating the probe further may perforate the esophagus. The esophagus is too narrow to correct a folded probe within the esophagus. The probe should be readvanced to the stomach, where the tip can be relaxed. If a folded TEE probe is suspected, chest radiography may be used to confirm the suspicion before further probe manipulation.

ANSWER 9:

A. Pleural effusion
B. Moderator band
C. Left inferior pulmonary vein
D. RA appendage

Image *A* shows a large echolucent space adjacent to the descending thoracic aorta (seen as a circle as the top of the image), consistent with a large left pleural effusion. Image *B* shows a 4-chamber view with an echodensity in the apex of the RV; this is the typical location for the moderator band. Image *C* shows two veins directed toward the transducer in a 90 degree image plane; these are consistent with a superior (on the right) and inferior (on the left) pulmonary vein—most likely the left pulmonary veins, although the right pulmonary veins may look similar. During an exam, right and left pulmonary veins are easily distinguished by rotating the probe toward the LA. Image *D* is a longitudinal view (at about 90 degrees) of the RA, atrial septum, and superior vena cava. The trabeculated space indicated by the arrow is the normal RA appendage.

4 Advanced Echocardiographic Modalities

STRESS ECHOCARDIOGRAPHY

Basic principles

- Physiologic abnormalities may be evident only when there is an increased cardiovascular demand.
- Cardiac workload can be increased with exercise or pharmacologic agents.
- Echocardiographic imaging before and immediately after (or during) stress is called stress echocardiography.

Key points:

□ Exercise duration, heart rate and blood pressure response to exercise, electrocardiogram (ECG) changes, and symptoms are all important components of the stress echocardiographic study.
□ The primary endpoint for an exercise stress test is inability to exercise further (often due to leg fatigue or dyspnea).
□ The primary endpoint for a pharmacologic stress test is reaching 85% of the patient's maximum predicted heart rate.
□ Other stress test endpoints are:
  - Abnormal symptoms
  - Marked ST changes on ECG
  - Hypertension or hypotension
  - An arrhythmia
  - A wall motion abnormality in 2 or more adjacent segments

Review the indications for the stress study

- Stress echocardiography is most often requested in patients with known or suspected coronary artery disease.
- Stress echocardiography also is increasingly utilized in patients with structural heart disease to assess hemodynamics at rest and with stress. (Table 4-1)

Key points:

□ Stress echocardiography most often is used for patients with suspected coronary artery disease to:
  - Detect the presence of coronary artery disease
  - Assess the location and severity of myocardial ischemia
  - Evaluate cardiac risk after revascularization
  - Identify viable myocardium (using a low-dose dobutamine stress protocol)
□ Stress echocardiography evaluates the functional effects of coronary disease but does not provide direct visualization of coronary anatomy. (Figure 4-1)

65

❐ Stress echocardiography (see Table 4-1) also is useful for evaluation of:
- Valve hemodynamics when aortic stenosis is accompanied by LV dysfunction, called low output aortic stenosis
- Pulmonary pressures with exercise in mitral valve disease (Figure 4–2)
- Dynamic outflow obstruction with hypertrophic cardiomyopathy
- Congenital heart disease, for example, aortic coarctation gradients with exercise

Choose the stress modality

- The choice of exercise versus pharmacologic stress depends on the patient's ability to exercise and the specific clinical indication.

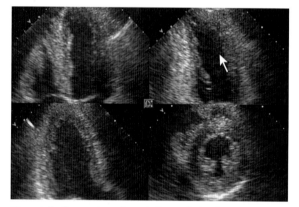

Figure 4–1. Stress echocardiography image display: A quad screen cine loop format is used to show the LV in apical 4-chamber (*upper left*), 2-chamber (*upper right*), long axis (*lower left*) and parasternal short axis (*lower right*) views. The same views are recorded at peak stress (with dobutamine) or immediately after stress (with treadmill exercise). The baseline and stress images are matched and placed side by side to facilitate recognition of changes in wall motion.

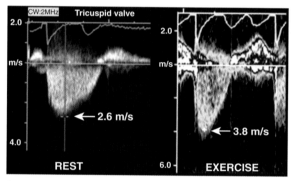

Figure 4–2. Stress echocardiography to evaluate pulmonary systolic pressure in a patient with rheumatic mitral stenosis. The tricuspid regurgitant jet, recorded with CW Doppler, increased from 2.6 m/s at rest to 3.8 m/s after exercise, corresponding to a rise in pulmonary pressure from 32 mm Hg to 63 mm Hg, which is abnormal and is an indication for mitral valvotomy when moderate to severe stenosis is present.

TABLE 4-1 Clinical Applications of Stress Echocardiography

Clinical Indication	Stress Modality	Protocol	Interpretation
Detection or evaluation of coronary artery disease	Exercise	• Use maximum treadmill exercise—provide highest workload, with image acquired immediately after exercise; or supine bicycle exercise (allows continuous imaging). Exercise protocol progressively increases in difficulty to achieve maximum workload using treadmill exercise (images acquired immediately after exercise) or supine bicycle exercise (allows continuous imaging during exercise.) • Compare rest and stress cine loop images of the LV in standard views.	• Normal wall motion at rest and a regional wall motion abnormality with stress indicates ischemia. • Abnormal regional wall motion at rest indicates prior infarction.
	Pharmacologic	• Dobutamine is infused beginning at low dose (5 or 10 µg/kg/min), increasing by 10 µg/kg/min every 3 minutes to a maximum dose of 40 µg/kg/min or target heart rate of 85% maximum predicted. • Atropine may also be used to achieve target heart rate. • Comparison of rest versus peak stress cine loop images of the LV in standard views.	• Normal wall motion at rest and a regional wall motion abnormality with stress indicate ischemia. • Abnormal regional wall motion at rest indicates prior infarction.

TABLE 4-1   Clinical Applications of Stress Echocardiography—cont'd

Clinical Indication	Stress Modality	Protocol	Interpretation
Myocardial viability	Dobutamine stress	• Dobutamine is infused beginning at low dose (5 µg/kg/min) and increasing to 10 µg/kg/min. • The stress test may be continued to evaluate for ischemia as above. • Images of the LV in cine loop format at baseline and low-dose dobutamine (increase in contractility with no change in heart rate) are compared.	• Viability is diagnosed when an area of hypokinesis or akinesis at rest shows improved wall motion at low-dose dobutamine. • If wall motion again worsens at higher dobutamine doses, ischemia also is present (the biphasic response to stress).
Post–cardiac transplant myocardial ischemia	Dobutamine stress	• Use standard dobutamine stress echo protocol. • Compare rest versus peak stress cine loop images of the LV in standard views.	• A new wall motion abnormality with stress is consistent with inducible ischemia. • Balanced ischemia (equal involvement of all major coronary arteries) or small-vessel disease may be missed on stress echocardiography.
Low output aortic stenosis	Dobutamine stress	• Measure stroke volume and ejection fraction as dobutamine is increased from 0 to 20 µg/kg/min in 5 µg/kg/min increments. • Measure AS velocity, mean gradient, and valve area at each stress level. • Stop for symptoms or when a hemodynamic endpoint is reached.	• Severe aortic stenosis is present if aortic velocity increases to at least 4 m/s or if valve area remains less than 1 cm^2 with a 20% or greater increase in stroke volume. • Failure of stroke volume or ejection fraction to increase by at least 20% is termed "lack of contractile reserve" and connotes a poor clinical outcome.
Mitral valve disease	Exercise stress	• Measure tricuspid regurgitant jet velocity at baseline and at peak exercise stress on maximum treadmill testing or with supine bicycle exercise. • The transmitral pulsed or CW Doppler velocity curve also may be evaluated at rest and with exercise. • Mitral regurgitation may be evaluated using CW and color Doppler (optional).	• The primary goal is to assess peak pulmonary systolic pressure with exercise (and change from baseline), calculated from the tricuspid regurgitant jet velocity. • With mitral stenosis, the transmitral velocity and mean gradient will increase as expected for the increase in flow rate; this measurement is rarely diagnostically useful. • With primary mitral regurgitation, severity may increase with exercise (e.g., with mitral prolapse) but quantitation at peak exercise is challenging. The change in pulmonary pressure is a surrogate for the increase in regurgitation.

Continued

TABLE 4-1   Clinical Applications of Stress Echocardiography—cont'd

Clinical Indication	Stress Modality	Protocol	Interpretation
Hypertrophic cardiomyopathy	Exercise stress	• Supine bicycle stress is preferred for evaluation of hypertrophic cardiomyopathy because it allows data recording at each stress level. • LV outflow velocity is recorded with pulsed and CW Doppler at baseline and with stress. • Mitral regurgitation also is evaluated with CW and color Doppler.	• Latent LV outflow obstruction is present when the resting subaortic gradient is < 30 mm Hg but increases to > 30 mm Hg with stress. • Separating the LV outflow signal from the higher-velocity mitral regurgitation signal can be challenging in some cases. • Useful features in identifying the origin of the Doppler signal are timing of flow onset relative to the QRS signal, shape of the velocity curve, delineation of a smooth dark edge to the velocity curve, and recordings showing separate LV outflow and mitral regurgitation CW Doppler flow curves.

AS, aortic stenosis; CW continuous wave; LV, left ventricle.

Key points:

❏ Exercise stress mimics normal physical activity of the patient but image acquisition may be limited.
❏ Treadmill exercise provides the most physiologic measures of exercise capacity.
❏ Supine bicycle exercise allows data acquisition at multiple exercise stages.
❏ Pharmacologic stress is preferred in patients unable to exercise (e.g., orthopedic limitations) and for some specific clinical indications (low output aortic stenosis and after cardiac transplantation)
❏ Pharmacologic stress allows optimal patient positioning and allows improved image acquisition but the total workload is lower and it does not mimic normal exertion.

Acquire the rest and stress data

■ For evaluation of coronary artery disease, cine loop quad screen images of the LV are acquired in standard image planes at rest and with stress.
■ For cardiac hemodynamics, the specific Doppler data recorded depends on the indication for the stress test.

Key points:

❏ A systematic approach to evaluation of regional wall motion is facilitated by comparing images in the same image plane, at the same depth, with the cine loop adjusted so rest and stress images are synchronized.
❏ Ensure correct triggering of the cine loops from the ECG signal before beginning the stress study.
❏ Experience is needed to quickly acquire images during bicycle or immediately following treadmill exercise stress.
❏ A physician should supervise stress studies for structural heart disease to ensure the needed hemodynamic information is recorded.
❏ Acquisition of Doppler data at high heart rates is challenging and requires a high degree of sonographer training, skill, and experience.

Interpret the study results

■ Evaluation of coronary disease depends on detection of a difference in regional wall motion between the baseline and stress images.
■ Hemodynamic data interpretation requires knowledge of the clinical implications of the data and is an evolving field of study.

Key points:

❏ Considerable experience is needed to reliably identify inducible ischemia on stress echocardiography.

❐ Each laboratory should periodically compare stress echocardiography results with coronary angiographic findings in their patient population to ensure reliability of the echocardiographic data.

❐ Examples of hemodynamic stress data that are useful in clinical decision making are shown in Table 4-1; it is likely there will be future refinements in the indications and clinical utility of stress testing for structural heart disease.

THREE-DIMENSIONAL ECHOCARDIOGRAPHY

■ Echocardiographic data can be acquired in a three-dimensional format by:
  • Integrating data from multiple two-dimensional images of known spatial location
  • Use of a transducer that acquires a volume of echocardiographic data.
  • Use of a transducer that simultaneously records more than one 2D image plane
  • Reconstruction of borders traced on 2D images in a 3D image format.

■ 3D echocardiography facilitates recognition of complex intracardiac spatial relationships.

Key points:

❐ Several types of 3D systems are available with instrumentation specific to each approach.

❐ Most clinical echocardiography laboratories continue to use 2D echocardiography as the primary diagnostic approach. Standards for a complete 3D TTE exam (typically performed as an adjunct to standard 2D imaging) are available. (Table 4-2)

❐ For each 3D volumetric realtime data set, cropping is used to view anatomy from both sides of three standard image planes:
  • Sagittal (similar to a long axis plane)
  • Coronal (similar to a 4-chamber plane)
  • Transverse (similar to a short axis view)

❐ A wide-angle acquisition is used for image data of the entire heart; narrow-angle acquisition may be helpful for examination of specific structures, such as the aortic valve.

❐ Proposed clinical applications of 3D echocardiography include:
  • a surgical view of the mitral valve in patients with mitral prolapse, facilitating surgical repair
  • evaluation of mitral valve anatomy before and after balloon valvotomy (Figure 4–3)
  • more complete visualization of the interatrial septum in patients undergoing percutaneous closure of an atrial septal defect
  • evaluation of complex congenital heart disease
  • more accurate measurement of ventricular volumes and ejection fraction
  • monitoring of transcutheter valve procedures, such as closure of paravalvulor leaks.

❐ Research applications of 3D echocardiography include:
  • studies on the mechanisms of functional mitral regurgitation
  • evaluation of regional myocardial function
  • changes in the size, shape, and function of the left and RV with pressure and/or volume overload

TABLE 4-2 Recommendations for Complete 3D Transthoracic Echocardiographic Study

Acquisition Mode	Ultrasound Window	Image Planes on Cropped Views	Imaging	Color Doppler
Wide angle	Parasternal	Coronal	Aortic valve	Aortic valve
		Sagittal	Mitral valve	Mitral valve
		Transverse	Tricuspid valve	Tricuspid valve
			Pulmonic valve	Pulmonic valve
Wide angle	Apical	Coronal	Left ventricle	Aortic valve
		Sagittal	Right ventricle	Mitral valve
		Transverse		Tricuspid valve
Wide angle	Subcostal		Left ventricle	Atrial septum
			Right ventricle	Ventricular septum
			Atrial septum	
Wide angle	Suprasternal		Aortic arch	Descending aorta

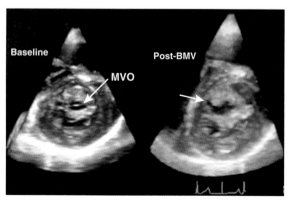

Figure 4–3. A realtime 3D echocardiographic image of rheumatic mitral stenosis showing the ovale-shaped mitral valve orifice (MVO) in diastole in a short axis orientation "looking" from the apex towards the mitral valve. After balloon mitral valvotomy (BMV), the medial commissure (*arrow*) shows improved opening. *Courtesy Edward A. Gill, MD; Harborview Medical Center, University of Washington, Seattle, WA.*

MYOCARDIAL MECHANICS

Basic principles

- LV function is incompletely described by simple measures such as ejection fraction or diastolic filling patterns.
- Myocardial strain, strain rate, and measures of synchrony attempt to provide an integrated, precise description of ventricular contraction and relaxation.

Key points:

- ☐ LV contraction occurs simultaneously in the longitudinal, radial, and circumferential directions.
- ☐ The LV apex and base move in opposite directions during contraction; this twisting motion is called torsion.

Tissue Doppler velocities

- Tissue Doppler measures the velocity of myocardial motion, displayed as a velocity curve for a single point or as a color display across the 2D image plane.
- Tissue Doppler velocities are measured relative to the position of the transducer, like all Doppler signals, so that accurate measurements depend on a parallel alignment between the Doppler beam and direction of motion.

Key points

- ☐ Recording tissue Doppler velocity at a single location, for example, adjacent to the mitral annulus for evaluation of diastolic function, provides a standard velocity versus time spectral display output.
- ☐ Tissue Doppler velocities also can be displayed for multiple points across the 2D image using a color display, analogous to color Doppler flow mapping for blood flow velocities.
- ☐ Tissue Doppler signals are high amplitude and low velocity. Recording requires adjusting the instrument settings with:
  - a low velocity range (usually +/− 0.2 m/s)
  - very low gain and wall filter settings
- ☐ Tissue Doppler velocity is recorded in the apical 4-chamber view with a 2-mm sample volume positioned in the septal myocardium about 1 cm apical from the mitral annulus. The lateral annulus can be used if septal motion is abnormal.
- ☐ The normal tissue Doppler velocity curve shows an early diastolic velocity (E') toward the apex, followed by a late diastolic velocity (A') reflecting atrial filling. In systole (S), the myocardial velocity is directed away from the apex with the velocity reflecting LV systolic function. (Figure 4–4)

Strain and strain rate

- Strain rate (SR) is the rate of change in myocardial length, normalized for the original length calculated from the difference in velocities at two myocardial sites (V_1 and V_2), and divided by the distance (D) between them:

$$SR = (V_2 - V_1)/D$$

- Strain is a measure of deformation of a material, defined as the difference between the original length (L_o) and final length (L), expressed as a percent of the original length:

$$Strain = [(L - L_o)/L_o] \times 100\%$$

Key points

- ☐ Using tissue Doppler, strain is typically measured from the apical view, reflecting longitudinal LV function, using 3 sample volumes placed about 12 mm apart.
- ☐ The tissue Doppler velocity curves should show a clear signal without aliasing and with avoidance of blood pool signals.
- ☐ The instrument calculates and displays strain rate in units of $seconds^{-1}$.
- ☐ Myocardial shortening (systole) is a negative strain rate. Lengthening (diastole) is a positive strain rate. Thus, the strain rate curve looks like a mirror image of a tissue Doppler velocity curve. (see Figure 4–4)

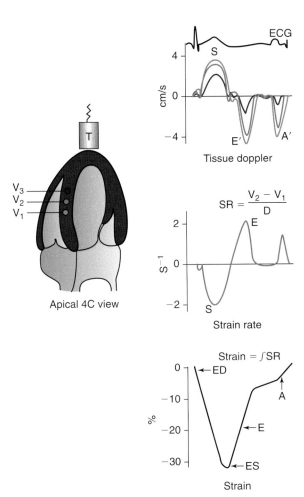

Figure 4–4. Schematic diagram of the derivation of strain rate and strain from myocardial tissue velocities. From the apical view at least three Doppler sample volumes are positioned in the myocardium about 12 mm apart. The three graphs on the right show one cardiac cycle, matched for timing as shown by the ECG at the top. The tissue Doppler tracings show mean velocity versus time with the line colors corresponding to each sample volume position. Strain rate is calculated for each time point at the change in velocity (V) between each two-sample volume positions, divided by the distance (D) between them. Strain is determined by integration of the strain rate to generate a curve similar to an LV volume curve with a rapid decrease in strain during ejection (ED to ES) and a rapid increase in strain in early diastole (E) with another increase in late diastole after atrial contraction (A).

❑ Peak systolic strain rate measures ventricular contractile function and is relatively insensitive to changes in loading conditions.
❑ Strain is calculated by integrating the strain rate curve over time.
❑ Strain is analogous to ejection fraction (change in length versus volume over time), and the strain curve is similar in shape to a ventricular volume curve.
❑ Like ejection fraction, peak systolic strain varies with preload, but can serve as an indicator of regional LV function.

Speckle tracking strain imaging

■ Speckle tracking uses small reflectors in the myocardium to track motion, allowing calculation of LV strain.
■ Unlike tissue Doppler, speckle tracking strain is not dependent on the angle between the ultrasound beam and direction of motion.

Key points

❑ Speckle tracking provides a direct measure of strain or the change in length of myocardium relative to the original length.
❑ Speckle tracking is displayed as a 2D color-coded image, alongside a graphic display of strain for different myocardial segments. (Figure 4–5)
❑ Longitudinal strain can be measured from apical views, circumferential strain from short axis views, and radial strain from various 2D views.

Dyssynchrony

■ Dyssynchrony is defined as spatial variation in the timing of LV contraction, most often seen in patients with a low ejection fraction.

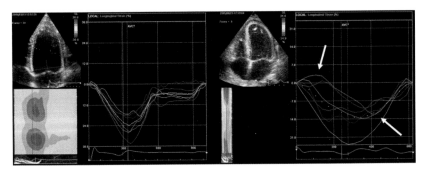

Figure 4–5. Speckle tracking echocardiography showing long-axis strains: The left panel shows the typical strain pattern from a normal LV. The right panel shows recordings from a patient with an anterior myocardial infarction. In the apical LV segments (*arrows*) there is lengthening during early systole and there is postsystolic shortening.

- Dyssynchrony is qualitatively easily appreciated on 2D imaging; various quantitative measures have been proposed.

Key points

- ❏ One measure of dyssynchrony is a difference > 130 ms in septal to posterior wall delay, defined as the interval between the QRS and the maximum inward motion of the myocardium. This measure is affected by other factors that alter septal motion.
- ❏ Interventricular dyssynchrony is reflected by a > 40 ms difference between the LV and RV pre-ejection periods (time from QRS to antegrade aortic or pulmonic flow).
- ❏ Tissue Doppler allows 2D display of dyssynchrony and measurement for multiple myocardial segments. Dyssynchrony is present when there is a difference of at least 65 ms in the tissue Doppler S-wave peaks between opposing LV walls in apical 4-chamber or long-axis views.

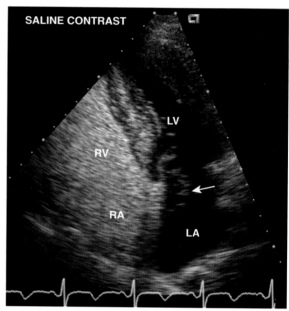

Figure 4–6. Intravenous injection of agitated saline provide opacification of the right heart chambers. A small amount of contrast is seen in the left atrium (*arrow*) consistent with the presence of patent foramen ovale.

CONTRAST ECHOCARDIOGRAPHY

- Intravenous injection of microbubbles to opacify the cardiac chambers or evaluate myocardial perfusion is called "contrast echocardiography."
- Agitated saline contrast opacifies the right heart and is used for detection of right to left intracardiac shunting based on the appearance of contrast in the left heart.
- Smaller microbubbles (1-5 μm diameter) transverse the pulmonary vasculature, allowing left heart chamber and myocardial opacification.

Key points:

- ❏ The most common use of right-sided contrast is to detect a patent foramen ovale, either on transthoracic or transesophageal imaging. (Figure 4–6)
- ❏ Left heart contrast typically is used to enhance LV endocardial border detection when transthoracic image quality is suboptimal. (Figure 4–7)
- ❏ Instrument settings to optimize left heart contrast images include:
  - a decrease in power output (to a mechanical index of about 0.5)
  - a lower transducer frequency
  - an increase in overall gain and dynamic range
  - focal depth at the mid- or near-field of the image

- ❏ When microbubble density is too high, excessive apical contrast results in shadowing of the rest of the ventricle. (Figure 4–8)
- ❏ A low microbubble density or high mechanical index results in a swirling appearance with inadequate LV opacification. (Figure 4–9)
- ❏ Left-sided contrast is contraindicated in patients with:
  - right to left or bidirectional shunts or
  - hypersensitivity to echo contrast
- ❏ Caution is needed (with blood pressure, arterial oxygen saturation, and ECG monitoring) in patients with:
  - pulmonary hypertension or
  - unstable cardiopulmonary conditions
- ❏ Assessment of myocardial perfusion by contrast echocardiography is not widely used for clinical diagnosis, although there is ongoing development of this approach.

INTRACARDIAC ECHOCARDIOGRAPHY

- Intracardiac echocardiography is performed in the cardiac catheterization or electrophysiology laboratory using a small high frequency transducer (5-10 MHz) on the tip of a catheter.
- ICE imaging is used to guide percutaneous interventions and complex electrophysiology procedures.

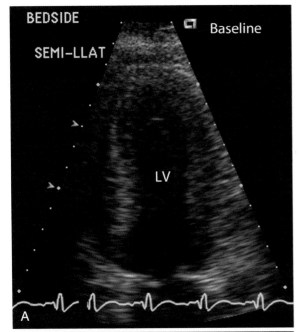

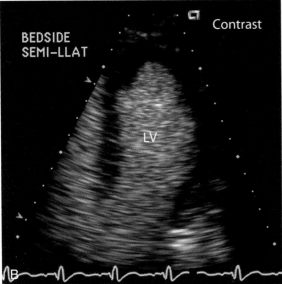

Figure 4–7. In this patient with suboptimal endocardial definition in the apical 4-chamber view (left), intravenous injection of a left heart contrast agent opacifies the left ventricle, providing improved evaluation of ventricular systolic function (right).

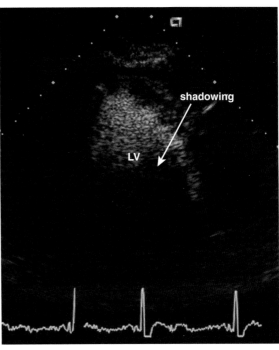

Figure 4–8. Shadowing of the LV by contrast in the apex is seen. Apical shadowing occurs when the volume or rate of contrast injection is too high.

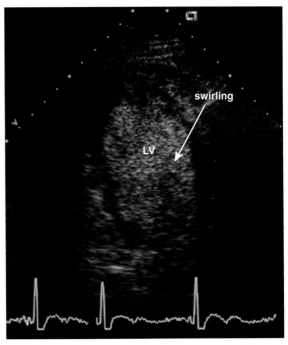

Figure 4–9. Swirling of ventricular contrast, with poor definition of the endocardium, is seen when the volume of contrast is too low or when the mechanical index is too high, which results in destruction of microbubbles.

Key points:

- ❏ ICE typically is performed by the physician doing the invasive procedure.
- ❏ Manipulation of the transducer-tipped catheter requires considerable experience in intracardiac procedures.
- ❏ Images are obtained primarily from the RA, allowing evaluation of the:
  - interatrial septum
  - LA, atrial appendage, and pulmonary veins
  - mitral valve and base of the LV
  - tricuspid valve and RV (Figure 4–10)
- ❏ Intracardiac echocardiography is used to guide procedures including:
  - atrial septal defect closure
  - patent foramen ovale closure
  - arrhythmia ablation procedures
  - other complex percutaneous procedures (Figure 4–11)
- ❏ Some procedures, such as balloon mitral valvuloplasty, can be monitored either by intracardiac, transesophageal, or transthoracic imaging.

INTRAVASCULAR ULTRASOUND

- ■ Intravascular ultrasound uses a high frequency transducer (30-50 MHz) on an intra-coronary catheter to visualize coronary artery atheroma.
- ■ Intravascular ultrasound allows assessment of the length, severity, and composition of the atherosclerotic plaque. (Figure 4–12)

Key points:

- ❏ Intravascular ultrasound typically is performed by the interventional cardiologist as part of a coronary intervention.

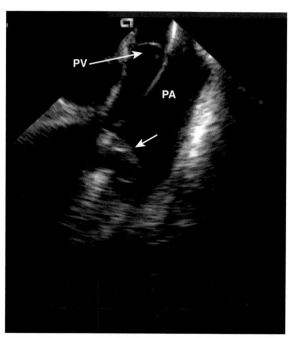

Figure 4–11. Intracardiac echocardiography is used to guide the position of a biopsy catheter. The intracardiac echocardiography transducer is in the right ventricular outflow tract. The biopsy catheter crosses the pulmonic valve with its tip attached to the mass (*arrow*) at the pulmonary artery bifurcation.

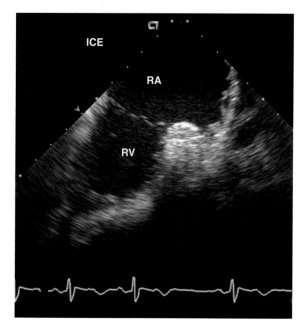

Figure 4–10. Intracardiac echocardiography with the catheter-tip transducer located in the RA. The trabeculated RA appendage, tricuspid valve, and RV are seen.

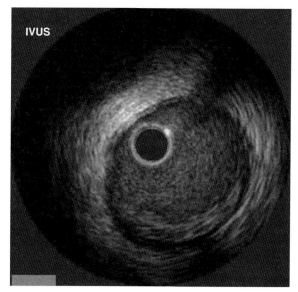

Figure 4–12. Intravascular ultrasound image recorded in the left anterior descending artery. The ultrasound catheter is the dark circle in the vessel lumen. With this high-frequency transducer, the blood appears light gray, with a denser crescent of tissue in the vessel due to atherosclerosis.

- ❑ The image depth is about 2-3 cm.
- ❑ A small, dedicated ultrasound system is used for image acquisition, recording, and analysis.

HANDHELD ECHOCARDIOGRAPHY

- ▪ The bedside use of small, portable ultrasound systems is called "Hand-held echocardiography."
- ▪ The capability of portable instruments ranges from simple 2D imaging to the full range of functions of a larger ultrasound system.

Key points:

- ❑ Appropriate education and training are essential for the appropriate use of handheld echocardiography.
- ❑ The most widely used applications of handheld echocardiography are:
  - evaluation for pericardial effusion
  - evaluation of ventricular global and regional systolic function
- ❑ Cardiologists also use handheld echocardiography for interim evaluation of patients with complex cardiac disease.

THE ECHO EXAM

Advanced Echocardiographic Modalities

Modality	Instrumentation	Clinical Utility	Special Training
Stress echocardiography	Cine loop images at rest and with stress Treadmill or bicycle exercise or pharmacologic stress	• Detection of myocardial ischemia • Low output aortic stenosis • Exercise PA pressures • LV outflow obstruction in hypertrophic cardiomyopathy	• Stress testing • Interpretation of images and Doppler data
3D echo	Volumetric or 2D image acquisition Various display formats	• Rapid acquisition for LV regional function • Mitral valve anatomy • Atrial septal defects	• Image acquisition and analysis
Tissue Doppler strain rate and strain	Tissue Doppler and 2D imaging to measure strain rate: $SR = (V_2 - V_1)/D$ Strain rate is integrated over time to calculate strain	• Strain rate: measure of ventricular contractility • Strain: measure of regional myocardial function	• Data acquisition and analysis • Clinical interpretation of data
Myocardial speckle tracking	Strain measured directly from change in distance between myocardial speckles (L) relative to original distance (L_0): $[(L - L_0)/L_0] \times 100\%$	• Myocardial speckle tracking is angle independent • Analysis can be performed after image acquisition	• Data acquisition and analysis • Clinical interpretation of data
Myocardial dyssynchrony	Multiple 2D, pulsed Doppler, and tissue Doppler methods	• Degree of dyssynchrony may predict response to dual chamber pacer therapy	• Data acquisition and analysis • Clinical interpretation of data
Contrast echo	Microbubbles for right- or left-heart contrast	• Detection of patent foramen ovale • LV endocardial definition	• Intravenous administration of contrast agents • Knowledge of potential risks
Intracardiac echo (ICE)	5-10 MHz catheter-like intracardiac probe	• Interventional procedures (ASD closure) • EP procedures	• Invasive cardiology training and experience
Intravascular ultrasound (IVUS)	30-50 MHz intracoronary catheter	• Degree of coronary narrowing and plaque morphology	• Interventional cardiology training
Handheld ultrasound	Small, inexpensive ultrasound instruments	• Bedside evaluation by MD for pericardial effusion, LV global and regional function	• At least level 1 echo training

2D, two-dimensional; 3D, three-dimensional; ASD, atrial septal defect; EP, electrophysiology; PA, pulmonary artery.

Diagram of the level of echocardiography training and the level of training in other skills for each of the echocardiographic modalities. All physicians perform physical examinations. Although handheld echocardiography extends the physical examination, at least basic training and experience are needed for accurate clinical use. Transthoracic echocardiography (TTE) is followed in level of training by transesophageal echocardiography (TEE). The practice of stress echocardiography, contrast echocardiography, and 3D echocardiography requires other skills in addition to echocardiography—for example, the safe performance of a stress study. Intravascular ultrasound typically requires advanced skills as an interventional cardiologist. Intracardiac echocardiography requires advanced invasive cardiology skills, preferably in combination with level 2 training in echocardiography given the complexity of the imaging data available with this modality.

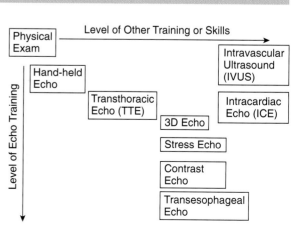

SELF-ASSESSMENT QUESTIONS

QUESTION 1

A 62-year-old male is referred for cardiac stress testing for symptoms of intermittent chest discomfort when he lifts or carries heavy loads. His past medical history includes tobacco use and medically treated hypertension. His baseline ECG shows normal sinus rhythm with criteria for LV hypertrophy.

The most appropriate test to obtain would be:

- A. Treadmill ECG stress test
- B. Exercise stress echocardiogram
- C. Dobutamine stress echocardiogram
- D. Cardiopulmonary exercise stress test

QUESTION 2

3D echocardiography has shown utility in imaging for all of the following conditions EXCEPT:

- A. Secundum ASD
- B. Rheumatic mitral stenosis
- C. Mitral valve prolapse
- D. Primary pulmonary hypertension

QUESTION 3

A 60-year-old male under evaluation for liver transplant undergoes a routine TTE. On the transmitral blood flow recording, the mitral peak E wave velocity was 1.4 m/s and the A-velocity was 0.4 m/s. The image below (Figure 4–13) is consistent with:

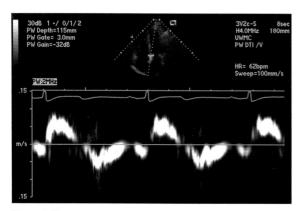

Figure 4–13.

- A. Decreased LV compliance
- B. Normal myocardial function
- C. Impaired LV relaxation
- D. Normal LA pressure

QUESTION 4

Exercise echocardiography may be a reasonable consideration in patients with:

- A. Symptomatic aortic stenosis
- B. Acute aortic dissection
- C. Recent myocardial infarction
- D. Severe systemic hypertension

QUESTION 5

The best option to improve image quality with microbubble transpulmonary contrast is:

- A. Decrease transmit frequency
- B. Concentrate microbubble solution
- C. Set focal depth in near field
- D. Increase mechanical index

QUESTION 6

Match the units to the echocardiographic modality

- A. 1/seconds
- B. centimeters
- C. dimensionless
- D. meters/second

    1. Strain
    2. Tissue Doppler
    3. Strain rate
    4. Speckle tracking

QUESTION 7

A transthoracic study was obtained in a 41-year-old patient with a history of recurrent dizziness. (Figure 4–14)

The image is most consistent with:

- A. Perimembranous VSD
- B. Anomalous coronary artery
- C. Secundum ASD
- D. Anomalous pulmonary return
- E. No intracardiac shunt

QUESTION 8

The following image, obtained after intravenous injection of agitated saline contrast, is most consistent with (Figure 4–15)

- A. Patent foramen ovale
- B. Supracristal ventricular septal defect
- C. Sinus venosus atrial septal defect
- D. Anomalous pulmonary return

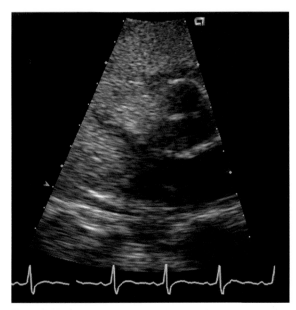

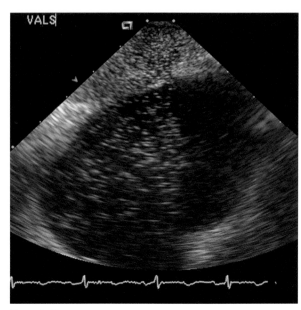

Figure 4–14.

Figure 4–15.

ANSWER 1: B

This patient has several cardiovascular risk factors and has exertional chest discomfort so further evaluation for coronary artery disease is indicated. The most appropriate next test is exercise stress echocardiography because the patient is ambulatory and his symptoms are provoked by physical activity. Echocardiographic imaging allows detection of ischemic myocardial based on the presence of a regional wall motion abnormality with stress, but not at rest. Exercise stress is preferred over pharmacologic (dobutamine) stress when it can be performed because additional data are obtained on exercise tolerance and the workload required for symptom provocation. A treadmill ECG test would not be helpful in this patient because of the abnormal baseline ECG, which increases the likelihood of a false positive study. A cardiopulmonary stress test concurrently measures oxygen consumption with the stress test but is not typically used for ischemia evaluation. Cardiopulmonary exercise testing is most useful to differentiate the pulmonary and cardiac components of exercise limitation in patients with symptoms of unclear etiology, to objectively measure exercise capacity in patient with chronic heart failure or congenital heart disease, and to measure exercise tolerance during cardiopulmonary rehabilitation.

ANSWER 2: D

Clinical applications for routine use of 3D echocardiography are still under investigation and, to date, 3D echocardiography is most often used as an adjunct to a standard 2D study. Improved spatial resolution with 3D imaging may allow for better understanding of the anatomical relationship of intracardiac structures. Current clinical applications of 3D echocardiography include guidance for procedures where spatial relationship is critical, such as imaging the interatrial septum during a patent foramen ovale or atrial septal defect closure, balloon placement for mitral valvuloplasty, and location of the prolapsing segment in mitral valve prolapse for surgical planning. Reliable 3D spectral Doppler imaging (i.e., to measure pulmonary arterial systolic pressures) is not yet available.

ANSWER 3: A

This is a tissue Doppler tracing of myocardial velocity sampled in the interventricular septum 1 cm below the mitral valve annulus. A low velocity range (usually +/− 0.2 m/s) with low gain and wall filter settings are used to optimize the signal from the moving tissue. This tracing shows a systolic velocity

toward the transducer, followed by an early diastolic tissue velocity (E') of 0.07 m/s (measured below the baseline) and a very small late diastolic atrial (A') velocity.

In conjunction with the transmitral blood flow pattern of an E velocity much higher than A velocity, these tissue Doppler findings are consistent with diastolic dysfunction and decreased LV compliance. In the setting of impaired LV relaxation, LV filling relies more heavily on the latter part of diastole, during atrial contraction, with an E/A ratio < 1 on both transmitral flow and tissue Doppler. In addition, the early filling mitral E wave velocity would not be as pronounced, and would be less than 1 m/s.

There also is evidence for an elevated (not normal) LA pressure. Given the mitral peak E wave velocity of 1.4 m/s, the E/E' ratio is markedly elevated at 20. LV diastolic dysfunction often is accompanied by an elevated left atrial pressure that is reflected in the ratio of early transmitral blood flow velocity (E) to the myocardial tissue Doppler peak (E') wave velocity. With higher transmitral E or with a lower myocardial peak E' velocity, this ratio increases. A ratio of over 15 is consistent with increased left atrial pressure.

ANSWER 4: C

In patients with a recent myocardial infarction who did not undergo coronary angiography, a submaximal stress test is appropriate 3-6 days after the initial event as it provides valuable prognostic information by risk stratifying patients on the basis of exercise tolerance and residual ischemia. Echocardiographic imaging also allows localization of the culprit vessel and the size of the ischemic territory at risk. Exercise echocardiography should not be done within 72 hours of an acute myocardial infarction in unrevascularized patients as it may provoke an arrhythmic event. Other contraindications to exercise testing include patients with uncontrolled arrhythmias, severe symptomatic aortic stenosis, and acute aortic dissection. In patients with severe systemic hypertension (systolic blood pressure > 200 mm Hg), blood pressure should be controlled, if necessary with medications, prior to stress testing.

ANSWER 5: A

Blood and microbubbles have different densities. The relative change in density causes a change in acoustic impedance that reflects transmitted ultrasound waves back to the transducer. However, microbubbles also are destroyed by strong ultrasound signals. Ultrasound machine settings that improve image quality during microbubble contrast by preserving micro-bubble integrity include decreasing acoustic power by decreasing the mechanical index (power output) and decreasing ultrasound transmit frequency. Image quality is also improved by increasing the focal depth from the transducer, but not to the point where attenuation occurs. Usually microbubble imaging is optimal with the focal depth set in the mid field. If ultrasound microbubble density is too high, as would occur with concentrating the microbubble solution, most of the ultrasound signal is reflected back to the transducer with shadowing of distal structures.

ANSWERS 6: 1C, 2D, 3A, 4C

Tissue Doppler measures velocity of myocardial motion; velocity is lower than the velocity of blood flow, but is still typically reported in units of either meters/second or centimeters/second. Strain rate is the rate of change in myocardial length, normalized for the original length. Strain rate is calculated from the difference in velocities at two myocardial sites (V_1, V_2) divided by the distance between them; the units are (meters/seconds)/meters. Thus, strain rate simplifies to (1/seconds). Strain is a measure of myocardial deformation. Strain of a myocardial segment is defined as the difference between baseline myocardial length (L_0) and final contraction length (L), relative to the original length, or $(L- L_0)/L_0$. The length units in the numerator and denominator cancel each other so that strain measurements are dimensionless. In clinical practice, strain is typically expressed as a percentage. Speckle tracking follows the motion of small reflectors in the myocardium, allowing calculation of LV strain at multiple sites, and is usually displayed as a 2D color-coded image. Because it measures strain, speckle tracking is also dimensionless.

ANSWER 7: C

This is an image from an agitated saline contrast study, taken from the parasternal short axis view. The aortic valve is the circular structure in the center of the image, the LA is in the lower right section of the image, and the RA and RV are seen opacified by saline contrast. There is a dark, negative washout of contrast that originates at the interatrial septum and goes toward the RA. This finding is consistent with flow of non-contrast blood from left to right across interatrial septum, consistent with a secundum atrial septal defect. If left atrial pressure is significantly higher than right atrial pressure, flow is predominantly left to right across the septum, with the right to left shunting. Anomalous takeoff of

the coronary arteries is not diagnosed with an agitated saline contrast study. Anomalous pulmonary vein return would return oxygenated blood from the pulmonary circulation back to the right heart, but not near the interatrial septum so that neither a positive or negative contrast jet would be seen. A perimembranous VSD would not be seen in this view, but could also cause a negative washout of contrast if present (would be seen best from a parasternal long-axis view or apical 4-chamber view).

ANSWER 8: A

This image was taken with intracardiac echocardiography during a percutaneous closure procedure for a patent foramen ovale. Saline contrast is seen opacifying the RA at the top of the image, with a small amount of contrast seen in the LA from passage across the interatrial septum, most consistent with a patent foramen ovale. During a Valsalva maneuver when right atrial pressure is transiently increased, microbubbles cross the interatrial septum and are seen in LA. The structure seen is the interatrial septum, and the image would not be consistent with a VSD or anomalous pulmonary return (which would not show right to left passage of contrast). A sinus venosus atrial septal defect lies closer to the insertion of the superior vena cava, which is not seen in this view.

In an image from the same patient later in the procedure, a closure device (arrow) is now seen bridging the septum. (Figure 4–16)

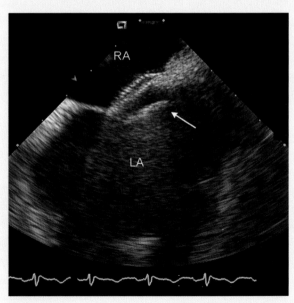

Figure 4–16.

5 Clinical Indications for Echocardiography

BASIC PRINCIPLES
  Understand the Reliability of Echocardiography for the Specific Diagnosis
  Integrate the Clinical Data and the Echocardiographic Findings
  Recommend Additional Diagnostic Testing as Appropriate
DIAGNOSTIC THINKING FOR THE ECHOCARDIOGRAPHER

ECHOCARDIOGRAPHY FOR COMMON SIGNS AND SYMPTOMS
  Murmur
  Chest Pain
  Heart Failure or Dyspnea
  Palpitations
  Embolic Event
  Fever/Bacteremia
THE ECHO EXAM
SELF-ASSESSMENT QUESTIONS

BASIC PRINCIPLES

■ The diagnostic value of echocardiography for a specific diagnosis depends both on the reliability of the echocardiographic data and on integration with other clinical information.

■ The framework for echocardiographic data acquisition and reporting is a structured diagnostic approach to the question posed by the requesting physician.

Key points:

❑ The echocardiographic study seeks to provide the appropriate data for clinical decision making depending on the patient's symptoms, signs, and known diagnoses.

❑ The list of possible diagnosis that might explain the clinical findings, called the differential diagnosis, is mentally constructed at the beginning of the echocardiographic study.

❑ As the study proceeds, some diagnoses are excluded while others may be suggested by specific findings.

❑ Pertinent positive data include abnormal echocardiographic findings.

❑ Pertinent negative data include normal echocardiographic findings that help narrow the differential diagnosis.

Step 1: Understand the reliability of echocardiography for the specific diagnosis

■ The accuracy of echocardiography describes the agreement between an echocardiographic measurement or diagnosis and an external reference standard, such as another imaging approach or clinical outcomes. (Figure 5–1)

■ The precision of an echocardiographic measurement is affected by variability in recording, measuring, and interpreting the echocardiographic data.

■ Expertise in image acquisition and interpretation both affect the reliability of echocardiographic data.

Key points:

❑ Sensitivity is the percent of patients with the diagnosis correctly identified by echocardiography.

❑ *Specificity* is the percent of patients without the diagnosis correctly identified by echocardiography.

❑ *Positive predictive value* (PPV) is the percent of patients with a positive echocardiogram who actually have the diagnosis.

❑ *Negative predictive value* (NPV) is the percent of patients with a negative echocardiogram who actually do not have the diagnosis.

❑ *Accuracy* indicates what proportion of all studies indicated a correct diagnosis.

❑ The positive and negative predictive value of a test depends on the prevalence of disease in addition to sensitivity and specificity.

❑ Each laboratory should periodically review the reproducibility of the echocardiographic measurements.

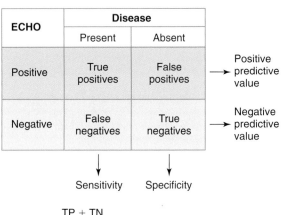

$$\text{Accuracy} = \frac{TP + TN}{\text{All tests}}$$

Figure 5–1. Sensitivity and specificity in comparison with positive and negative predictive value. Predictive values depend on the prevalence of disease in the population. *TP*, true positives; *TN*, true negatives.

❑ The effect of variability is minimized when images from sequential studies are compared side by side.

Step 2: Integrate the clinical data and the echocardiographic findings (Figure 5–2)

■ The likelihood ratio indicates the probability of disease in a patient with a positive or negative echocardiographic finding; a positive likelihood ratio greater than 10 or a negative likelihood ratio less than 0.1 indicate an excellent diagnostic test.

■ Pre- and post-test probability estimates integrate the likelihood of disease before the echocardiogram is performed with the echocardiographic results.

■ The threshold approach to clinical decision making indicates that diagnostic testing, such as echocardiography, is most helpful in patients where the results will change the subsequent:
- Therapy *or*
- Diagnostic strategy

Key points:

❑ The positive likelihood ratio is calculated as the true positive rate divided by the false positive rate. The negative likelihood ratio is the false negative rate divided by the true negative rate.

❑ The pretest probability of disease is the probability of disease before echocardiography is done—for example, consideration of cardiac risk factors and symptoms in a patient scheduled for stress echocardiography provides an estimate of the probability of coronary artery disease.

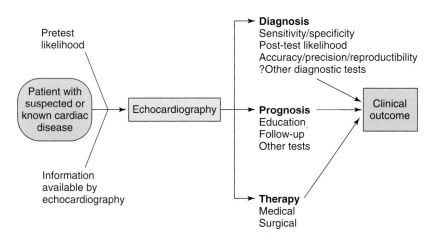

Figure 5–2. Flow chart illustrating the impact of echocardiographic results on diagnosis, prognosis, and therapy. The effects of echocardiography on clinical outcome are the best measure of the usefulness of the test result.

❑ Echocardiography is most helpful when the pretest likelihood of disease is intermediate and echocardiography has a high accuracy for the diagnosis.
  • When the pretest likelihood of disease is very low, an abnormal echocardiographic finding often is a false positive result.
  • Conversely, when the pretest likelihood of disease is very high, the failure to demonstrate the disease on echocardiography often is a false negative.
❑ With the threshold approach, the upper threshold is the point where the risk of the test is higher than the risk of treating the patient; for example, additional diagnostic testing should not delay surgical intervention for an acute ascending aortic dissection.
❑ The lower threshold for transthoracic echocardiography occurs only with a very low probability of disease; the major potential adverse effect is a false positive result leading to further inappropriate testing or therapy.

Step 3: Recommend additional diagnostic testing as appropriate

■ The interpretation of the echocardiogram lists the pertinent positive and negative findings along with any confirmed diagnoses.
■ The differential diagnosis of equivocal findings is indicated and appropriate additional diagnostic testing is recommended when the echocardiographic results are not diagnostic.

Key points:

❑ Echocardiography provides qualitative and quantitative information on cardiac structure and function and often provides a definitive diagnosis.
❑ Positive findings are more helpful than negative findings; for example, a dissection flap seen on transthoracic echocardiography is diagnostic for a dissection but its absence does not exclude this possibility.
❑ A non-cardiac cause for symptoms is likely when the echocardiogram is normal.
❑ The echocardiographer often needs to assist in choosing the optimal diagnostic approach (e.g., transthoracic or transesophageal echocardiography [TEE], stress echocardiography, contrast study, etc.) based on the indication for the study.
❑ Additional diagnostic studies, with either another echocardiographic modality or an alternate imaging approach, are recommended after review of the echocardiographic exam.

DIAGNOSTIC THINKING FOR THE ECHOCARDIOGRAPHER

■ The echocardiographer needs:
  • clinical data to estimate the pretest likelihood of disease before starting the exam
  • an understanding of pertinent positive and negative findings for each clinical indication
  • knowledge of the reliability of echocardiography for each diagnosis
  • ability to integrate the echocardiographic findings with the clinical data
■ The Echo Exam section summarizes the approach by anatomic diagnosis.
■ Examples of the approach to common clinical indications for echocardiography are discussed in the next section.

ECHOCARDIOGRAPHY FOR COMMON SIGNS AND SYMPTOMS

Murmur

■ The echocardiographic differential diagnosis for a murmur is based on an anatomic approach with evaluation of all four valves and a search for an intracardiac shunt. (Figure 5–3)
■ Most patients referred to echocardiography for a murmur on auscultation have a benign flow murmur.

Key points:

❑ The echocardiography request form may not specify the type of murmur (e.g., systolic or diastolic), so a systemic echocardiographic exam is essential.
❑ Normal physiologic regurgitation rarely accounts for an audible murmur.
❑ The most common pathologic causes for a murmur in adults are aortic valve stenosis and mitral valve regurgitation.
❑ Murmurs typically are due to high-velocity intracardiac flows (e.g., aortic stenosis or mitral regurgitation) because low-velocity flows (e.g., tricuspid regurgitation with normal pulmonary pressures) are not usually audible with a stethoscope.
❑ Conditions that cause increased cardiac output (e.g., anemia or pregnancy) may cause a murmur due to high velocity transvalvular flow in patients with otherwise anatomically normal valves.
❑ Congenital heart disease may first be diagnosed in an adult based on finding a murmur. In

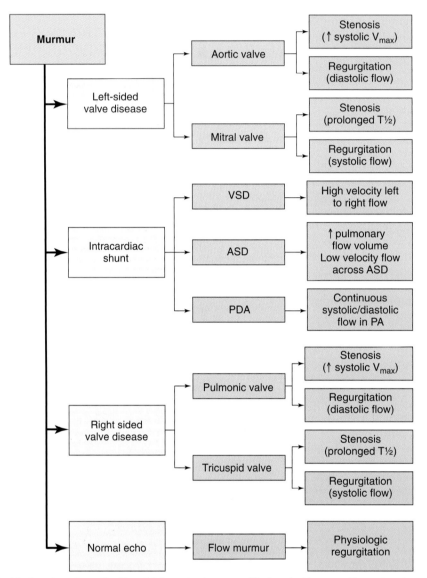

Figure 5–3. Flow chart for the echocardiographic differential diagnosis of a murmur. The flow chart is arranged by anatomy because the echocardiographer often is not provided information about the type of murmur or other clinical findings. The basic echocardiographic examination includes measurement of antegrade flows and evaluation for regurgitation of all four valves. Additional evaluation for murmur includes careful interrogation of flow in the pulmonary artery to detect a patent ductus arteriosus or increased flow due to an atrial septal defect. Flow in the septal region is examined with color and CW Doppler to exclude a ventricular septal defect. Normal physiologic amounts of mitral and tricuspid regurgitation are not audible and do not explain the presence of a murmur. *ASD*, atrial septal defect; *PA*, pulmonary artery; *PDA*, patent ductus arteriosus, $T\frac{1}{2}$, pressure half time; V_{max}, maximum antegrade velocity; *VSD*, ventricular septal defect.

patients with an atrial septal defect, the murmur is due to increased pulmonary blood flow volume, not to flow across the atrial septum.

Chest pain

■ The echocardiographic differential diagnosis for chest pain is based on the major clinical diagnoses that are of immediate clinical concern. (Figure 5–4)

■ When the echocardiogram does not establish a diagnosis, further evaluation may be needed emergently.

Key points:

❏ Acute chest pain is a medical emergency because the differential diagnosis includes acute coronary syndromes and aortic dissection, both of which require immediate treatment.

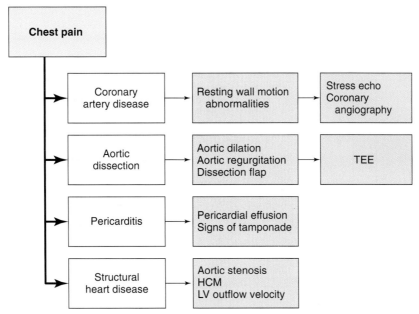

Figure 5–4. Echocardiographic approach to evaluation of chest pain. The primary goal in the acute setting is to exclude life-threatening conditions, such as an acute coronary syndrome or acute aortic dissection. With both acute and chronic chest pain, further diagnostic evaluation often is needed. *HCM,* hypertrophic cardiomyopathy; *LV,* left ventricular; *TEE,* transesophageal echocardiography.

- An abnormal echocardiographic finding, such as anterior wall hypokinesis, may prompt further diagnostic and therapeutic interventions, such as coronary angiography.
- An acute pulmonary embolism, if large enough, may show signs of right heart strain and increased pulmonary pressures. A smaller pulmonary embolism may have no significant findings on echocardiography.
- Even when the transthoracic echocardiogram is normal, further evaluation may be needed— for example, TEE or chest computed tomography (CT) in a patient with suspected aortic dissection.
- Normal resting wall motion does not exclude the possibility of significant coronary artery disease. Wall motion is abnormal only after infarction or with ongoing ischemia—for example, with unstable angina or on stress testing.
- The presence of a pericardial effusion is consistent with pericarditis, although not all patients with pericarditis have an effusion.
- In a patient with aortic dissection, pericardial fluid may be due to rupture of the aorta into the pericardial space.
- With significant LV outflow obstruction, the increase in LV myocardial wall stress and oxygen demand results in angina-type chest pain.

Heart failure or dyspnea

- Symptoms of dyspnea, edema, and decreased exercise tolerance are non-specific, with a wide differential diagnosis that includes cardiac and non-cardiac conditions.
- Heart failure, defined as the inability of the heart to supply adequate blood flow at a normal filling pressure, is the clinical consequent of several types of heart disease (Figure 5–5).

Key points:

- LV systolic dysfunction may be due to a cardiomyopathy, coronary disease with prior infarction, long-standing valvular heart disease, or congenital heart disease.
- Diastolic dysfunction typically accompanies systolic dysfunction; predominant diastolic dysfunction is seen with hypertensive heart disease, hypertrophic cardiomyopathy, and infiltrative myocardial disease.
- Constrictive pericarditis often presents as right heart failure, with ascites and peripheral edema.
- Heart failure occurs in patients with valvular heart disease, even when LV function is normal, due to obstruction of blood flow (e.g., mitral stenosis) or elevated pulmonary diastolic pressure (e.g., mitral regurgitation).
- Pulmonary hypertension due to left heart disease, pulmonary vascular disease, or

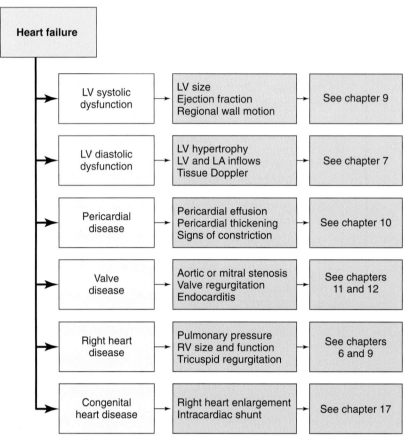

Figure 5–5. Echocardiographic approach to patients referred for heart failure. A systemic echocardiographic study will include the 2D views and Doppler flows to identify each of these possible diagnoses. In addition, the sonographer should mentally "check off" each of these conditions as the exam progresses to ensure that the entire differential diagnosis is considered. If the echocardiographic study is normal, a non-cardiac cause of symptoms is likely. *LA,* left atrial; *LV,* left ventricular; *RV,* right ventricular.

underlying lung disease leads to right heart failure with a dilated hypokinetic RV, sometimes called cor pulmonale.

❑ Heart failure in patients with congenital heart disease may be due to ventricular dysfunction, obstructive or regurgitant lesions, or intracardiac shunts.

❑ When "heart failure" is present with a normal echocardiographic study, non-cardiac causes for the patient's symptoms should be considered.

Palpitations

■ Palpitations are the patient's awareness of a forceful, rapid, or irregular heart rhythm.

■ The primary approach to evaluation of palpitations includes resting and ambulatory ECG monitoring.

■ Echocardiography allows evaluation of any underlying anatomic abnormalities associated with the cardiac arrhythmia.

Key points:

❑ Echocardiography typically is normal in patients with a supraventricular arrhythmia and no prior cardiac history.

❑ Conditions associated with supraventricular arrhythmias include:
  • ebstein's anomaly in patients with pre-excitation syndromes
  • prior surgery for congenital heart disease

❑ Atrial fibrillation often is associated with hypertensive heart disease, mitral valve disease, and LV systolic dysfunction.

❑ The prevalence of atrial fibrillation increases with age (present in about 4% of people older than 60 years of age).

❑ LA thrombi are associated with atrial fibrillation but are not reliably visualized on transthoracic echocardiography; TEE imaging is more accurate for diagnosis of atrial thrombi.

❑ Echocardiography often is abnormal in patients with ventricular arrhythmias. Quantitative evaluation of LV systolic function is particularly important in these patients. Diseases that affect the RV, such as RV dysplasia, also may present with palpitations.

Embolic event

- An intracardiac thrombus or mass may result in a systemic embolic event.
- Aortic atheroma is present in 20% of patients with an embolic event.
- The presence of a patent foramen ovale or atrial septal aneurysm has been associated with an increased prevalence of systemic embolic events.

Key points:

- ❏ A systematic transthoracic examination is the first step in evaluation for a potential cardiac source of embolus, but TEE is a more sensitive diagnostic approach.
- ❏ Conditions associated with systemic embolic events include:
  - atrial fibrillation
  - LA thrombus
  - prosthetic heart valves
  - valvular vegetations (bacterial or non-bacterial thrombotic endocarditis)
  - patent foramen ovale
  - aortic atheroma

- LV thrombus (e.g., after anterior myocardial infarction)
- left-sided cardiac tumors (atrial myxoma, valve fibroelastoma)
- ❏ In patients with a systemic embolic event, a cardiac source must be presumed to the cause when there is atrial fibrillation, a prosthetic valve, an intracardiac thrombus, or a tumor.
- ❏ A cause–effect relationship between the cardiac finding and embolic event is more difficult to establish in individual patients with common conditions, such as a patent foramen ovale or aortic atheroma.
- ❏ Diagnosis of a patent foramen ovale is based on demonstration of right to left shunting at rest or after Valsalva maneuver, following right heart agitated saline contrast. TEE is more sensitive than transthoracic echocardiography for detection of a patent foramen ovale, which is present in about 30% of normal individuals.

Fever/Bacteremia

- Echocardiography is the primary approach to diagnosis of endocarditis in patients with bacteremia. (Figure 5–6)
- In most patients, transthoracic echocardiography is the initial approach, but TEE is more sensitive for detection of valvular vegetations.

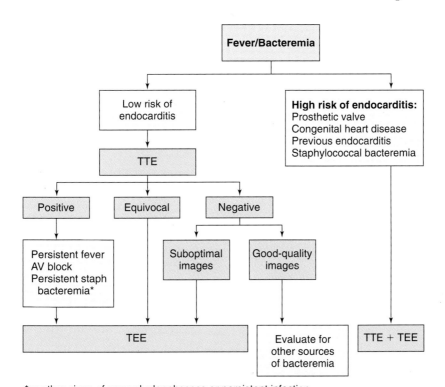

*or other signs of paravalvular abscess or persistent infection.

Figure 5–6. Flow chart for a suggested approach to evaluation of patients with fever and/or bacteremia who are referred for echocardiography. *AV,* atrioventricular; *TEE,* transesophageal echocardiography; *TTE,* transthoracic echocardiography.

- Complications of endocarditis (e.g., abscess, fistula) are best evaluated by TEE.
- Patients with an intracardiac device (pacer, defibrillator, or chronic indwelling intravascular line such as a hemodialysis catheter) should undergo echocardiography to exclude a lead infection.

Key points:

- ❏ Detection of valvular vegetations is a major criterion for diagnosis of endocarditis.
- ❏ Specificity of transthoracic echocardiography for detection of a vegetation is high (i.e., the finding of a vegetation is diagnostic) but sensitivity is low; therefore, failure to demonstrate vegetations does not "rule out" the diagnosis.

- ❏ When bacteremia or other clinical signs of endocarditis are present, TEE is appropriate unless the likelihood of endocarditis is very low and image quality is high on transthoracic imaging.
- ❏ Both TTE echocardiography and TEE are appropriate with suspected prosthetic valve endocarditis because posterior structures are shadowed by the prosthetic valve on transthoracic imaging, whereas anterior structures are shadowed on TEE imaging.
- ❏ Detection of vegetations is enhanced by scanning across the valve, using multiple images planes and using non-standard views, on both TTE and TEE imaging.

THE ECHO EXAM

Indications for Echocardiography

Clinical Diagnosis	Key Echo Findings	Limitations of Echo	Alternate Approaches
VALVULAR HEART DISEASE			
Valve stenosis	Etiology of stenosis, valve anatomy Transvalvular ΔP, valve area Chamber enlargement and hypertrophy LV and RV systolic function Associated valvular regurgitation	Possible underestimation of stenosis severity Possible coexisting coronary artery disease	Cardiac catheterization MRI
Valve regurgitation	Mechanism and etiology of regurgitation Severity of regurgitation Chamber enlargement LV and RV systolic function PA pressure estimate	TEE may be needed to evaluate mitral regurgitant severity and valve anatomy (especially before MV repair)	Cardiac catheterization MRI
Prosthetic valve function	Evidence for stenosis Detection of regurgitation Chamber enlargement Ventricular function PA pressure estimate	Imaging prosthetic valves limited by shadowing and reverberations TEE needed for suspected prosthetic MR due to "masking" of LA on TTE	Cardiac catheterization Fluoroscopy
Endocarditis	Detection of vegetations (TTE sensitivity 70%-85%) Presence and degree of valve dysfunction Chamber enlargement and function Detection of abscess Possible prognostic implications	TEE more sensitive for detection of vegetations (>90%) Definitive diagnosis of endocarditis also depends on bacteriologic criteria TEE more sensitive for abscess detection	Blood cultures and clinical findings also are diagnostic criteria for endocarditis
CORONARY ARTERY DISEASE			

Acute myocardial infarction	Segmental wall motion abnormality reflects "myocardium at risk"
	Global left ventricular function (EF)
	Complications:
	   Acute MR vs. VSD
	   Pericarditis
	   LV thrombus, aneurysm or rupture
	   RV infarct
		Coronary artery anatomy itself not directly visualized	Coronary angio (cath or CT)
			Radionuclide or PET perfusion imaging

Angina	Global and segmental LV systolic function Exclude other causes of angina (e.g., AS, HCM)	Resting wall motion may be normal despite significant CAD Stress echo needed to induce ischemia and wall motion abnormality	Coronary angio (cath or CT) Radionuclide or PET perfusion imaging ETT

Continued

Indications for Echocardiography—cont'd

Clinical Diagnosis	Key Echo Findings	Limitations of Echo	Alternate Approaches
Pre-/ post-revascularization	Assess wall thickening and endocardial motion at baseline Improvement in segmental function post-procedure	Dobutamine stress and/ or contrast echo needed to detect viable but non-functioning myocardium	MRI Coronary angio (cath or CT) Radionuclide or PET perfusion imaging Contrast echocardiography
End-stage ischemic disease	Overall left ventricular systolic function (EF) PA pressures Associated MR Left ventricular thrombus RV systolic function		Coronary angio (cath or CT) Radionuclide or PET perfusion imaging MRI for myocardial viability
CARDIOMYOPATHY Dilated	Chamber dilation (all four) LV and RV systolic function (qualitative and EF) Coexisting atrioventricular valve regurgitation PA systolic pressure LV thrombus	Indirect measures of LVEDP Accurate EF may be difficult if image quality is poor	Radionuclide EF LV and RV angiography
Restrictive	LV wall thickness LV systolic function LV diastolic function PA systolic pressure and central venous pressure	Must be distinguished from constrictive pericarditis	Cardiac catheterization with direct, simultaneous RV and LV pressure measurement after volume loading
Hypertrophic	Pattern and extent of LV hypertrophy Dynamic LVOT obstruction (imaging and Doppler) Coexisting MR Diastolic LV dysfunction		
Hypertension	LV wall thickness and chamber dimensions LV mass LV systolic function Aortic root dilation, AR		
PERICARDIAL DISEASE	Pericardial thickening Detection, size, and location of PE 2D signs of tamponade physiology Doppler signs of tamponade physiology	Diagnosis of tamponade is a hemodynamic and clinical diagnosis Constrictive pericarditis is a difficult diagnosis Not all patients with pericarditis have effusion	Intracardiac pressure measurements for tamponade or constriction MRI or CT to detect pericardial thickening

Indications for Echocardiography—cont'd

Clinical Diagnosis	Key Echo Findings	Limitations of Echo	Alternate Approaches
AORTIC DISEASE Aortic root dilation	Etiology of aortic dilation Accurate aortic root diameter measurements Anatomy of sinuses of Valsalva (especially Marfan syndrome) Associated aortic regurgitation		CT, MRI, aortography
Aortic dissection	2D images of ascending aorta (PLAX, PSAX), aortic arch (SSN), descending thoracic (A2C), and proximal abdominal (SC) aorta Imaging of dissection "flap" Associated aortic regurgitation Ventricular function	TEE more sensitive (97%) and specific (100%) Cannot assess distal vascular beds	Aortography CT MRI TEE
CARDIAC MASSES LV thrombus	High sensitivity and specificity for diagnosis of left ventricular thrombus Suspect with apical wall motion abnormality or diffuse left ventricular systolic dysfunction	Technical artifacts can be misleading 5 MHz or higher frequency transducer and angulated apical views needed	LV thrombus may not be recognized on radionuclide or contrast angiography
LA thrombus	Low sensitivity for detection of LA thrombus, although specificity is high Suspect with LA enlargement, MV disease	TEE needed to detect LA thrombus reliability	TEE
Cardiac tumors	Size, location, and physiologic consequences of tumor mass	Extracardiac involvement not well seen Cannot distinguish benign from malignant, or tumor from thrombus	TEE CT MRI (with cardiac gating) Intracardiac echo
PULMONARY HYPERTENSION	Estimate of PA pressure Evidence of left heart disease to account for increased PA pressures Right ventricular size and systolic function (cor pulmonale) Associated TR	Indirect PA pressure measurement Unable to determine pulmonary vascular resistance accurately	Cardiac catheterization
CONGENITAL HEART DISEASE	Detection and assessment of anatomic abnormalities Identify intracardiac shunt Quantitation of physiologic abnormalities Chamber enlargement Ventricular function	No direct intracardiac pressure measurements Complicated anatomy may be difficult to evaluate if image quality is poor (TEE helpful)	MRI with 3D reconstruction Cardiac catheterization TEE 3D echo

2D, two-dimensional; 3D, three-dimensional; A2C, apical two-chamber; angio, angiography; AS, aortic stenosis; CAD, coronary artery disease; cath, cardiac catheterization; CT, computed tomography; EF, ejection fraction; ETT, exercise treadmill test; HCM, hypertrophic cardiomyopathy; LA, left atrium; LV, left ventricle; LVEDP, left ventricular end-diastolic pressure; LVOT, left ventricular outflow tract; MHz, megahertz; MR, mitral regurgitation; MRI, magnetic resonance imaging; MV, mitral valve; ΔP, pressure gradient; PA, pulmonary artery; PE, pericardial effusion; PET, position emission tomography; PLAX, parasternal long axis; PSAX parasternal short axis; RV, right ventricle; SC, subcostal; SSN, suprasternal notch; TEE, transesophageal echocardiography; TR, tricuspid regurgitation; TTE, transthoracic echocardiography; VSD, ventricular septal defect.

Select the best diagnostic modality option available for the clinical scenario presented.

    A. Transthoracic echocardiography (TTE)
    B. Dobutamine stress echocardiography (DSE)
    C. Transesophageal echocardiography (TEE)
    D. Intracardiac echocardiography (ICE)
    E. Exercise stress echocardiography
    F. No further diagnostic testing indicated

QUESTION 1

A 49-year-old female with symptomatic rheumatic mitral stenosis is undergoing evaluation for percutaneous mitral valvuloplasty.

QUESTION 2

A 30-year-old gravid woman in her 35th week of pregnancy is seen for routine follow-up. She is asymptomatic from a cardiopulmonary standpoint but is noted to have a grade II/VI mid-systolic murmur on physical examination.

QUESTION 3

A 56-year-old woman with a history of embolic stroke undergoing periprocedure evaluation for percutaneous closure of a recently diagnosed secondum atrial septal defect.

QUESTION 4

A 26-year-old man with a history of endocarditis and bioprosthetic aortic valve replacement due to illicit drug use presents with fever and bacteremia. Electrocardiogram demonstrates a prolonged PR interval compared with previous ECGs.

QUESTION 5

A 40-year-old man with hypertrophic cardiomyopathy presents with several episodes of exertional presyncope. A TTE performed 1 month ago demonstrated a LV outflow tract (LVOT) velocity of 1.8 m/s after Valsalva maneuver, with a maximal diastolic septal wall thickness of 18 mm.

QUESTION 6

A 74-year-old woman with a history of mechanical mitral valve replacement presents with blood tests showing subtherapeutic anticoagulation and new onset dyspnea.

QUESTION 7

A 60-year-old asymptomatic man presents with severe back pain and left arm numbness. An urgent TTE demonstrates normal LV size and function with a normally functioning bicuspid aortic valve. Pulmonary pressures are normal, and there is no pericardial effusion.

QUESTION 8

A 42-year-old with non-Hodgkin's lymphoma presents with sinus tachycardia and hypotension. Electrocardiogram demonstrates low voltage in the precordial leads.

QUESTION 9

A 65-year-old man with type 2 diabetes mellitus is undergoing preoperative evaluation for bilateral femoral artery bypass surgery.

QUESTION 10

A 68-year-old sedentary woman has been recently diagnosed with a cardiac murmur. The patient denies exertional cardiopulmonary symptoms. A transthoracic echocardiogram demonstrates normal LV size and function. There is bileaflet mitral valve prolapse with severe mitral regurgitation. There are no other significant valvular abnormalities. Pulmonary pressures are at the upper limits of normal.

ANSWERS

ANSWER 1: C, TEE

Patients with symptomatic rheumatic mitral stenosis are candidates for percutaneous mitral valvuloplasty. In addition to TTE, before valvuloplasty, TEE is indicated to evaluate severity of mitral regurgitation and LA thrombus. There is an increased likelihood of success with favorable valve anatomy (less leaflet calcification, less leaflet thickening, and less involvement of the subvalvular apparatus). Valvuloplasty may significantly increase regurgitation, particularly if the valve leaflets are thickened or calcified and leaflet tearing occurs during the procedure. Also, during the procedure, the catheter is in the LA, where a LA thrombus may dislodge if present. Therefore, valvuloplasty is contraindicated if there is greater than moderate regurgitation or there is an LA thrombus at baseline. TTE may be adequate to evaluate mitral regurgitation severity but is not adequate to exclude LA appendage thrombus. This patient has symptomatic mitral stenosis, and further provocation with stress testing (dobutamine or bicycle) is not indicated. ICE may be used intraprocedurally during the valvuloplasty, but TEE is first indicated to determine if the patient is a candidate for the procedure.

ANSWER 2: F, No Further Testing

In the last trimester of pregnancy, intravascular volume increases significantly. Increased antegrade flow over the cardiac valves increases turbulent flow and commonly produces a benign systolic flow murmur seen in more than 80% of pregnant women. Postpartum, volume status normalizes and the benign murmur typically resolves. Rather than echocardiographic testing, routine postpartum clinical follow-up with cardiac auscultation to determine if the murmur is still present is indicated.

ANSWER 3: D, ICE

ICE allows for optimal visualization of the interatrial septum and atria. This modality is advantageous for invasive cardiac procedures because it may be performed concurrently during the case. Common application of ICE includes use during percutaneous closure of atrial septal defects or during electrophysiology procedures to determine intracardiac catheter position. TEE may be performed during invasive procedures, but optimal image plane may be limited by the anatomic constraints of transducer positioning in the esophagus. TTE is less optimal during invasive procedures because it is difficult to perform while the patient is sterilely draped.

ANSWER 4: C, TEE

Clinical suspicion for endocarditis is high in this patient with bacteremia, and additional diagnostic testing is indicated. The presence of atrioventricular nodal block raises concern for a paravalvular abscess with intramyocardial extension affecting conduction pathways. TTE is inadequate for definitive evaluation of paravalvular abscess, particularly in a patient with a prosthetic aortic valve, because reverberations and acoustic shadowing from the prosthetic valve may obscure or limit visualization of a paravalvular abscess. An aortic paravalvular abscess may extend into the septum, affecting the conduction system, but may also extend into the posterior aortic annulus, adjacent to the anterior mitral valve leaflet. With TEE, there are no interposed ribs or lung tissue between the transducer and the heart, so image quality is improved and posterior cardiac structures are better visualized compared with TTE. This patient presents with an acute infectious process, and cardiac stress testing (dobutamine or bicycle) is not indicated.

ANSWER 5: E, Exercise Stress Echocardiography

This patient presents with presyncope, and further diagnostic testing is indicated. Repeat TTE is unlikely to demonstrate a significant interval change from a prior study completed only 1 month prior. Patients with hypertrophic cardiomyopathy may develop LV outflow tract obstruction that only manifests with physical activity. If there is concurrent systolic anterior motion of the mitral valve with physical activity, LV outflow obstruction may be exacerbated. Provoked LVOT gradients reflect true peak stress gradients when measured in real time. Exercise may be performed using a standard treadmill protocol or with a supine bicycle. With treadmill exercise, echocardiographic data are recorded at baseline and immediately after exercise. Bicycle stress ergometry allows continuous concurrent echocardiographic imaging during exercise because the patient lies recumbent. With some systems, an integrated stress bed can be maneuvered to allow for optimal patient positioning. TEE is not optimal for patients with hypertrophic cardiomyopathy because TEE is a resting study and the LVOT jet is difficult to align in a parallel manner with the transducer due to the physical constraints of the esophagus on the transducer.

ANSWER 6: C, TEE

Assessment of prosthetic mitral valve function by TTE alone is relatively limited because the LA is a posterior structure situated in the far field of the imaging plane. The prosthetic material in mechanical valves is a strong specular reflector, blocking ultrasound penetration distal to the valve. For TTE, acoustic shadowing of the LA prohibits evaluation of mitral prosthetic regurgitation. With TEE, the transducer is placed posterior to the heart and the LA is in the near field. Mitral regurgitation can be more definitively assessed. Also, TEE reduces reverberation artifact of the prosthetic material and valve occluders are generally better seen, which allows for better evaluation for adherent thrombus or vegetation. In this case, stress testing (bicycle or dobutamine stress) is not indicated.

ANSWER 7: C, TEE

Despite the TTE that demonstrates normal LV size and function, the presenting symptoms of severe back pain and left arm numbness warrant further diagnostic evaluation. A bicuspid aortic valve may be associated with an ascending aortopathy, which predisposes to potential aortic aneurysm and rupture. For most of these patients, dilation is limited to the proximal aorta. When aortic dissection is suspected, definitive imaging modalities include TEE, CT, or cardiac magnetic resonance imaging. An aortic process should be excluded before any other diagnostic testing, such as cardiac stress testing (bicycle or dobutamine stress).

ANSWER 8: A, TTE

To determine potential etiologies of hypotension, TTE is useful in evaluation of LV function, central venous pressure, and pericardial tamponade. In this case, the clinical history and clinical status suggest a pericardial effusion that is hemodynamically significant. This is further supported by low voltage on the ECG in the precordial leads. TTE is diagnostic for a pericardial effusion. Hemodynamic significance of the effusion (tamponade) physiology may be evidenced by external compression of the RV, respiratory variation in flow velocities across the mitral and tricuspid valves, and increased central venous pressure.

ANSWER 9: B, DSE

Preoperative evaluation for patients with significant cardiovascular risk factors typically includes provocative stress testing to identify myocardial ischemia. Resting studies such as TTE or TEE do not provide evaluation of the cardiac response to stress, as would potentially be encountered intraoperatively. An exercise stress study (treadmill or bicycle stress) is preferred over pharmacologic testing when possible because it provides an evaluation of the cardiac response to physiologic stress. However, given that the patient in this case scenario is undergoing preoperative evaluation for bilateral lower peripheral artery disease, it is unlikely that the workload achieved would be adequate to provide a maximal stress study.

ANSWER 10: E, Exercise Stress Echocardiography

Surgical indications for valve repair or replacement in a patient with mitral regurgitation are predicated on the presence of cardiopulmonary symptoms attributable to the valve lesion. In the absence of symptoms, other surgical indicators include evidence of the adverse hemodynamic effect of the regurgitant volume load, manifested as a decline in LV systolic function or LV enlargement. In this case, the patient's LV size and function are normal and she denies cardiopulmonary symptoms but is noted to be sedentary. In cases where there is significant mitral regurgitation but the patient does not meet surgical criteria, an increase in pulmonary pressures during provocative stress testing suggests that the hemodynamic effect of the regurgitation is significant and earlier surgical intervention is indicated. Exercise testing also allows the clinical provider to objectively gauge the exercise tolerance of a patient who has an unclear functional status (the patient is sedentary in this case) rather than evaluate the patient with pharmacologic testing, as would occur with DSE. The TTE in this case was diagnostic for the severity and mechanism of mitral regurgitation, and additional imaging of the mitral valve with TEE is not needed at this time.

6 Left and Right Ventricular Systolic Function

LEFT VENTRICULAR SYSTOLIC FUNCTION

Step 1: Measure Left Ventricular Size

Left ventricular chamber dimensions

■ Two-dimensional (2D) guided M-mode measurement of LV minor axis internal dimensions at end-diastole and end-systole *or*
■ 2D measurement of LV minor axis internal dimensions

Key Points:

❑ LV internal dimensions are measured from the parasternal window because the ultrasound beam is perpendicular to the blood–myocardial interface, providing high axial resolution. (Figure 6–1)
❑ The parasternal long axis view allows verification that measurements are perpendicular to the long axis of the LV. An oblique angle may not be recognized in short axis views.
❑ 2D imaging in long and short axis views is used to ensure the dimension is measured in the minor axis of the ventricle (not at an oblique

angle, which would overestimate size). (Figure 6–2)
❑ The rapid sampling rate of M-mode (compared with the slow frame rate of 2D imaging) provides more accurate identification of the endocardial borders. (Figure 6–3)
❑ End-diastolic measurements are made at the onset of the QRS complex; end-systolic measurements are made at the minimum chamber size, just before aortic valve closure.
❑ Measurements are made from the leading edge of the septal endocardial to the leading edge of the posterior LV wall.
❑ The posterior LV wall is identified on M-mode as the steepest, most continuous line. Identification of the endocardial border on 2D images is less reliable. (Figure 6–4)
❑ Measurements of LV internal dimensions and wall thickness are made at the level of the mitral valve chords just apical to the mitral leaflet tips.

Left ventricular chamber volumes

■ Endocardial borders are traced in apical 4-chamber and 2-chamber views at end-diastole and end-systole. (Figure 6–5)

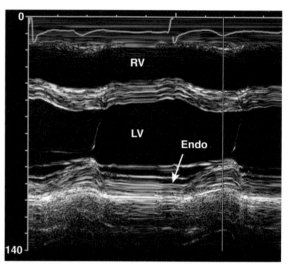

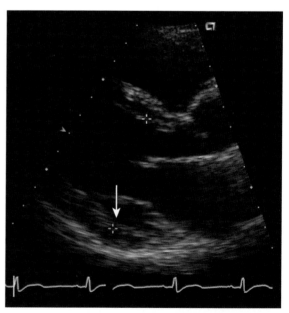

Figure 6-1. Parasternal long-axis view showing 2D measurement of LV internal dimension at end-diastole (onset of the QRS) from the septal endocardium to the posterior wall endocardium at the level of the mitral valve chords. This minor axis dimension is measured perpendicular to the long axis of the left ventricle.

Figure 6-3. When the M-mode bean can be aligned perpendicular to the long axis of the LV, based on 2D long and short-axis views, the advantage of the M-mode recording is a high temporal sampling rate. The rapid motion of the septal and posterior wall endocardium allows precise measurements. The endocardium (Endo) typically is the most continuous line with the steepest slope in systole. Measurement of the end-systolic dimension (maximal posterior motion of the septum, or minimal LV dimension) is shown by the vertical line.

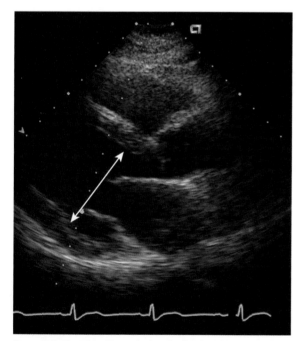

Figure 6-2. Parasternal long-axis view showing that a M-mode measurement of LV dimensions, along the *dotted line,* would overestimate ventricular size because the sample line is oblique compared to the minor axis dimension, shown by the *arrow.*

Figure 6-4. Identification of the posterior wall endocardium on a still frame end-systolic 2D image can be difficult, as shown in this example.

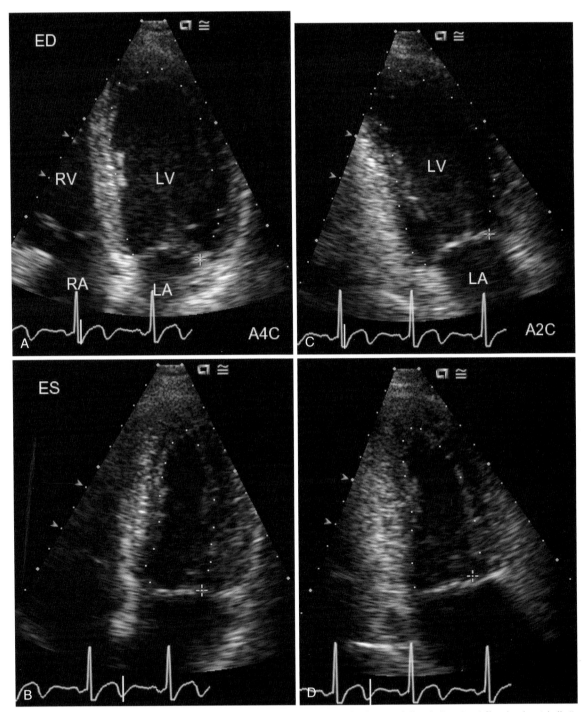

Figure 6–5. LV volumes and ejection fraction are calculated based on tracing endocardial borders at end-diastole (*top, A* and *C*) and end-systole (*bottom, B* and *D*) in both apical 4-chamber (*left, A* and *B*) and apical 2-chamber views (*right, C* and *D*). Identification of endocardial borders is optimized by playing the cine loop to show endocardial motion.

- Volumes are calculated by the ultrasound system using the biplane method of disks.
- LV end-diastolic and end-systolic volumes are indexed by dividing by body surface area. (Tables 6-1 and 6-2)

Key Points:

❑ Care is needed to obtain images from a true apical position; use of a steep left lateral decubitus position with an apical cutout in the stretcher allows optimal transducer positioning.

❑ Depth is adjusted so the mitral annulus just fits on the image; gain and processing curves are adjusted to optimize endocardial definition.

❑ Left-sided echo contrast enhances recognition of endocardial borders when image quality is poor.

TABLE 6-1 Left Ventricular Dimension Measurements

	TTE 2D	TTE—2D-Guided M-Mode	TEE
Transducer position	Parasternal	Parasternal	Transgastric
Image plane	Long axis	Long and short axis	2-chamber view (rotation angle 60-90 degrees)
Measurement position in LV chamber	Perpendicular to LV long axis in center of LV Biplane imaging or rotation between long and short axis views helps ensure centered measurement	Perpendicular to LV long axis in center of LV Correct M-line orientation often requires moving transducer up an interspace	Perpendicular to LV long axis in center of LV Ensuring centered measurement is more difficult on TEE
Measurement site along LV length	Just apical to mitral leaflet tips (chordal level)	Just apical to mitral leaflet tips (chordal level)	At junction of basal ⅓ and apical ⅔ of LV
Measurement technique	White–black interface	Leading edge to leading edge	White–black interface
Timing in cardiac cycle **End-diastole** **End-systole**	Onset of QRS Frame just before mitral valve closure, *or* Maximum LV volume Minimum LV volume *or* Frame just before aortic valve closure	Onset of QRS Minimum LV volume	Onset of QRS Frame just before mitral valve closure *or* Maximum LV volume Minimum LV volume *or* Frame just before aortic valve closure
Advantages	Feasible in most patients Measurements can be made perpendicular to LV long axis	High sampling rate facilitates identification of endocardium Reproducible	Data can be obtained intraoperatively to monitor preload Ultrasound beam is perpendicular to endocardium from TG view, improving border recognition
Disadvantages	Endocardial and epicardial borders may be difficult to accurately identify Slow frame rate compared with M-mode	M-line measurements should only be made if perpendicular LV measurement is possible Requires more attention to transducer and M-line position	Image plane may be oblique Wall thickness measured in TG short axis view

2D, two-dimensional; TEE, transesophageal; TG, transgastric; TTE, transthoracic echocardiography.

TABLE 6-2 Left-Sided Heart Chamber Sizes in Adults

		Normal	Abnormal Mild	Moderate	Severe
LV minor axis ED dimension (2D or guided M-mode)	Women	3.9–5.3 cm	5.4–5.7 cm	5.8–6.1 cm	≥6.2 cm
		2.4–3.2 cm/m²	3.3–3.4 cm/m²	3.5–3.7 cm/m²	≥3.8 cm/m²
	Men	4.2–5.9 cm	6.0–6.3 cm	6.4–6.8 cm	≥6.9 cm
		2.2–3.1 cm/m²	3.2–3.4 cm/m²	3.5–3.6 cm/m²	≥3.7 cm/m²
LV ED volumes (2D)	Women	56–104 mL	105–117 mL	118–130 mL	≥131 mL
	Men	67–155 mL	156–178 mL	179–201 mL	≥202 mL
	Indexed for BSA	35–75 mL/m²	76–86 mL/m²	87–96 mL/m²	≥97 mL/m²
LV minor axis ES dimension (2D or guided M-mode)		2.1–4.0			
	Indexed for BSA	1.4–2.1 cm/m²			
LV ES volumes (2D)	Women	19–49 mL	50–59 mL	60–69 mL	≥70 mL
	Men	22–58 mL	59–70 mL	71–82 mL	≥83 mL
	Indexed for BSA	12–30 mL/m²	31–36 mL/m²	37–42 mL/m²	≥43 mL/m²
Ejection fraction		≥55%	45%–54%	30%–44%	<30%
LV wall thickness	Women	0.6–0.9 cm	1.0–1.2 cm	1.3–1.5 cm	≥1.6 cm
	Men	0.6–1.0 cm	1.0–1.3 cm	1.4–1.6 cm	≥1.7 cm
LV mass (2D method)	Women	66–150 g	151–171 g	172–192 g	≥193 g
		44–88 g/m²	89–100 g/m²	101–112 g/m²	≥113 g/m²
	Men	96–200 g	201–227 g	228–254 g	≥255 g
		50–102 g/m²	103–116 g/m²	117–130 g/m²	≥131 g/m²
LA diameter	Women	2.7–3.8 cm	3.9–4.2 cm	4.3–4.6 cm	≥4.7 cm
		3.0–4.0 cm	4.1–4.6 cm	4.7–5.2 cm	≥5.2 cm
LA volume index	Men	22 ± 6 mL/m²	29–33 mL/m²	34–39 mL/m²	≥40 mL/m²

2D, two-dimensional; ED, end-diastolic; ES, end-systolic.
Data from Lang RM et al: JASE 2005;18:1440-1463 and other sources (for end-systolic dimensions).

□ End-diastolic tracings are made at the onset of the QRS (first frame on digital cine loop); end-systole is defined as minimal LV volume and is identified visually by frame-by-frame viewing of the images. (Figure 6–6)

□ Volumes are more reflective of the degree of LV dilation than linear dimensions.

□ The most common limitation of this approach is a foreshortened apical view, resulting in under-estimation of ventricular volumes. (Figure 6–7)

□ Body surface area may not be the ideal measure of body size but is widely used clinically.

Left ventricular wall thickness

■ 2D guided M-mode measurement of LV septal and posterior wall thickness at end-diastole

■ 2D measurement of LV wall thickness

Key Points:

□ LV wall thickness is measured from the parasternal window because the ultrasound beam is perpendicular to the blood–myocardial interface, providing high axial resolution. (Figure 6–8)

□ The rapid sampling rate of M-mode (compared with the slow frame rate of 2D imaging) provides more accurate identification of the endocardial borders.

□ Wall thickness of both the septum and posterior wall is measured at the level of the mitral valve chordae at end-diastole.

□ The septal wall thickness measurement does not include trabeculations on the right ventricular side of the septum and does not mistake the mid-septal stripe for the right-sided endocardium.

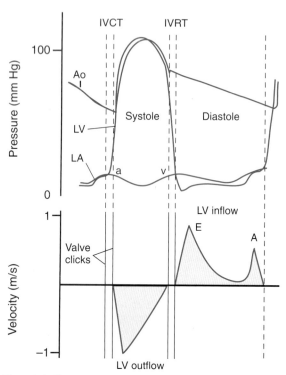

Figure 6–6. The cardiac cycle. Left ventricular *(LV)*, aortic *(Ao)*, and left atrial *(LA)* pressures are shown with the corresponding Doppler left ventricular outflow and inflow velocity curves. The isovolumic contraction time *(IVCT)* represents the time between mitral valve closure and aortic valve opening, while the isovolumic relaxation time *(IVRT)* represents the time between aortic valve closure and mitral valve opening.

❒ The posterior LV wall thickness is measured from the endocardium to the posterior epicardium.

Left ventricular mass and wall stress

■ LV wall thickness measurements usually are sufficient for clinical care.
■ LV mass and wall stress can be calculated from 2D images and LV pressures, if needed.

Key Points:

❒ LV mass is calculated from endocardial and epicardial border tracing in a short axis view at the papillary muscle level and measurement of LV length. (Figure 6–9)
❒ LV wall stress can be calculated based on tracing LV endocardial and epicardial borders and measuring LV systolic pressure.
❒ Wall thickness of both the septum and posterior wall is measured at the level of the mitral valve chordae at end-diastole.
❒ LV mass and wall stress calculations are mainly useful for research studies and are rarely needed for clinical decision making.
❒ Color Doppler strain rate imaging may be helpful as clinical guidelines are developed.

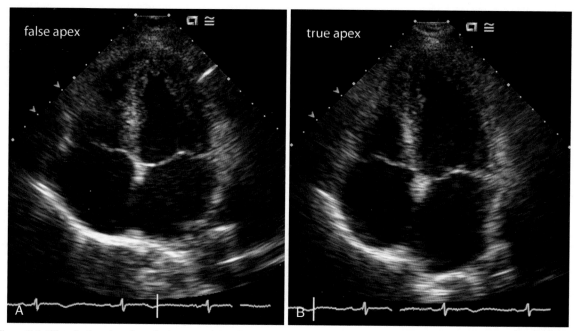

Figure 6–7. When the transducer is on the true apex of the left ventricle, the chamber is ellipsoid, compared with a foreshortened view (A) where the ventricle appears more spherical with a "false apex." LV volumes will be underestimated in a foreshortened view and apical wall motion abnormalities may be missed. This potential error is avoided by moving the transducer down an interspace and laterally to the true apex (B).

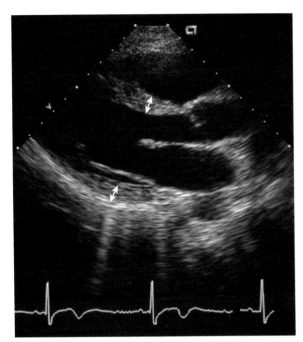

Figure 6–8. Parasternal long-axis view for measurement of LV wall thickness. The ultrasound beam is perpendicular to the blood–myocardial interface from this window, allowing accurate identification of the walls.

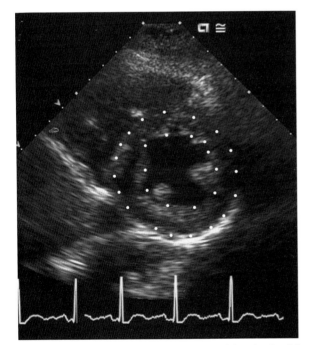

Figure 6–9. To calculate LV mass, the endocardial and epicardial borders are traced in a parasternal short axis view. This provides a mean wall thickness that is used in the LV mass calculations. In clinical practice, the diagnosis of LV hypertrophy typically is based on a single linear measurement of wall thickness or quantitative assessment in multiple views. 2D quantitation of LV mass is used mainly for research applications.

This advanced topic is discussed in other text-books (e.g., see Otto: *The Practice of Clinical Echocardiography*, 4th ed.).

Step 2: Measure left ventricular ejection fraction

- LV ejection fraction is visually estimated based on parasternal and apical views.
- LV ejection fraction is quantitated using the apical biplane method by tracing endocardial borders at end-diastole and end-systole in apical 4- and 2-chamber views. (Figure 6–10)
- When the visual estimate and measured ejection fraction are similar, the measurement is reported; when there is disagreement, the measurement is repeated or only the visual estimate is reported (if image quality precludes accurate border tracing).

Key Points:

❑ LV ejection fraction is visually estimated based on parasternal short axis and apical 4-chamber, 2-chamber, and long axis views. Estimates by an experienced observer are very reliable.

❑ LV ejection fraction (EF) is calculated from end-diastolic volume (EDV) and end-systolic volume (ESV) as:

$$EF = [(EDV - ESV)/EDV] \times 100\%$$

❑ When the visual estimate disagrees with the measured EF, the traced endocardial borders are reviewed to ensure the correct transducer positioning and image planes and accurate identification of the endocardium. (Figure 6–11)

❑ When image quality is suboptimal, left-sided contrast may enhance identification of endocardial borders.

Biplane apical

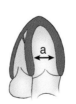

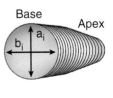

Figure 6–10. Illustration of the apical biplane formula for LV volume calculations showing the 2D echocardiographic views and measurements on the left and the geometric model on the right. Endocardial borders are traced in apical 4-chamber and 2-chamber views, which are used to define a series of orthogonal diameters (*a* and *b*). A "Simpson's rule" assumption based on stacked disks is used to calculate volume.

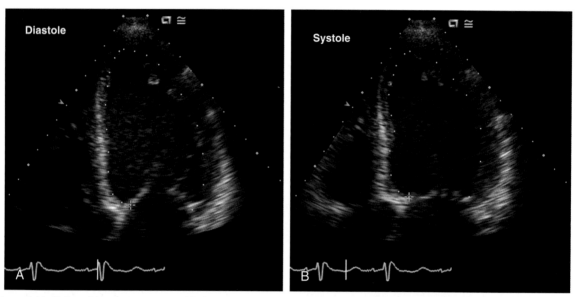

Figure 6–11. Endocardial borders were retraced by the physician interpreting this study to ensure that the calculated ejection fraction was accurate when the visual estimate appeared different from the initial measurements. The endocardial borders at end-diastole (*A*) and end-systole (*B*) in the apical 4-chamber view are shown in this patient with severely reduced systolic function and a calculated ejection fraction of 16%.

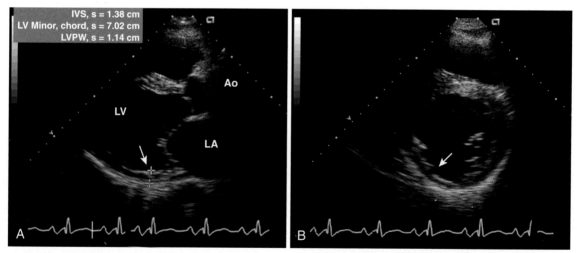

Figure 6–12. In these parasternal long axis (*A*) and short axis (*B*) views, the inferior and inferior-lateral (or posterior) LV walls are thin compared with the septum, consistent with a previous inferior myocardial infarction.

❑ When quantitation of ejection fraction is not needed or is limited by image quality, the visual estimate is reported, along with a descriptive scale as follows:
Normal (EF ≥ 55%)
Mildly reduced (EF 45%-54%)
Moderately reduced (EF 30%-44%)
Severely reduced (EF < 30%)

Step 3: Evaluate regional ventricular function

■ Regional (or segmental) ventricular function is evaluated as detailed in Chapter 8.

■ Wall motion and thickening for each myocardial segment is graded as normal, hypokinetic, akinetic or dyskinetic.
■ Any areas of thinning and increased echogenicity (consistent with scar) are noted. (Figure 6–12)

Key Points:

❑ The presence of wall motion abnormalities in a pattern corresponding to coronary artery perfusion suggests ischemic cardiac disease.
❑ In a short axis view, the inferior wall may normally flatten along the diaphragm in diastole (with normal systolic motion); this normal

pattern should not be mistaken as a wall motion abnormality.

- ❏ Optimal endocardial definition is needed to evaluate regional function.
- ❏ Wall thickening, as well as endocardial motion, should be evaluated for each myocardial segment.

Step 4: Calculate left ventricular stroke volume and cardiac output

- Stroke volume calculations are not a routine part of every examination but are helpful when ventricular function is abnormal and when valve regurgitation or an intracardiac shunt is present.
- Stroke volume (SV in cm³ or mL) is the product of the cross-sectional area of flow (CSA in cm²) multiplied by the velocity-time integral (VTI in cm) of flow at that site (Figure 6–13):

$$SV = CSA \times VTI$$

- Stroke volume can be calculated at any site where diameter and velocity can be measured but most often is measured in the LV outflow tract (LVOT), just proximal to the aortic valve.
- Cardiac output (CO in L/min) is stroke volume (mL) times heart rate (beats/min), divided by 1000 mL/L:

$$CO = [SV\,(mL) \times heart\ rate\,(beats/min)]/1000\ mL/L$$
$$= L/min$$

Key Points:

- ❏ LVOT diameter (D) is measured from a parasternal long-axis view in mid-systole, from inner edge to inner edge, immediately adjacent to the base of the aortic valve leaflets. (Figure 6–14)
- ❏ Cross-sectional area (CSA) is calculated as the area of a circle:

$$CSA = \pi\,(radius)^2 = 3.14\,(D/2)^2$$

- ❏ LV outflow velocity is recorded using pulsed Doppler, with a 2- to 3-mm sample volume length, from the apical window with the sample volume just proximal to the aortic valve. (Figure 6–15)
- ❏ A visible aortic valve closing (but not opening) click on the Doppler tracing ensures correct sample volume placement.
- ❏ The modal velocity (darkest part of the velocity curve) is traced to obtain the velocity-time integral.
- ❏ The velocity-time integral represents the "stroke distance" or the length of the cylinder of blood ejected by the LV on each beat.
- ❏ A similar approach can be used to calculate stroke volume across the mitral annulus or the pulmonic valve.
- ❏ In adults, normal stroke volume is about 80 mL and normal cardiac output is about 6 L/min.

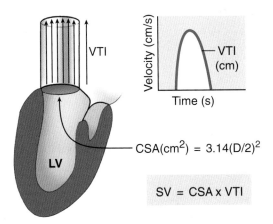

Figure 6–13. Doppler stroke volume calculation. The cross-sectional area (CSA) of flow is calculated as a circle based on a 2D echo diameter (D) measurement. The length of the cylinder of blood ejected through this cross-sectional area on a single beat is the velocity-time integral (VTI) of the Doppler curve. Stroke volume (SV) then is calculated as CSA × VTI.

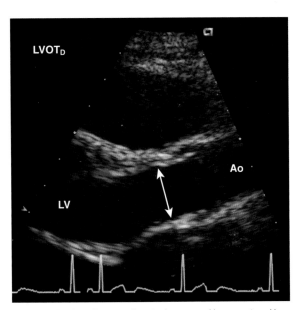

Figure 6–14. LV outflow tract diameter is measured in a parasternal long axis view (for axial resolution) in mid-systole using zoom mode. The diameter is measured at the base of the open aortic valve leaflets from the inner edge of the septal endocardium to the inner edge of the anterior mitral leaflet, as shown.

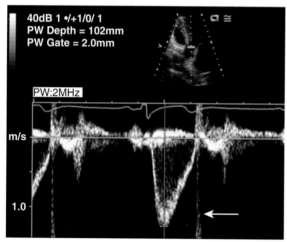

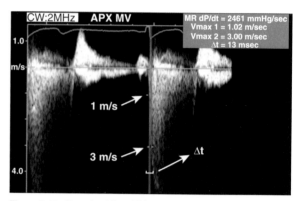

Figure 6–16. The rate of rise of LV pressure in early systole is calculated by measuring the time integral between 1 and 3 m/s on the mitral regurgitant Doppler velocity curve. This time in seconds is divided by the pressure difference corresponding to a change in velocity from 1 to 3 m/s (32 mm Hg). In this example, the *dP/dt* is 32 mm Hg divided by 0.013 sec (13 milliseconds), which equals 2461 mm Hg/sec.

Figure 6–15. The LV outflow velocity curve is recorded from the apical window, so the ultrasound beam is parallel to the direction of flow, with the 2- to 3-mm sample volume on the left ventricular side of the valve. Appropriate positioning is confirmed by the presence of an aortic valve closing click (*arrow*) but no opening click. The Doppler curve should show a narrow band of velocities with a clearly defined peak. The velocity-time integral is measured by tracing the modal velocity of the systolic flow signal.

Step 5: Calculate left ventricular *dP/dt*

- The rate of rise of ventricle pressure, or change in pressure *(dP)* over time *(dt)*, is a load-independent measure of ventricular function.
- LV *dP/dt* can be calculated from the rise in velocity of the mitral regurgitant jet. (Figure 6–16)
- This measurement is useful in selected patients with evidence of ventricular dysfunction or with significant mitral regurgitation.

Key Points:

❏ The time interval *(dt)* between the points on the mitral regurgitant velocity curve at 1 and 3 m/s is measured in seconds. (Figure 6–17)
❏ The pressure difference *(dP)* between 1 and 3 m/s, calculated using the Bernoulli equation, is:

$$4(3)^2 - 4(1)^2 = 32 \text{ mm Hg}$$

❏ Thus, *dP/dt* is 32 mm Hg divided by the time interval in seconds.
❏ A normal *dP/dt* is more than 1000 mm Hg/sec.

Step 6: Other measures of left ventricular systolic function

- Other signs of LV systolic function that are not independently diagnostic may aid in recognition of abnormal function and prompt quantitative evaluation of ventricular function.

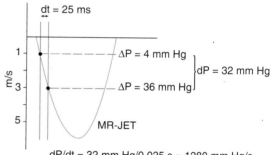

Figure 6–17. Schematic diagram showing measurement of *dP/dt* from the mitral regurgitation velocity curve. The points where the velocity reaches 1 m/s and 3 m/s are identified and the time interval *(dt)* between these two points is measured as shown. The pressure difference *(dP)* between 1 m/s (4 mm Hg) and 3 m/s (36 mm Hg) is 32 mm Hg, so *dP/dt* is calculated as shown.

- These findings include increased E-point septal separation, decreased aortic root anterior-posterior motion, and decreased mitral annular apical motion.

Key Points:

❏ The distance between the most anterior motion of the mitral leaflet and the most posterior motion of the septum normally is only 0 to 5 mm. An increased mitral E-point to septal separation occurs with LV dilation or systolic dysfunction, aortic regurgitation, or mitral stenosis. This finding is best appreciated on M-mode tracings. (Figure 6–18)
❏ The movement of the aortic root in an anterior-posterior direction on M-mode reflects the

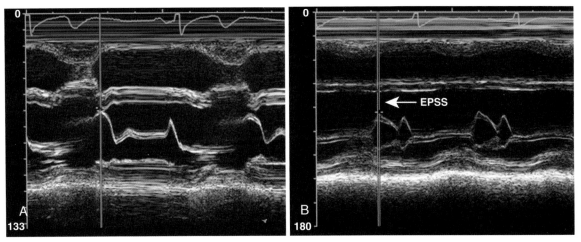

Figure 6–18. The vertical distance between the maximum anterior motion of the mitral leaflet (*E-point*) and the maximum posterior motion of the septum, or E-point septal separation (*EPSS*), reflects LV size and systolic function. The normal EPSS is less than 5 mm. A larger separation indicates LV dilation or systolic dysfunction. The EPSS also is increased with aortic regurgitation due to impingement of the regurgitant jet on the anterior mitral leaflet and with mitral stenosis, due to restricted motion of the mitral leaflet. Examples of a normal (*A*) and increased (*B*) E-point separation (due to a low LV ejection fraction) are shown.

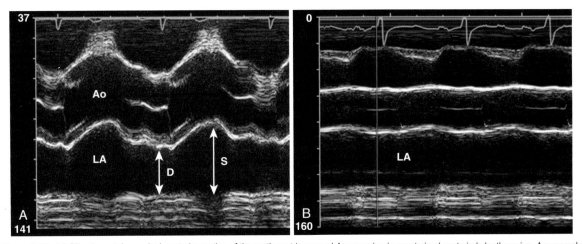

Figure 6–19. LA filling in systole results in anterior motion of the aortic root because LA expansion is constrained posteriorly by the spine. An example of normal aortic root motion on M-mode in a patent with normal LA filling and emptying and a normal cardiac output (*A*) is compared with the reduced aortic root motion seen in a patient with severe left ventricular dysfunction (*B*) and reduced LA filling and emptying. Conversely, aortic root motion may be increased when significant mitral regurgitation is present.

filling and emptying of the left atrium, which is confined between the aortic root and spine. A decrease in atrial filling/emptying, for example, with a low forward stroke volume, results in decreased motion of the aortic root. (Figure 6–19)

☐ Ventricular contraction occurs along the long axis of the ventricle, in addition to circumferential shortening. The mitral annulus moves apically with longitudinal contraction of the LV, with the magnitude of motion reflecting ventricular function. Reduced apical motion of the annulus (<8 mm) indicates an ejection fraction less than 50%. (Figure 6–20)

RIGHT VENTRICULAR SYSTOLIC FUNCTION (TABLE 6-3)

Step 1: Evaluate right ventricular chamber size and wall thickness

■ Right ventricular size and wall thickness are evaluated from multiple views, including parasternal short axis and RV inflow views, apical 4-chamber view, and subcostal 4-chamber view.

■ RV size is graded qualitatively based on the relative size of the right and left ventricle:

• normal (RV < LV, with RV apex more basal than LV apex)

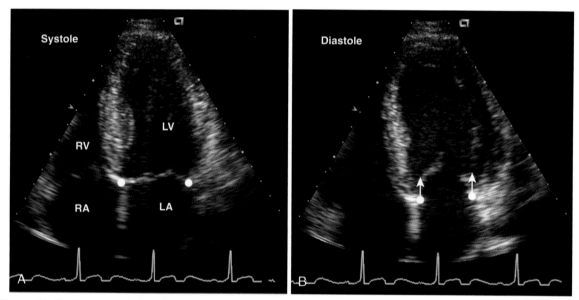

Figure 6–20. The distance the mitral annulus moves toward the LV apex in systole, as indicated by the arrow, reflects the longitudinal shortening of the ventricle. This measurement is similar to the tissue Doppler systolic velocity at the annulus.

TABLE 6-3 Right Heart Chamber Sizes in Adults				
			Abnormal	
	Normal	**Mild**	**Moderate**	**Severe**
RV ED diameter*	2.7–3.3 cm	3.4–3.7	3.8–4.1	≥4.2
RV ED length*	7.1–7.9 cm	8.0–8.5	8.6–9.1	≥9.2
RV ED outflow tract diameter†	2.5–2.9 cm	3.0–3.2	3.3–3.5	≥3.6
RV free wall thickness‡	<0.5 cm			
Tricuspid annular excursion from systole to diastole	1.5–2.0 cm			
RV fractional area change (4-chamber view)	32%–60%	25%–31%	18%–34%	≤17%
RA minor axis dimension§	1.7–2.5 cm/m²	2.6–2.8	2.9–3.1	≥3.2
Pulmonary artery diameter	1.5–2.1 cm	2.2–2.5	2.6–2.9	≥3.0

*Measured in 4-chamber view, with length from annulus to apex and diameter measured midway between tricuspid annulus and RV apex.
†Measured in short-axis view at the aortic valve level from the RV free wall to the aortic valve (inner edge to inner edge).
‡Measured in subcostal view at R wave peak (end-diastole) at level of tricuspid valve chords.
§Minor axis dimension measured in 4-chamber view.
ED, end-diastolic.
Data from Lang RM et al: JASE 2005;18:1440-1463.

- mildly enlarged (enlarged but RV < LV)
- moderately enlarged (RV = LV)
- severely enlarged (RV > LV)
■ RV wall thickness is evaluated qualitatively, or free wall thickness can be measured.

Key Points:

❏ The best views for evaluation of RV size are an apical 4-chamber view tilted toward the RV and a subcostal 4-chamber view. (Figure 6–21)

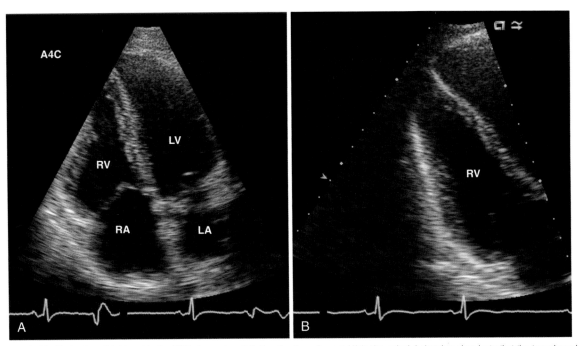

Figure 6–21. Evaluation of right ventricular (*RV*) size and systolic function is performed (*A*) in the apical 4-chamber view (note that the transducer is correctly located over the LV apex) and (*B*) in a zoom view with the transducer tilted toward the RV.

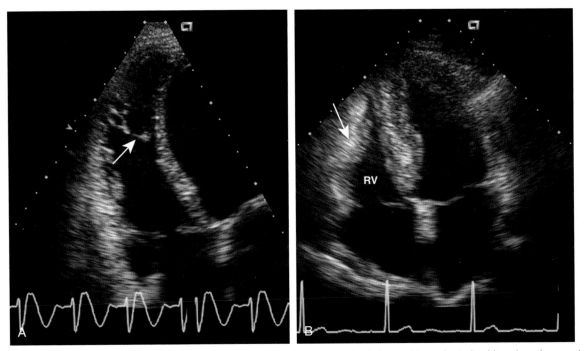

Figure 6–22. The RV free wall normally is thinner than the LV wall, although prominent trabeculations and the moderator band (arrow) may be appreciated, as seen in a patient with mild RV dilation (*A*). An increased thickness of the RV free wall (*B*) is seen in a patient with pulmonary hypertension.

- ❏ RV size may be overestimated if the apical view is foreshortened, if the transducer is medial to the LV apex, or if the free wall of the RV is not well visualized.
- ❏ The subcostal view provides the most reliable estimate of RV size because the ultrasound beam is perpendicular to the RV free wall and ventricular septum.
- ❏ RV hypertrophy is seen when the RV free wall is more than 5 mm or when the RV wall appears as thick as the LV wall. (Figure 6–22)

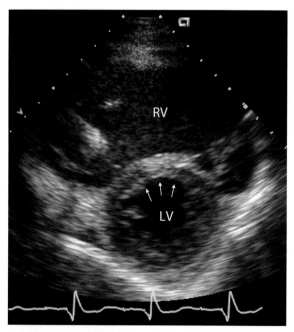

Figure 6–23. With right ventricular volume overload, the RV is enlarged and septal motion is flat in diastole. However, in systole (shown here) the contour of the septum is normal, with a circular shape of the LV in short axis.

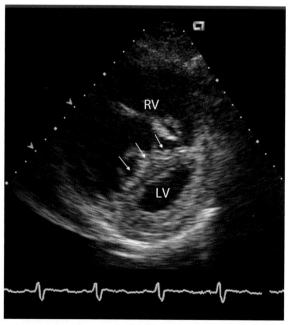

Figure 6–24. In contrast to volume overload, RV pressure overload results in septal flattening in both diastole and in systole, as seen on this end-systolic image.

Step 2: Examine the pattern of ventricular septal motion

- Ventricular septal motion is evaluated in 2D parasternal long and short-axis images.
- M-mode evaluation of ventricular septal motion may be helpful in some cases.

Key Points:

- ☐ With right ventricular volume overload, the ventricular septum is flattened in diastole, but in systole the LV assumes the normal circular configuration. (Figure 6–23)
- ☐ With RV pressure overload, the ventricular septum remains flattened or reversed in systole so that the LV assumes a D shape in the short axis view. (Figures 6–24 and 6–25)
- ☐ The pattern of ventricular septum motion is also altered by conduction abnormalities, previous cardiac surgery, and pericardial disease.

Step 3: Estimate right ventricular systolic contraction

- RV systolic function is assessed from multiple views, including parasternal short axis and RV inflow views, the apical 4-chamber view, and the subcostal 4-chamber view.

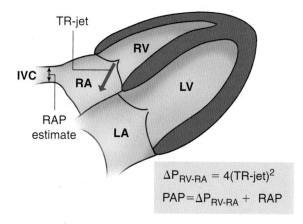

$$\Delta P_{RV\text{-}RA} = 4(TR\text{-jet})^2$$

$$PAP = \Delta P_{RV\text{-}RA} + RAP$$

Figure 6–25. Pulmonary artery pressure (*PAP*) can be calculated non-invasively based on the velocity in the tricuspid regurgitant (*TR*) jet and the respiratory variation in inferior vena cava (*IVC*) size as an estimate of right atrial pressure (*RAP*).

- RV systolic function is graded qualitatively as normal, mildly, moderately, or severely reduced.

Key Points:

- ☐ The best views for evaluation of RV systolic function are an apical 4-chamber view tilted toward the RV and a subcostal 4-chamber view.

- ❑ RV systolic function can be graded in comparison to LV systolic function.
- ❑ If LV systolic function is reduced and the RV looks similar to the LV, the degree of dysfunction is similar.
- ❑ The subcostal view provides the most reliable estimate of RV systolic function because the ultrasound beam is perpendicular to the RV free wall and ventricular septum.

Step 4: Calculate pulmonary systolic pressure

- ■ Non-invasive calculation of pulmonary systolic pressures is possible in more than 80% of transthoracic echocardiograms.
- ■ The RV-to-RA systolic pressure gradient is calculated from the maximum velocity in the tricuspid regurgitant (TR) jet using the Bernoulli equation:

$$\Delta P_{RV-RA} = 4 \left(V_{TR\,peak} \right)^2$$

- ■ Right atrial pressure (RAP), estimated from the size and respiratory variation in the inferior vena cava, is added to this pressure gradient to determine right ventricular systolic pressure. (Table 6-4)

Key Points:

- ❑ In the absence of pulmonic valve stenosis, right ventricular and pulmonary systolic pressures are the same.
- ❑ When pulmonic stenosis is present, pulmonary systolic pressure is calculated by subtracting the RV-to-pulmonary artery gradient from the estimated RV systolic pressure.
- ❑ A diligent search for the highest tricuspid regurgitant jet velocity includes CW Doppler recording from parasternal and apical views. The highest signal obtained is the most parallel to jet direction.
- ❑ Signal strength may be enhanced by repositioning the patient or having the patient hold their breath at end expiration or in mid-inspiration.
- ❑ The Doppler scale, gain, and wall filters are adjusted to show a gray-scale spectrum with a dense outer edge and smooth systolic curve. (Figure 6–26)
- ❑ Estimation of RA pressure (RAP) from the respiratory variation in the inferior vena cava is only useful in spontaneously breathing patients. In ventilated patients, a measured central venous pressure is used or an estimated range of pulmonary pressures is provided. (Figure 6–27)

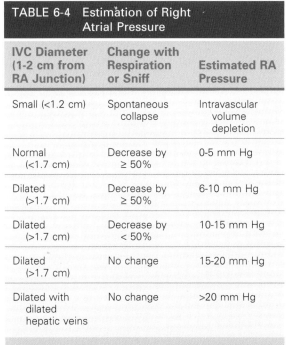

TABLE 6-4	Estimation of Right Atrial Pressure	
IVC Diameter (1-2 cm from RA Junction)	**Change with Respiration or Sniff**	**Estimated RA Pressure**
Small (<1.2 cm)	Spontaneous collapse	Intravascular volume depletion
Normal (<1.7 cm)	Decrease by ≥ 50%	0-5 mm Hg
Dilated (>1.7 cm)	Decrease by ≥ 50%	6-10 mm Hg
Dilated (>1.7 cm)	Decrease by < 50%	10-15 mm Hg
Dilated (>1.7 cm)	No change	15-20 mm Hg
Dilated with dilated hepatic veins	No change	>20 mm Hg

Adapted from Kircher BH, Himelmann RB, Schiller NG: Am J Caridol 1990;66:493; and Lang RM, Bierig M, Devereux RB, et al: J Am Soc Echocardiogr 2005;18:1440.

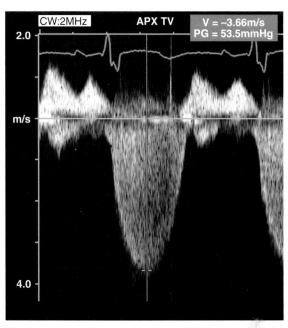

Figure 6–26. Tricuspid regurgitant jet recorded with CW Doppler showing a smooth velocity curve with a dark edge and a well-defined peak velocity. Although these characteristics are consistent with a high signal-to-noise ratio, they do not exclude to the possibility of underestimation of velocity due to a non-parallel intercept angle between the flow direction and Doppler beam.

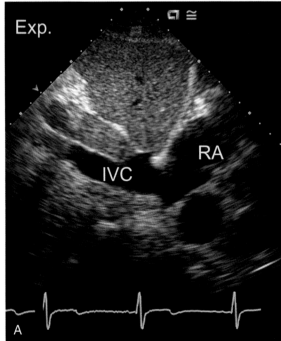

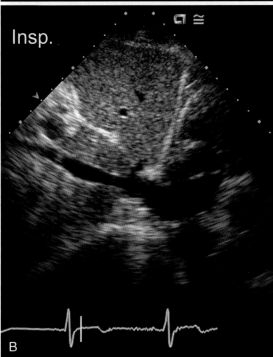

Figure 6–27. RA pressure is estimated from zoom views of the inferior vena cava from the subcostal window. The size of the inferior vena cava at the caval–RA junction during expiration (1.8 cm in this case) and the change in size during inspiration or with a sniff (>50% in this case) indicate a RA pressure of 5-10 mm Hg. (see Table 6–4)

Step 5: Consider the cause of an elevated pulmonary systolic pressure

- Pulmonary hypertension may be due to left-sided heart disease, resulting in an elevated LA pressure and consequent increase in pulmonary pressure.
- Pulmonary hypertension also may be due to a pulmonary arterial disease, lung disease, or pulmonary embolism, or may be due to multiple factors with a systemic disease. (Table 6-5)

Key Points:

- ❏ The definition of pulmonary arterial hypertension is mean pulmonary artery pressure more than 25 mm Hg at rest with a pulmonary capillary wedge pressure less than 15 mm Hg.
- ❏ In patients with left-sided heart disease, typically both LA and pulmonary pressures are elevated.
- ❏ If pulmonary systolic pressure is elevated and there is no obvious left-sided heart disease, careful evaluation of LV diastolic function is appropriate.
- ❏ An elevation in pulmonary pressure greater than expected for the degree of left heart disease suggests primary pulmonary vascular disease or lung disease.

TABLE 6-5	Classification of Pulmonary Hypertension	
Classification	**Examples**
Pulmonary arterial disease	Idiopathic
	Heritable
	Drug or toxin induced
	Portal hypertension
	Connective tissue disease
Left heart disease	Mitral stenosis
	Mitral regurgitation
	LV systolic dysfunction
	LV diastolic dysfunction
	Aortic valve disease
Lung disease or hypoxia	Chronic obstructive lung disease
	Sleep apnea
	Interstitial lung disease
Chronic pulmonary thromboembolism	Recurrent pulmonary emboli
Multifactorial	Systemic disorders (e.g., vasculitis)
	Myeloproliferative disorders
	Metabolic disorders

THE ECHO EXAM

Ventricular Systolic Function

	TTE	TEE
Indications	A standard echo exam includes measures of LV and RV size and global and regional systolic function	Non-diagnostic TTE Intraoperative and procedural TEE monitoring Whenever TEE is performed for other indications
LV size and wall thickness	2D or M-mode LV internal dimensions and wall thickness. LV volumes calculated from the apical biplane method.	Linear dimensions can be measured on TG short axis views. LV volumes can be calculated by the biplane method, but may be underestimated if the LV is foreshortened.
LV ejection fraction	Biplane method using 4C and 2C·views, taking care to image from tip of LV apex	Biplane method using TEE 4C and 2C views, taking care to include LV apex by angulation of the image plane
LV regional wall motion	Apical 4C, 2C, and long axis views plus parasternal long and short-axis views	TEE 4C, 2C and long-axis views plus TG short axis view Apical wall motion difficult to assess
Doppler cardiac output	LVOT and transmitral flows from apical approach PA flow from parasternal views	Transmitral flow in 4C view PA flow from high TEE view LVOT flow sometimes obtained from TG long axis view but intercept angle may be non-parallel
LV dP/dt	CW Doppler mitral regurgitant jet	CW Doppler mitral regurgitant jet
RV size and systolic function	Apical and subcostal 4C views plus parasternal long and short axis views	TEE 4C view plus transgastric short axis and RV inflow views
PA pressure estimates	TR jet may be recorded from parasternal and apical views with dedicated CW Doppler transducer.	TR jet may be recorded on TEE 4C or short-axis views, but underestimation may occur due to a non-parallel intercept angle.

2C, two-chamber; 2D, two-dimensional; 4C, four-chamber; CW, continuous wave; dP/dt, rate of change in pressure over time; LVOT, left ventricular outflow tract; PA, pulmonary artery; TEE, transesophageal echocardiography; TG, transgastric; TR, tricuspid regurgitation; TTE, transthoracic echocardiography.

Technical Details

Parameter	Modality	View	Recording	Measurements
Ejection fraction	2D	Apical 4-chamber and 2-chamber	Adjust depth, optimize endocardial definition, harmonic imaging, contrast if needed	Careful tracing of endocardial borders at end-diastole and end-systole in both views
dP/dt	CW Doppler	MR jet, usually from apex	Patient positioning and transducer angulation to obtain highest-velocity MR jet, decrease velocity scale, increase sweep speed	Time interval between 1 and 3 m/s on Doppler MR velocity curve
PA pressures	CW Doppler	Parasternal and apical	Patient positioning and transducer angulation to obtain highest-velocity TR jet	Estimate of RA pressure from size and appearance of IVC

Continued

Technical Details—cont'd

Parameter	Modality	View	Recording	Measurements
Cardiac output	2D and pulsed Doppler	Parasternal LVOT diameter	Ultrasound beam perpendicular to LVOT with depth decreased and gain adjusted to see mid-systolic diameter	LVOT diameter from inner edge to inner edge in mid-systole, adjacent and parallel to aortic valve
		Apical LVOT velocity-time integral	LVOT velocity from anterior angulated A4C view with sample volume just on LV side of aortic valve	Trace modal velocity of LVOT spectral Doppler envelope

2D, two-dimensional; A4C, apical four-chamber; CW, continuous wave; *dP/dt*, rate of change in pressure over time; IVC, inferior vena cava; LVOT, left ventricular outflow tract; MR, mitral regurgitation; PA, pulmonary artery; TR, tricuspid regurgitation.

EXAMPLE

A 68-year-old man with a recent inferior myocardial infarction now is hypotensive. Echocardiography shows:

LV wall thickness (diastole)	8 mm
LV end-diastolic dimension	50 mm
LV end-systolic dimension	33 mm
Apical biplane	
End-diastolic volume	106 mL
End-systolic volume	62 mL
Time interval between 1 and 3 m/s on MR jet	34 msec
LV segmental wall motion	Akinesis of basal and mid–left ventricular segments of inferior and inferior-lateral walls
RV size	Moderately increased
RV systolic function	Severely decreased
TR-jet velocity (V_{TR})	2.7 m/s
IVC	
Diameter	2.0 cm
Inspiratory change	< 50%
LV outflow tract diameter ($LVOT_D$)	2.3 cm
LVOT velocity-time integral (VTI_{LVOT})	11 cm
Heart rate (HR)	88 bpm

INTERPRETATION

The left ventricle is normal to small in size, based on diastolic dimensions and volumes, with a mildly reduced ejection fraction and regional wall motion abnormalities consistent with a recent inferior myocardial infarction. Ejection fraction is calculated from the apical biplane volumes as:

$$EF = (EDV - ESV)/EDV \times 100\%$$
$$= (106\,mL - 62\,mL)/106\,mL \times 100\% = 42\%$$

Qualitative evaluation of ejection fraction is used only when image quality is too poor for tracing endocardial borders. *Left ventricular dP/dt* is calculated from the time interval between 1 and 3 m/s on the MR jet signal (dt) as:

$$dP/dt = \left[4(V_2)^2 - 4(V_1)^2\right]/dt = \left[4(3)^2 - 4(1)^2\right]/dt$$
$$= [36 - 4\,mm\,Hg]/.034\,s = 941\,mm\,Hg/s$$

which is mildly reduced (normal > 1000 mm Hg/s).

RV size and systolic function are graded qualitatively. The findings of a moderately dilated RV with severe systolic dysfunction in this patient are consistent with right ventricular infarction accompanying the inferior LV infarction, because the coronary artery that supplies the LV inferior wall also often supplies the RV free wall.

Right atrial pressure is moderately elevated (estimate 10-15 mm Hg) as shown by the < 50% respiratory change in the diameter of a dilated inferior vena cava (see Table 6–4).

Pulmonary systolic pressure (PAP) is calculated from the tricuspid regurgitant jet velocity (V_{TR}) and estimate of right atrial pressure (RAP) as:

$$PAP = 4(V_{TR})^2 + RAP = 4(2.7)^2 + 10$$
$$= 29 + 10 = 39\,mm\,Hg$$

This is consistent with mild pulmonary hypertension.

Cardiac output (CO) is calculated using the LVOT diameter to calculate the circular cross-sectional area of flow:

$$CSA_{LVOT} = \pi(LVOT_D/2)^2 = 3.14(2.3/2)^2 = 4.2\,cm^2$$

Stroke volume across the aortic valve (cm^3 = mL), then, is:

$$SV_{LVOT} = (CSA_{LVOT} \times VTI_{LVOT})$$
$$= 4.2\,cm^2 \times 11\,cm = 46\,cm^3$$

Cardiac output is:

$$CO = SV \times HR$$
$$= 46\,mL \times 88\,beats/min$$
$$= 4020\,mL/min\ or\ 4.02\,L/min$$

Cardiac index (CI) is:

$$CI = CO/BSA = 4.02\,L/min/1.8\,m^2 = 2.23\,L/min/m^2$$

The low cardiac index (normal > 2.5 $L/min/m^2$) is due to the right ventricular infarction resulting in reduced LV preload in combination with mild LV systolic function.

As an internal check of the consistency of the echocardiographic data, stroke volume and cardiac output can also be calculated from the 2D apical biplane volume data:

$$SV = EDV - ESV = 106\,mL - 62\,mL = 44\,mL$$

$$CO = SV \times HR = 44\,mL \times 88\,beats/min$$
$$= 3872\,mL/min\ or\ 3.87\,L/min$$

The differences between stroke volumes and cardiac outputs calculated by the two methods (Doppler and 2D) is consistent with normal measurement error. If significant mitral regurgitation were present, transaortic Doppler stroke volume would be less than the 2D apical biplane stroke volume (see Chapter 12).

SELF-ASSESSMENT QUESTIONS

QUESTION 1

Echocardiography is performed in a 27-year-old woman with chronic dyspnea. There was no significant respiratory change in inferior vena cava diameter. There are no other significant valvular abnormalities. (Figure 6–28)

Based on this data, what is the estimated pulmonary systolic pressure?

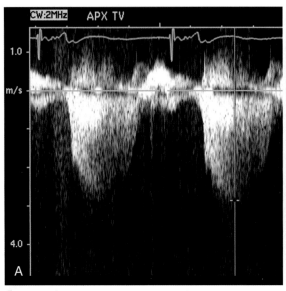

Figure 6–28.

A.   25 mm Hg
B.   50 mm Hg
C.   75 mm Hg
D.   100 mm Hg

QUESTION 2

A transthoracic study is obtained in a patient with a history of non-Hodgkin's lymphoma who presents with decreased exercise tolerance (Figure 6–29). The image is *most* consistent with:

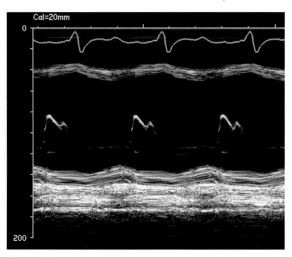

Figure 6–29.

A.   Pericardial effusion
B.   Dilated cardiomyopathy
C.   Pericardial constriction
D.   Pulmonary hypertension
E.   Restrictive cardiomyopathy

QUESTION 3

Which of the following is the *least* useful measure of LV systolic function:

A.   Strain rate
B.   Fractional shortening
C.   B-bump
D.   Mitral dP/dt
E.   Ejection fraction

QUESTION 4

Echocardiography is ordered in a patient with a familial cardiomyopathy. Results from the current and prior studies are shown here:

	Current	Prior
LV end-diastolic dimension (EDD)	7.4 cm	7.2 cm
LV end-systolic dimension (ESD)	5.1 cm	5.0 cm
LV EDV	200 mL	310 mL
LV ESV	110 mL	200 mL
Ejection fraction	45%	35%

Based on these results, you conclude that:

A. LV systolic function has improved
B. Fractional shortening has increased
C. LV size has increased
D. Additional imaging is needed

QUESTION 5

Calculate the LV stroke volume (SV), cardiac output (CO), fractional shortening (FS), and ejection fraction (EF) of the following patient:

Heart rate	70 bpm
Blood pressure	132/50 mm Hg
LV EDD	5.0 cm
LV diastolic area 4-chamber	36 cm²
LV diastolic area 2-chamber	36 cm²
LV EDV	125 mL
LV ESD	3.7 cm
LV systolic area 4-chamber	20 cm²
LV systolic area 2-chamber	22 cm²
LV ESV	53 mL
LVOT diameter	2.3 cm
LVOT velocity-time integral	18 cm

QUESTION 6

A 48-year-old man with a murmur is referred for echocardiography, and the following Doppler signal is recorded (Figure 6–30). The time interval between the two marked points is 50 ms. Based on this data:

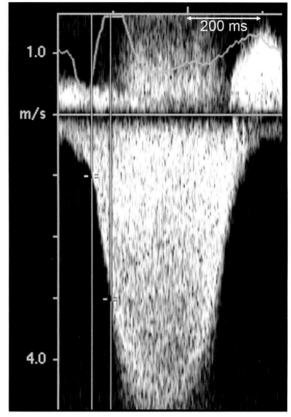

Figure 6–30.

A. Mitral valve area is 4.4 cm²
B. LA pressure is 20 mm Hg
C. LV dP/dt is 640 mm Hg/sec
D. Isovolumic relaxation time is 50 ms
E. Aortic stenosis maximum gradient is 100 mm Hg

QUESTION 7

A transthoracic study is obtained in a patient with complaints of dyspnea. The tracing seen below was obtained from the apical 4-chamber view.

Based on the image (Figure 6–31), you conclude there is:

A. Normal RV systolic function
B. Pericardial tamponade
C. Primary pulmonary hypertension
D. Decreased LV systolic function
E. Paced rhythm

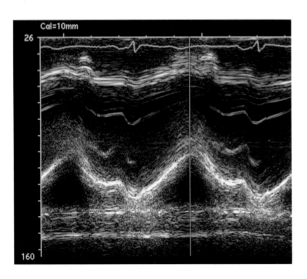

QUESTION 8

Which of the following *least* affects septal myocardial motion?

    A. Pericardial constriction
    B. Left bundle branch block
    C. Coronary artery bypass surgery
    D. Pacing for sinoatrial exit block
    E. Primary pulmonary hypertension

QUESTION 9

A 30-year-old man with a dilated cardiomyopathy presents with decompensated heart failure and volume overload. He is referred for echocardiography. Which of the following echocardiographic findings is *most* likely present?

    A. Pulmonic regurgitant end-diastolic velocity 1.2 m/s
    B. Mitral regurgitant vena contracta 6 mm
    C. LV *dP/dt* 1218 mm Hg/sec
    D. LV end-diastolic volume 70 mL/m^2

QUESTION 10

Which of the following clinical findings is *least* likely to be associated with an increased tricuspid regurgitant jet velocity?

    A. Severe mitral stenosis
    B. Primary pulmonary hypertension
    C. Severe tricuspid regurgitation
    D. Pulmonic stenosis

ANSWERS

ANSWER 1: B

The tricuspid regurgitant jet velocity is 3.0 m/s, corresponds to a 36 mm Hg systolic pressure difference between the RV and RA. The inferior vena cava is severely dilated and shows no respiratory variation consistent with severely elevated RA pressures of at least 20 mm Hg. Thus, the best estimate of RV systolic pressure, which equals pulmonary systolic pressure in the absence of pulmonic stenosis, is 56 mm Hg.

ANSWER 2: B

This is an M-mode tracing recorded from the parasternal long axis view of the heart. The ventricular chamber size is severely dilated with the marks on the vertical axis each representing 2 cm. The tracing is taken just apical to the mitral valve leaflet tips (seen along the mid-portion of the image), opening in diastole and closing in systole. The end-diastolic dimension is about 9 cm and the end-systolic dimension is about 7 cm. There is a large separation between the anterior mitral valve leaflet and the anterior septum consistent with severe LV enlargement and systolic dysfunction. In the far field, beyond the posterior wall, a pericardial effusion is not seen. Septal and posterior wall thickening and endocardial motion are severely reduced, consistent with dilated cardiomyopathy, but are synchronous throughout the cardiac cycle. The echolucent space anterior to the LV is the RV. With pericardial constriction, findings include parallel dense echoes in the posterior pericardial region and abnormal septal motion with rapid posterior motion in early diastole followed by a flat septum in mid- to late diastole, reflecting the pattern of rapid early diastolic LV filling with pericardial constriction. This image is not consistent with either myocardial restriction or pericardial constriction. With restrictive cardiomyopathy, wall thickness typically is increased with a small chamber size. Pulmonary hypertension is unlikely given the normal RV size and wall thickness.

ANSWER 3: C

The B-bump is the M-mode finding of delayed mitral valve closure seen as a change in slope of the closure line between atrial contraction and full mitral closure. The presence of a B-bump is specific (but not sensitive) for increased LV diastolic pressure and is not a measure of LV systolic function. Strain rate is the rate of change in myocardial length along a particular segment, normalized for the original length. Strain rate is calculated from the difference in velocities at two myocardial sites divided by the distance between them. Velocities at myocardial sites with poor systolic function would be lower than at sites with normal

systolic function. The fractional shortening is measured from the parasternal long axis LV dimensions and is the relative change in diameter between the end-systolic (LV ESD) and end-diastolic (LV EDD) left ventricular dimensions, measured as $100 \times$ (LV EDD − LV ESD)/LV EDD. The initial slope of the mitral regurgitant jet *(dP/dt)* measures the relative change in transmitral pressure over time. In patients with LV systolic dysfunction, the LV does not generate a transmitral gradient as rapidly as a normally functioning LV, and the slope of the mitral regurgitation (MR) jet decreases. A slope of less than 1000 mm Hg/sec is consistent with systolic dysfunction. Ejection fraction is the most commonly used measure of LV systolic function, although not ideal as it is affected by loading conditions.

ANSWER 4: D

The data provided are incongruent. The LV chamber linear minor axis dimensions are comparable between the current and the prior studies, with a similar fractional shortening, measured as:

$$100 \times (\text{LV EDD} - \text{LV ESD})/\text{LV EDD}$$

The minimal interval change in LV minor axis chamber dimensions seen in this patient likely reflects measurement variability. These measurements are typically made in a parasternal long axis view from 2D guided M-mode or 2D images and some difference between studies is expected due to physiologic variability or to slight variation in aligning the measurement perpendicular to the LV long axis. However, there is a large discrepancy between studies in measured LV volume and ejection fraction. The smaller diastolic and systolic LV volumes, despite no change in LV chamber size, suggests systematic measurement error. This is commonly encountered with apical views that foreshorten the LV, which excludes the apex from volume measurements, decreases measured LV volumes, and often erroneously raises ejection fraction calculations. When reviewing echocardiography studies, it is critical to review images from the previous study in a side-by-side comparison with the current study, to ensure comparable image planes, rather than relying only on the calculated volumes and ejection fraction. In this case, additional imaging is needed, either to eliminate foreshortening of the apex or, if image quality remains inadequate, with use of transpulmonary microbubble contrast to optimize endocardial border definition for more accurate LV tracing.

ANSWER 5:

The stroke volume is the volume of blood ejected from the LV during systole on a single beat. Stroke volume is calculated as the product of the velocity-time integral and the cross-sectional area at the point of interrogation. For calculation of stroke volume in the LVOT, the cross-sectional area of flow is calculated as $\pi(\text{Diameter}_{LVOT}/2)^2$, which is then multiplied by the LV outflow tract VTI_{LVOT}. Thus:

$$\text{Stroke volume} = 3.14(1.15 \text{ cm})^2 \times 18 \text{ cm}$$
$$= 75 \text{ cm}^3 = 75 \text{ mL}$$

Stroke volume can also be calculated as the difference between LV end-diastolic and end-systolic volumes, similar to the Doppler method calculation:

$$\text{Stroke volume} = \text{EDV} - \text{ESV} = 125 \text{ mL} - 53 \text{ mL} = 72 \text{ mL}$$

Cardiac output is the volume of blood pumped by the LV during 1 minute and so is calculated by multiplying stroke volume times heart rate:

$$\text{Cardiac output} = \text{SV} \times \text{heart rate}$$
$$= 72 \text{ mL} \times 70 \text{ bpm}/(1000 \text{ mL/L})$$
$$= 5.1 \text{ L/min}$$

Fractional shortening is the percent change in LV minor axis dimensions between systole and diastole, or:

$$\text{Fractional shortening} = (\text{LV EDD} - \text{LV ESD})/$$
$$\text{LV EDD} \times 100\%$$
$$= (5.0 \text{ cm} - 3.7 \text{ cm})/5.0 \text{ cm}$$
$$\times 100\% = 0.26 \text{ or } 26\%$$

which is in the low normal range.

Ejection fraction is more commonly reported than the fractional shortening and is more clinically robust because it considers the entire LV, not a single minor axis dimension. EF is calculated as the percent change in LV volume between systole and diastole:

$$\text{EF} = (\text{EDV} - \text{ESV})/\text{EDV} \times 100\%$$
$$= (125 \text{ mL} - 53 \text{ mL})/125 \text{ mL} \times 1005 = 58\%$$

ANSWER 6: C

This is a Doppler tracing of mitral regurgitation; diagnostic features include a systolic velocity of more than 4 m/s, consistent with the high LV-to-LA pressure gradient and the Doppler signal timing relative to the QRS on the ECG tracing. The markers are placed at 1 and 3 m/s, corresponding to a LV-to-LA pressure difference of 36 mm Hg − 4 mm Hg, or a 32 mm Hg change in pressure over a 50 ms time interval. The rate of rise of LV pressure *(dP)* over time *(dt)* is:

$$dP/dt = 32 \text{ mm Hg}/0.05 \text{ sec} = 640 \text{ mm Hg/sec}$$

A normal rate of pressure rise is more than 1000 mm Hg/sec. This case is consistent with LV systolic dysfunction, most likely with functional mitral regurgitation. Mitral regurgitation is at least moderate based on the density of the CW Doppler signal relative to the density of antegrade flow. In patients with mitral stenosis, mitral valve area is measured

from the diastolic transmitral Doppler signal (not the systolic regurgitant signal) based on the time interval between the peak transmitral pressure and half the peak transmitral pressure (the pressure half-time [PHT]). Mitral valve area is calculated as 220/PHT. In patients with aortic stenosis, transaortic gradient is calculated from the maximum transaortic velocity using the Bernoulli equation ($4V_{AV}^2$). The peak velocity of the mitral regurgitant jet reflects the instantaneous pressure difference between the LV and LA, not the absolute LA pressure. The isovolumic relaxation time is the time interval between aortic valve closure and mitral valve opening and serves as a measure of LV diastolic relaxation. Isovolumic relaxation time is measured from a pulsed Doppler tracing taken from the apical 5-chamber view positioned midway between the aortic and mitral valves.

ANSWER 7: A

This is an M-mode tracing taken from the apical 4-chamber view with the ultrasound beam directed through the tricuspid valve annulus (Figure 6–31, *B*). The M-mode beam first traverses the apex of the LV chamber, the ventricular septum (the proximal band of echoes), and the RV chamber before the rapidly moving tricuspid annulus. The tricuspid annular plane systolic excursion (TAPSE) toward the apex is a measure of RV systolic function with apical systolic displacement over 3 cm, as seen in this case, consistent with normal RV systolic function.

With the M-mode ultrasound beam positioned at the tricuspid valve annulus, the pericardial space and LV are not optimally seen. Pericardial tamponade and LV systolic dysfunction cannot be excluded from this view. In primary pulmonary hypertension, RV systolic pressure is increased, often with decreased RV systolic function, and a concordant decrease in the TAPSE. Based on the ECG tracings, this patient does not have a paced rhythm. Additionally, there is no pacer lead seen in the RV on the M-mode tracing.

ANSWER 8: D

With sinoatrial exit block, the sinus node generates an electrical impulse, but conduction of the impulse to the atrium is impaired. If atrioventricular node conduction is preserved, therapy for sinoatrial exit block is an atrial pacer. If no atrial electrical activity is detected, the pacer delivers a paced beat to the right atrium, which then conducts normally through the atrioventricular node and bundle of His. Myocardial activation and septal motion are therefore normal. In pericardial constriction, there is rapid early diastolic filling followed by limited septal motion in late diastole. In addition, with constriction, the fixed space for cardiac motion often results in respiratory-dependent shifting of septal motion from right to left

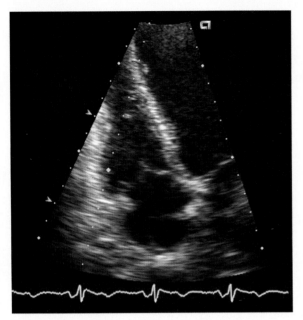

Figure 6–31.

with transient increases in preload, as occurs with inspiration. Ventricular conduction abnormalities (left bundle branch block, right bundle branch block, or ventricular pacing) alter the sequence of ventricular contraction. Initial activation with a RV apical lead will lead to dyssynchronous contraction of the RV free wall relative to the septum and LV and to abnormal septal motion. Cardiac surgery typically results in abnormal septal motion anteriorly during systole, although septal thickening is normal, possibly due to a fixed anterior cardiac surface after thoracotomy. Pressure overload of the right ventricle, as occurs with severe pulmonary hypertension, results in septal flattening with a leftward septal shift throughout the cardiac cycle.

ANSWER 9: B

Functional mitral regurgitation is common in dilated cardiomyopathy. LV dilation leads to apical tethering of the mitral valve leaflets and poor leaflet coaptation. With progressive volume overload and worsening LV dilation, mitral regurgitation often worsens. The vena contracta is the narrowest diameter of a regurgitant jet. A mitral valve vena contracta of 0.6 cm is consistent with at least moderate mitral regurgitation. Pulmonic regurgitant end-diastolic velocity provides an estimate of RV diastolic pressure, based on the pulmonary artery-to-RV diastolic pressure difference of $4(V_{PV\,peak})^2$ added to the RA pressure estimate, inferred from inferior vena cava size and respiratory variation. A pulmonic end-diastolic velocity of 1.2 m/s suggests a pulmonary artery-to-RV diastolic pressure difference of only 6 mm Hg, with an RV diastolic pressure of only 11 mm Hg, assuming a normal RA pressure, which is not consistent with decompensated heart failure. In patients with LV systolic function, the slow rate of rise in LV systolic pressure is reflected in a slow rate of rise in the mitral regurgitant jet velocity, allowing calculation of LV dP/dt, with a dP/dt less than 1000 mm Hg/sec indicating LV systolic dysfunction; a slope of more than 1200 mm Hg/sec is consistent with normal LV systolic dysfunction. A LV end-diastolic indexed volume of 70 mL/m² is normal; for both women and men, a value of about 75 mL/m² is consistent with only mild LV dilation and a volume more than 100 mL/m² is consistent with severe LV dilation. A normal LV volume, as was seen in this case, is unlikely with decompensated dilated cardiomyopathy.

ANSWER 10: C

The peak tricuspid regurgitant jet velocity reflects the peak systolic RV-to-RA gradient. This gradient is calculated as $4(V_{TR})^2$ based on the Bernoulli principle. The severity of tricuspid regurgitation, per se, does not affect the RV-to-RA pressure gradient. For example, severe tricuspid regurgitation may be present with a normal right heart and pulmonary pressures, resulting in low-velocity back and forth flow across the unrestricted orifice. Conversely, a high-velocity tricuspid regurgitant jet is present when RV systolic pressure is elevated, even if the volume of regurgitation is small. Thus, clinical conditions that increase RV systolic pressure, such as pulmonary hypertension or pulmonic valve stenosis, result in a high-velocity tricuspid regurgitant jet. Severe mitral stenosis is associated with elevated LA pressure and pulmonary hypertension, which is reflected in an increased TR jet velocity.

7 Ventricular Diastolic Filling and Function

STEP-BY-STEP APPROACH
  Measure Left Ventricular Inflow Velocities
  Record Left Atrial Inflow
  Record Tissue Doppler at the Mitral Annulus
  Measure the Isovolumic Relaxation Time
  Consider Other Useful Measurements
  Integrating the Data
    Normal Diastolic Function
    Factors That Affect Left Ventricular Diastolic
    Filling Independent of Diastolic Function

Mild Diastolic Dysfunction (Impaired Relaxation)
Moderate Diastolic Dysfunction
  (Pseudo-Normalization)
Severe Diastolic Dysfunction (Decreased
  Compliance)
Left Atrial Pressure Estimates
THE ECHO EXAM
SELF-ASSESSMENT QUESTIONS

Basic principles

- Diastolic dysfunction often occurs in association with abnormal imaging findings, for example LV hypertrophy or impaired systolic function.
- Diastolic dysfunction may be the earliest sign of cardiac disease with Doppler findings antedating clinical or imaging signs of ventricular dysfunction.
- Chronic elevation of LV diastolic pressure often leads to LA enlargement which is a key element in evaluation of LV diastolic dysfunction.

STEP-BY-STEP APPROACH

Step 1: Measure left ventricular inflow velocities

- LV inflow velocities are recorded at the mitral leaflet tips and at the mitral annulus. (Figure 7–1)
- Standard measurements are E velocity and deceleration time and A velocity and duration. (Figure 7–2)
- The normal pattern of a higher E than A velocity is reversed with impaired early diastolic relaxation, but the pattern may be "pseudo-normalized" with more severe diastolic dysfunction.

Key points:

- ❏ LV inflow velocities are recorded at the mitral leaflet tips (highest velocity signal) in the apical

4-chamber view using pulsed Doppler with a sample volume of 2 to 2.5 mm in length.
- ❏ The Doppler scale, baseline and gain, are adjusted to show a clear velocity curve.
- ❏ Low wall filter settings allow accurate measurements that require identification of where the velocity signal intersects the baseline. (Figure 7–3)
- ❏ Recordings at the leaflet tips are used to measure E and A velocity and deceleration slope. Recordings at the annulus are used to measure A duration.
- ❏ Recording LV inflow at the mitral leaflet tips with the patient performing a Valsalva maneuver results in a decrease in preload. The decrease in preload may unmask impaired relaxation in patients with superimposed elevated filling pressures.

Step 2: Record left atrial inflow

- LA inflow velocities are recorded in the right superior pulmonary vein from an apical 4-chamber view on transthoracic echocardiography (TTE) or in any pulmonary vein on transesophageal echocardiography (TEE). (Figure 7–4)
- Standard measurements are peak systolic velocity, peak diastolic velocity, and the atrial velocity peak and duration (a_{dur}). (Figure 7–5)
- A PV_a greater than 0.35 m/s and an a_{dur} 20 ms longer than transmitral A duration indicate an elevated LV end-diastolic pressure.

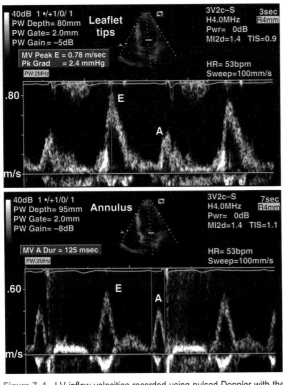

Figure 7–1. LV inflow velocities recorded using pulsed Doppler with the sample volume at the mitral leaflet tips (*top*) and at the mitral annulus (*bottom*).

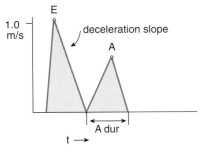

Figure 7–2. Schematic diagram showing basic measurements from the LV inflow curve; the early (*E*) diastolic peak velocity, the velocity after atrial (*A*) contraction, the early diastolic deceleration slope, and the duration of the A velocity (from the recording at the annulus).

Key points:

❐ LA inflow velocities from the transthoracic approach may be difficult to record due to poor signal strength at the depth of the pulmonary vein.

❐ Color flow imaging may be helpful in locating the pulmonary vein and optimizing sample volume position. The 2- to 3-mm length sample volume should be at least 1 cm into the pulmonary vein. (Figure 7–6)

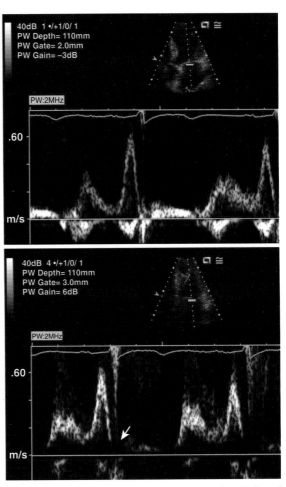

Figure 7–3. Example of LV inflow recorded at the annulus with the wall filters set at a low level (indicated by the *1*) to allow accurate timing measurements (*top*). When the wall filter is inappropriately high (level is set at 4), the intersection of the Doppler signal with the baseline is no longer seen, making accurate measurement difficult (*bottom*).

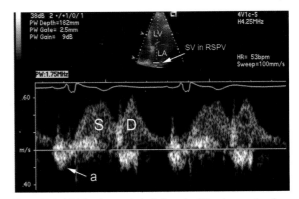

Figure 7–4. LA inflow is recorded with the pulsed Doppler sample volume positioned in the right superior pulmonary vein (RSPV) from an apical 4-chamber approach. With atrial contraction, there is a small atrial reversal velocity (*a*), with a normal pattern of systolic (*S*) and diastolic (*D*) inflow into the atrium.

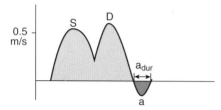

Figure 7–5. Schematic of measurements for pulmonary vein flow showing atrial (*a*) reversal peak and duration and peak systolic (*S*) and diastolic (*D*) filling velocities.

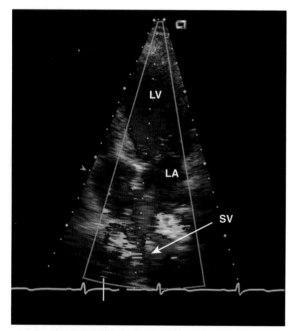

Figure 7–6. Identification of the right superior pulmonary vein from the transthoracic apical 4-chamber view may be enhanced with color Doppler imaging. The pulsed Doppler sample volume (*arrow*) is positioned about 1 cm into the pulmonary vein for optimal data quality.

☐ The Doppler scale, baseline, and gain are adjusted to show a clear spectral signal.
☐ Low wall filter settings allow accurate measurements that require identification of where the velocity signal intersects the baseline.

Step 3: Record tissue Doppler at the mitral annulus

■ Tissue Doppler myocardial velocities are recorded at the mitral annulus from a TTE apical approach. (Figure 7–7)
■ Standard measurements are the early myocardial velocity (E′) and atrial myocardial velocity (A′). (Figure 7–8)
■ An E′/A′ ratio more than 1.0 is normal, with a reduced ratio indicating impaired early diastolic relaxation.

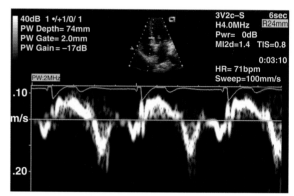

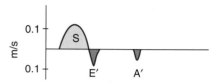

Figure 7–7. Doppler myocardial tissue velocities are recorded at the septal side of the mitral annulus using a small sample volume, with the velocity scale reduced (note that the velocity range is only 0.2 m/s), the wall filters at a low level (setting = 1) , and the gain reduced to a very low level (setting = –17 dB).

Figure 7–8. Schematic diagram of tissue Doppler measurements. The typical early (*E*) and late (*A*) tissue Doppler velocities are seen in diastole directed away from the transducer (as the ventricle fills). In systole, there is a velocity component toward the transducer corresponding to systolic contraction of the ventricle.

■ A ratio of the transmitral E velocity to the tissue Doppler E′ velocity greater than 15 predicts an LV end-diastolic pressure more than 15 mm Hg.

Key points:

☐ In the apical 4-chamber view, a small (2 mm) sample volume is positioned in the myocardium about 1 cm from the mitral annulus. (Figure 7–9)
☐ The tissue Doppler instrument settings include a velocity scale of about 0.2 m/s, low gain settings, low velocity scale, and low wall filters.
☐ Tissue Doppler recordings at the septal side of the annulus are more reproducible than signals from the lateral wall. (Figure 7–10)
☐ The E′ and A′ velocities are less dependent on preload than the transmitral flow velocities.

Step 4: Measure the isovolumic relaxation time

■ Pulsed Doppler is used to show the time interval between aortic valve closure and mitral valve opening (the isovolumic relaxation time). (Figure 7 11)

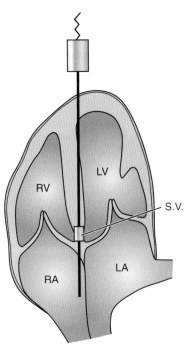

Figure 7–9. Schematic diagram showing position of sample volume for Doppler tissue velocity recording. In the apical 4-chamber view, the sample volume is placed about 1 cm apical to the medial mitral annulus.

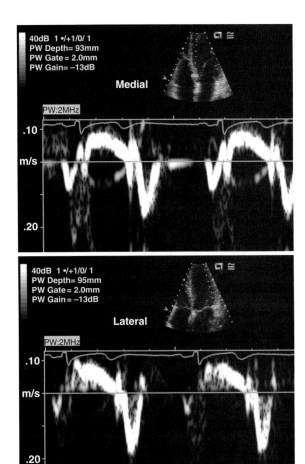

Figure 7–10. Although tissue Doppler velocities can be recorded both from the medial side of the annulus (*top*) and the lateral side (*bottom*), the medial annular signal tends to be more reliable for evaluation of diastolic dysfunction.

■ The IVRT (normal 50-100 ms) is prolonged with impaired relaxation but is shortened with severe diastolic dysfunction and impaired compliance. (Figure 7–12)

Key points:

❐ In an anteriorly angulated 4-chamber view, a 2- to 3-mm sample volume is positioned midway between aortic and mitral valves to show both LV ejection and LV filling velocity curves. (Figure 7–13)

❐ The wall filters are set at a low level to identify the end of aortic outflow and onset of mitral inflow at their intersection with the baseline.

❐ The time interval is measures in milliseconds (ms).

Step 5: Consider other useful measurements

■ The diastolic slope of the apical color M-mode recording of LV inflow (the propagation velocity) reflects the rate of LV diastolic relaxation. (Figure 7–14)

■ The rate of decline in velocity of the mitral regurgitant jet at end-systole reflects the early diastolic rate of decline in LV pressure. (Figure 7–15)

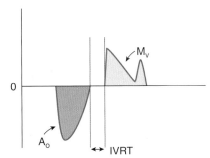

Figure 7–11. The isovolumic relaxation time (IVRT) is measured from aortic valve closure to mitral valve opening on the Doppler tracing, corresponding to the phase of the cardiac cycle where LV pressure is rapidly declining, but LV volume is constant.

Key points:

❐ These additional measures may be helpful in selected cases:

• Propagation velocity is measured from an apical view using a narrow sector, a depth that just

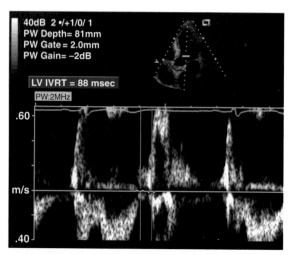

Figure 7–12. Measurement of IVRT as the time interval between the end of aortic antegrade flow and the onset of diastolic inflow across the mitral valve. The scale and wall filters have been adjusted to optimize identification of the onset and end of flow, at their intersection with the baseline. A rapid sweep speed (100 mm/s) is used to improve the accuracy of the measurement. In this patient, the IVRT is normal at 88 ms (normal 50-100 ms).

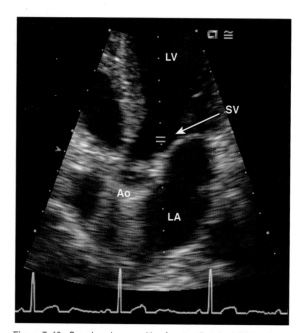

Figure 7–13. Sample volume position for recording the IVRT is shown. In an apical 4-chamber view angulated anteriorly to include the aortic valve, the sample volume is positioned so that it is on the LV side of the anterior mitral leaflet in systole (to record LV outflow) and on the atrial side in diastole (to record LV inflow).

includes the mitral annulus, with the aliasing velocity set to 0.5 to 0.7 m/s, at a fast (100-200 mm/s) sweep speed.

- The early diastolic −dP/dt is measured from the mitral regurgitant CW Doppler curve by measuring the time interval between 3 and 1 m/s and dividing by 32 mm Hg (analogous to

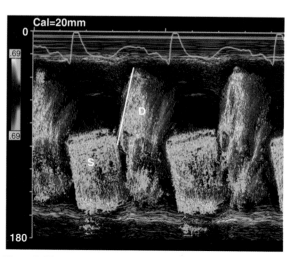

Figure 7–14. Color M-mode propagation velocity. LV inflow is recorded from an apical view using a color Doppler M-mode beam aligned along the center of the mitral annulus. Thus, the vertical axis is distance from the LA (at about 160 mm depth on the scale) to the apex (at the top of the scale) with the horizontal axis indicating time, using an electrocardiogram (ECG) for timing of the cardiac cycle. Flow toward the transducer in diastole represents LV filling with the slope of the edge of this signal (*line*) reflecting the velocity of the movement of blood from the annulus to the apex.

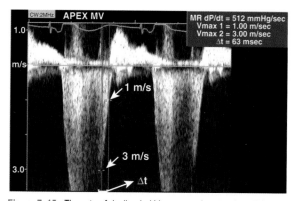

Figure 7–15. The rate of decline in LV pressure (or negative *dP/dt*) can be measured from the mitral regurgitant jet velocity as velocity decelerates, analogous to measurement of positive *dP/dt* from the rate of acceleration in velocity. The pressure difference between 1 and 3 m/s (32 mm Hg) is divided by the time interval (in seconds) measured between these points on the velocity curve at 1 and 3 m/s to give the −*dP/dt* in mm Hg/s.

measurement of +*dP/dt* from the early systolic part of the mitral regurgitant velocity curve).

Step 6: Integrating the data

- Measurement of LA size (diameter and/or indexed volume) is useful in the assessment of diastolic function. Chronically elevated LV filling pressure leads to increased LA chamber size.
- Based on integration of data from LA size, LV filling velocities, LA filling velocities, tissue Doppler, and IVRT, diastolic dysfunction can be detected and graded. (Figure 7–16)

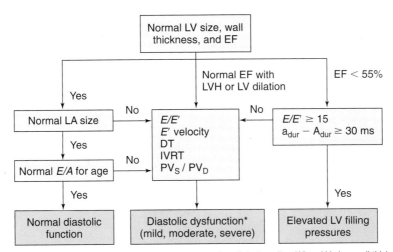

Figure 7–16. Suggested algorithm for evaluation of diastolic dysfunction on routine clinical studies. When LV size, wall thickness, and ejection fraction are normal, further evaluation of diastolic function is needed only if there is left atrial enlargement or an abnormal E/A ratio for age. In patients with ventricular hypertrophy or dilation with a normal ejection fraction, diastolic function should be fully evaluated, particularly if there is a clinical concern that diastolic dysfunction may account for symptoms. When ejection fraction is reduced, the first step is to evaluate for elevated filling pressures. If simple criteria for elevated filling pressures are not present, a more complete evaluation of diastolic function is appropriate.

■ The clinical interpretation of the data also takes several other factors into consideration, including severity of mitral regurgitation, LV systolic function, LV wall thickness, and clinical signs and symptoms.

Normal diastolic function (Figure 7–17)

❐ Normal LA size.
❐ Transmitral flow shows an E/A velocity ratio between 1 and 2.
❐ The E deceleration time is 150 to 200 ms
❐ The tissue Doppler E′/A′ ratio is 1 to 2.
❐ The pulmonary vein systolic to diastolic flow ratio is 1 or more.
❐ The pulmonary vein a-velocity is less than 0.35 m/s and duration is less than 20 ms longer than transmitral A duration.

Factors that affect left ventricular diastolic filling independent of diastolic function

❐ At a higher heart rate (shorter diastolic filling time), the A velocity may be increased as it is superimposed on the E deceleration slope. (Figure 7–18)
❐ The transmitral E/A ratio decreases with age, reversing at about age 50 years. Similarly, the pulmonary vein diastolic flow declines, so that the systolic to diastolic ratio increases with age.
❐ A higher preload increases the transmitral E velocity; hypovolemia results in a lower velocity—with Valsalva maneuver, E velocity falls transiently due to reduced venous return. (Figure 7–19)

❐ Increased transmitral volume flow due to mitral regurgitation increases the transmitral E velocity.
❐ Atrial contractile function affects LV filling, LA filling, and tissue Doppler signals. (Figure 7–20)

Mild diastolic dysfunction (impaired relaxation) (Figure 7–21)

❐ Increased LA diameter and volume.
❐ Impaired relaxation is typical of mild diastolic dysfunction, due, for example, to hypertensive heart disease, ischemic disease, or an early infiltrative cardiomyopathy.
❐ The decreased rate of early diastolic filling is associated with a reduced E velocity (reduced E/A ratio), a reduced E′/A′ ratio on tissue Doppler, reduced pulmonary vein diastolic flow, and a prolonged IVRT.
❐ LV filling pressure may be normal with mild diastolic dysfunction, so pulmonary vein atrial velocity and duration are normal.

Moderate diastolic dysfunction (pseudo-normalization) (Figure 7–22)

❐ LV relaxation is impaired and LV filling pressures are elevated with moderate diastolic dysfunction—for example, due to dilated, hypertrophic, or restrictive cardiomyopathy.
❐ In addition to the findings seen with mild diastolic dysfunction, there is evidence for elevated filling pressures, including a higher peak (>0.35 m/s) and duration of the pulmonary

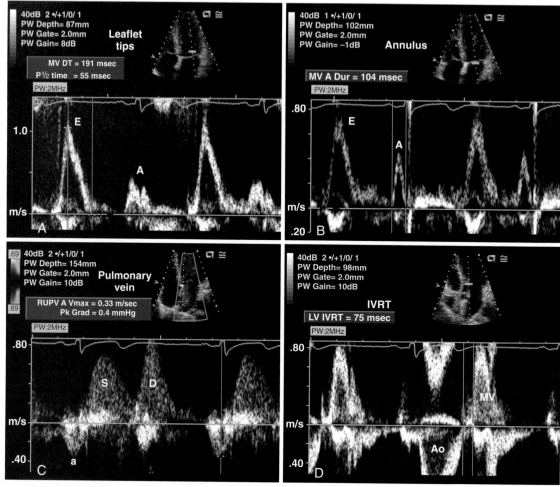

Figure 7–17. An example of normal diastolic function. *A,* The LV inflow curve at the mitral leaflet tips shows a normal E and A velocity with a deceleration time of 191 msec. *B,* Inflow recorded at the annulus shows the duration of the atrial flow curve (104 msec) is the same as the duration of atrial reversal in the pulmonary vein recording (*C*). The pulmonary vein flow also shows normal systolic and diastolic inflow signals. *D,* The IVRT is normal at 75 msec.

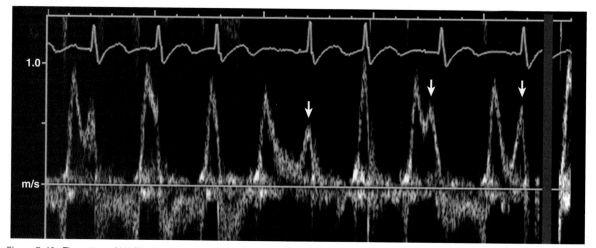

Figure 7–18. The pattern of LV filling across the mitral valve in this patient with a variable R-R interval illustrates the effect of the duration of diastolic filling on the E/A ratio. The E/A ratio is >1 on the longer R-R interval but the A velocities (*arrows*) are higher when superimposed on the E deceleration slope on the shorter R-R intervals. There is fusion of the E and A velocities on the shortest diastolic intervals.

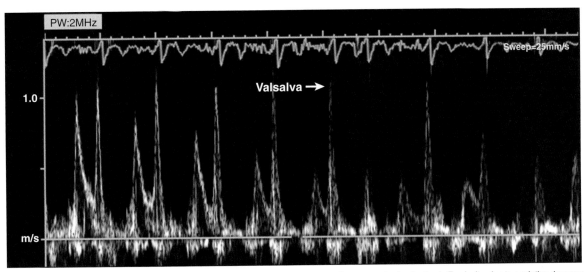

Figure 7–19. LV inflow recorded at a slow sweep speed during the Valsalva maneuver shows a gradual reduction in E velocity, due to a relative decrease in LV preload, but no change in A velocity. Thus, E/A ratio is dependent on preload.

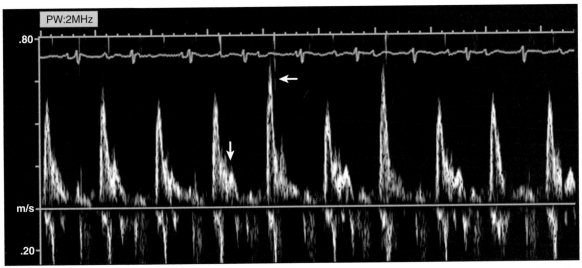

Figure 7–20. In this patient with third-degree atrioventricular (AV) block, the height of the E velocity varies with the timing of atrial contraction. When atrial contraction occurs in mid- to late diastole, a separate A velocity is seen (*vertical arrow*), but when atrial contraction occurs in early diastole, a higher (summated) E velocity is seen (*horizontal arrow*).

vein a-velocity, an increased E/E′ ratio (>15), and a shorted E velocity deceleration time.

☐ The LV filling velocity shows an apparently normal E/A ratio of 1 to 2 (pseudo-normal) that is distinguished from a true normal by the tissue Doppler showing an E′/A′ less than 1 and a shortened E velocity deceleration time.

☐ The change in the transmitral flow pattern with Valsalva maneuver also can be used to identify a pseudo-normal transmitral flow pattern; the E velocity decreases with pseudo-normalization.

Severe diastolic dysfunction (decreased compliance) (Figure 7–23)

☐ Severe diastolic dysfunction is characterized by decreased compliance, in addition to impaired relaxation, an enlarged LA and an elevated filling pressure.

☐ Decreased compliance means there is a greater increase in LV pressure for a given increase in LV volume compared with a normal ventricle.

☐ Although the E/A ratio is more than 2 and the E′/A′ ratio is more than 1, severe diastolic dysfunction is differentiated from normal by the

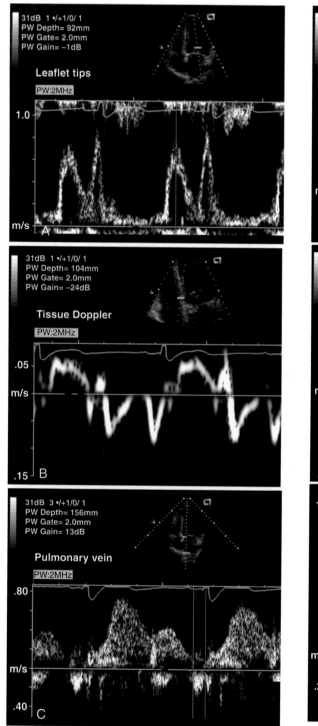

Figure 7–21. Mild diastolic dysfunction with impaired early diastolic relaxation is characterized by: (A) an E/A ratio less than 1 on the LV inflow curve; (B) a tissue Doppler early to late diastolic velocity ratio less than 1; and (C) a pulmonary vein flow curve with a reduced diastolic inflow curve but a relatively normal atrial reversal velocity and duration.

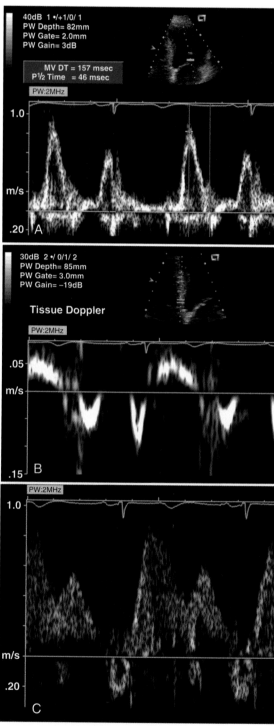

Figure 7–22. Moderate diastolic dysfunction (pseudo-normalization) is characterized by (A) a mitral inflow curve with an E/A velocity between 1 and 2 but a relatively steep deceleration time (>150 msec), and (B) a tissue Doppler E'/A' less than 1. Typically, the pulmonary vein flow signal shows greater systolic than diastolic flow and a prolonged duration and increased velocity of the atrial reversal. However, in this case the pulmonary venous flow signal (C) does not show these features, suggesting the degree of diastolic function falls between mild-moderate and moderate (pseudo-normal) as shown in the classification in the Echo Exam section.

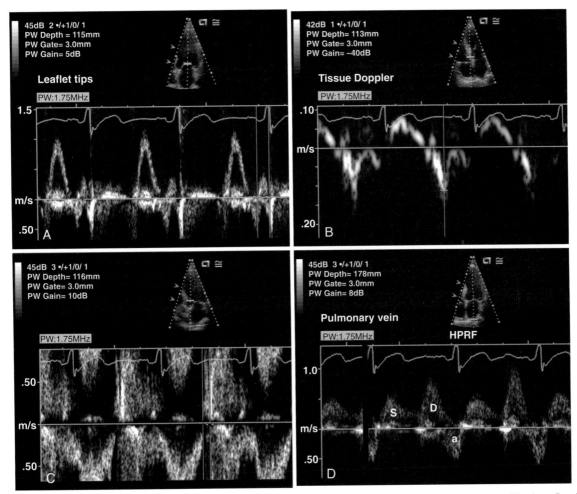

Figure 7–23. Severe diastolic dysfunction is characterized by (*A*) a LV inflow curve with an E/A > 2 and a short deceleration time; (*B*) a tissue Doppler E′/A′ more than 1; (*C*) a short IVRT; and (*D*) reduced systolic flow compared with diastolic flow in the pulmonary vein with a pulmonary vein a-reversal that is prolonged (>20 msec longer than transmitral A duration) and increased in velocity (≥0.35 m/s).

higher E/A ratio, shorter IVRT, decreased deceleration time (<150 ms), blunted pulmonary vein systolic flow, and increased pulmonary a-wave velocity and duration.

❑ The E′ velocity is very low (<5 cm/s) with severe diastolic dysfunction.

LA pressure estimates

❑ Exact measurement of LA (or LV filling) pressure is not possible with echocardiography, but there are several parameters that suggest significant elevation of LA pressures:
- Pulmonary vein atrial reversal velocity (PV_a) more than 0.35 m/s. (Figure 7–24)
- Pulmonary vein atrial reversal duration (a_{dur}) at least 20 ms longer than transmitral A duration (A_{dur}) recorded at the mitral annulus
- Ratio of transmitral E velocity to myocardial tissue E′ velocity more than 15. (Figure 7–25)

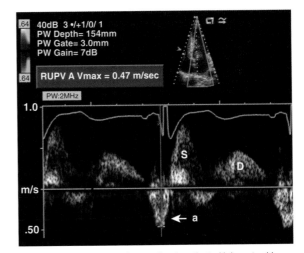

Figure 7–24. Pulmonary vein recording in patient with hypertrophic cardiomyopathy and severe diastolic dysfunction. The diastolic inflow velocity is reduced compared with systolic flow. The atrial reversal duration is prolonged with an elevated velocity of 0.47 m/s. These findings suggest markedly elevated LV filling pressures.

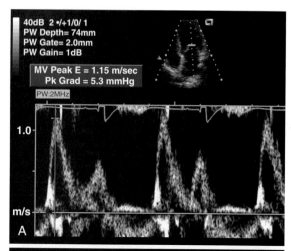

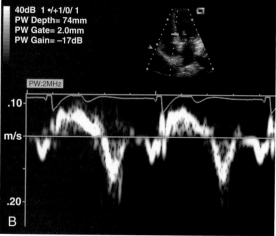

Figure 7–25. Another marker of an elevated LV filling pressure is a ratio of the transmitral E velocity to myocardial tissue Doppler velocity more than 15. In this example, the ratio is 1.15:0.15 = 7.7, suggesting normal filling pressures.

- Pulmonary venous diastolic flow deceleration time less than 175 ms
- E velocity deceleration time less than 140 ms
- E/A ratio more than 2

❏ When more than one parameter is consistent with elevated LA pressure, the diagnosis is more certain.

❏ In patients with atrial fibrillation, parameters of diastolic function that do not rely on atrial contraction may be helpful, including deceleration time, the E/E′ ratio, and the IVRT.

❏ With mitral valve stenosis or regurgitation, evaluation of LV diastolic function and LA pressure are problematic because transmitral filling reflects mitral valve hemodynamics, rather than LV diastolic function.

THE ECHO EXAM

Diastolic Dysfunction
Quantitation of Diastolic Function

Parameter	Modality	TTE View	TEE View	Recording	Measurements
LV inflow at leaflet tips	Pulsed Doppler	A4C with 2–3 mm sample volume positioned at mitral leaflet tips	High TEE 4-chamber view with sample volume at leaflet tips	Parallel to flow Normal expiration Low wall filters	E = Early diastolic filling velocity (m/s) A = Filling velocity after atrial contraction (m/s) E/A ratio DT = Deceleration time (msec)
LV inflow at annulus	Pulsed Doppler	A4C with 2 mm sample volume at mitral annulus	High TEE 4-chamber view with sample volume at mitral annulus	Parallel to flow Normal expiration Low wall filters	A_{dur} = duration of atrial filling velocity in msec
Myocardial tissue Doppler	Pulsed Doppler	A4C with 2–3 mm sample volume placed within basal segment of septal wall	High TEE 4-chamber view with 2–3 mm sample volume placed within basal segment of septal wall	Very low gain settings Low wall filters Low velocity scale	E' = Early diastolic filling velocity (m/s) A' = Filling velocity after atrial contraction (m/s) E/E' = ratio of left ventricular inflow E velocity to tissue Doppler E' velocity
IVRT	Pulsed Doppler	Anteriorly angulated A4C with 3–5 mm sample volume midway between aortic and mitral valves	High TEE 4-chamber view angulated toward aortic valve with a 2–3 mm sample volume midway between aortic and mitral valves	Clear aortic closing click Clear onset of transmitral flow Low wall filters	IVRT = isovolumic relaxation time (msec)
Pulmonary venous inflow	Pulsed Doppler (color to guide location)	Right superior pulmonary vein in A4C view using color flow to visualize flow	Left superior pulmonary vein from high TEE view (all four veins can be used)	2 mm sample volume positioned 1–2 cm into pulmonary vein	PV_S = peak systolic velocity PV_D = peak diastolic velocity PV_a = peak atrial reversal velocity a_{dur} = pulmonary vein atrial reversal duration

A4C, apical 4-chamber; IVRT, isovolumic relaxation time; TEE, transesophageal echocardiography.

Diastolic Dysfunction

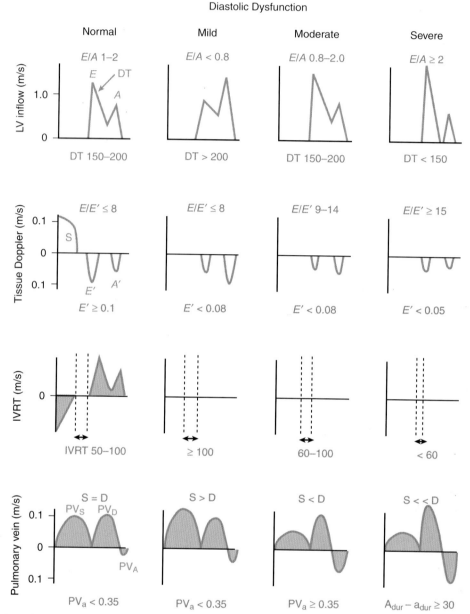

Diagram comparing typical Doppler findings in patients with normal, mild, moderate, and severe diastolic dysfunction. The top row shows LV inflow with early (E) and atrial (A) phases of diastolic filling, the second row shows tissue Doppler recorded at the septal side of the mitral annulus with the myocardial early (E') and atrial (A') velocities and the expected ratio of E/E', the third row shows the isovolumic relaxation time (IVRT), and the bottom row shows the pulmonary vein (PV) inflow pattern with systolic (S) and diastolic (D) antegrade flow and the pulmonary vein atrial (PV$_a$) reversal of flow.

Classification of Diastolic Dysfunction

	Normal	Mild	Moderate	Severe*
Pathophysiology		↓ Relaxation	↓ Relaxation & ↑ LV-EDP	↓ Compliance & ↑↑ LV-EDP
E/A ratio	1–2	<0.8	0.8-2.0††	≥2.0
DT (ms)	150–200	>200	150–200	<140
E' velocity (cm/s)	≥10	<8	<8	<5
E/E' ratio	≤8	<8	9–14	≥15
IVRT (ms)	50–100	≥100	60–100	≤60
PV S/D	≅1	S > D	S < D	S << D
PV_a (m/s)	<0.35	<0.35†	≥0.35	≥0.35
$a_{dur} - A_{dur}$ (ms)	<20	<20†	≥30	≥30

*An additional grade of irreversible severe dysfunction is characterized by the absence of a decrease in E velocity with the strain phase of the Valsalva maneuver.

†Pulmonary vein a duration and velocity may be increased if filling pressures are elevated.

††E/A with Valsalva is less than 1.0.

LV-EDP, left ventricular end-diastolic pressure.

Modified from Canadian Consensus Guidelines: Rakowki H et al: J Am Soc Echocadiogr 1996;9:736–760; Yamada H et al: J Am Soc Echocardiogr 2002;15:1238-1244; Redfield MM: JAMA 2003;289:194–202; Lester SJ et al: J Am Coll Cardiol 2008;51:679–689.

EXAMPLE

A 62-year-old man with amyloidosis has an echocardiogram that shows a symmetric increase in wall thickness with an ejection fraction of 52%. The following parameters of diastolic function are recorded.

E velocity	1.0 m/s
A velocity	0.6 m/s
Deceleration time (DT)	160 msec
A_{dur}	130 msec
E'	0.07 m/s
E'/A' ratio	<1
IVRT	40 msec
PV_S /PV_D	<1
PV_a	0.4 m/s
a_{dur}	155

The E/A ratio is more than 1 but the E'/A' ratio is less than 1, indicating a pattern of pseudo-normalization suggestive of moderate diastolic dysfunction with decreased compliance. Moderate diastolic dysfunction is confirmed by the short IVRT and relatively short deceleration time.

There also is evidence of elevated filling pressures with an equivocal E/ E' ratio of 14, but a PV_a more than 0.35 m/s and with the duration of pulmonary vein atrial flow minus the duration of atrial flow at the mitral annulus more than 20 msec.

SELF-ASSESSMENT QUESTIONS

QUESTION 1

Echocardiogram (Figure 7–26) is requested in a 72-year-old woman with hypertension. Both pulsed wave Doppler tracings of LV inflow shown below were recorded in the same patient a few minutes apart during the same study, with the sample volume positioned at the leaflet tips.

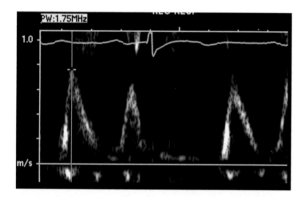

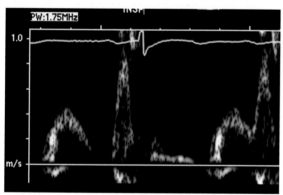

Figure 7–26.

The interval change in the Doppler signals is accounted for by:

A. Recumbent leg lift
B. Paced rhythm
C. Amyl nitrate
D. Atrial fibrillation
E. Valsalva maneuver

QUESTION 2

Which of the following, if present, *least* affects echocardiographic Doppler assessment of LV diastolic function?

A. Pulmonary hypertension
B. Atrial fibrillation
C. Mitral regurgitation
D. Mitral stenosis

QUESTION 3

Which of the following patients most likely has severe diastolic dysfunction?

A. Cardiac transplant recipient, E/A = 2.4
B. Hypertension, indexed LA volume 24 mL/m^2
C. Dilated cardiomyopathy, EF 15%
D. Inferior wall infarct, EF 50%, E/E′ = 19

QUESTION 4

A TTE (Figure 7–27) is completed on a patient with a history of exertional dyspnea.

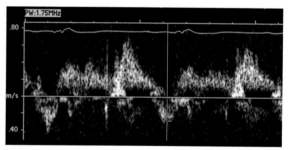

Figure 7–27.

Of the following, an additional finding you would *most* expect on the echocardiogram study is:

A. E velocity deceleration time 100 msec
B. LA volume 48 ml
C. Tissue E′ velocity 0.14 m/s
D. Tricuspid regurgitant jet velocity 2.1 m/s

QUESTION 5

In the evaluation of LV diastolic function, the Doppler E/A ratio should be recorded from the apical window using pulsed wave Doppler with the sample volume positioned at the:

A. Mitral valve annulus
B. Midpoint of the mitral leaflets
C. Mitral leaflet tips
D. Mid-LV chamber

QUESTION 6

Review the image shown below (Figure 7–28).

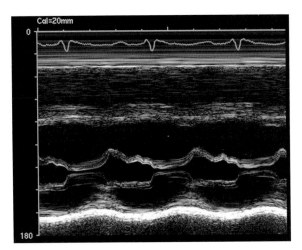

Figure 7–28.

Which feature of the image is *most* helpful in evaluating LV diastolic pressure?

A. Late diastole mitral leaflet motion
B. Peak early mitral valve diastolic displacement
C. Duration of diastolic leaflet excursion
D. E-point septal separation

QUESTION 7

What feature of the color Doppler M-mode tracing below (Figure 7–29) is most useful in LV diastolic assessment?

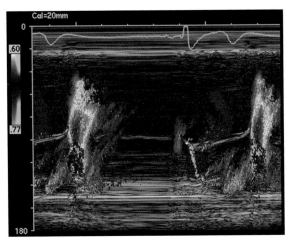

Figure 7–29.

A. Signal duration
B. Maximal signal distance from mitral valve
C. Slope of signal from mitral valve opening
D. Signal intensity

For questions 8 to 11, match the images below with the most likely diagnosis.

A. Normal diastolic function
B. Impaired LV relaxation
C. Pseudo-normal (moderate diastolic dysfunction)
D. Restrictive LV filling

QUESTION 8

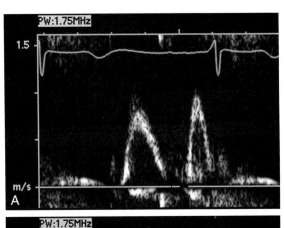

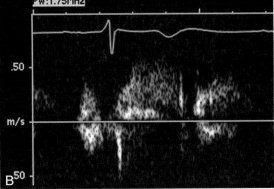

Figure 7–30.

QUESTION 9

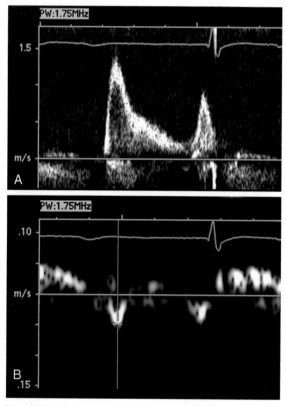

Figure 7–31.

QUESTION 10

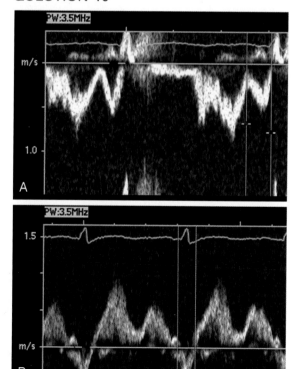

Figure 7–32.

QUESTION 11

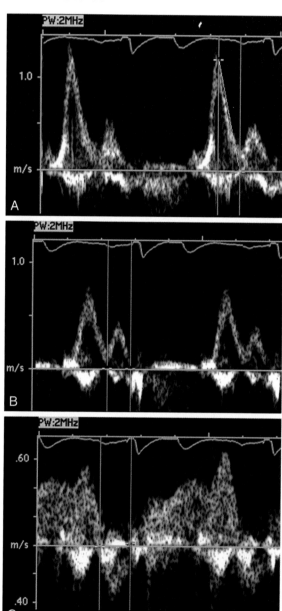

Figure 7–33.

ANSWERS

ANSWER 1: E

The first image shows a normal E/A ratio, which could be consistent with normal LV filling or a pseudo-normal filling pattern. The second Doppler tracing is recorded during Valsalva's maneuver, which causes a transient decrease in preload and a reduction in the volume of transmitral flow. With abnormal diastolic function, there is a relatively greater reduction in flow in early diastole (lower E velocity), which results in E/A reversal due to a relatively larger contribution of atrial contraction to LV filling, although the absolute value of the A velocity may be unchanged or may increase slightly. With relaxation of Valsalva, the transmitral filling pattern returns to baseline. Thus, these findings are consistent with a pseudo-normalized LV inflow pattern. This diagnosis was confirmed on the tissue myocardial velocity recording (Figure 7–34), which shows a low E' velocity and low E'/A' ratio. With normal diastolic function, both E and A velocities decrease in parallel with Valsalva maneuver, E/A ratio remains normal, and the E' velocity and E'/A' ratio remain normal.

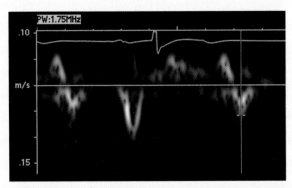

Figure 7–34.

A recumbent leg lift would transiently increase preload, the opposite effect of a Valsalva maneuver. The rhythm is not paced, nor is it atrial fibrillation. The ventricular rate is the same in both images, and the late diastolic filling due to atrial contraction is seen just before each QRS signal on the tracings. Amyl nitrate administration would transiently decrease LV afterload and would not significantly change the transmitral inflow pattern.

ANSWER 2: A

Pulmonary hypertension does not cause LV diastolic dysfunction or affect Doppler parameter of LV diastolic function, although pulmonary hypertension may be a consequence of LV diastolic dysfunction and increased LA pressure. In contrast, atrial fibrillation results in the loss of the atrial contribution to diastolic filling and absence of the A wave, making evaluation of diastolic dysfunction more challenging. Pulmonary vein flow patterns are also not reliable because the absence of atrial contraction is associated with a lower pulmonary vein systolic inflow velocity and absence of a pulmonary vein a-velocity. However, the transmitral E to myocardial velocity E' ratio (E/E' ratio) can still be used in atrial fibrillation to gauge LA pressure. With either mitral stenosis or regurgitation, transmitral flow velocities reflect mitral valve dysfunction, not LV diastolic function. With mitral stenosis, the increase in transmitral gradient is due to valve obstruction, rather than reflecting LV diastolic pressure. Pulmonary vein flow patterns reflect the increase in LA pressure due to valve obstruction, not to LV diastolic dysfunction. With mitral regurgitation, the increased transmitral volume flow is reflected in an increased transmitral E velocity. Systolic pulmonary vein flow may be reversed due to severe mitral regurgitation.

ANSWER 3: C

Of these clinical scenarios, the patient with dilated cardiomyopathy and an EF of 15% is most likely to have severe diastolic dysfunction. Patients with severe systolic dysfunction inherently have myocardial dysfunction, both systolic and diastolic, with decreased myocardial compliance. LV diastolic pressure and, as a consequence, LA pressure are elevated. The cardiac transplant recipient likely has normal diastolic function because donor hearts usually come from younger, previously healthy individuals and the Doppler LV inflow pattern is comparable to a young individual, with a relatively higher E/A ratio. In young hearts, the majority of LV inflow occurs early in diastole with a relatively small contribution of LV filling by atrial contraction. So, a ratio of 2.4 in a cardiac transplant recipient is not surprising. Hypertension may be associated with LV diastolic dysfunction, typically due to decreased LV relaxation and reversal of the E/A ratio. However, in this case, the indexed LA volume is 24 ml/m^2, which is normal. Patients with LV diastolic dysfunction or increased LA pressure almost always have significant LA dilation, so that a normal LA size excludes severe diastolic dysfunction. Tissue myocardial velocity sampled in a region of akinesis, such as an inferoseptal myocardial infarction, will lead to low myocardial velocities in this region and an erroneously elevated E/E' ratio. In the case of a right coronary artery distribution infarction, the tissue myocardial velocity should be sampled from a remote, non-infarcted zone such as the lateral wall.

ANSWER 4: A

This is a pulmonary venous tracing in a patient with a restrictive diastolic LV filling pattern and elevated LA pressure. The systolic wave is blunted with a dominant diastolic wave. The pulmonary vein atrial wave duration is prolonged, with a higher peak velocity of 0.35 m/s. These findings are all consistent with increased LA pressure. A restrictive LV filling pattern is reflected by a short transmitral E velocity deceleration time, increased LA volume, shortened isovolumic relaxation time, and low tissue myocardial Doppler E′ wave velocity. With elevated LA pressure, there is rapid equalization of transmitral pressure early in diastole; the deceleration time would be shortened to less than 140 ms and the IVRT would be shortened to less than 60 ms. There typically is at least moderate LA enlargement, with an LA volume greater than 65 mL or a LA volume indexed to body surface area (BSA) of at least 34 mL/m^2. The tissue myocardial E′ velocity usually is decreased, with a peak velocity less than 0.05 m/s and an E/E′ ratio of greater than 15. Patients with severe diastolic dysfunction typically have at least mildly increased pulmonary pressures as a result of increased left-sided pressures. A tricuspid regurgitant jet peak velocity of 2.1 m/s corresponds to a pulmonary arterial systolic pressure of only 18 mm Hg over RA pressure.

ANSWER 5: C

LV inflow (E and A) velocities are recorded at the narrowest point along the inflow stream, at the mitral leaflet tips. The LV inflow Doppler tracing is recorded from the apical 4-chamber view using pulsed Doppler. The highest, or peak, velocity signal for both the E and A waves and the E wave deceleration slope are measured for evaluation of diastolic function. In contrast, the mitral atrial, or A, wave duration is measured from pulsed Doppler samples taken at the mitral valve annulus. For volume flow rate calculations, tracing the modal velocity of the inflow signal recorded at the annulus is recommended. Spectral Doppler measurements at the midpoint of the LV leaflets or in the mid-LV chamber are not used in standard echocardiographic studies.

ANSWER 6: A

This is an M-mode tracing taken from the parasternal long-axis view at the mitral valve leaflet tips. In the mid-portion of the image, the anterior and posterior mitral valve leaflets are seen separating and opening during diastole; they are also seen coming together and closing during systole. Diastolic motion of the anterior mitral valve leaflet reflects early diastolic anterior motion concurrent with early filling (E). There is a later anterior motion concurrent with atrial

contraction and late diastolic filling (A). Just before systole, there is a very late anterior displacement, or "bump," in the motion of the anterior mitral valve leaflet (see Figure 7–35).

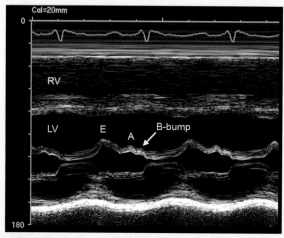

Figure 7–35.

This point between the A and C (closure) points is called an AC shoulder or a B-bump and is indicative of elevated LV end-diastolic pressure, with delayed mitral leaflet closure. The peak early mitral valve diastolic anterior displacement and E-point septal separation are a reflection of LV chamber size and systolic function. With dilated cardiomyopathy, apical tethering of the mitral valve leaflet tips may hinder leaflet excursion and increase the distance between the anterior mitral valve leaflet and the interventricular septum. Both systolic and diastolic dysfunction often coexist in patients with dilated cardiomyopathy; however, LV diastolic pressure may or may not be significantly elevated, depending on volume status and medical therapy. The duration of diastolic leaflet excursion reflects the time in the cardiac cycle spent in diastole, which is primarily dependent on heart rate rather than diastolic function. With changes in heart rate, the duration of systole is relatively constant; diastole is longer at slower heart rates and shorter at faster heart rates.

ANSWER 7: C

This is a color Doppler M-mode tracing of transmitral flow along the center of the mitral annulus taken from an apical view. With the mitral valve open in diastole, flow toward the transducer (or LV apex) is recorded. The slope of the color Doppler signal from the point of valve opening (color propagation velocity [Vp]) reflects the velocity of LV inflow from the mitral valve plane to the apex. A steep slope is consistent with normal diastolic function and a flatter slope suggests diastolic dysfunction with a higher LV diastolic pressure. The maximal signal distance from the mitral valve is the distance where LV inflow velocities were detected, which is a function of Doppler color flow instrument parameters, not diastolic function. The color signal duration corresponds to the duration of diastole, and signal intensity reflects the color Doppler scale, gain, and signal strength; neither of these reflects LV diastolic function.

ANSWER 8: B

The LV inflow Doppler image shows reversal of the peak E/A velocities. The E wave deceleration slope is prolonged, consistent with impaired LV relaxation. The second image shows the pulmonary vein inflow. The systolic wave is dominant and the pulmonary atrial reversal wave is short with a low peak velocity, implying normal LA pressure.

ANSWER 9: C

The LV inflow Doppler image shows a normal E/A velocity ratio of about 1.8. The E wave deceleration slope is shortened, consistent with rapid equalization of transmitral pressure gradient during mitral valve opening. The second image shows the septal tissue myocardial velocity. E′ is reduced at 0.05, indicating decreased myocardial motion. The E/E′ ratio of 28 suggests severely increased LA pressure.

ANSWER 10: A

These are images taken during a TEE study. Because the transducer is placer posterior to the heart, in the esophagus, flow into the LV is directed away from the transducer and flow entering the left atrium from the pulmonary veins is directed toward the transducer. The image B is of pulmonary venous flow with both anterograde flow in systole and diastole and a small reversal of flow during atrial contraction. The systolic wave is dominant on the pulmonary venous tracing. The image A is of transmitral flow at the level of the mitral annulus. Although the LV inflow pattern at the mitral valve tips is not shown, the Doppler sample at the mitral annulus level indicates that the early filling velocity is greater than the atrial filling velocity. The pulmonary venous atrial wave duration is shorter than the mitral atrial duration, suggesting normal LA pressure. The findings, in sum, support a diagnosis of normal diastolic function.

ANSWER 11: D

The LV inflow Doppler velocity signal (A) at the mitral valve leaflet tips shows an increased E/A velocity ratio of 1.4 m/s to 0.5 m/s, or about 2.8. The E wave deceleration slope is shortened, consistent with rapid equalization of transmitral pressure gradient during mitral valve opening. The Doppler flow signal in panel B shows the transmitral flow at the mitral annulus. Doppler sampling at the mitral annulus is used for the mitral atrial wave duration. Comparison of the peak early diastolic wave velocities from the mitral valve tips and mitral annulus shows the difference in velocities, highlighting the necessity for careful attention to Doppler sample placement when interpreting images. Pulmonary vein inflow is shown in panel C. The diastolic wave is dominant, with blunting of the systolic wave. The pulmonary atrial reversal wave is prolonged relative to the mitral atrial wave duration, with a high peak pulmonary atrial wave velocity, implying increased LA pressure.

8 Ischemic Cardiac Disease

REVIEW OF CORONARY ANATOMY AND LEFT VENTRICULAR WALL SEGMENTS

■ Evaluation of coronary disease by echocardiography is based on visualization of endocardial motion and wall thickening.
■ For description of regional myocardial function, the left ventricle (LV) is divided into segments that correspond to the coronary artery blood supply. (Figure 8–1)
■ Myocardial infarction results in thinning and akinesis of the affected regions. With myocardial ischemia, wall motion may be normal at rest.
■ The ostia of the right and left main coronary arteries often can be identified, but direct visualization of distal coronary anatomy by echocardiography is limited. (Figures 8–2 and 8–3)

Key points

❑ The ventricle is divided into basal, mid-ventricular, and apical segments, plus the tip of the apex.
❑ A distal coronary stenosis results in apical abnormalities; a mid-coronary lesion results in mid-ventricular and apical wall motion changes; and proximal coronary disease results in abnormalities that extend from the base to the apex.
❑ In the short axis plane, the LV is divided into six segments: anterior, anterior-lateral, inferior-lateral, inferior, inferior-septal, and anterior-septal.
❑ The left anterior descending coronary supplies the entire anterior wall and anterior septum and typically extends to supply the apical segment of the inferior septum and the tip of the apex.

140

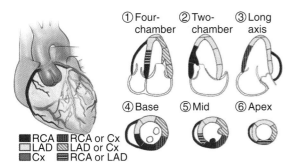

Figure 8–1 Typical coronary artery distribution of blood flow shown in the apical and parasternal short-axis views. *RCA*, right coronary artery; *LAD*, left anterior descending; *Cx*, circumflex. *From Lang RM, Bierig M, Devereux RB, et al: Chamber Quantification Writing Group; American Society of Echocardiography's Guidelines and Standards Committee; European Association of Echocardiography. Recommendations for chamber quantification. J Am Soc Echocardiogr 2005;18(12):1440-1463.*

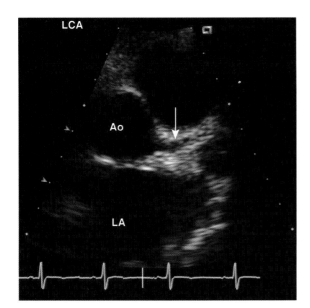

Figure 8–2. The left main coronary artery (*LCA, arrow*) visualized on TTE arising from the aorta (*Ao*) anterior to the left atrium (*LA*) in a transthoracic parasternal short-axis view just above to the aortic valve plane.

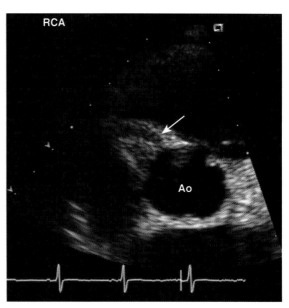

Figure 8–3. The right coronary artery (*RCA, arrow*) is seen in a transthoracic parasternal short-axis view arising from the aorta (*Ao*) by slight adjustment of the image plane.

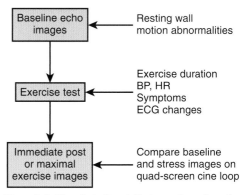

Figure 8–4. Flow chart of treadmill stress echocardiography.

□ The right coronary artery supplies the basal and mid-ventricular segments of the inferior septum and the entire inferior wall and sometimes supplies the inferior-lateral wall.

□ The circumflex coronary artery supplies the entire anterior-lateral and inferior-lateral walls.

STEP-BY-STEP APPROACH

Stress echocardiography

Basic principles

■ LV global and regional function is normal at rest, even when significant coronary artery disease is present.

■ With an increase in myocardial oxygen demand, myocardial ischemia is evidenced by reversible regional hypokinesis or akinesis.

■ The basis of stress echocardiography is a comparison of images of the LV acquired at rest and after induction of myocardial ischemia, either with exercise or pharmacologic intervention. (Figures 8–4 and 8–5)

Key points

□ The accuracy of stress echocardiography correlates with the stress load achieved. Typically, the goal is a peak heart rate at least 85% of the patient's maximum predicted heart rate.

□ Comparison of resting and stress images is facilitated by acquiring images in a cine loop format,

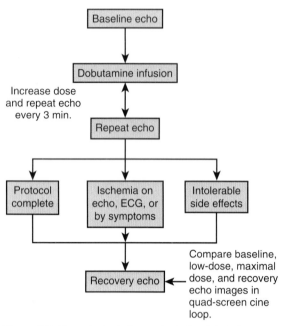

Figure 8–5. Flow chart of the protocol for dobutamine stress echocardiography.

TABLE 8-1 Qualitative Scale for Assessment of Segmental Wall Motion on Echocardiography

Score*	Wall Motion	Definition
1	Normal	Normal endocardial inward motion and wall thickening in systole
2	Hypokinesis	Reduced endocardial motion and wall thickening in systole
3	Akinesis	Absence of inward endocardial motion or wall thickening in systole
4	Dyskinesis	Outward motion or "bulging" of the segment in systole, usually associated with thin, scarred myocardium

*A score of 0 may be used for hyperkinesis, defined as increased endocardial inward motion and wall thickening in systole.

gated from the onset of the QRS to include the same number of frames for each image.

❏ Because ischemia may be induced with the stress protocol, appropriate medical supervision and monitoring is essential for patient safety and to promptly treat any complications of the procedure.

Step 1: Prepare for the stress echo

■ The patient is instructed to hold beta-blocking medications the day before and day of the stress test.
■ The reason for the stress study and the patient history is reviewed, followed by a directed physical examination.
■ Informed consent is obtained for both exercise and pharmacologic stress echo.
■ Patient monitoring includes continuous 12-lead ECG monitoring (with a recording at each stress stage) and intermittent blood pressure measurement under the supervision of a qualified medical professional, in a procedure room with resuscitation equipment and medications readily available.
■ When needed, an intravenous line is placed for infusion of dobutamine and/or use of contrast echocardiography.

Key points

❏ Any potential contraindications or risk factors for the stress study are identified and discussed with the referring health care provider before beginning the test.

❏ The risks and benefits of the stress echo study are discussed with the patient, in the context of the patient's medical history and cardiac function.
❏ Because the cardiac sonographer's attention is focused on image acquisition, patient monitoring typically is performed by an additional health care professional.
❏ The rationale for a pharmacologic versus exercise stress echo is reviewed. Usually, exercise stress is preferred because of the additional information gained regarding hemodynamics and symptoms.
❏ Pharmacologic (usually dobutamine) stress echo is preferred in patients unable to walk on a treadmill or use a supine bicycle due to orthopedic or vascular problems and in some specific patient subgroups, such as those who have undergone heart transplantation.

Step 2: Evaluate regional and global left ventricular systolic function at rest

■ Left ventricular global and regional function is evaluated in parasternal long- and short-axis views and in apical 4-chamber, 2-chamber, and long-axis views. (Figure 8–6)
■ The function for each myocardial segment is graded as hyperdynamic, normal, hypokinetic, akinetic, or dyskinetic based on the degree of endocardial motion and wall thickening. (Table 8-1)

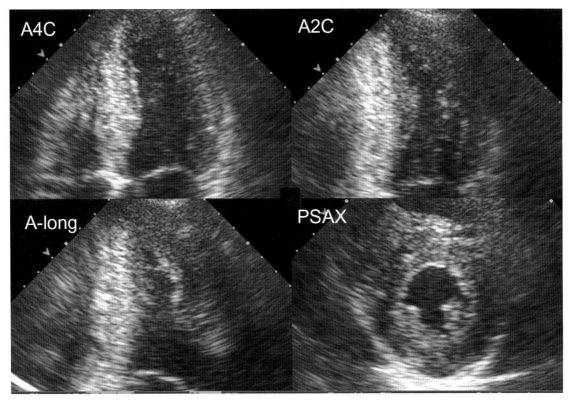

Figure 8–6. Images of the LV are recorded at baseline using a cine loop quad-screen format, with apical 4-chamber (*A4C*), apical 2-chamber (*A2C*) and apical (or parasternal) long-axis (*A-long*) and parasternal short-axis (*PSAX*) views. Several beats are acquired and the best image saved. The cine loop only includes systole, to allow matching with the stress images. Images are again acquired at peak stress (with dobutamine) or immediately post stress (with exercise) in the same image planes. The rest and exercise images are then matched by view to allow comparison of the same myocardial segments on side-by-side views. Because a set number of frames is recorded and there is little change in the duration of systole with stress, the rest and exercise images move at the same speed, despite the difference in heart rates.

■ Overall LV ejection fraction is visually estimated or (preferably) measured using the apical biplane approach.

Key points

❑ The four standard views (with the long axis in apical or parasternal, whichever is best) are recorded in cine loop format A beat with clear definition of endocardial borders and optimal image plane alignment chosen for each view.

❑ Depth is reduced to maximize LV image size, including the mitral annulus but not the LA. The same depth and sector width is used for the stress images.

❑ If endocardial definition is suboptimal, left-sided echo contrast is used to improve evaluation of regional endocardial motion. (Figure 8–7)

❑ The electrocardiographic leads and gain are adjusted to show a clear signal with an adequate QRS height for accurate electrocardiography gating. (Figure 8–8)

Step 3: Perform the stress protocol

Exercise stress

■ Any standard exercise protocol can be used with electrocardiographic and blood pressure monitoring.

■ Upright treadmill exercise provides the highest workload, but images can only be obtained after exercise, so rapid image acquisition is essential.

■ Supine bicycle exercise provides a lower workload, but images can be acquired during exercise using a dedicated stress echo stretcher and bicycle.

Key points

❑ With treadmill exercise, ensuring the patient can rapidly move from the treadmill to the echo stretcher is important.

❑ In addition to echo images, the heart rate and blood pressure response to exercise, patient symptoms, arrhythmias, and ST segment

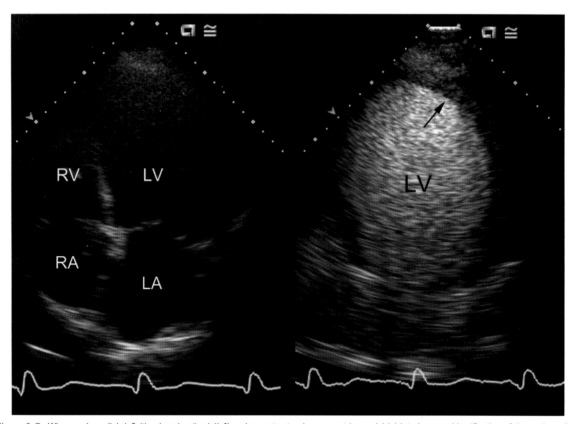

Figure 8–7. When endocardial definition is suboptimal (*left*), echo contrast enhancement is used (*right*) to improve identification of the endocardium (*arrow*) and evaluation of regional and global function with stress echocardiography.

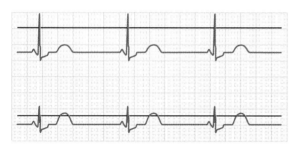

Figure 8–8. Schematic of an appropriate electrocardiographic signal with little noise and a QRS height greater than the T wave, allowing accurate triggering for digital image acquisition and an example with the T wave equal in height to the QRS signal so that both signals will trigger image acquisition, resulting in very short cine loops that do not include the full cardiac cycle.

changes are important clinical parameters. (Figure 8–9)

❏ The endpoint for a maximal exercise stress study is when the patient cannot exercise further due to shortness of breath, leg fatigue, or other symptoms.

❏ The exercise test also is stopped for any decline in blood pressure, significant arrhythmias, excessive increase in blood pressure, or significant ST-segment depression.

Dobutamine stress

■ A typical dobutamine stress protocol is to infuse intravenous dobutamine beginning at 5 (if there are resting wall motion abnormalities) or 10 mcg/kg/min, with an increase by 10 mcg/kg/min every 3 minutes to a maximum dose of 40 mcg/kg/min.

■ Atropine in increments of 0.25 mg (maximum 1 mg total) may be added to achieve target heart rate, if needed.

■ The primary endpoint is a heart rate 85% of maximum predicted heart rate for age.

■ Other endpoints include:
  • Maximum dose allowed by protocol
  • Definite wall motion abnormality in two or more adjacent segments
  • Fall in systolic blood pressure to less than 100 mm Hg or increase in blood pressure to more than 200 mm Hg
  • Diastolic blood pressure more than 120 mm Hg
  • Significant arrhythmia
  • Patient discomfort

Key points

❏ Careful monitoring of heart rate, blood pressure, electrocardiographic findings, and symptoms is needed.

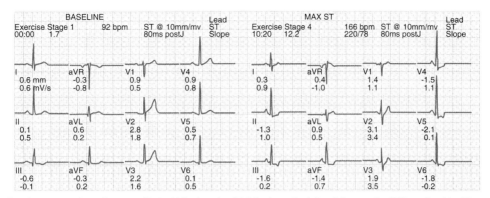

Figure 8–9. Exercise stress echocardiogram, with the 12-lead resting ECG leads on the left and the exercise ECG on the right. The numbers below each averaged ECG lead show the amount of ST depression (in mm) and the slope of the ST segment for each lead. In this 42-year-old man with multiple cardiac risk factors and chest pain symptoms, there is a 1.5- to 2-mm flat ST depression in the inferior and lateral leads consistent with myocardial ischemia.

TABLE 8-2 Patterns of Wall Motion with Dobutamine Stress Echo

	Normal	Ischemia	Stunned or Hibernating	Infarction
Baseline	Normal	Normal	Hypokinetic or Akinetic	Hypokinetic or Akinetic
Low dose	Normal	Normal	Improved	Hypokinetic or Akinetic
High dose	Hyperkinetic	Hypokinetic or Akinetic	Hypokinetic or Akinetic	Hypokinetic or Akinetic

- ❏ Maximum predicted heart rate is roughly 220 minus the patient's age.
- ❏ About 10% of patients will have a fall in blood pressure; this does not indicate coronary disease but may necessitate ending the dobutamine infusion.
- ❏ ST-segment depression with dobutamine is not diagnostically useful. ST-segment elevation is rare but is predictive of significant coronary disease.
- ❏ Both ventricular and atrial arrhythmias may be precipitated by dobutamine and require prompt cessation of dobutamine infusion.
- ❏ When needed, the effects of dobutamine can be reversed with a rapidly acting intravenous beta blocker, such as esmolol.
- ❏ Improvement in wall motion at low-dose dobutamine of a myocardial segment that is abnormal at rest is evidence for myocardial viability.
- ❏ A biphasic response is when a myocardial segment that is abnormal at rest shows increased wall thickening at low-dose dobutamine (viability) and then worsening of wall motion at high dose (ischemia). (Table 8-2)

Step 4: Evaluate regional and global left ventricular systolic function at peak heart rate

- ■ Cine loop images of the ventricle are acquired at (or immediately after) peak stress using the same four image planes as the baseline images (see Figure 8–6).
- ■ The image depth, sector width, and electrocardiography gating on the stress images are the same as on the baseline images.
- ■ Rest and exercise images are compared side by side in the cine loop format. (Figure 8–10)

Key points

- ❏ With exercise stress, the images are obtained as quickly as possible after exercise.
- ❏ With pharmacologic stress, images are acquired at each dosage stage, as well as at peak dose and heart rate.
- ❏ If endocardial definition is suboptimal, left-sided echo contrast is used to improve evaluation of regional endocardial motion.

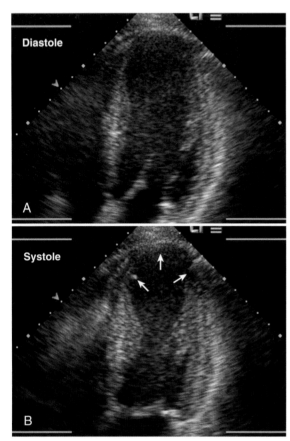

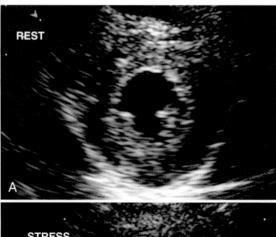

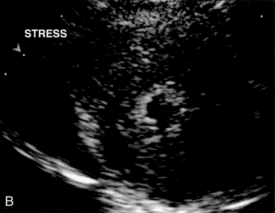

Figure 8–10. Resting myocardial wall motion was normal in this 56-year-old man with exertional chest discomfort. The immediate post-stress images with the apical 4-chamber view at end diastole (*A*) and end systole (*B*) show akinesis of the apical lateral wall and inferior septum. These findings are consistent with inducible ischemia in the territory of the distal left anterior descending coronary artery.

Figure 8–11. These parasternal short-axis end-systolic images at rest (*A*) and maximum-dose dobutamine (*B*) demonstrate the normal decrease in ventricular size with dobutamine stress.

- Several cine loops are quickly acquired in each view with subsequent selection of the best image to compare to the baseline images.
- Using electrocardiography gating and the same cine loop length for rest and exercise images results in a similar timing of contraction on both images.
- The normal response to exercise or dobutamine stress is hyperkinesis of all segments with a decrease in ventricular chamber size. (Figure 8–11)
- Each myocardial segment is graded as hyperkinetic, normal, hypokinetic, akinetic, or dyskinetic.

Step 5: Monitor patient recovery

- The patient is monitored until all symptoms or wall motion abnormalities (if any) resolve and heart rate has returned to normal (<100 bpm).
- If symptoms or wall motion abnormalities were seen at peak-dose dobutamine, heart rate may be slowed more rapidly with a short-acting beta blocker.

Key points

- Ischemia is reversible so that stress-induced wall motion abnormalities quickly resolve as heart rate declines.
- Post-stress images are recorded to document that LV global and regional function has returned to baseline on completion of the study.
- If ischemia is induced, as evidenced by chest discomfort or wall motion abnormalities, a short-acting beta blocker, such as esmolol, is used to reduce heart rate and relieve symptoms.

Step 6: Review and interpretation of the stress study

- Baseline and stress echocardiographic images are reviewed in a side-by-side cine loop format using a systemic approach to grading wall motion for each myocardial segment.

- The stress study interpretation depends on integration of clinical (symptoms, exercise duration), hemodynamic (blood pressure, heart rate), electrocardiographic (ST changes and arrhythmias), and echocardiographic data.

Key Points

- ❏ The stress echo report includes the following minimal elements:
  - Exercise duration or maximum dobutamine/atropine dose
  - Heart rate and blood pressure at baseline and maximal stress
  - Electrocardiographic ST-segment changes or arrhythmias
  - Symptoms
  - Resting global and regional LV systolic function
  - Global and regional LV systolic function at maximal stress
  - Integration of these data to indicate study quality (images and maximum stress achieved), the likelihood of coronary disease, and the probable affected vessels
- ❏ The maximum stress achieved is a key element in interpretation; typically the study is considered non-diagnostic unless the maximum heart rate is at least 85% of the maximum predicted heart rate for that patient.
- ❏ An inducible wall motion abnormality is defined as hypokinesis or akinesis of a segment that was normal at rest. Failure of a normal segment to become hyperkinetic also is evidence of ischemia.
- ❏ Echocardiographic evidence of an inducible wall motion abnormality in one or more adjacent segments is consistent with coronary artery disease, with the probable affected coronary artery identified from the location of the wall motion abnormality. (Figure 8–12)
- ❏ With three-vessel coronary disease, instead of a regional wall motion abnormality, the only finding may be the absence of hyperkinesis and failure of ventricular size to decrease appropriately
- ❏ Symptoms of chest discomfort accompanied by inducible wall motion abnormalities are consistent with ischemia; symptoms occurring simultaneously with normal regional function suggest non-cardiac chest pain.

Acute coronary syndromes

Basic principles

- Acute coronary syndromes include patients with:
  - ST-segment elevation myocardial infarction (STEMI)

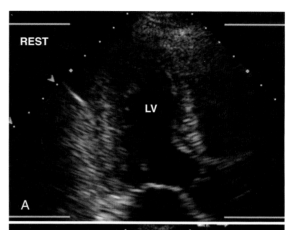

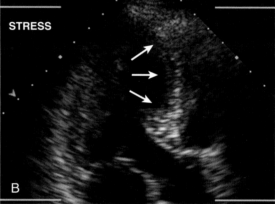

Figure 8–12. Example of inducible ischemia with the apical long axis view showing normal wall motion on this end-systolic image at rest, with akinesis of the mid and apical segments of the anterior septum with exercise stress (*arrows*).

TABLE 8-3	Medically Urgent Causes of Acute Chest Pain

Acute coronary syndrome
Acute ST-elevation myocardial infarction (STEMI)
Non-ST elevation myocardial infarction (NSTEMI)
Unstable angina
Aortic dissection
Pulmonary embolus
Acute pericarditis
Esophageal rupture (Boerhaave's syndrome)

  - Non–ST-segment elevation myocardial infarction (NSTEMI)
  - Unstable angina
- Other causes of acute chest pain that require immediate intervention (Table 8-3) are:
  - Aortic dissection
  - Pericarditis
  - Pulmonary embolism

Step 1: Evaluate regional ventricular function

- A regional wall motion abnormality in a patient with chest pain indicates myocardial infarction or ischemia.
- In a patient with prior coronary disease, it may be difficult to distinguish pre-existing regional dysfunction from acute dysfunction.
- Regional ventricular function may be normal between episodes of chest pain in patients with unstable angina.

Key points

- ❑ Echocardiographic evaluation of wall motion is most helpful when the electrocardiogram (ECG) is non-diagnostic; prompt revascularization is appropriate in patients with ST-elevation myocardial infarction.
- ❑ A remote transmural myocardial infarction results in akinesis, myocardial thinning, and increased echogenicity, consistent with scar. (Figure 8–13)
- ❑ However, with a prior non–ST-elevation or reperfused myocardial infarction, wall thickness may be relatively normal.
- ❑ Normal regional myocardial function simultaneous with chest pain symptoms indicates a very low likelihood of an acute coronary syndrome.

Step 2: Estimate or measure ejection fraction

- Evaluation of overall LV systolic function is clinically useful in management of patients with acute chest pain.

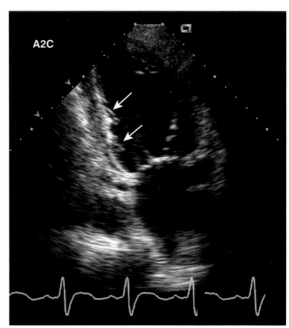

Figure 8–13. The inferior wall is thinned, bright, and akinetic in the 2-chamber view in a patient with a prior ST-elevation inferior myocardial infarction.

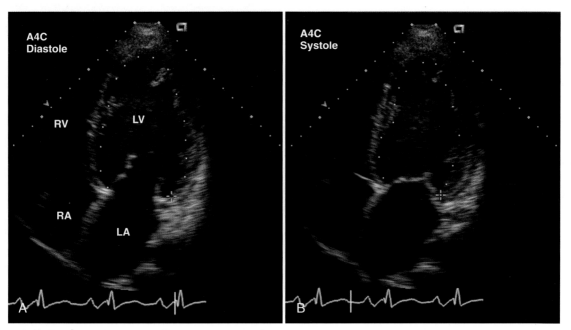

Figure 8–14. This patient with a prior non–ST-elevation myocardial infarction has relatively normal wall motion when the apical 4-chamber diastolic and systolic images are compared. Apical hypokinesis is present.

■ Hospitalization and further evaluation often is needed in patients with a reduced ejection fraction, even when due to causes other than acute coronary syndrome.

Key points

❏ Measurement of ejection fraction using the apical biplane approach is preferred when endocardial definition is adequate and there are no time constraints. (Figure 8–14)

❏ In urgent situations, a visual estimate of ejection fraction based on parasternal short-axis and apical 4-chamber, 2-chamber, and long-axis views is appropriate.

❏ Left-sided echo contrast may be helpful for definition of both global and regional LV systolic function when image quality is suboptimal.

Step 3: Consider alternate causes of chest pain

■ Echocardiography may suggest other causes of chest pain when LV function is normal.

■ Often additional imaging approaches are needed for further evaluation when the clinical diagnosis remains unclear.

Key points

❏ Evidence of aortic dilation and aortic regurgitation in a patient with acute chest pain prompts further evaluation for aortic dissection by transesophageal echocardiography (TEE) or cardiac computed tomographic imaging.

❏ Although a pulmonary embolus is rarely visualized on echocardiography, findings of pulmonary hypertension and RV dilation or dysfunction suggest this diagnosis be considered.

❏ A pericardial effusion is consistent with the diagnosis of pericarditis but also may be seen with acute aortic dissection (with rupture into the pericardium) and with numerous systemic diseases (see Chapter 10).

Step 4: Evaluate cardiac hemodynamics

■ Echocardiographic evaluation of cardiac hemodynamics is helpful in selected patients with acute chest pain.

Key Points

❏ Ischemia or infarction often is accompanied by diastolic dysfunction with evidence of elevated left atrial pressure on the Doppler LV and LA filling curves (see Chapter 7).

❏ Pulmonary pressures may be elevated due to elevated left-sided filling pressures.

❏ Cardiac output can be measured using the LV outflow tract diameter and flow velocity integral (see Chapter 6).

Complications of acute myocardial infarction

■ Echocardiography provides rapid, accurate bedside diagnosis of mechanical complications of acute myocardial infarction.

■ Mechanical complications of myocardial infarction present as recurrent chest pain, new systolic murmur, heart failure, cardiogenic shock, or systemic embolic event.

■ Arrhythmias associated with acute myocardial infarction may occur in the absence of significant structural abnormalities.

Step 1: Evaluation of the patient with recurrent chest pain after myocardial infarction

■ Recurrent chest pain after myocardial infarction may be due to recurrent ischemia, pericarditis, or non-cardiac chest pain.

■ Echocardiographic evaluation focuses on segmental wall motion and detection of a pericardial effusion.

Key Points

❏ Comparison of regional wall motion with previous studies may allow detection of recurrent ischemia in the peri-infarct region or in the distribution of a different coronary artery. However, coronary angiography often is needed for definitive diagnosis.

❏ The presence of a pericardial effusion is consistent with the diagnosis of pericarditis but also may be seen with acute aortic dissection (with rupture into the pericardium) or with LV rupture.

❏ LV rupture may present as transient chest pain; this diagnosis should be considered when pericardial effusion is present in a patient with a history of myocardial infarction, particularly if the episode of chest pain was accompanied by hypotension. (Figure 8–15)

Step 2: Evaluation of the patient with a new systolic murmur after myocardial infarction

■ The differential diagnosis of a new murmur that develops after myocardial infarction is:
- Ventricular septal defect due to rupture of the septal myocardium *or*
- Acute mitral regurgitation due to papillary muscle rupture or dysfunction

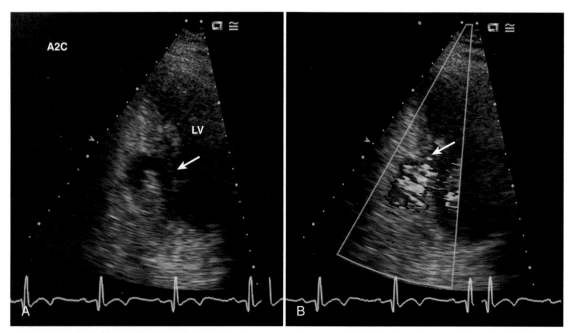

Figure 8–15. LV rupture in this patient with an inferior myocardial infarction is seen in the apical 2-chamber view (*A2C*) with an area of discontinuity in the inferior wall (arrrow) and with color Doppler showing flow into a narrow-necked pseudo-aneurysm. The myocardial rupture is contained by pericardial adhesions, which form the wall of the pseudo-aneurysm.

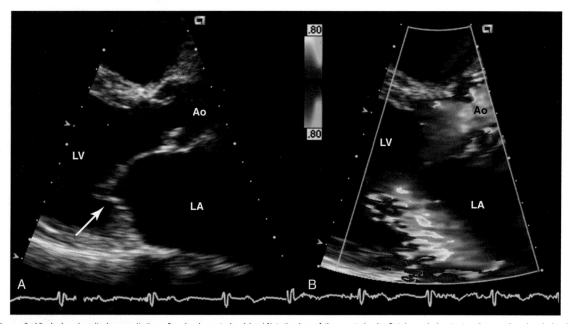

Figure 8–16. Ischemic mitral regurgitation often is characterized by (*A*) tethering of the posterior leaflet (arrow) due to traction on the chords by the ischemic myocardium underlying the papillary muscle, resulting in a "tented" appearance of the closed valve at end-systole and (*B*) a posterior-laterally directed jet of mitral regurgitation as the anterior leaflet fails to coapt completely with the relatively immobile posterior leaflet.

■ Imaging focuses on evaluation of segmental wall motion and detection of a pericardial effusion with Doppler evaluation for the cause of the murmur.

Key Points

❑ Mitral regurgitation after myocardial infarction most often is due to ischemia or infarction of the papillary muscle or underlying inferior-lateral LV wall, resulting in "tethering" of the mitral leaflets with inadequate systolic coaptation. (Figures 8–16 and 8–17)

❑ With partial or complete papillary muscle rupture, acute severe mitral regurgitation occurs, with pulmonary edema and cardiogenic shock.

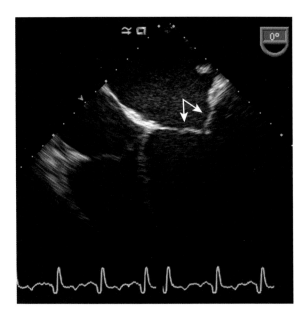

Figure 8–17. Transesophageal 4-chamber view in patient with LV dilation and systolic dysfunction due to severe three-vessel coronary disease. This mid-systolic image shows the tenting (or tethering) of the mitral leaflets due to lateral displacement of the papillary muscles in the dilated ventricle. This restriction of leaflet motion resulted in inadequate leaflet apposition and moderate mitral regurgitation.

- ❐ TEE often is needed to define the mechanism and evaluate the severity of ischemic mitral regurgitation.
- ❐ Ventricular septal defects that develop after myocardial infarction are detected using color Doppler showing a flow disturbance on the RV side of the septum. Often the defect can be visualized on 2D imaging. Continuous wave (CW) Doppler interrogation provides information on the LV-to-RV systolic pressure difference. (Figure 8–18)
- ❐ With a ventricular septal defect, oxygen saturation is increased from the right atrium (RA) to the RV due to shunting of oxygenated blood from the left to RV across the ventricular defect. If a right-sided heart catheter is in position, measurement of oxygen saturations may be helpful when the diagnosis is unclear.

Step 3: Evaluation of the patient with hypotension or cardiogenic shock after myocardial infarction

- ■ Hypotension after myocardial infarction may be due to RV infarction, LV systolic dysfunction, or myocardial rupture with pericardial tamponade.
- ■ Echocardiographic evaluation focuses on evaluation of global left and RV systolic function and detection of a pericardial effusion.

Key Points

- ❐ RV infarction often accompanies an inferior myocardial infarction. The typical presentation is hypotension that responds to volume loading. Echocardiography shows a dilated hypocontractile RV, despite normal pulmonary pressures. (Figure 8–19)
- ❐ With a large or recurrent myocardial infarction, LV systolic function may be significantly reduced, resulting in pulmonary edema and hypotension. Echocardiography allows measurement (or estimation) of ejection fraction and assessment of regional ventricular function.
- ❐ Myocardial ischemia or infarction is typically accompanied by diastolic dysfunction, often with elevated LV filling pressures. Diastolic dysfunction may lead to pulmonary congestion, but rarely is it the primary cause of hypotension.
- ❐ LV rupture due to myocardial infarction may result in acute cardiac tamponade and death. However, in some cases the myocardial rupture is contained by a pericardial thrombus and adhesions.
- ❐ A contained LV rupture is called a pseudo-aneurysm because its wall consists of pericardium (not myocardium). (Figure 8–20)
- ❐ Typical characteristics of a pseudo-aneurysm are a narrow neck compared with its widest diameter and an abrupt transition at an acute angle between the normal myocardium and the aneurysm. Often the pseudo-aneurysm is lined with thrombus.
- ❐ Most pseudo-aneurysms require urgent surgical intervention to repair the ventricular rupture. True aneurysms typically are treated medically.

Step 4: Evaluation for late complications of myocardial infarction

- ■ Late complications of myocardial infarction include LV aneurysm, thrombus, and systolic dysfunction.
- ■ Echocardiographic examination includes evaluation of global and regional myocardial function, calculation of ejection fraction, assessment of diastolic dysfunction, and a diligent search for apical thrombus.

Key Points

- ❐ Adverse ventricular remodeling after myocardial infarction results in thinning and scar formation in areas of infarction, overall LV dilation, and a reduction in ejection fraction. Adverse remodeling is prevented, to some extent, by appropriate medical therapy.

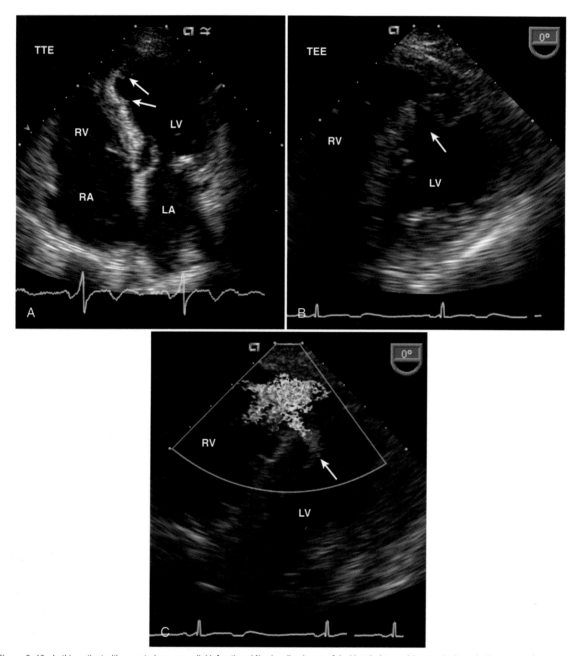

Figure 8–18. In this patient with an anterior myocardial infarction, (A) a localized area of dyskinesis (arrows) is seen in the apical segment of the septum in the 4-chamber view on transthoracic echocardiography (TTE), (B) with an area of frank discontinuity in the septum (arrow) seen on the transgastric short-axis view on transesophageal imaging (TEE). (C) Color Doppler confirms the post-myocardial infarction ventricular septal defect with a narrow jet of flow from the left ventricle (LV) into the right ventricle (RV).

❏ The myocardial thickness in diastole, wall thickening during systole, and endocardial motion are graded for each myocardial segment.

❏ An aneurysm is defined as a discrete area of the LV (usually the apex) with a diastolic contour abnormality and systolic dyskinesis. (Figure 8–21)

❏ LV ejection fraction is calculated using the biplane apical approach. Single plane or M-mode evaluation of LV function may be inaccurate due to regional ventricular dysfunction.

❏ Apical thrombus is best visualized in standard and oblique apical views. Identification of thrombus is enhanced by use of a higher-frequency transducer and a shallow image depth. (Figure 8–22)

❑ Apical trabeculation is distinguished from thrombus by the lack of mobility, linear appearance, and attachments to the LV wall.

❑ Left-sided ultrasound contrast may be helpful when it is difficult to distinguish apical trabeculation from thrombi. (Figure 8–23)

End-stage ischemic disease

■ End-stage ischemic disease, colloquially called "ischemic cardiomyopathy" has many features in common with a dilated cardiomyopathy or ventricular dysfunction due to valvular heart disease (see The Echo Exam as the end of the chapter).

■ The echocardiographic features most helpful in diagnosis of end-stage ischemic disease are:
  • Definite regional wall motion abnormalities with areas of thinning and akinesis (Figure 8–24)
  • Normal RV size and systolic function (unless RV infarction has occurred)
  • Absence of evidence for primary valvular heart disease

Step 1: Evaluate global left ventricular systolic and diastolic function

■ Overall LV systolic function is evaluated by calculation of an apical biplane ejection fraction.

■ LV diastolic function is evaluated as described in Chapter 7.

Key points

❑ Calculation of a biplane ejection fraction is performed whenever possible. If endocardial definition is suboptimal, left-sided contrast echocardiography provides better visualization of LV function.

❑ Most patients with end-stage ischemia disease have diastolic dysfunction, as well as systolic dysfunction.

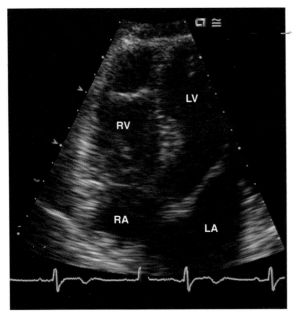

Figure 8–19. Right ventricular (*RV*) dilation and (in real time) hypokinesis in a patient with an inferior myocardial infarction, is consistent with RV infarction as seen in this apical 4-chamber view.

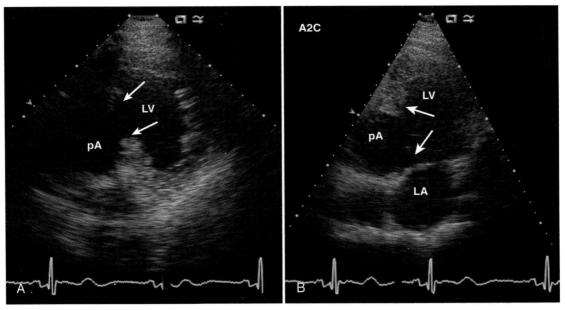

Figure 8–20. A chronic LV pseudo-aneurysm (*pA*) is characterized by a narrow neck (*arrows*) relative to the maximum diameter of the pseudo-aneurysm, as seen in (A) a short-axis view of the left ventricle (*LV*) and (B) in the apical 2-chamber (*A2C*) view. There is an abrupt transition from the normal myocardial thickness to the aneurysm and the pseudo-aneurysm has an irregular echodensity consistent with thrombus lining the cavity.

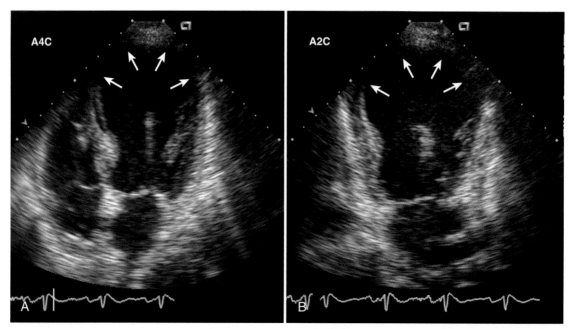

Figure 8–21. This apical true aneurysm shows a diastolic contour abnormality with a gradual, smooth transition from normal myocardial thickness to the thin scarred myocardial of the aneurysm and with systolic dyskinesis as shown by the arrows in the (A) apical 4-chamber (*A4C*) and (B) 2-chamber (*A2C*) end-diastolic images.

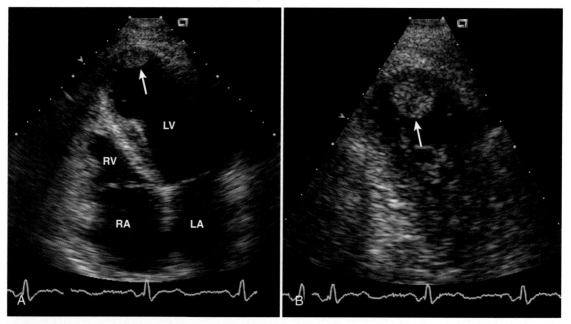

Figure 8–22. (A) This apical echodensity that protrudes into the chamber in an area of dyskinesis is consistent with an apical thrombus. (B) The zoomed image using a higher-frequency transducer and an oblique image plane through the apex, helps confirm that these echoes represent a thrombus, and not prominent trabeculation or an imaging artefact.

- ❏ Early in the disease course, diastolic dysfunction is characterized by impaired relaxation.
- ❏ However, as systolic function deteriorates, LV filling pressures may increase, LV compliance decreases, and the increased ventricular volumes result in a rightward shift along the LV diastolic pressure–volume curve.

Step 2: Evaluate regional left ventricular systolic function

- ■ Regional function is evaluated by grading each myocardial segment as normal, hypokinetic, akinetic, or dyskinetic.
- ■ Any areas of thin, scarred myocardium are noted.

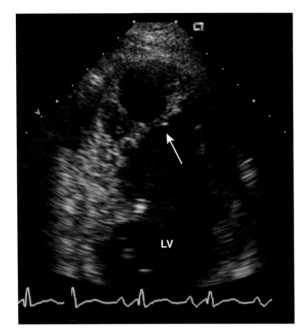

Figure 8–23. The apical trabeculation seen in this apical 2-chamber view is distinguished from thrombus by similar echodensity to myocardium, a linear structure that connects to the myocardium at both ends and the absence of an underlying wall motion abnormality.

Key points

❏ A discrete area of scarring or dyskinesis is consistent with coronary disease, rather than a primary cardiomyopathy.

❏ In both end-stage ischemic disease and primary cardiomyopathy, ventricular function typically is best preserved for the inferior-lateral and lateral basal segments of the LV.

Step 3: Evaluate right ventricular size and systolic function

■ RV size and systolic function are qualitatively evaluated as discussed in Chapter 6.

■ RV systolic function typically is normal in patients with end-stage ischemic disease, so that the RV appears small and hypercontractile compared with the dilated, hypokinetic LV. (Figure 8–25)

Key points

❏ When the RV is proportionate to the LV, the degree of RV dilation is similar to the degree of LV dilation.

❏ When RV systolic function appears similar to LV function, the degree of dysfunction is the same for both ventricles.

❏ RV function may be impaired in patients with coronary disease and a prior RV infarction.

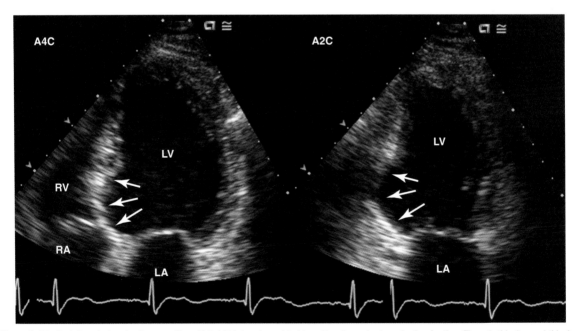

Figure 8–24. End-stage ischemic disease with a dilated LV chamber, global hypokinesis, and a low ejection fraction. There is thinning and thinning, increased echogenicity and dyskinesis (arrows) of the basal inferior septum (apical 4-chamber, A4C, view) and inferior wall (A2C view) on these end-systolic images, consistent with old infarction and myocardial scar.

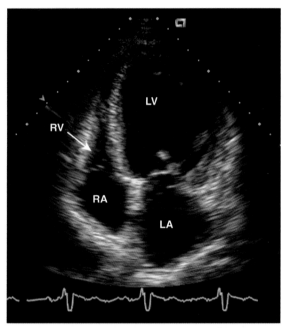

Figure 8–25. In patients with heart failure due to end-stage ischemic disease, RV size and systolic function often are normal (unless concurrent RV infarction has occurred). Compared to the dilated and hypokinetic LV, the normal RV appears relatively small and hyperdynamic.

Step 4: Estimate cardiac hemodynamics

- Pulmonary artery systolic pressure is estimated from the velocity of the tricuspid regurgitant jet and the appearance and respiratory variation of the inferior vena cava, as discussed in Chapter 6.
- Evidence for elevated left atrial pressure includes a prolonged and high-velocity pulmonary vein a-reversal and a high ratio of transmitral flow to tissue Doppler velocity in early diastole (See Chapter 7.)

Key points

- ❐ Pulmonary pressures may be elevated due to LV dysfunction, leading to chronic elevation of LA pressure and consequent pulmonary hypertension.
- ❐ Evidence for elevated filling pressures may no longer be present after optimization of medical therapy.

Step 5: Identify and evaluate any associated valve disease

- LV dilation and systolic dysfunction due to chronic valve disease may be difficult to distinguish from a primary cardiomyopathy or end-stage ischemic heart disease.
- LV systolic dysfunction of any cause often is accompanied by significant mitral valve regurgitation due to displacement of the papillary muscle, leaflet tethering, and annular dilation.

Key points

- ❐ Primary mitral valve disease is characterized by abnormalities of the valve leaflets or chordae—for example, myxomatous or rheumatic valve disease.
- ❐ With secondary mitral regurgitation, the mitral valve apparatus is anatomically normal but geometric relationships are altered by the dilated LV.
- ❐ Mitral regurgitation due to ischemic heart disease may improve with medical or interventional approaches for relief of ischemia.
- ❐ Coronary angiography may be needed to determine the contribution of coronary disease to the clinical cardiac dysfunction.

THE ECHO EXAM

Myocardial Ischemia

STRESS ECHO MODALITIES

Treadmill exercise
Supine bicycle
Dobutamine

DIGITAL CINE LOOP VIEWS

Short axis mid-cavity
Apical 4-chamber
Apical 2-chamber
Apical long-axis

INTERPRETATION

Exercise duration
Heart rate and blood pressure
Symptoms
Wall motion at rest and with stress
EF at rest and with stress

UTILITY

Diagnosis of coronary artery disease
Severity of disease
    Number of vessels involved
    Extent of myocardium at risk
Overall LV systolic function
Diastolic LV function
Clinical prognosis

End-Stage Ischemic Disease

LEFT VENTRICULAR SYSTOLIC DYSFUNCTION

Decreased ejection fraction
Decreased *dP/dt*
Regional pattern may be seen

RIGHT VENTRICULAR SYSTOLIC DYSFUNCTION

May be present with right ventricular (RV) infarction or
    elevated pulmonary pressures

MITRAL REGURGITATION (MR)

Diverse mechanisms of ischemic MR
    LV dilation and systolic dysfunction
    Regional wall motion abnormality
    Papillary muscle dysfunction or rupture
Quantitate severity (see Chapter 12)

LEFT VENTRICULAR ANEURYSM

Diastolic contour abnormality with dyskinesis
Thrombus formation

MEDICAL LIBRARY
MORRISTON HOSPITAL

Differentiation of Left Ventricular Systolic Dysfunction Due to End-Stage Ischemic Disease from Dilated Cardiomyopathy or Chronic Valvular Disease			
Findings	**End-Stage Ischemic Disease**	**Dilated Cardiomyopathy**	**Chronic Valvular Disease**
LV ejection fraction	Moderately to severely depressed	Moderately to severely depressed	Moderately to severely depressed
Segmental wall motion abnormalities	May be present	Absent	Absent
RV systolic function	Normal	Decreased	Variable
Pulmonary artery pressures	Elevated	Elevated	Elevated
Mitral regurgitation	Moderate	Moderate	Moderate/severe
Aortic regurgitation	Not significant	Not significant	Moderate/severe

Echo Views for Wall Motion

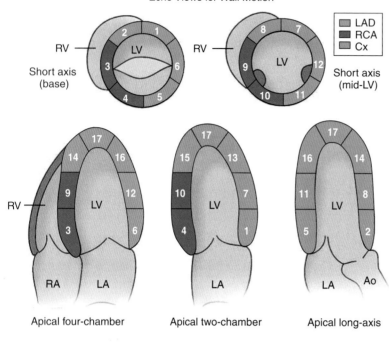

Echocardiographic views for wall motion evaluation. In the short-axis view, at the base and midventricular levels, the LV is divided into the anterior (1, 7), anterior-septal (2, 8), inferior septal (3, 9), inferior (4, 10), inferolateral (5, 11), and anterolateral (6, 12) segments. In the apical region there are four segments: anterior (13), septal (14), inferior (15), and lateral (16), plus the tip of the apex (17). The territory of the LAD artery is indicated in green, the RCA in red, and the left Cx coronary artery in yellow.

Stress Echocardiography

Parameter	Modality	View	Recording	Interpretation
Resting regional wall motion	2D	PSAX mid-cavity level A4C A2C Apical long axis	Depth that includes only LV Optimize endocardial definition Use contrast if needed	Select optimal image from series of digital cine loops
Stress regional wall motion	2D	PSAX mid-cavity level A4C A2C Apical long axis	Same depth as baseline Optimize endocardial definition Use contrast if needed	Compare optimal baseline and stress images in same views
Clinical and hemodynamic data		Symptoms Heart rate and rhythm Blood pressure	Continuous during exam Report values at each stage of stress	Maximal work load affects accuracy of echo results for detection of ischemia
LV systolic function	2D and Doppler	Ejection fraction *dP/dt*	Biplane apical ejection fraction CW Doppler MR jet	

PSAX, parasternal short axis view; A4C, apical 4-chamber view; A2C, apical 2-chamber view; EF, ejection fraction; MR, mitral regurgitation

Acute Myocardial Infarction

Detection of wall motion abnormalities
Evaluation of recurrent chest pain
Assessment of the response to reperfusion
Complications of acute myocardial infarction
    LV systolic dysfunction
    LV thrombus
    Aneurysm formation
    Acute mitral regurgitation
    Ventricular septal defect
    LV rupture (pseudo-aneurysm)
    Pericardial effusion

SELF-ASSESSMENT QUESTIONS

QUESTION 1

A 72-year-old woman presents with symptoms of transient right middle cerebral artery ischemia. Her medical history includes recent myocardial infarction and placement of a drug-eluting stent in the left anterior descending artery 2 weeks ago. Medications include aspirin, metoprolol, clopidogrel, lisinopril, and atorvastatin. A TTE (Figure 8–26) is completed.

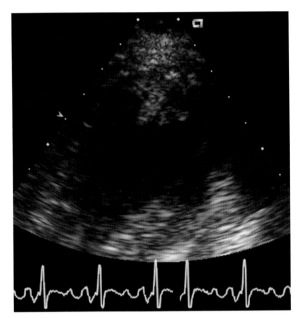

Figure 8–26.

You refer the patient for:

A. Patent foramen ovale closure
B. Pulmonary artery thrombectomy
C. Atrial myxoma resection
D. Warfarin therapy

QUESTION 2

A 54-year-old man is taken to the emergency department with chest pain lasting 2 hours. His blood pressure is 90/60 mm Hg with a heart rate of 106 bpm. Physical examination reveals jugular venous distention to 16 cm and bibasilar lung crackles. There is a systolic murmur at the cardiac apex radiating toward the left axilla and trace pedal edema. Transthoracic echocardiogram reveals a hypokinetic inferior wall with an ejection fraction of 42%. The RV is mildly dilated with systolic dysfunction. There is moderate mitral regurgitation. The tricuspid regurgitant jet velocity is 3.4 m/s and the inferior vena cava

diameter measures 2.1 cm, with minimal inspiratory collapse.

What is the most appropriate next step?

A. Right heart catheterization
B. Coronary angiography
C. Chest computed tomography
D. Transesophageal echocardiography

QUESTION 3

A 68-year-old man presents for dobutamine stress echocardiography. Image quality was not optimal and transpulmonary microbubble contrast was used. Resting LV function is normal, with an ejection fraction of 60%. The end-systolic images in the apical 4-chamber view at rest (Figure 8–27, *top*) and at peak dobutamine infusion (Figure 8–27, *bottom*) are presented.

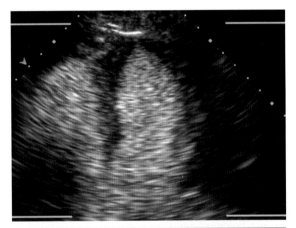

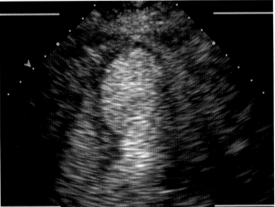

Figure 8–27.

The LV response to dobutamine in this case is best described as:

A. Akinetic
B. Biphasic
C. Hyperdynamic
D. Tethered

QUESTION 4

A 58-year-old man is preparing for hospital discharge after a myocardial infarct. He had presented with stuttering chest discomfort over 3 to 4 days and subsequently received a drug-eluting stent in the right coronary artery. Before discharge, a transthoracic echocardiogram is completed (Figure 8–28). Images from the subcostal short-axis view are shown.

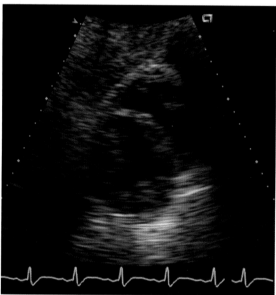

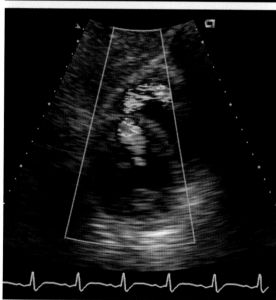

Figure 8–28.

Based on the images provided, which of the following additional findings would you expect on the echocardiogram?

A. Pulmonary to systemic shunt ratio = 2.4
B. Septal E' velocity = 0.1m/s
C. Tricuspid regurgitant velocity = 2.1m/s
D. Wall motion score index = 1

QUESTION 5

A 68-year-old woman presents to the emergency department with precordial chest discomfort that developed suddenly during a protracted argument with her estranged son. The patient has hypertension but is a non-smoker. Physical examination reveals flat neck veins. Her blood pressure is 158/98 mm Hg. Her lungs are clear and no murmurs are heard. The ECG shows diffuse ST elevation and her troponin is mildly elevated at 2.5 ng/mL (normal <0.5 ng/mL) with a normal B-type natriuretic peptide level. Transthoracic echocardiography demonstrates a maximal dimension of the ascending aorta at 3.8 cm and preserved sinotubular junction. There is hyperdynamic function of the basal LV segments; the rest of the LV is akinetic. There is no valvular dysfunction and no pericardial effusion. Estimated pulmonary systolic pressure is 40 to 45 mm Hg.

Which of the following is the most likely diagnosis?

A. Aortic dissection
B. Apical myocardial infarction
C. Pulmonary embolism
D. Stress cardiomyopathy

QUESTION 6

A 68-year-old woman presents with decreased responsiveness and failure to thrive. Her family relates a recent history of exertional dyspnea and she had been bedbound for the last several weeks. Before this, she had been able to participate in family outings. On physical examination, her blood pressure was 82/46 mm Hg and her heart rate 90 bpm. A grade III/VI holosystolic murmur at the apex is present and radiates toward the axilla. Her electrocardiogram shows Q waves in leads II III and aVF. A TTE is performed. An image from the apical 2-chamber view is shown (Figure 8–29).

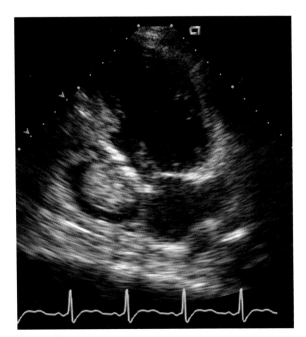

Figure 8-29.

The most likely diagnosis is LV:

A. Aneurysm
B. Pseudo-aneurysm
C. Septal rupture
D. Papillary muscle rupture

QUESTION 7

Which of the following is the earliest manifestation of myocardial ischemia detectable during stress echocardiography?

A. Anginal chest discomfort
B. ECG horizontal ST depression
C. Regional coronary hypoperfusion
D. Segmental wall motion abnormality

QUESTION 8

Which of the following patients will derive the most diagnostic value from stress echocardiography?

A. A 30-year-old woman with palpitations and normal resting ECG who now has fleeting chest pain on deep inspiration
B. An 80-year-old man who underwent coronary bypass surgery 13 years ago and now has recurrent typical angina
C. A 72-year-old diabetic woman with jaw pain and chest pressure that increases with activity and improves with rest
D. A 56-year-old man who had a coronary stent placed 1 year ago and now has chest pain at rest

QUESTION 9

A 74-year-old woman presents for evaluation for preoperative cardiovascular risk assessment for an upcoming hip replacement. In addition to her chronic hip pain, she describes left-sided chest pressure that occurs when walking slowly to her bus stop. Her symptoms stop once she is on the bus and resting. Her past medical history includes only medically treated hypertension. She is a non-smoker. Her physical examination is unremarkable.

Which diagnostic test is the best option for this patient?

A. No testing needed
B. Coronary angiography
C. Dobutamine stress echocardiogram
D. Treadmill stress echocardiogram

QUESTION 10

Which of the following factors most lowers the sensitivity of a treadmill stress echocardiography?

A. Delayed transpulmonary microbubble contrast
B. Increased LV wall thickness
C. Increased treadmill to stretcher transfer time
D. Multivessel coronary disease
E. Prolonged exercise duration

QUESTION 11

Which of the following provides the greatest advantage of bicycle ergometry over treadmill exercise for stress echocardiography?

A. Achieved maximal workload
B. Familiarity as a form of exercise
C. Increased dependence on patient cooperation
D. Timing of stress image acquisition

QUESTION 12

A 64-year-old woman undergoes treadmill stress echocardiography. End-systolic images at rest (Figure 8-30, *top*) and immediately after stress (Figure 8-30, *bottom*) are provided.

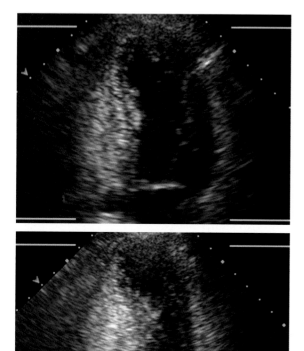

Figure 8–30.

Based on the images, what coronary distribution is most likely affected?

A.   Left anterior descending
B.   Right coronary artery
C.   Left main artery
D.   Left circumflex artery

ANSWERS

ANSWER 1: D

This is an anteriorly angulated 4-chamber view of the LV apex. There is a large apical thrombus. Thrombus formation occurs with blood stasis. A recent left anterior descending artery infarction likely resulted in anteroapical akinesis. Blood stasis in the akinetic apex can lead to thrombus formation, which can subsequently embolize peripherally, as occurred in this case. Warfarin therapy is indicated for 3 to 6 months, with a follow-up echocardiogram to monitor resolution of the thrombus. An embolic stroke can also result from a paradoxical embolus via a patent foramen ovale (PFO). However, in this case therapy for the LV thrombus is indicated, regardless of whether a PFO is present. In patients with a recurrent stroke despite warfarin therapy in whom a PFO is identified, closure of the PFO to reduce the risk of a paradoxical embolus may be considered. A pulmonary artery embolism does not pose increased risk of stroke and is not seen on this image. The image also is not typical of a myxoma and the mass is in the LV.

ANSWER 2: B

This symptomatic patient is presenting with cardiogenic shock and an echocardiogram with evidence of an inferior wall infarct. Patients with inferior wall ischemia may develop mitral regurgitation due to infarct involvement of the posterolateral papillary muscle. In this patient, ischemia has involved the RV as well, exacerbating hemodynamic instability. Prompt coronary angiography with percutaneous revascularization should restore coronary blood flow and improve myocardial function in ischemic regions. If the posterolateral papillary muscle is frankly infarcted, necrosis and rupture of the papillary muscle can occur, which is an indication for urgent mitral valve replacement. Right heart catheterization provides a direct intravascular measurement of pulmonary pressures and cardiac output. In this case, the transthoracic study was diagnostic for mitral regurgitation, regional wall motion abnormality, and pulmonary hypertension; additional diagnostic information from a right heart catheterization is not needed. Chest computed tomography allows for evaluation of the aorta and great vessels to assess for aortic aneurysm, dissection, and pulmonary embolism. This patient's clinical presentation, with cardiogenic shock and heart failure, is most consistent with an acute coronary syndrome rather than an acute aortic process or pulmonary embolism. Transesophageal echocardiography provides improved visualization of posterior structures such as the mitral valve. In this case, the regional wall motion abnormalities and significant mitral regurgitation were adequately identified by transthoracic imaging, and a transesophageal echocardiogram would provide little additional information.

ANSWER 3: A

This is an abnormal stress echocardiogram. The resting image shows a normal LV contour and wall thickness consistent with normal endocardial motion for all myocardial segments in systole. At peak stress, there is a contour abnormality of the apical $\frac{2}{3}$ of the inferior septum and the entire apex consistent with lack of systolic inward motion, whereas the basal $\frac{2}{3}$ of the lateral wall shows increased inward motion compared with the baseline image. All segments returned to normal function during recovery. Thus, this stress image is consistent with ischemia, with exercise-induced akinesis in the LV septum and apex. Subsequent coronary angiography demonstrated a 90% occlusion of the right coronary artery and an 80% occlusion of the left anterior descending artery.

A biphasic response describes the LV response of hibernating myocardium to low-dose dobutamine. In patients with severe LV dysfunction and akinetic regions at rest, an increase in contractility of the akinetic zones at very low doses of dobutamine (approximately 5 mcg/kg/min) followed by akinesis at higher infusion doses (approximately 20-30 mcg/kg/min) is consistent with a "biphasic" response. This response is the effect of ischemic but not infarcted myocardium, which responds with increased inotropy at a very low dose of dobutamine but becomes akinetic at higher doses due to an increased oxygen demand that exceeds the ischemic threshold of the myocardium. A hyperdynamic response refers to increased endocardial motion of the LV and a decrease in systolic cavity size, which is normal and consistent with no impairment in coronary flow (not seen in this case). In patients with a transmural infarct, a resting regional wall motion abnormality is present and there is no augmentation of wall thickening with dobutamine. Normal myocardium adjacent to infarcted tissue may have decreased systolic motion due to "tethering" from the akinetic, infarcted region. In this case, resting LV function was normal without infarction at baseline.

ANSWER 4: A

This is a subcostal short-axis view of the heart. The liver is seen on the left of the image with the heart on the right showing a short-axis view of the mid LV and RV. The interventricular septum is thin, bright, and scarred, consistent with prior infarct. Color Doppler imaging shows flow toward the transducer across the infarct, consistent with ventricular septal rupture. The ratio of the stroke volume in the pulmonary artery (Qp) to the stroke volume in the LV outflow tract (Qs) would be increased, representing the additional volume of flow across the defect from the higher-pressure LV into the RV. Ischemic ventricular septal rupture is a rare complication after a myocardial infarct and typically occurs several days after the infarct event. Most patients present with acute cardiac symptoms and hypotension, but some patients are relatively asymptomatic initially. The rupture may be evident as a systolic murmur on physical examination; echocardiography usually is diagnostic. The treatment is surgical, or more recently percutaneous, closure of the defect because mortality is more than 90% without intervention.

A septal E′ velocity of 0.1 m/s implies normal septal tissue velocity. With a septal infarct, myocardial velocity should be severely reduced, generally less than 0.05 m/s. With the left to right shunt, pulmonary pressures should be increased, whereas a tricuspid jet velocity of only 2.1 m/s implies normal pulmonary pressures. The wall motion score index is a quantitative measure of regional wall motion, based on the mean wall motion score for all myocardial segments, using a grade of 1 and 4, where 1 is normal motion, 2 is hypokinetic, 3 is akinetic, and 4 is dyskinetic. Thus, a wall motion score index of 1 implies normal LV function in all segments and is not consistent with a myocardial infarction.

ANSWER 5: D

This elderly woman most likely has stress cardiomyopathy, an acute cardiac syndrome also called Takotsubo cardiomyopathy or transient apical ballooning. The clinical presentation is acute chest pain or dyspnea after significant emotional or physiologic stress. The clinical manifestation is transient akinesis or dyskinesis of the apical and mid-ventricular segments of the LV that extend beyond a single epicardial coronary distribution. An end-systolic image from this patient's ventriculogram is presented (Figure 8–31).

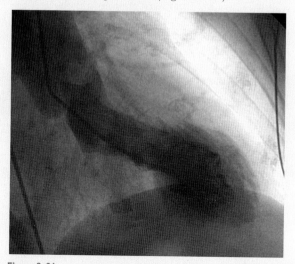

Figure 8-31.

Angiography demonstrates absence of obstructive coronary disease. Stress cardiomyopathy, although rare, has a strong female predominance (>90%). Catecholamine excess in the setting of microvascular disease has been implicated. Other findings include ST-segment elevation on ECG that exceeds biomarker measurement of necrosis. Outcome of stress cardiomyopathy is generally good, and LV functional recovery is likely with supportive care. Pericarditis should be considered in the differential of this patient. However, the wall motion abnormalities observed would be out of proportion to acute pericarditis, even if myopericarditis were present. Also, although not a definitive exclusion criteria, the absence of pericardial fluid lowers likelihood of pericarditis. Aortic dissection is a diagnosis of exclusion. The patient's ascending aorta is mildly dilated, a consequence of her history of medically treated hypertension. Transthoracic echocardiography can visualize the proximal portion of the ascending aorta relatively well but often does not provide the image quality adequate to definitively exclude dissection. However, the pattern of LV dysfunction is not typical for dissection, which can present with regional wall motion abnormalities if the dissection flap involves a coronary artery ostium, or may show aortic regurgitation if there is retrograde dissection to the aortic valve. Although pulmonary embolism is also in the differential diagnosis for this patient, the echocardiogram is compelling for a primary myocardial process. This patient has no known history of coronary disease. Although the echocardiogram findings might be consistent with multivessel disease (more than one epicardial coronary distribution), they are discordant, with the relatively low serum biomarker values for myocardial necrosis. Therefore, stress cardiomyopathy, rather than epicardial coronary occlusion with apical myocardial infarction, is the more likely diagnosis.

ANSWER 6: B

This patient has an LV pseudo-aneurysm, which is a rare complication of myocardial infarction. The apical 2-chamber view shows a thinned and akinetic basal inferior wall with an abrupt transition between the basal infarct and the normal myocardial thickness of the mid-inferior wall. In the mid-portion of the infarct is a small echolucent region, consistent with a myocardial rupture, and there is a large thrombus in a contained space adjacent to the infarct. These findings (abrupt transition of myocardial thickness, narrow neck, contained thrombus) are all consistent with LV pseudo-aneurysm. Because an LV pseudo-aneurysm is an LV rupture that has been contained by adherent pericardium, prompt surgical intervention is needed.

A true LV aneurysm is defined as a diastolic contour abnormality of the LV with dyskinesis in systole. The walls of a true aneurysm consist of thin, scarred myocardium (not pericardium as with a pseudo-aneurysm) and there is a smooth transition from normal to infarcted myocardium with a wide neck of the aneurysm. Thrombus may be present in either a true or pseudo-aneurysm and so does not distinguish between them. The differential diagnosis of a new murmur after myocardial infarction also includes mitral regurgitation, due to papillary muscle dysfunction or rupture, or ventricular septal rupture, with left to right flow across the defect. Neither of those complications is evident on this image.

ANSWER 7: D

The sequential progression of myocardial ischemia during stress echocardiography is initiated by relative regional hypoperfusion distal to a coronary occlusion provoked by increased myocardial oxygen demand. With regional hypoperfusion, metabolic changes occur within the affected myocardium. After this, there are alterations in LV diastolic function. With continued ischemia, there is onset of impaired systolic function in the ischemic region. Only with prolonged ischemia do characteristic electrocardiographic changes, such as horizontal ST depression, and typical angina manifest. However, on standard stress echocardiography, regional coronary hypoperfusion cannot be visualized, so the earliest change seen is a segmental wall motion abnormality. Although evaluation of diastole during stress echocardiography is conceptually possible, practical application of diastolic interrogation is difficult to routinely implement.

ANSWER 8: D

Patient D has known coronary disease with symptom onset in a time frame consistent with re-stenosis. Thus, although his pain is atypical because it occurs at rest, stress echocardiography is reasonable to determine if symptoms are provoked with increased myocardial oxygen demand. The diagnostic value of any testing modality is greatest when it significantly increases likelihood for a significant coronary lesion (based on a positive result) or lowers likelihood with a negative result. Therefore, the greatest clinical utility for stress echocardiography is in those with an intermediate pretest probability of disease, based on symptom profile and cardiovascular risk factors. In patients with a low pretest probability of disease, a positive test is more likely to be a false positive and thus not helpful in decision making. Similarly, in individuals with a high pretest probability of disease, a negative result likely is a false negative and further testing will still be appropriate. Patient A is young, with non-anginal symptoms; the pretest likelihood of disease is so low that counseling and reassurance, without diagnostic testing, is indicated. Patient B has known coronary disease with recurrent typical angina

and thus has a very high likelihood of a new significant coronary stenosis. As a diabetic, patient C is in a high-risk subset and presents with classic exertional angina. Both patients B and C have a high pretest probability of disease and thus would more likely benefit from direct coronary angiography because a negative result on a stress echocardiogram in a patient with ongoing symptoms is likely a false negative.

ANSWER 9: C

This patient ha exertional symptoms that are concerning for angina. Her cardiovascular risk factors include an older age and hypertension. She is under evaluation for hip replacement. Given her symptoms, cardiovascular diagnostic testing is reasonable. In patients who are able to exercise adequately, treadmill stress is preferred over pharmacologic testing. This allows assessment of exercise tolerance and determination of the threshold where symptoms are provoked. Exercise duration is a good prognostic marker. However, in patients whose physical limitations may hinder maximal exertion, pharmacologic stress is a reasonable alternative. In this case the patient is scheduled for hip surgery, and exercise performance on the treadmill will likely be hindered. Coronary angiography allows for direct visualization of intraluminal occlusion but does not assess for the hemodynamic significance of blockages. The primary focus of preoperative cardiovascular assessment is to determine the cardiac response to the physiologic stress of anesthesia and surgery. Assessing the cardiac response to a stressor, rather than just identifying intraluminal occlusion, is more appropriate for risk assessment.

ANSWER 10: C

Because induced regional wall motion abnormalities may resolve quickly once adequate oxygen supply is reestablished, rapid post-stress imaging to identify myocardial dysfunction is critical. Images should be obtained 90 seconds after completion of exercise, ideally within 60 seconds, to increase likelihood of detecting abnormalities. We have the patient practice the transfer from the treadmill to the imaging stretcher before beginning the test to ensure the patient understands the sequence of events and is comfortable with the process.

Transpulmonary microbubble contrast allows for improved endocardial border definition in patients for whom image quality is suboptimal, which improves the sensitivity of stress echocardiography. A delay in transit time would not significantly affect LV opacification. Increased LV wall thickness, or LV hypertrophy, can lead to false positive electrocardiographic findings but does not affect echocardiographic identification of myocardial dysfunction. Exercise duration only affects test sensitivity if the patient fails to achieve an adequate workload; in this situation, there is no evident wall motion abnormality because oxygen delivery to the myocardial segment does not fall below the ischemic threshold. However, prolonged exercise duration indicates a fit individual and does not limit sensitivity of the stress test. In general, the sensitivity of stress echocardiography is higher with multivessel compared with single vessel coronary disease because the area of ischemic myocardium is larger. However, with "balanced" ischemia in all myocardial beds, a discrete wall motion abnormality may not be evident; instead there is a lack of the normal decrease in chamber size and increase in endocardial motion with stress. As long as the echocardiographer recognizes these findings by comparing stress images to rest images, sensitivity of stress echocardiography for multivessel disease remains high.

ANSWER 11: D

Bicycle ergometry allows for echocardiographic imaging during exercise stress. Acquisition of peak stress images from the apical window can be obtained during active exercise. For treadmill stress, imaging at peak stress during active exercise is procedurally difficult, and imaging is performed after exercise cessation once the patient transfers from the treadmill to the imaging bed. Thus, bicycle ergometry offers the advantage of optimizing imaging without the "all-or nothing" constraints of a narrow, immediate post-treadmill stress time window. However, treadmill stress is generally favored over bicycle ergometry because of the familiarity of walking as a form of exercise. Also, there is widespread availability of treadmills given treadmill electrocardiography testing as an established diagnostic modality. With bicycle ergometry, exercise workload is effort driven. Resistance of the bicycle is increased at preset intervals; patients keep up with the resistance and maintain a consistent cadence during the protocol. For treadmill protocols, the treadmill automatically increases speed and incline at each stage and the patient only has to match increases to continue the protocol. Because maintaining consistent achievement of maximal

workload is more patient dependent with bicycle ergometry than with treadmill protocols, maximal workload is more variable. Patients performing upright treadmill exercise are generally able to achieve a higher workload, increasing the likelihood of attaining hemodynamic targets. Additionally, with supine bicycle ergometry, patients may feel awkward because the lower extremities are supported against gravity and may prematurely cease exercise if leg fatigue precedes maximal workload.

ANSWER 12: A

The images provided are from the apical 2-chamber view. The descending thoracic aorta is seen in cross section adjacent to the base of the posterior mitral valve leaflet to the left of the heart. At rest, the chamber size is small and the myocardial walls are thick along the entire left ventricle, consistent with normal wall motion. After peak stress, the anterior wall and apex appear thin relative to the inferior wall, reflecting lack of systolic wall thickening consistent with ischemia. There is hyperdynamic function of the non-ischemic myocardium, with increased myocardial thickening of the inferior wall and a decrease in overall LV chamber size. These findings are most consistent with occlusion of a left anterior descending artery that "wraps around" and supplies the LV apex.

The posterior descending coronary artery, which most often arises from the right coronary artery, does not typically serve the entire apex, and involvement of the anterior wall is more suggestive of a left anterior descending artery lesion. The myocardial regions supplied by the left circumflex artery are the postero-lateral and anterolateral segments. These are best seen on the apical 4-chamber and apical long-axis views, which are not included on the images provided. A left main coronary occlusion would cause ischemia in both the left anterior descending artery and left circumflex artery (whose myocardial distribution is not shown). With a left main coronary occlusion, the myocardial ischemic burden is significant and LV dilation with stress, rather than compensatory hyperdynamic function of nonischemic segments, is typically seen.

9 Cardiomyopathies, Hypertensive and Pulmonary Heart Disease

CARDIOMYOPATHIES

General step-by-step approach

An overall approach to patients with a known or suspected cardiomyopathy is reviewed, followed by specific features of each type of cardiomyopathy.

Step 1: Measure LV chamber size and systolic function

LV chamber size

■ Two-dimensional or 2D guided M-mode measurement of LV minor axis internal dimensions at end-diastole and end-systole. (Figure 9–1)
■ Apical biplane calculation of end-diastolic and end-systolic ventricular volumes. (Figure 9–2)

Key points

❏ LV internal dimensions are measured from the parasternal window because the ultrasound beam is perpendicular to the blood–myocardial interface, providing high axial resolution.

❏ 2D imaging in long- and short-axis views is used to ensure that the dimension is measured in the minor axis of the ventricle (not at an oblique angle, which would overestimate size).

❏ On 2D images, the white–black (tissue–blood) interface is used to measure LV dimensions.

❏ The rapid sampling rate of M-mode (compared with the slow frame rate of 2D imaging) provides more accurate identification of the endocardial borders. (Figure 9–3)

❏ Two-dimensional guided M-mode measurements are most accurate when the ultrasound beam can be aligned perpendicular to the LV wall of interest.

❏ For sequential studies, measurements should be made with the same method at the same location.

❏ Apical biplane ventricular volumes are indexed to body surface area.

LV systolic function

■ LV ejection fraction (EF) is calculated using the apical biplane approach.

167

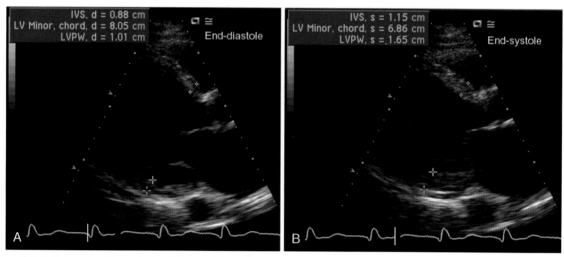

Figure 9–1. In the parasternal long-axis view, LV minor axis internal dimensions are measured at (A) end-diastole (onset of the QRS) and (B) end-systole (minimal LV volume just before aortic valve closure) from the septum to the posterior wall at the level of the mitral valve chords. The dimension is measured perpendicular to the long axis of the ventricle. Because the ultrasound beam is perpendicular to the myocardial–blood interface, the endocardium appears as a distinct edge, although, as in this example of a patient with a dilated ventricle, the septal endocardium typically is more clearly defined that the posterior wall endocardium, due to muscular trabeculations and overlying chords.

- LV dP/dt is calculated from the mitral regurgitation velocity curve. (Figure 9–4)
- Forward cardiac output is measured in the LV outflow tract.
- Regional ventricular function is evaluated qualitatively as normal, hypokinetic, or akinetic for each myocardial segment. (see Chapter 8)

Key points

- ❑ Ejection fraction measured by the apical biplane method is compared with the visually estimated ejection fraction.
- ❑ The traced endocardial borders are reviewed for accuracy and retraced if the estimated and measured ejection fractions differ by more than 10 ejection fraction units.
- ❑ Echo-contrast is used to enhance identification of endocardial borders when image quality is suboptimal.
- ❑ Measured ejection fraction is reported whenever possible. The estimated ejection fraction is reported only if endocardial borders cannot be traced accurately.
- ❑ Ejection fraction is an imperfect measure of contractility because it is affected by loading conditions. Even so, ejection fraction is useful for clinical decision making.
- ❑ LV dP/dt and forward stroke volume are other useful parameters of LV systolic function. (see Chapter 6)
- ❑ Indirect qualitative indicators of LV systolic dysfunction include M-mode findings of reduced aortic root motion and increased E-point septal separation. (Figure 9–5)

Evaluate for other cause of LV dilation and systolic dysfunction

- A cardiomyopathy is defined as a primary disease of the myocardium in the absence of coronary or valvular disease.
- Evaluate for evidence for other causes of LV dilation and dysfunction, specifically valve disease (aortic stenosis, mitral regurgitation, or aortic regurgitation) and coronary artery disease.

Key points

- ❑ LV dilation and dysfunction due to coronary disease with myocardial infarction or hibernation can be difficult to distinguish from a primary cardiomyopathy (see Chapter 8).
- ❑ Mitral regurgitation may be a cause or a consequence of LV dilation and dysfunction. When more than mild mitral regurgitation (vena contracta > 3 mm) is present, careful quantitative evaluation may be helpful (see Chapter 12). (Figure 9–6)
- ❑ The degree of aortic valve leaflet opening is reduced when LV dysfunction is present, making it difficult to separate severe aortic stenosis resulting in LV dysfunction from moderate aortic stenosis with coincidental LV dysfunction. (see Chapter 11). (Figure 9–7)

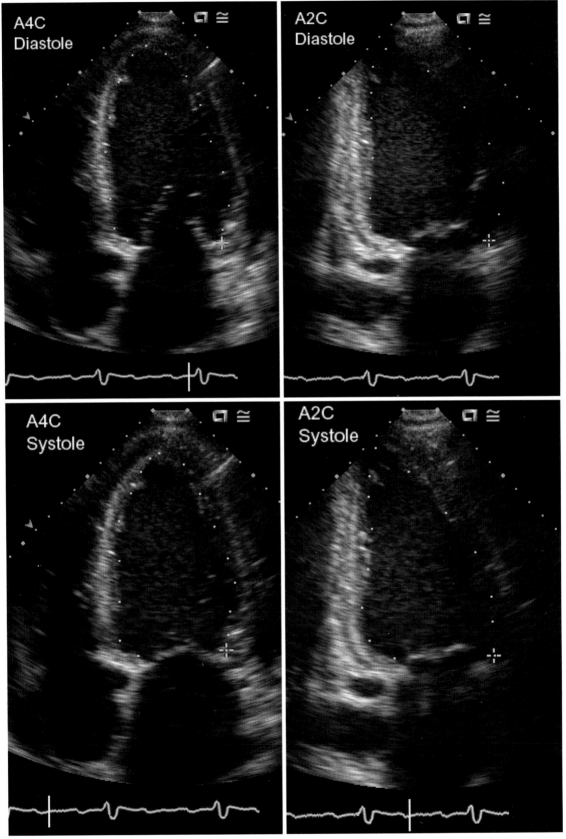

Figure 9–2. Apical biplane calculation of ejection fraction is based on tracing endocardial borders at end-diastole (*A*) and end-systole (*B*) in the 4-chamber view (*A* and *B*) and in the 2-chamber view (*C* and *D*). Foreshortened apical views are avoided by positioning the patient in a steep left lateral position with an apical cutout in the stretcher to allow the transducer to be positioned on the true apex and after moving the transducer down one or more interspaces.

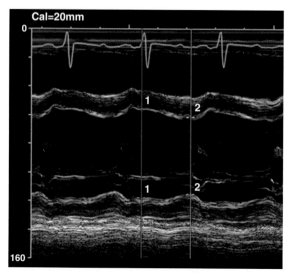

Figure 9–3. M-mode tracing of the LV recorded using 2D echocardiography to ensure the M-line is perpendicular to the long-axis of the LV in the parasternal long axis view and in the middle of the chamber in the short-axis view. The rapid sampling rate of the M-mode recording (time on the horizontal axis) provides more accurate identification and measurement of septal and posterior wall thickness and ventricular chamber dimensions at end-diastole (*1,* onset of QRS) and end-systole (*2,* maximum posterior motion of septum).

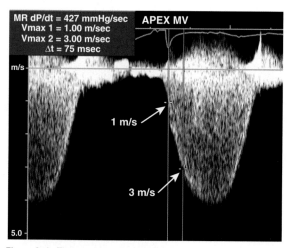

Figure 9–4. The rate of increase in velocity of the mitral regurgitant jet is markedly reduced in early systole. The calculated *dP/dt* of 427 mm Hg/s indicated severely reduced LV contractility.

Step 2: Evaluate for the presence and pattern of ventricular hypertrophy

Presence and severity of LV hypertrophy

- 2D guided M-mode measurement of LV wall thickness. (Figure 9–8)
- Calculation of LV mass in selected cases

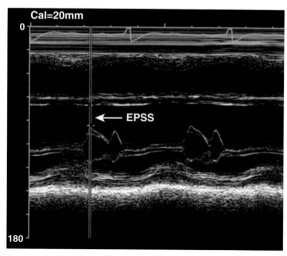

Figure 9–5. M-mode tracing at the level of the mitral valve shows a marked increase in the E-point septal separation (EPSS) consistent with severe LV systolic dysfunction.

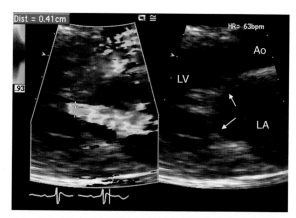

Figure 9–6. Mitral regurgitation in a patient with dilated cardiomyopathy due to tethering of the leaflets (*arrows*) with central regurgitant jet. The vena contracta width of 4 mm is consistent with moderate regurgitation.

Key Points

☐ Two-dimensional guided M-mode measurement of LV wall thickness at end-diastole (onset of the QRS) is adequate in most cases.

☐ Calculation of LV mass from traced 2D endocardial and epicardial borders is largely limited to research applications (see Figure 6–9).

Pattern of LV hypertrophy

- Long-axis, short-axis, and apical views are used to evaluate the pattern of ventricular hypertrophy (Figures 9–9 and 9–10).

Key points

☐ Two-dimensional imaging allows evaluation of the pattern of hypertrophy in all myocardial segments.

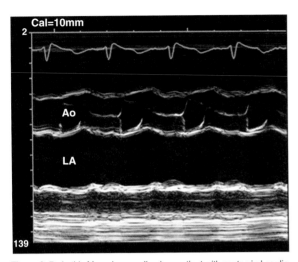

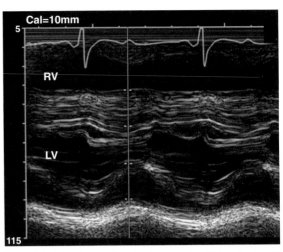

Figure 9–7. In this M-mode recording in a patient with acute viral cardio-myopathy, the aortic tracing shows reduced anterior-posterior motion of the root due to a reduced cardiac output. In addition, the aortic valve leaflets do not remain fully opened during systole due to low transaortic flow.

Figure 9–8. M-mode recording showing concentric LV hypertrophy with increased wall thickness and a small LV chamber. The rapid sampling rate of the M-mode recording allows more accurate identification of the endocardial and epicardial LV walls.

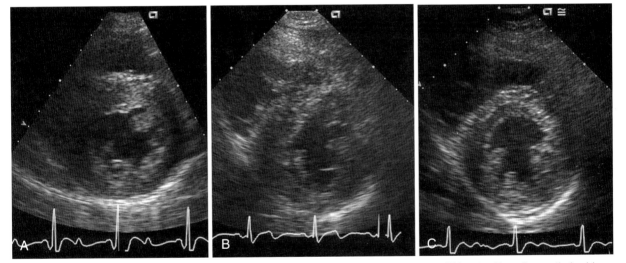

Figure 9–9. Parasternal short-axis images in three different patients showing (A) concentric LV hypertrophy, (B) hypertrophic cardiomyopathy involving the septum and anterior wall with sparing of the inferior-lateral and lateral walls, and (C) apical hypertrophic cardiomyopathy with hypertrophy of the inferior, posterior, and lateral walls but a relatively normal septum and anterior wall.

❏ When hypertrophy is concentric, LV wall thickness measurements at one site adequately represent the degree of hypertrophy.

❏ When hypertrophy is asymmetric, measurements at key sites are reported, particularly the septal thickness in patients with hypertrophic cardiomyopathy.

❏ Two-dimensional guided M-mode measurements are most accurate when the ultrasound beam can be aligned perpendicular to the LV wall of interest. Otherwise, 2D measurements at end-diastole are reported.

Step 3: Assess LV diastolic function (see chapter 7)

■ LV and LA inflow patterns. (Figure 9–11)
■ Tissue Doppler at the mitral annulus. (Figure 9–12)
■ Isovolumic relaxation time (IVRT). (Figure 9–13)

Key points

❏ Systolic LV dysfunction typically is accompanied by some degree of diastolic dysfunction.

❏ Classification of the degree of diastolic dysfunction as mild (impaired relaxation) versus severe

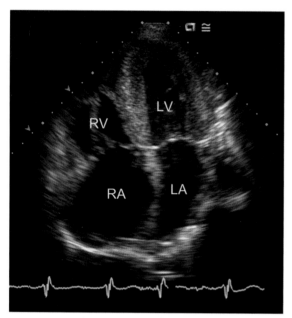

Figure 9–10. Concentric LV hypertrophy in an apical 4-chamber view shows equal thickness of the septum and lateral wall.

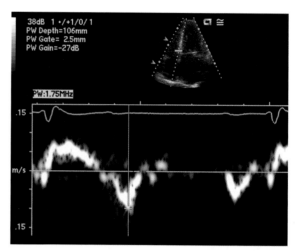

Figure 9–12. Tissue Doppler at the mitral annulus shows an E′ less than 0.10 m/s, with an E′ greater than A′, in the same patient as Figure 9–11. The ratio of transmitral E velocity to tissue Doppler E′ velocity is 2.2/0.10 = 22, which is severely elevated, consistent with a high LA pressure.

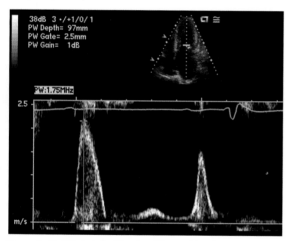

Figure 9–11. LV diastolic filling in a 62-year-old patient with a dilated cardiomyopathy showing an increased E/A ratio with a steep early diastolic deceleration slope. The E > A in this patient older than age 50, in association with a steep deceleration slope, suggests severe LV diastolic dysfunction with elevated filling pressures.

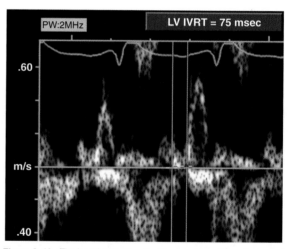

Figure 9–13. The isovolumic relaxation time, measured from the end of aortic ejection flow to the onset of mitral inflow, is normal at 75 ms in this patient with dilated cardiomyopathy.

(decreased compliance) is used in clinical decision making.

❏ LV filling pressures are estimated whenever systolic dysfunction is present.

Step 4: Estimate pulmonary artery pressures (see chapter 6)

■ Pulmonary systolic pressure is estimated from the tricuspid regurgitant jet velocity and estimated RA pressure. (Figures 9–14 and 9–15)

■ Other signs of pulmonary hypertension include a short time to peak velocity in the pulmonary artery velocity curve, paradoxical septal motion, and a high end-diastolic pulmonic regurgitant velocity

Key points

❏ Pulmonary pressures often are elevated in patients with heart failure due to a cardiomyopathy.

❏ Pulmonary pressures may be reduced with effective medical therapy, in conjunction with a decrease in LA (or LV filling) pressure.

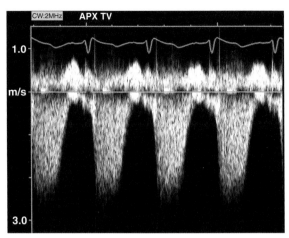

Figure 9–14. This tricuspid regurgitant jet velocity has a peak somewhere around 2.5 m/s. This signal is not ideal because the peak is not well defined. This likely is due to the position of the ultrasound beam relative to the jet and the use of color coding (instead of gray scale) for the spectral display, which often obscures the peak velocity with superimposed noise. However, the peak velocity of about 2.4 m/s indicates a RV–to–RA systolic pressure difference of 23 mm Hg.

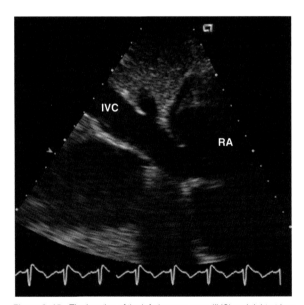

Figure 9–15. The junction of the inferior vena cava (IVC) and right atrium (RA) is visualized from the subcostal window for estimating RA pressure. In this patient, the IVC diameter is about 2.5 cm and collapses less than 50% with inspiration, consistent with an RA pressure of 10 to 15 mm Hg.

❑ When pulmonary pressures are elevated disproportionately to the degree of left-sided heart dysfunction, concurrent primary pulmonary disease or pulmonary thromboembolism may be present.

Step 5: Evaluate RV size and systolic function (see chapter 6)

■ RV size and systolic function are assessed from parasternal, apical, and subcostal views. (Figure 9–16)

Key points

❑ RV systolic dysfunction may be due to primary myocardial disease affecting both ventricles or to the effects of pulmonary hypertension.
❑ Qualitative assessment of RV size and function takes into account the degree of LV dilation and dysfunction. If there is severe LV dilation and dysfunction and the RV appears similar in size and function, then severe RV dilation and dysfunction also is present.
❑ RV lengthwise systolic shortening or tricuspid annular plane systolic excursion (TAPSE) is less than 2 cm when moderate or severe RV dysfunction is present.

Step 6: Evaluate the severity of mitral and tricuspid regurgitation (see chapter 12)

■ Mitral and tricuspid regurgitation often are present in patients with a cardiomyopathy.
■ Regurgitant severity is evaluated using standard approaches, starting with the color Doppler vena contracta and the continuous wave (CW) Doppler velocity curve.
■ The mechanism of regurgitation is evaluated using 2D imaging from multiple views.

Key points

❑ Mitral and tricuspid regurgitation due to LV dilation and dysfunction are common.
❑ The mechanism of atrioventricular valve regurgitation is "tethering" of the mitral leaflets resulting in incomplete systolic coaptation. This also has been described as an increased angle between the papillary muscles so that the leaflets are "pulled apart" relative to the mitral annulus. (Figure 9–17)
❑ The degree of annular dilation is variable, with a variable contribution to the degree of mitral regurgitation.
❑ Mitral regurgitant severity may decrease with effective medical or resynchronization therapy for heart failure.

Step 7: Evaluate LA size (see chapter 2)

■ LA size typically is increased either due to chronic elevation of LV filling pressures or to coexisting mitral regurgitation. (see Figure 2–22)

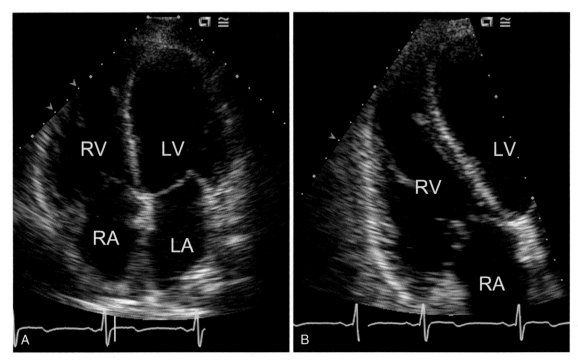

Figure 9–16. The RV is imaged from the apical 4-chamber view (A) by tilting the transducer toward the RV and narrowing the sector (B).

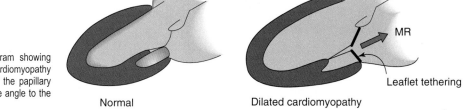

Figure 9–17. Schematic diagram showing leaflet tethering with dilated cardiomyopathy due to lateral displacement of the papillary muscles, resulting in an oblique angle to the mitral annulus.

Normal   Dilated cardiomyopathy

■ LA size can be evaluated qualitatively, using a simple anterior-posterior dimension, or by calculation of atrial volume from apical views.

Key points

❐ LA anterior-posterior dimension is measured in a long-axis view at end-systole (maximum LA dimension).
❐ Although atrial volumes are predictive of clinical outcome, simpler measures of atrial size suffice for clinical decision making in many cases.
❐ When clinically indicated, LA volume is calculated from tracing the LA border at end-systole in apical 4-chamber and 2-chamber views. LA volume then is indexed for body size.

❐ RA size also may be increased and is evaluated qualitatively (as mild, moderately, or severely dilated) in comparison to the other cardiac chambers.

Additional steps

Dilated cardiomyopathy

■ Evaluate for LV apical thrombus (Figure 9–18).
■ Differentiate from end-stage coronary disease. (Table 9-1)
■ Differentiate LV dysfunction due to severe mitral regurgitation from a primary cardiomyopathy with secondary mitral regurgitation. (Table 9-2)
■ Ensure an accurate ejection fraction calculation.

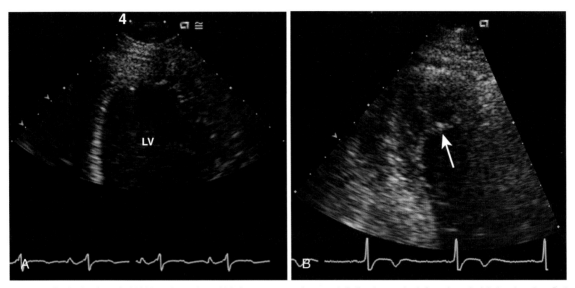

Figure 9–18. Evaluation for apical LV thrombus using a high-frequency transducer and shallow image depth from the apical 4-chamber view. Both of these examples show normal apical trabeculation, which is distinguished from thrombus by the linear appearance with attachments to the myocardial wall.

TABLE 9-1 Differentiation of Left Ventricular Systolic Dysfunction Due to End-Stage Ischemic Disease from Dilated Cardiomyopathy

Findings	End-Stage Ischemic Disease	Dilated Cardiomyopathy
LV ejection fraction	Moderate to severely depressed	Moderate to severely depressed
Segmental wall motion abnormalities	May be present	Absent
RV systolic function	Normal	Decreased
Pulmonary artery pressures	Elevated	Elevated
Other tests	Coronary disease on angiography or chest CT	No significant coronary disease

CT, computed tomography.

TABLE 9-2 Differentiation of LV Systolic Dysfunction Due to Dilated Cardiomyopathy from Primary Mitral Regurgitation

Findings	Dilated Cardiomyopathy	Chronic Mitral Regurgitation
Left ventricular ejection fraction	Moderate to severely depressed	Moderate to severely depressed
Segmental wall motion abnormalities	Absent	Absent
Right ventricular systolic function	Decreased	Variable
Pulmonary artery pressures	Elevated	Elevated
Mitral regurgitation	Moderate	Moderate to severe
Mitral valve anatomy	• Dilated annulus • Abnormal papillary muscle—annular angle • Leaflet tethering	• Primary leaflet involvement • Rheumatic changes *or* • Leaflet prolapse or flail segment

Key points

- ❑ Decision making for placement of an automated implanted defibrillator is based on the calculated EF, with the breakpoint typically at an EF less than 35% after optimal medical therapy.
- ❑ Examination for LV apical thrombus includes oblique views of the LV apex using a high-frequency transducer and shallow image depth.
- ❑ Transesophageal echocardiography (TEE) is not useful to evaluate for apical thrombus due to the distance of the apex from the transducer and the likelihood that the true apex may be missed from this approach.
- ❑ LV systolic dysfunction due to coronary disease and to a primary cardiomyopathy may look similar on echocardiography. Both may show wall motion that is best preserved at the inferior-lateral base.
- ❑ Features that suggest end-stage coronary disease include: definite evidence for myocardial infarction (segmental thinning and akinesis) and normal RV size and systolic function. However, direct visualization of coronary anatomy by conventional catheter or computed tomographic (CT) angiography typically is needed.
- ❑ Stress echocardiography is difficult to interpret with significant resting LV systolic dysfunction with a suboptimal sensitivity and specificity for detection of ischemia.
- ❑ Dyssynchrony evaluation is being studied as one possible approach to patient selection for biventricular pacing therapy.

Hypertrophic cardiomyopathy

Step 1: LV hypertrophy

- ■ Describe the anatomic pattern of hypertrophy. (Figure 9–19)
- ■ Evaluate the end-diastolic wall thickness of the basal posterior wall.
- ■ Measure the maximal end-diastolic septal thickness. Wall thickness measurements should be taken from both long-axis and short-axis views of the ventricle.

Key points

- ❑ The most common pattern of hypertrophy involves the ventricular septum with a normal posterior LV wall.
- ❑ Apical hypertrophy may be missed unless echo-contrast is used to opacify the ventricle, because the endocardial border in the mid-LV may be difficult to visualize. (Figure 9–20)
- ❑ Even with atypical patterns of hypertrophy, the basal posterior wall thickness typically is normal.

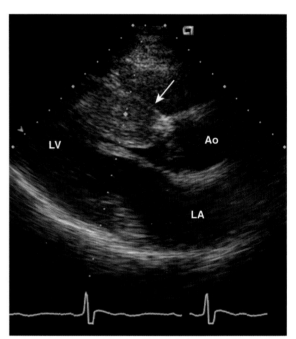

Figure 9–19. Hypertrophic cardiomyopathy in a parasternal long-axis view at end diastole showing marked increased thickness of the interventricular septum with a normal thickness of the posterior wall.

- ❑ Maximal septal thickness is a predictor of sudden death risk. Septal thickness is measured at end-diastole, taking care to exclude RV trabeculations from the measurement.
- ❑ Screening of first-degree relatives is recommended when hypertrophic cardiomyopathy is diagnosed, because early detection and treatment can prevent sudden death.

Step 2: Dynamic subaortic outflow obstruction

- ■ Evaluate dynamic subaortic outflow obstruction.
- ■ Evaluate the mechanism and severity of mitral regurgitation.

Key points

- ❑ Subaortic obstruction is due to systolic anterior motion (SAM) of the mitral leaflet and a hypertrophied septum. (Figure 9–21)
- ❑ The Doppler velocity curve peaks in late systole, instead of in mid-systole as seen with valvular obstruction. (Figure 9–22)
- ❑ The level of obstruction is established with pulsed or high pulse repetition frequency Doppler, with CW Doppler used to measure the maximum velocity.
- ❑ The severity of obstruction varies with loading conditions, increasing when afterload is decreased or when ventricular volume is reduced.

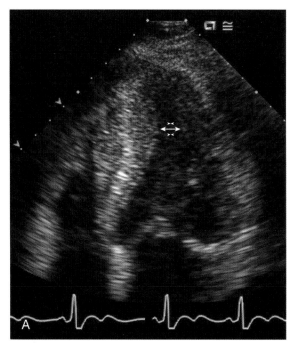

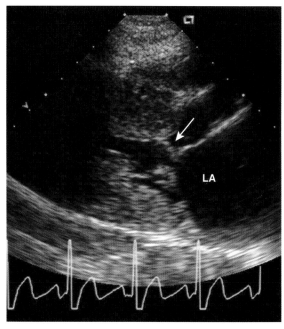

Figure 9–21. Hypertrophic cardiomyopathy in a parasternal long-axis view, showing systolic anterior motion of the mitral leaflet (*arrow*) causing dynamic subaortic obstruction.

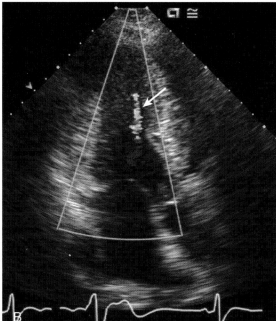

Figure 9–20. Apical 4-chamber view (*A*) in a young woman with hypertrophic cardiomyopathy showing the small chamber (*double arrow*) and thick walls at the apex on a diastolic frame. In systole, the long-axis view (*B*) shows flow acceleration at the midventricular level (*arrow*), instead of the subaortic obstruction seen with more typical basal septal hypertrophy.

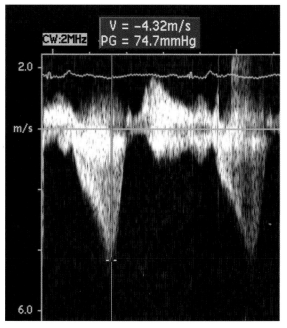

Figure 9–22. CW Doppler recording from an apical approach of outflow velocity in a patient with hypertrophic cardiomyopathy. This waveform is consistent with dynamic obstruction with a late-peaking high-velocity systolic signal. The level of obstruction is not defined using CW Doppler because the signal includes velocities from the entire length of the ultrasound beam. A step-by-step pulsed Doppler evaluation moving the sample volume from the LV toward the aortic valve allows localization of the site of obstruction.

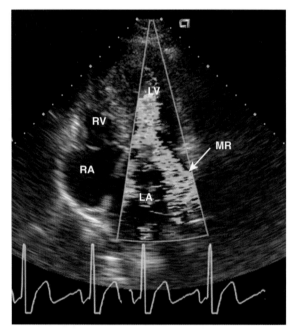

Figure 9–23. Mitral regurgitation (MR) in a patient with hypertrophic cardiomyopathy and dynamic subaortic obstruction. The mitral regurgitant posterior-lateral jet direction is demonstrated in this apical 4-chamber view.

❏ Exercise testing may be used to evaluate the change in outflow obstruction with exertion; latent obstruction is defined as an increase in subaortic velocity to at least 2.7 m/s with exercise.

❏ Mitral regurgitation may be due to SAM of the mitral leaflet, resulting in inadequate coaptation with a typical posterior-directed regurgitant jet. (Figure 9–23)

Step 3: Distinguish from hypertensive heart disease and normal aging changes

■ Hypertensive heart disease may be mistaken for hypertrophic cardiomyopathy.

■ LV hypertrophy in a patient with a clinical history of hypertension is nearly always due to hypertensive heart disease.

■ With aging, dilation and tortuosity of the ascending aorta result in an increased angle between the basal septum and aortic root, with "bulging" of the septum into the LV outflow tract (LVOT).

Key points

❏ Hypertension results in concentric LV hypertrophy; even the basal posterior wall is thickened.

❏ Dynamic outflow obstruction may occur with hypertensive heart disease, but the location of obstruction is mid-ventricular and systolic

anterior motion (SAM) occurs in the mitral chordal region, instead of at the leaflet level.

❏ Age-related bulging of the basal septum can be difficult to distinguish from hypertrophic cardiomyopathy; diagnosis depends on associated echocardiographic and clinical findings, as well as genetic and family studies.

Restrictive cardiomyopathy

■ Perform a more detailed evaluation of LV diastolic function. (Figure 9–24)

■ Differentiate restrictive cardiomyopathy from constrictive pericarditis. (see Chapter 10)

Key points

❏ Restrictive cardiomyopathy is a primary disease of the myocardium, often related to an infiltrative or inflammatory process.

❏ Restrictive cardiomyopathy is characterized by predominant diastolic, rather than systolic, dysfunction so that detailed evaluation of diastolic function is helpful.

❏ Restrictive cardiomyopathy and constrictive pericarditis result in similar changes in ventricular filling but can be differentiated based on several features. (see Table 10–2)

❏ LV systolic dysfunction may also be present, especially late in the disease course.

❏ Pulmonary systolic pressure usually is moderately to severely elevated.

Other cardiomyopathies

■ Arrhythmogenic RV dysplasia (ARVD) is a genetic cardiomyopathy with fibrofatty replacement of the RV resulting in arrhythmias, dilation, and systolic dysfunction.

■ LV noncompaction is characterized by areas of prominent trabeculation and hypokinesis, typically located in the LV apex and mid-LV segments of the lateral and inferior walls. (Figure 9–25)

■ Chagas disease is due to a parasitic infection. It results in apical aneurysm formation in about 50% of patients and global hypokinesis in those with advanced disease.

■ Tako-tsubo cardiomyopathy is an acute stress-related cause of heart failure with apical dilation and dyskinesis (apical "ballooning").

HYPERTENSIVE HEART DISEASE

■ Evaluation of the patient with hypertensive heart disease follows the general approach outlined for a patient with a cardiomyopathy. (Figure 9–26)

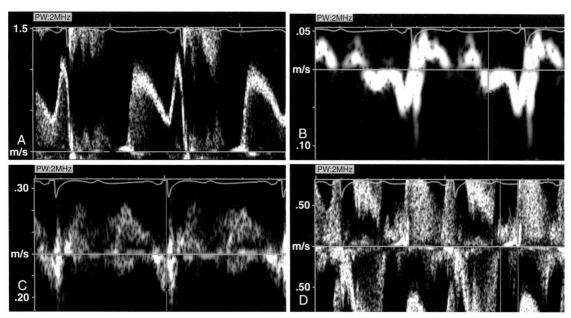

Figure 9–24. Evaluation of diastolic function in a patient with a restrictive cardiomyopathy includes (*A*) transmitral flow, (*B*) tissue Doppler velocity at the mitral annulus, (*C*) pulmonary vein flow, and (*D*) the isovolumic relaxation time. These tracings show impaired diastolic relaxation (transmitral and tissue Doppler E < A, prolonged deceleration time, and prolonged IVRT). LA pressure also may be elevated with an E/E′ > 30, even though the pulmonary venous a-wave is low velocity and short in duration.

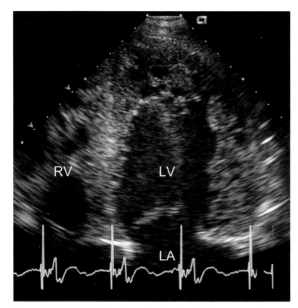

Figure 9–25. Apical 4-chamber view showing LV noncompaction, particularly in the apex.

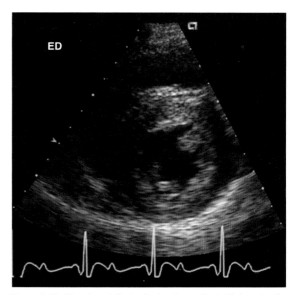

Figure 9–26. Parasternal short-axis view in a patient with hypertensive heart disease showing a small ventricular cavity and concentric hypertrophy in early diastole.

■ Blood pressure should be recorded at the time of every echocardiographic examination.

Key points

❏ Hypertension results in LV hypertrophy with impaired diastolic relaxation.

❏ Prolonged poorly controlled hypertension may eventually result in more severe diastolic dysfunction and in superimposed systolic dysfunction.

❏ Effective treatment of hypertension results in regression of LV hypertrophy.

❏ LV hypertrophy may be accompanied by dynamic mid-cavity obstruction due to a small, thick-walled, hyperdynamic ventricle. (Figure 9–27)

❏ Obstruction may only be present or may increase with hypovolemia or hyperdynamic states (such as anemia, fever, sepsis, etc.)

❏ Aortic valve sclerosis and mitral annular calcification are typically seen in patients with hypertensive heart disease. (Figure 9–28)

❏ Hypertension, like aging, is associated with dilation and increased tortuosity of the ascending aorta, resulting in a more acute angle between the ventricular septum and the aortic root, sometimes mistaken for focal basal septal thickening. (Figure 9–29)

POST-TRANSPLANT HEART DISEASE

■ Evaluation of the patient after heart transplantation follows the general approach outlined for a patient with a cardiomyopathy.

■ Early after heart transplantation, the major issues are surgical (e.g., pericardial effusion) and

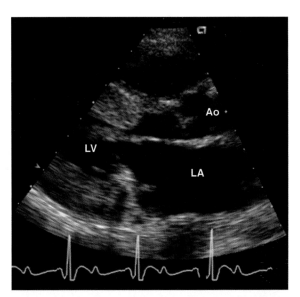

Figure 9–28. Parasternal long-axis view in a patient with hypertension showing mild ventricular hypertrophy, aortic valve sclerosis, and mild mitral annular calcification.

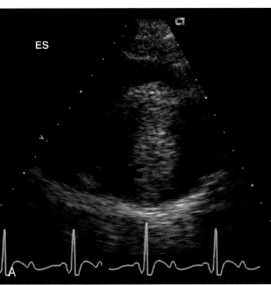

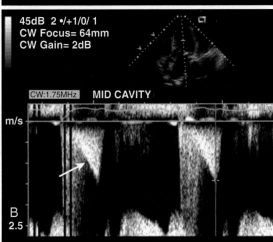

Figure 9–27. In the same patient as in Figure 9–26, (A) the end-systolic parasternal short-axis view shows complete obliteration of the chamber at end-systole; (B) CW Doppler shows a late-peaking systolic velocity of 1.4 m/s, consistent with mid-cavity obstruction due to a small, thick-walled chamber with normal systolic function.

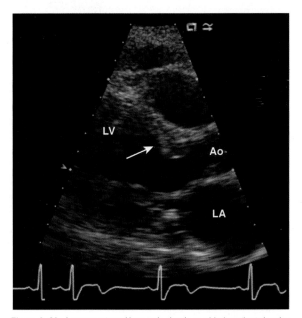

Figure 9–29. Low parasternal long-axis view in an elderly patient showing prominence of the base of the septum (sometimes called a "septal knuckle"; *arrow*) due to an increased angle between the long axes of the aorta and LV. Mild mitral annular calcification is present, but there is no evidence of LV hypertrophy.

myocardial preservation (e.g., RV and LV systolic function).

■ Echocardiographic signs of transplant rejection include diastolic and systolic LV dysfunction.

■ After transplant, long-term follow-up of patients includes dobutamine stress echocardiography for detection of graft coronary artery disease.

Key points

❑ The clinical history is reviewed regarding the type of surgical anastomoses (bicaval versus atrial level suture lines). (Figure 9–30)

❑ Biatrial enlargement is typical after heart transplantation, with sometimes massive atrial enlargement with biatrial anastomotic suture lines.

❑ Complications of percutaneous myocardial biopsy include (1) cardiac perforation resulting in pericardial effusion and tamponade and (2) tricuspid valve damage resulting in regurgitation.

❑ Detection of rejection based on diastolic dysfunction is challenging, and this approach is used only by experienced transplant centers.

❑ New systolic dysfunction, even if mild, may indicate acute rejection and requires prompt evaluation by the transplant team.

❑ When dobutamine stress echocardiography is performed after heart transplantation, atropine is unlikely to increase heart rate due to cardiac denervation.

PULMONARY HEART DISEASE

■ Pulmonary hypertension in the absence of significant left-sided heart disease indicates primary pulmonary or pulmonary vascular disease.

■ The effects of pulmonary hypertension on the right heart result in pulmonary heart disease (or cor pulmonale). (Figure 9–31)

■ New onset of increased pulmonary pressures in a patient with acute chest pain or shortness of breath suggests the possibility of acute pulmonary embolism.

Step-by-step approach

Step 1: Estimate pulmonary pressure

■ Pulmonary systolic pressure is determined based on the velocity in the tricuspid regurgitant jet and the estimated RA pressure (see Chapter 6). (Figure 9–32)

■ Additional signs of pulmonary hypertension also are evaluated.

Key points

❑ When 2D echocardiography findings show right heart dysfunction, a diligent search for the

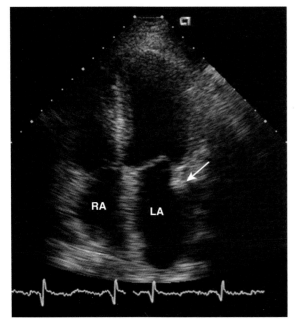

Figure 9–30. In this patient with biatrial anastomoses at heart transplantation. The enlarged left and right atria, caused by suturing of the native and donor atrium (arrow shows suture line), are seen in the apical 4-chamber view.

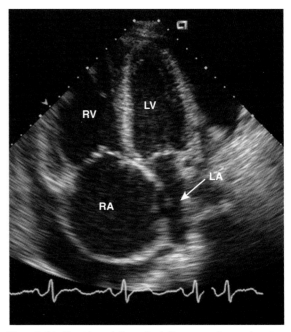

Figure 9–31. Cor pulmonale in a patient with severe pulmonary hypertension resulting in severe RV hypertrophy and dilation and severely reduced RV systolic function. The RA is severely enlarged, with bulging of the atrial septum from right to left, suggesting that RA pressure is higher than LA pressure. A moderate pericardial effusion also is seen.

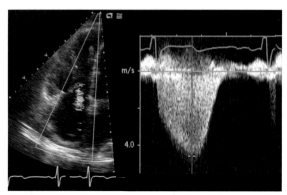

Figure 9–32. Tricuspid regurgitant jet recorded with CW Doppler from an apical window. This recording shows a well-defined peak velocity with a dark band of velocities along the outer edge of the velocity curve, consistent with a good-quality signal. Even though color Doppler was used to guide placement of the CW ultrasound beam, a non-parallel intercept angle cannot be excluded with certainly. However, this velocity indicates an RV–to–RA systolic pressure difference of 70 mm Hg, consistent with severe pulmonary hypertension.

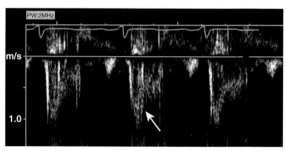

Figure 9–33. Pulsed Doppler recording of antegrade flow in the pulmonary artery from the parasternal RV outflow view, in the same patient as Figure 9–32, shows a short time to peak velocity and a mid-systolic notch (*arrow*) in the velocity curve, which are specific for severe pulmonary hypertension.

highest-velocity tricuspid regurgitant jet is especially important.

❏ Other findings that suggest pulmonary hypertension include a short time to peak velocity and mid-systolic deceleration of the pulmonary artery velocity curve and paradoxical septal motion (Figure 9–33).

❏ The velocity of the tricuspid regurgitant jet reflects the systolic pressure difference between the RV and RA, not the volume of regurgitation. Thus, severe pulmonary hypertension may be present with only mild tricuspid regurgitation.

❏ Overestimation of pulmonary pressures is avoided by using a gray-scale velocity display, increasing the high-pass (or wall) filter and adjusting the gain level appropriately. The low-intensity linear signals outside the edge of the velocity envelope are not included in the velocity measurement.

❏ Pulmonary vascular resistance (PVR in Wood units) can be estimated from the tricuspid regurgitant peak velocity (V_{TR}) and the velocity-time integral of flow in the RV outflow tract (VTI_{RVOT}) using the equation:

$$PVR = 10 \; (V_{TR}/VTI_{RVOT})$$

Step 2: Evaluate RV size and systolic function

■ The RV responds to chronic pressure overload with dilation of the chamber, in addition to hypertrophy of the wall, often accompanied by systolic dysfunction.

■ RV size is compared with LV size and graded as mildly, moderately, or severely enlarged (Figure 9–34).

■ RV systolic function is qualitatively evaluated as mildly, moderately, or severely reduced.

■ The pattern of ventricular septal motion is evaluated in a parasternal short-axis view.

Key points

❏ If the LV is normal in size, the RV is severely dilated if the 2D area in a 4-chamber view is larger than the LV; moderately dilated if equal to the LV; and mildly dilated if greater than normal but not equal to the LV.

❏ If the LV is dilated or hypovolemic, estimates of RV size are adjusted accordingly.

❏ RV size and systolic function are evaluated based on parasternal, apical, and subcostal views.

❏ RV size and function often are best evaluated from the subcostal window because the RV is seen in oblique image planes from the parasternal view and the RV free wall may be difficult to visualize on apical views.

❏ Elevated RV pressure results in flattening of the ventricular septum during both systole and diastole, whereas right heart volume overload results in flattening mostly during diastole.

Step 3: Evaluate the severity of tricuspid regurgitation

■ Pulmonary hypertension often results in dilation of the tricuspid annulus with inadequate leaflet coaptation and tricuspid regurgitation.

■ Tricuspid regurgitant severity is evaluated based on the vena contracta width of the regurgitant jet, the density of the CW Doppler velocity curve, and the pattern of flow in the hepatic veins.

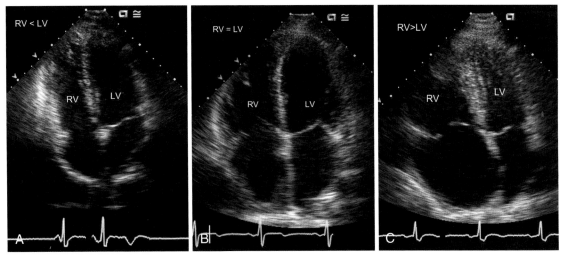

Figure 9-34. Examples of estimating RV size compared with the LV in the apical 4-chamber view. *A,* The LV and RV are normal size. The transducer is slightly over the RV apex to show the entire RV chamber buit RV size is less than LV size. *B,* Moderate RV dilation with the RV chamber size about the same as the LV. In addition, the RV apex extends beyond the LV apex (instead of being about ⅔ of the LV basal-apical distance). *C,* Severe RV enlargement with an RV that is larger in area than the LV and an RV apex at the same level as the LV. In addition, RV free wall thickness is increased, indicating RV pressure overload and hypertrophy.

Key points

- ❑ Vena contracta width is best measured in the parasternal RV inflow view; a width greater than 7 mm indicates severe regurgitation.
- ❑ The density of the CW Doppler signal is compared with antegrade flow: Equal density indicates severe regurgitation.
- ❑ The normal hepatic vein pattern of systolic flow into the RA is reversed when tricuspid regurgitation is severe. However, systolic flow reversal also may be seen when the patient is not in sinus rhythm, even when regurgitation is not severe.

Step 4: Exclude other causes of pulmonary hypertension or right heart enlargement

- ■ Pulmonary hypertension and right heart enlargement also may be due to left-sided heart disease or congenital heart disease.

- ■ Right heart enlargement without severe pulmonary hypertension is seen with volume overload due to valve regurgitation or a left to right shunt.

Key points

- ❑ Left-sided or congenital heart disease results in secondary pulmonary hypertension, which is easily distinguished from primary pulmonary disease.
- ❑ Right-sided volume overload in the absence of an obvious atrial septal defect or severe right-sided valve regurgitation prompts TEE examination to exclude a sinus venous atrial septal defect or partial anomalous pulmonary venous return.

THE ECHO EXAM

Cardiomyopathies, Hypertensive Heart Disease, and Pulmonary Heart Disease
Echo Differential Diagnosis of Heart Failure

Ischemic disease
Valvular disease
Hypertensive heart disease
Cardiomyopathy
  Dilated
  Hypertrophic
  Restrictive
  Other
Pericardial disease
  Constriction
  Tamponade
Pulmonary heart disease

Cardiomyopathies: Typical Features

	Dilated	Hypertrophic	Restrictive	Athlete's Heart
LV systolic function	Moderate to severely ↓	Normal	Normal	Normal
LV diastolic function	May be abnormal	Abnormal	Abnormal	Normal
LV hypertrophy	↑ LV mass due to LV dilation with normal wall thickness	Asymmetric LV hypertrophy	Concentric LV hypertrophy	Normal wall thickness
Chamber dilation	All four chambers	LA and RA dilation if MR is present	LA and RA dilation	LV dilation
Outflow tract obstruction	Absent	Dynamic LV outflow tract obstruction may be present	Absent	Absent
LV end-diastolic pressure	Elevated	Elevated	Elevated	Normal
Pulmonary artery pressures	Elevated	Elevated	Elevated	Normal

MR, mitral regurgitation.

Differentiation of Cause of Increased Wall Thickness

	Hypertensive Heart Disease	Hypertrophic Cardiomyopathy	Restrictive Cardiomyopathy
LV hypertrophy	Present	Present	Present
Pattern of hypertrophy	Concentric	Asymmetric	Concentric
Clinical history of hypertension	Present	Absent	Absent
Outflow obstruction	Mid-LV cavity obliteration	Dynamic subaortic obstruction	Absent
RV hypertrophy	Absent	May be present	Present
Pulmonary hypertension	Mild	Mild	Moderate
LV systolic function	Normal initially but may be reduced late in disease course	Normal	Normal initially but may be reduced late in disease course
LV diastolic function	Abnormal	Abnormal	Abnormal

Echo Approach to the Cardiomyopathies

Modality	Echo Views and Flows	Measurements
Imaging	LV size and systolic function	EDV and ESV Apical biplane EF
	Degree and pattern of LV hypertrophy	LV mass
	Evidence for dynamic outflow tract obstruction	SAM of the mitral valve Aortic valve mid-systolic closure
	RV size and systolic function	
	LA size	LA volume
Doppler echo	Associated valvular regurgitation	Measure vena contracta; quantitate if more than mild
	LV diastolic function	Standard diastolic function evaluation with classification of severity and estimate of LV EDP
	LV systolic function	dP/dt from MR jet Calculation of cardiac output
	Pulmonary pressures	TR jet and IVC for PA systolic pressure Evaluate PR jet for PA diastolic pressure Estimate pulmonary resistance
	Color, pulsed, and CW Doppler to quantitate outflow obstruction	Maximum outflow tract gradient

CW, color Doppler; echo, echocardiography; EDP, end-diastolic pressure; EDV, end-diastolic volume; EF, ejection fraction; ESV, end-systolic volume; IVC, inferior vena cava; MR, mitral regurgitation; PA, pulmonary artery; PR, pulmonic regurgitation; SAM, systolic anterior motion; TR, tricuspid regurgitation.

SELF-ASSESSMENT QUESTIONS

QUESTION 1

A 62-year-old patient who underwent cardiac transplantation 12 years ago for a familial cardiomyopathy is referred for echocardiography. The following measurements are recorded:

LV dimension, end-diastole/ end-systole	5.0 cm/3.5 cm
Ejection fraction	62%
LA dimension	5.2 cm
Tricuspid regurgitant jet	2.1 m/s

His LV inflow (Figure 9–35, *A*), tissue Doppler (Figure 9–35, *B*), and LA inflow velocities (Figure 9–35, *C*) are shown.

These findings are most consistent with:

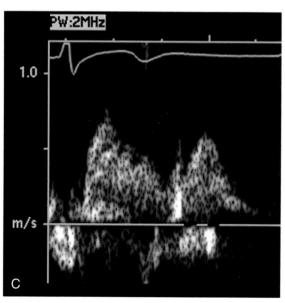

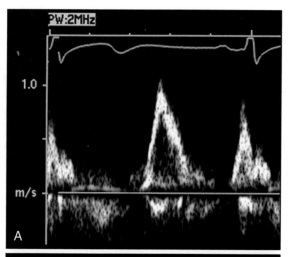

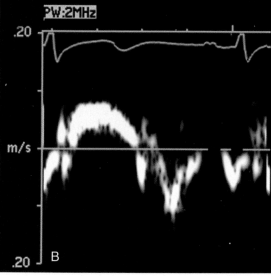

Figure 9–35.

A. Transplant rejection
B. Coronary vasculopathy
C. Pericardial constriction
D. Normal heart

QUESTION 2

A 75-year-old woman presents to establish care. A murmur is heard on examination; an image from the TTE is shown here (Figure 9–36).

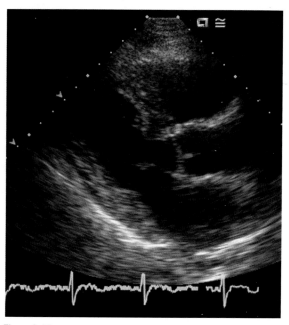

Figure 9–36.

A. Hypertrophic cardiomyopathy
B. Hypertensive heart disease
C. Aortic stenosis
D. Amyloid heart disease

QUESTION 3

A 28-year-old woman presents with palpitations and decreased exercise tolerance. A Doppler tracing from the TTE is shown here (Figure 9–37).

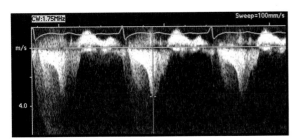

Figure 9–37.

The most appropriate next test for this patient is:

A. Exercise stress testing
B. Right heart catheterization
C. Transesophageal echocardiography (TEE)
D. Coronary angiography

QUESTION 4

A 66-year-old woman with primary pulmonary hypertension confirmed by right heart catheterization is referred for echocardiography to determine if there has been interval improvement in pulmonary pressures since starting medical therapy. On her prior study, comment was made that peak tricuspid regurgitant jet was faint and unmeasurable. To evaluate RV pressure, you recommend:

A. Pulmonary valve Doppler velocity recording
B. Qp/Qs measurement
C. 2D imaging inferior vena cava
D. Doppler tracing pulmonary branches

QUESTION 5

A patient is referred for echocardiography for a newly diagnosed systolic murmur. The following M-mode tracings were obtained (Figure 9–38).

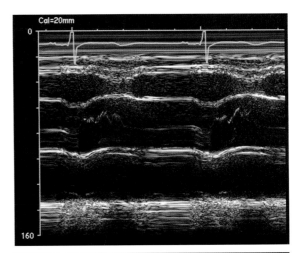

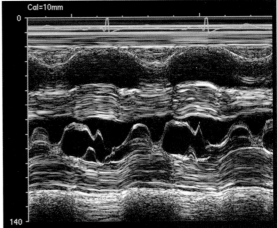

Figure 9–38.

These images are most consistent with:

A. Mitral valve prolapse
B. Dilated cardiomyopathy
C. Hypertrophic cardiomyopathy
D. Aortic stenosis

QUESTION 6

A 58-year-old female with no prior cardiac history presents to your clinic with progressive dyspnea over several months. Physical examination shows a blood pressure of 110/70 mm Hg, jugular venous distension to 10 cm, and 2+ pedal edema. Cardiac examination shows a normal S1 and S2 with an S4 gallop. An image from the apical 4-chamber view is shown here (Figure 9–39).

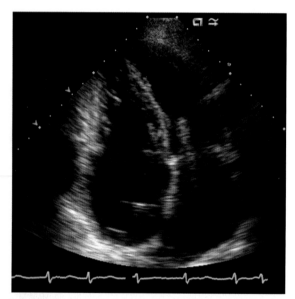

Figure 9–39.

The most likely diagnosis in this patient is:

A. Dilated cardiomyopathy
B. Restrictive cardiomyopathy
C. Hypertensive heart disease
D. Normal heart

QUESTION 7

You are asked to review an ECG (Figure 9–40) from a 37-year-old patient who has familial dilated cardiomyopathy. The prior study, performed 2 years ago, documented:

LV end-diastolic dimension	6.3 cm
LV ejection fraction	46%
Pulmonary systolic pressure	40 mm Hg
Mitral regurgitation	Moderate
Tricuspid regurgitation	Mild

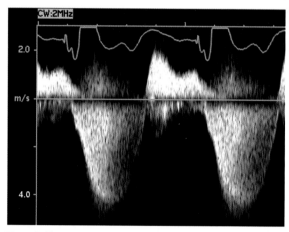

Figure 9–40.

Based on the Doppler tracing, the most likely interval change is:

A. Mitral regurgitation decreased
B. Pulmonary pressures increased
C. Ejection fraction decreased
D. Aortic stenosis increased

QUESTION 8

A 50-year-old man presents to the emergency room with sudden-onset chest pain and dyspnea. The electrocardiogram (ECG) shows occasional ectopic beats and non-specific ST-T wave changes. Troponin I is mildly elevated at 1.6 ng/ml. A TTE is obtained. LV ejection fraction is measured at 65% by the apical biplane method and no regional wall motion abnormalities are seen. Urgent coronary angiographic examination does not find critical intracoronary lesions. The following image is recorded (Figure 9–41).

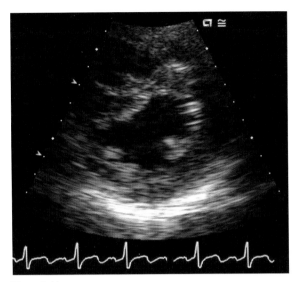

Figure 9–41.

The most likely diagnosis is:

A. Takotsubo cardiomyopathy
B. Pulmonary embolism
C. Transmural myocardial infarction
D. Cardiac tamponade

QUESTION 9

A 43-year-old woman is referred by her primary care physician for management of a dilated cardiomyopathy. Diagnostic evaluation done at the time of her initial presentation included a coronary angiogram, which showed the absence of coronary artery disease. A TTE is obtained (Figure 9–42).

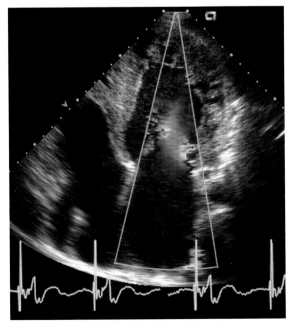

Figure 9–42.

The image is consistent with:

A. Ebstein's anomaly
B. Takotsubo cardiomyopathy
C. Constrictive pericarditis
D. LV noncompaction

QUESTION 10

A 64-year-old man is referred for exertional dyspnea. A 12-lead ECG shows low-voltage QRS complexes with non-specific ST-T wave abnormalities. A coronary angiogram documented absence of coronary artery disease. An echocardiogram is obtained (Figure 9–43).

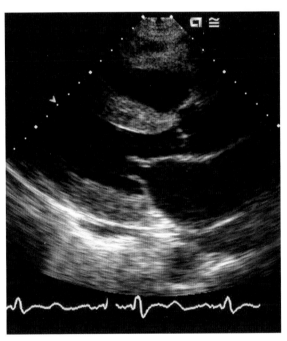

Figure 9–43.

The image is consistent with:

A. Hypertrophic cardiomyopathy
B. LV noncompaction
C. Amyloid heart disease
D. Cardiac tamponade

QUESTION 11

A 36-year-old man with known hypertrophic cardio-myopathy is evaluated with echocardiography. The following Doppler tracings are obtained (Figure 9–44). Which feature of the Doppler signal is most helpful in distinguishing which is the LV outflow gradient and which is mitral regurgitation?

A. Duration of flow
B. Maximum velocity
C. Shape of velocity curve
D. Accompanying diastolic flow velocity
E. Color imaging of jet direction

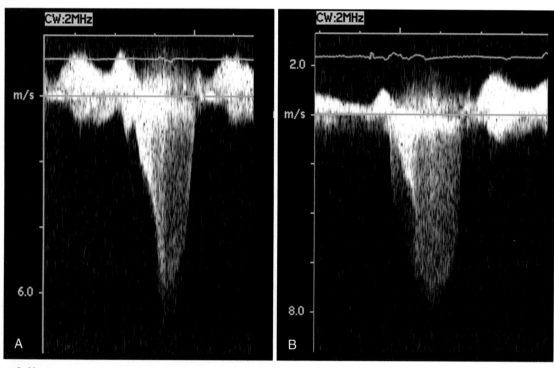

Figure 9–44.

ANSWER 1: D

The tissue Doppler signal (*B*) demonstrates a normal myocardial E' velocity, implying normal myocardial motion and a normal E/E'' ratio (normal LA pressure). Cardiac donor hearts usually come from younger, previously healthy donors, so the age of the heart is younger than patient age in this case. Periodic echocardiography is routinely utilized to monitor for post-transplant complications. The Doppler LV inflow pattern (*A*) seen in this case is comparable to a young individual, with a relatively higher E/A ratio. In young hearts, vigorous contraction of a normal ventricle "pulls" blood into the LV and the majority of LV inflow occurs early in diastole, with a relatively small contribution of LV filling by atrial contraction. Left atrial enlargement was the result of suturing the native and donor atria rather than increased LA pressure.

Echocardiographic markers of cardiac transplant rejection are usually absent in the early stages. However, with progression, myocardial inflammation may lead to increased wall thickness (hypertrophy), evidence of diastolic dysfunction with restrictive ventricular filling, and, in advanced cases, systolic dysfunction. Coronary vasculopathy would manifest with regional wall motion abnormalities in the myocardial distributions affected by the vasculopathy. With diffuse microvascular disease, systolic dysfunction may be global in nature. Post-transplant pericardial constriction is rare given that the native pericardium typically is not resewn after transplant.

ANSWER 2: B

The parasternal long-axis view demonstrates normal LV chamber size at end-diastole. There is prominence of the basal septum, a common finding in the elderly, particularly in those with longstanding hypertension. With increasing age there is thought to be straightening of the proximal ascending aorta, which tethers the proximal ventricular septum anteriorly, producing the septal "knuckle." In these patients, to keep the aortic root in view and horizontal in the image plane, the LV may be oriented more vertically than expected in a standard parasternal long-axis view, as seen in this case. Septal thickening in hypertensive heart disease is focal, usually limited to the base of the septum; significant hemodynamic obstruction of LV outflow is rare.

With hypertrophic cardiomyopathy, an increase in myocardial thickness may be seen at any point along the length of the septum. Although the basal septum is most prominently affected, there usually is more severe septal compared to hypertensive heart disease. In some cases of hypertrophic cardiomyopathy, there

is hemodynamic obstruction of LV outflow. The aortic valve is shown closed in diastole with thin, normal-appearing leaflets; aortic stenosis is not present. Amyloid heart disease is a myocardial infiltrative disorder that causes diffuse, concentric thickening throughout the myocardium.

ANSWER 3: A

This patient has hypertrophic cardiomyopathy, and the most appropriate next test is stress echocardiography. Spectral Doppler data from the LV outflow tract shows overlap of two Doppler signals. The denser signal is a late-peaking systolic signal consistent with dynamic outflow obstruction. Superimposed on this velocity curve is a faint mitral regurgitation signal that starts at the onset of the QRS signal and with a higher peak velocity, reflective of the high-pressure gradient between the LV and LA in systole. The LV outflow tract signal shows a delay in the start of the signal, compared with the superimposed mitral regurgitation, because of the isovolumic contraction time. The LV outflow tract Doppler peak velocity is 3.4 m/s at rest, consistent with moderate obstruction, but some patients have even greater obstruction with exercise. If a significant increase in velocity is identified with exercise stress testing (a velocity > 4 m/s), relief of LV outflow obstruction is indicated, either surgically or via percutaneous septal ablation.

This Doppler tracing, with superimposed LV outflow tract and mitral regurgitation signals, is not consistent with a tricuspid regurgitant jet, so there is no reason to suspect pulmonary hypertension or need for right heart catheterization based on these data. TEE imaging is not needed at this point because the transthoracic study is diagnostic for hypertrophic cardiomyopathy. Concurrent atherosclerotic disease is unlikely in this 28-year-old; therefore, coronary angiography is not indicated.

ANSWER 4: A

This patient's peak tricuspid regurgitant jet was faint and unmeasurable, making estimation of RV systolic pressure by echocardiography limited on repeat studies. Some centers advocate the use of contrast to increase the strength of the Doppler signal. Another approach is to estimate pulmonary pressure based on other intracardiac flow signals. In the absence of pulmonic stenosis, the RV end-diastolic pressure gradient can be estimated from the pulmonic regurgitant jet. The RV diastolic pressure is calculated as $4V^2$, where V is the peak end-diastolic velocity measured from the pulmonic valve Doppler regurgitant jet. Analogous to the PA systolic pressure estimate, the

PA diastolic pressure is the sum of the pulmonary artery–to–RV diastolic pressure difference and the RA pressure estimate, which is made based on the diameter of the inferior vena cava. In this example, assuming a RA pressure of 10 mm Hg, estimated RV diastolic pressure is 19 + 10 = 29 mm Hg, which is moderately elevated. The shape of the antegrade pulmonary flow signal also reflects pulmonary pressure, with a short time to peak velocity seen with more severe pulmonary hypertension.

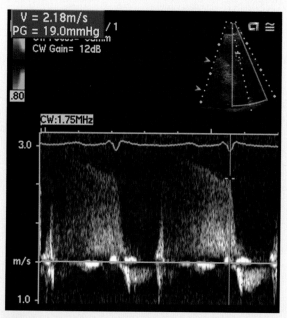

Figure 9–45.

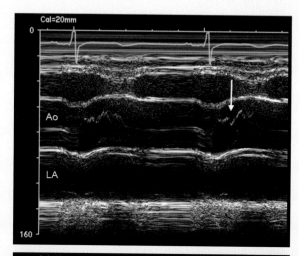

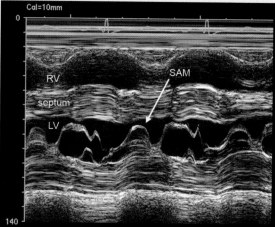

Figure 9–46.

The pulmonary to systemic flow ratio (Qp/Qs ratio) is a calculation of the comparative volume flow rates between the RV and LV, which allows quantitation of the severity of an intracardiac shunt but does not provide information on pulmonary or RV pressures. The diameter of the inferior vena cava, as assessed by 2D imaging, provides an estimate of right atrial pressure (not RV pressure, the question in this case). Antegrade Doppler tracing of the pulmonary branches would provide hemodynamic data for the pressure gradient at the point of interrogation (i.e., PA branch stenosis) and would not provide data on RV chamber pressure in systole.

ANSWER 5: C

A newly diagnosed systolic murmur is a common clinical indication for echocardiography. M-mode tracings across the aortic valve (Figure 9–46, top) and mitral valve (Figure 9–46, bottom) for this patient were shown. The M-mode tracing of the aortic valve shows mid-systolic closure (*arrow*), consistent with dynamic subaortic late systolic LV outflow obstruction.

The M-mode tracing at the mitral valve level shows a severely thickened septum and systolic anterior motion of the anterior mitral valve leaflet (*arrow*). These echocardiographic findings are consistent with hypertrophic cardiomyopathy. A systolic murmur is common in hypertrophic cardiomyopathy, due to high-velocity flow in the LV outflow tract.

The murmur of mitral valve prolapse is due to mitral regurgitation. M-mode tracings of the mitral valve leaflets in mitral valve prolapse would show late systolic posterior buckling into the LA. Patients with dilated cardiomyopathy often have significant functional mitral regurgitation due to dilation of the valve annulus and resultant poor leaflet coaptation. M-mode tracings of these patients show enlargement of the LV and increased E-point septal separation. In calcific aortic stenosis, there is thickening and calcification of the aortic valve leaflets with reduced systolic opening of the leaflets The aortic valve leaflets in this M-mode tracing appear thin and mobile, not consistent with valvular aortic stenosis.

ANSWER 6: B

The echocardiogram shows normal LV and RV chamber sizes. There is severe biatrial enlargement at end-diastole. (The atrioventricular valves are open.) There is a central venous catheter tip in the right atrium. The clinical presentation of restrictive cardiomyopathy is typically one of right heart failure, with increased central venous pressure and pedal edema, as was seen in this case. Although atrial size may be increased in dilated cardiomyopathy, the disproportionate biatrial enlargement relative to ventricular size supports a diagnosis of restrictive cardiomyopathy and is not consistent with a normal heart. A dilated cardiomyopathy would show either LV dilation or both LV and RV dilation with decreased ventricular function. In patients with systemic hypertension, increased afterload on the heart may lead to concentric LV hypertrophy. With hypertensive heart disease, coexistent diastolic dysfunction with increased left atrial pressure is common, but the extent of atrial enlargement is not as severe as that seen in restrictive cardiomyopathy.

ANSWER 7: C

This is a CW Doppler tracing of the mitral regurgitant jet. Mitral regurgitation is a systolic flow, which can be differentiated from LV outflow by the absence of isovolumic contraction time following the QRS (from the ECG tracing). The initial rate of increase in velocity versus time (or slope) of the mitral regurgitant jet provides a quantitative measure of LV function, based on the instantaneous pressure difference between the LA and LV. With normal systolic function, there is a rapid rate of rise of LV pressure with a corresponding rapid rate of rise in mitral regurgitant jet velocity. The rate of change in pressure over time (dP/dt) is quantitated from the mitral regurgitant jet by measuring the time interval between measured velocities of 1 m/s and 3 m/s. This value in seconds is then used in the equation:

$$dP/dt = 32 \, \text{mmHg}/time$$

where 32 mm Hg is the pressure difference between the time points with a velocity of 1 m/s (4 mm Hg) and 3 m/s (36 mm Hg). With normal systolic function, dP/dt is more than 1000 mm Hg/s. In this case, the dP/dt is only 512 mm Hg/sec, consistent with severe systolic dysfunction. Given that the prior ejection fraction was 46%, an interval decline in ejection fraction is the most likely change. The mitral regurgitant jet signal is dense and comparable to the antegrade density. This is consistent with at least moderate mitral regurgitation. It is unlikely that mitral regurgitation has decreased since the last study. Pulmonary pressures cannot be evaluated on this tracing (e.g., this is not a tricuspid regurgitant jet). The Doppler signal is not consistent with aortic stenosis because there is no delay after the QRS complex, which would be seen with aortic flow due to isovolumic contraction time.

ANSWER 8: B

This parasternal short-axis view shows diastolic interventricular septal flattening, consistent with RV enlargement. The echocardiogram and acute clinical presentation are most consistent with pulmonary embolism with acute RV strain. Although increased cardiac biomarkers suggest acute myocardial injury, LV systolic function is preserved without regional wall motion abnormalities. Coronary angiography is negative, excluding a transmural myocardial infarction with occlusion of a major epicardial artery. The clinical presentation of Takotsubo cardiomyopathy is chest pain or dyspnea following a significant emotional or physiologic stress, manifested as transient akinesis of the apical and mid-LV segments with regional wall motion abnormalities that extend beyond a single epicardial coronary arterial distribution. Normal LV chamber size and systolic function, as was seen in this case, is not consistent with Takotsubo cardiomyopathy. There is no pericardial effusion seen on the image provided to suggest cardiac tamponade.

ANSWER 9: D

The apical 4-chamber view shows prominent LV apical trabeculations consistent with LV noncompaction. There is an ICD wire seen in the right atrium. LV noncompaction is a congenital defect of myocardial development with failure of apical trabeculations to compact and solidify. Advanced cases of LV noncompaction can lead to progressive systolic dysfunction. In congenital Ebstein's anomaly, the tricuspid valve leaflets are attached or tethered to the RV walls, resulting in apical displacement of the valve coaptation plane with "atrialization" of a segment of the RV chamber. Takotsubo cardiomyopathy, or "transient apical ballooning syndrome," is an acute cardiac syndrome presenting with chest pain or dyspnea following a significant emotional or physiologic stress. On imaging there is transient akinesis of the apical and mid-LV segments, with regional wall motion abnormalities that extend beyond a single epicardial coronary arterial distribution. Takotsubo cardiomyopathy has a strong female predominance (>90%), and angiography demonstrates absence of obstructive coronary disease. In constrictive pericarditis, the thickened pericardium encases both the ventricles and atria; biventricular systolic function is usually relatively preserved, with only mildly increased biatrial size. Other findings in constrictive pericarditis include increased central venous pressure and respiratory variation in atrioventricular valve flow.

ANSWER 10: C

This parasternal long-axis view of the heart shows diffuse, concentric LV thickening at end-diastole and LA enlargement. The myocardium appears bright and echodense. There is a trivial, posterior pericardial effusion. These findings are consistent with an infiltrative myocardial disorder, such as amyloid heart disease. Other echocardiographic findings consistent with an infiltrative disorder include pulmonary hypertension and evidence for diastolic dysfunction with decreased LV compliance and elevated left atrial pressure. Generally, systolic function is relatively preserved until the late stages of the disease. With hypertrophic cardiomyopathy, myocardial thickening is more concentrated in the septum compared with the posterior wall, with hemodynamic obstruction of LV outflow in more severe cases. LV noncompaction is a congenital defect of myocardial development with prominence of LV apical trabeculations. The echocardiogram is not consistent with cardiac tamponade; the effusion is trivial in size and does not appear hemodynamically significant.

ANSWER 11: B

It can be challenging to separate the velocity signal from the mitral regurgitant jet from the LV outflow signal in patients with hypertrophic cardiomyopathy when dynamic obstruction is present. All the listed features can be helpful, but maximum velocity, when both signals are recorded, is most reliable. The mitral regurgitant velocity must be higher than the LV outflow velocity because the LV to LA pressure difference is always higher than the LV to aortic pressure difference. However, the signals may overlap because the CW Doppler beam width is relatively broad and the jet direction may be similar, with an anteriorly directed mitral regurgitant jet due to the mitral leaflets separating as the anterior leaflet moves anteriorly in systole. The duration of flow can be helpful because LV outflow starts only after isovolumic contraction, whereas mitral regurgitation starts at mitral valve closure. However, this sign can be misleading if mitral regurgitation only occurs with systolic anterior motion of the mitral leaflets; in that situation there may be simultaneous onset of flow. The shape of the LV outflow curve usually is late-peaking with a "dagger" shape, compared with the more rounded holosystolic signal of mitral regurgitation, but this sign is not reliable because some obstructive flows will appear more rounded. Mitral inflow signals accompany both high-velocity systolic jets because beam width include mitral inflow in both cases. Color imaging with guided CW Doppler recordings may be helpful, but overlap still occurs with the wide CW Doppler beam.

10 Pericardial Disease

STEP-BY-STEP APPROACH

Pericardial effusion

- There are numerous causes for accumulation of fluid in the pericardial space. (Table 10-1)
- A pericardial effusion may be asymptomatic or may be associated with pericarditis or with tamponade physiology.
- Pericarditis is a clinical diagnosis based on the triad of typical pericardial pain, a pericardial rub, and diffuse ST elevation on the electrocardiogram (ECG). (Figure 10–1)
- Tamponade physiology is present when systemic blood pressure or cardiac output is reduced due to compression of the cardiac chambers by the pericardial fluid.

Key points

- In patients with pericarditis, the effusion ranges from absent to large in size.
- The presence of a pericardial rub does not correlate with the size of the effusion.
- In a patient with a large pericardial effusion and hypotension or a low cardiac output, tamponade physiology likely is present, even if other echocardiographic signs are not seen.

Step 1: Record the patient's blood pressure and heart rate

- The first step in echocardiographic evaluation of a patient with suspected pericardial disease is to measure and record blood pressure and heart rate (as for any echocardiographic examination).
- Pulsus paradoxus is a decline in the systolic blood pressure by more than 20 mm Hg with inspiration. (Figure 10–2)

Key points

- Hypotension and tachycardia are non-specific but are seen in patients with tamponade physiology.
- To measure pulsus paradoxus, the blood pressure cuff is deflated until the first Korotkoff sound is intermittently heard during expiration. The cuff is then slowly deflated until the Korotkoff sound is heard on every beat. The difference between these two pressures is the paradoxical pulse.

❑ A physician should be present for the echocardiographic study when the patient is hemodynamically compromised (i.e., hypotension or significant tachycardia).

Step 2: Evaluate for the presence of pericardial fluid

■ An echo-free space adjacent to the heart is consistent with a pericardial effusion. (Figure 10–3)

TABLE 10-1	Differential Diagnosis of Pericardial Disease

I. Infections
   A. Postviral pericarditis
   B. Bacterial
   C. Tuberculosis
   D. Parasitic (Echinococcus, amebiasis, toxoplasmosis)
II. Malignant
   A. Metastatic disease (e.g., lymphoma, melanoma)
   B. Direct extension (lung carcinoma, breast carcinoma)
   C. Primary cardiac malignancy
III. "Inflammatory"
   A. Post-myocardial infarction (Dressler's syndrome)
   B. Uremia
   C. Collagen-vascular disease
   D. Post-cardiac surgery
   E. Radiation
IV. Intracardiac-pericardial communications
   A. Blunt or penetrating chest trauma
   B. Post-catheter procedures (electrophysiology studies, percutaneous coronary intervention, valvuloplasty, endomyocardial biopsy)
   C. Pacer lead or IV line perforation
   D. Left ventricular rupture post-myocardial infarction
   E. Aortic dissection

■ The pericardial sac extends completely around both the LV and RV, from the apex to the base, and extends around the RA to the bases of the superior and inferior vena cava.

■ The pericardial sac extends posterior to the LA, between the pulmonary vein orifices (the oblique sinus of the pericardium), and there is a small cuff of pericardial space around the base of the great vessels (the transverse sinus). (Figure 10–4)

Key points

❑ An isolated anterior, relatively echo-free space usually is due to the normal epicardial fat pad. With an effusion, the echo-free space usually is seen both anteriorly and posteriorly. (Figure 10–5)

❑ A pericardial effusion is seen anterior to the descending thoracic aorta, whereas a pleural effusion extends posteriorly to the descending aorta. (Figure 10–6)

❑ Fluid adjacent to the RA in the apical 4-chamber view may be due to pericardial or pleural fluid. The specific diagnosis is based on evidence of pericardial or pleural fluid in other views. (Figure 10–7)

❑ If the pericardial fluid contains thrombus or fibrinous debris, the effusion may be echogenic instead of echolucent. (Figure 10–8)

Step 3: Evaluate the distribution of pericardial fluid

■ Effusions may be circumferential or loculated so that evaluation in multiple views from parasternal, apical, and subcostal windows is essential.

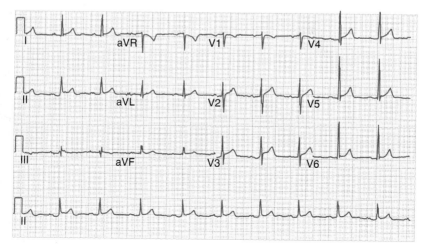

Figure 10–1. This 12-lead ECG shows diffuse upsloping ST elevation and PR segment depression, consistent with pericarditis in this 42-year-old man with a 2-week history of persistent dull chest pain and a pericardial rub on physical examination.

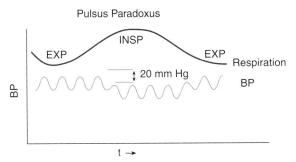

Figure 10–2. This schematic shows that with inspiration (INSP), systolic blood pressure (BP) falls by at least 20 mm Hg when pulsus paradoxus is present.

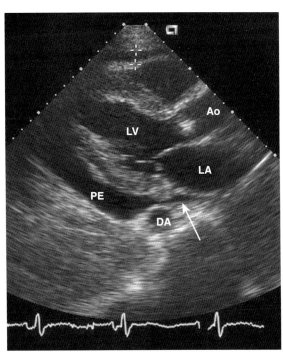

Figure 10–4. Pericardial fluid is seen posterior to the LA (arrow) in the oblique sinus of the pericardium in this parasternal long-axis view. This is clearly a pericardial effusion (PE), not pleural fluid, as it tracks anteriorly to the descending aorta (DA).

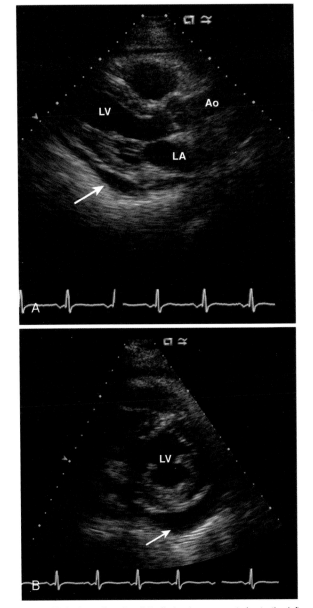

Figure 10–3. A small pericardial effusion is seen posterior to the left ventricle in both the parasternal long-axis view (A) and in the short-axis view at the mid-ventricular level (B).

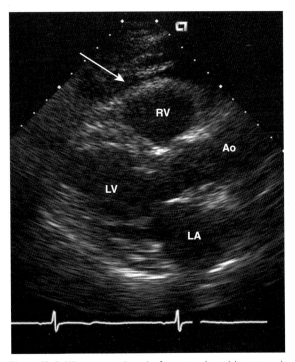

Figure 10–5. When an anterior echo free space (arrow) is seen, as in this parasternal long-axis view, without evidence for posterior effusion, the most likely diagnosis is normal epicardial adipose tissue or a "fat pad."

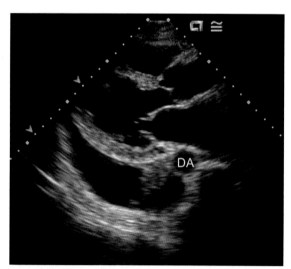

Figure 10–6. A large left pleural effusion is seen in this parasternal long-axis view. The pleural effusion extends posterior to the descending thoracic aorta (*DA*).

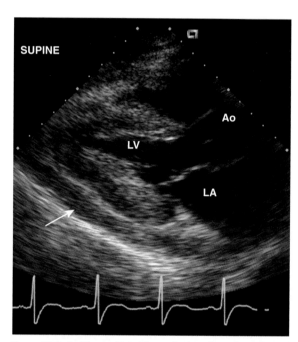

Figure 10–8. In this parasternal long-axis view, the pericardial space (*arrow*) is filled with echo-dense material, consistent with hematoma, tumor, or fibrinous debris.

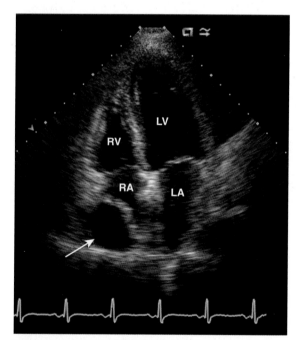

Figure 10–7. Fluid (*arrow*) adjacent to the RA seen in the apical 4-chamber view most likely is pericardial, although pleural effusion also may extend adjacent to the RA in this view.

■ Loculation of fluid due to adhesions often is seen after cardiac surgery or trauma or with malignant effusions.

Key points

❏ Loculated fluid may be missed unless multiple views are examined; sometimes TEE is needed

to identify loculated fluid posterior to the LA. (Figure 10–9)

❏ Loculated fluid occasionally may be mistaken for a normal cardiac chamber, for example when loculated fluid compresses the LA or RA. (Figure 10–10)

Step 4: Estimate the size of the pericardial effusion

■ A small amount of pericardial fluid is normal, appearing as a trivial or absent effusion on echocardiography.

■ The volume of an abnormal pericardial effusion ranges from 50 mL to more than 1 liter.

■ The size of the effusion is qualitatively graded as small, moderate, or large.

Key points

❏ A small effusion on 2D imaging can be confirmed by the M-mode finding of flat motion of the parietal pericardium with systolic separation of the epicardium. (Figure 10–11)

❏ There is no precise approach to estimation of pericardial fluid volume by echocardiography.

❏ One useful approach is to consider the effusion small if the distance between the epicardium and pericardium is less than 0.5 cm, moderate if 0.5 to 2 cm, and large if more than 2 cm. (Figure 10–12)

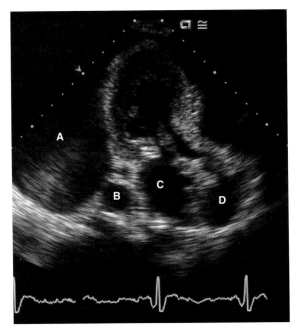

Figure 10–9. This apical long-axis view was obtained in a 58-year-old woman after renal transplantation with an enlarged heart on chest radiograph. The large left pleural effusion (*A*) is identified based on its relationship to the descending thoracic aorta (*B*). There is a space that most likely is the LA (*C*) and another space that may be the ascending aorta (*D*). However, the space labeled *D* seems unusual in size and shape for the aorta and raises the concern of a loculated effusion. In addition, a loculated effusion can fill the space normally occupied by the LA. The location of the mitral annular calcification and the shape of the basal posterior wall are worrisome for a compressed LA. Color flow imaging would be helpful for confirming whether the LA is compressed. The structure labeled *D* should be imaged from other views and interrogated with color and pulsed Doppler.

❑ With loculated effusions, size is described in a similar fashion along with the location of the fluid.
❑ Evaluation from the subcostal view is especially important because this approach often is used for pericardiocentesis. (Figure 10–13)

Tamponade physiology

■ Pericardial pressure depends on both the volume and rate of accumulation of pericardial fluid.
■ Tamponade physiology occurs when pericardial pressure exceeds intracardiac pressure.
■ With tamponade physiology, cardiac output and blood pressure are reduced due to impaired cardiac filling due to compression of the cardiac chambers.
■ Pulsus paradoxus is an excessive fall (>20 mm Hg) in systolic blood pressure with inspiration, due to the fall in cardiac output with inspiration.

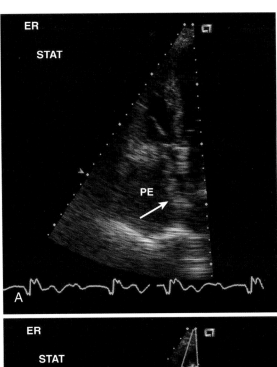

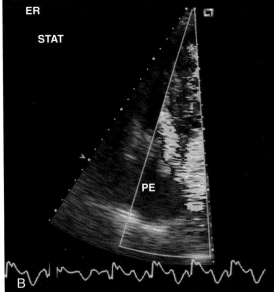

Figure 10–10. In an apical 4-chamber orientation, the sector has been narrowed to focus on the right side of the heart. The RV is small, with a catheter seen in the chamber. *A*, The area normally occupied by the RA consists primarily of loculated pericardial effusion (PE) with the RA free wall (*arrow*) compressed so that is almost touches the interatrial septum. *B*, Color Doppler confirms the severe compression of the RA with a very narrow flow stream into the RV.

Key points

❑ Tamponade physiology may occur with a rapidly accumulating moderate-sized effusion (for example, with aortic dissection or trauma) but may not occur even with very large effusions if the rate of increase in size was gradual.

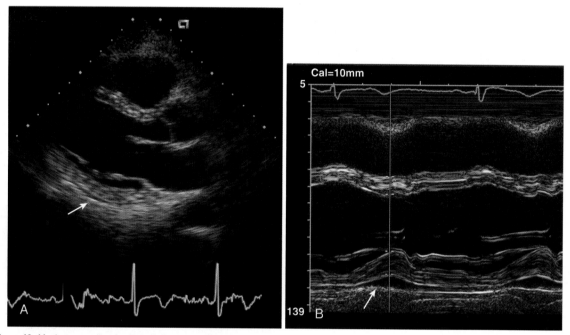

Figure 10–11. A very small pericardial effusion is seen (*A*) on 2D imaging posterior to the left ventricle. (*B*) The M-mode tracing demonstrates the small effusion more clearly with flat motion of the parietal pericardium so that there is a more prominent posterior echo-free space in systole than diastole.

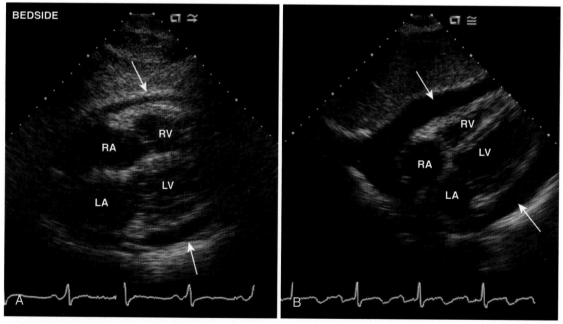

Figure 10–12. The size of a pericardial effusion is graded qualitatively, but measurement of the distance between the epicardium and pericardium is helpful. On a subcostal view, both these patients have circumferential pericardial effusion, with a moderate effusion (*A*) showing between 0.5 and 2 cm maximal pericardial separation compared to more than 2 cm with a large effusion (*B*).

❐ Thin-walled, low-pressure cardiac chambers (e.g., the RA) are compressed at lower pericardial pressures than thicker-walled chambers (e.g., the right ventricle [RV]).

❐ Cardiac compression is most evident during the phase of the cardiac cycle when the chamber pressure is low (e.g., systole for the atrial chambers, diastole for the RV).

❐ With inspiration, intrathoracic pressure falls, resulting in increased filling of the right heart. If total cardiac volume is fixed (as with tamponade physiology), the increased filling of the right

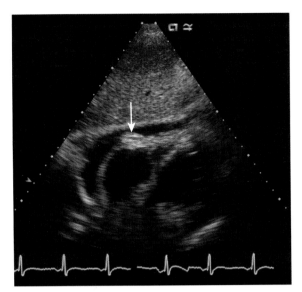

Figure 10–13. The subcostal window is key in evaluation of pericardial effusions because this approach often is used for drainage of pericardial fluid. In this patient, the effusion between the liver and right side of the heart is seen. The normal adipose tissue at the right atrioventricular groove (*arrow*) often is well seen when a pericardial effusion is present. If pericardiocentesis is planned, a transducer position where the effusion is closer to the site of needle entry, with less intervening hepatic tissue, is preferred. This effusion is only small to moderate in size, so many clinicians would defer pericardiocentesis.

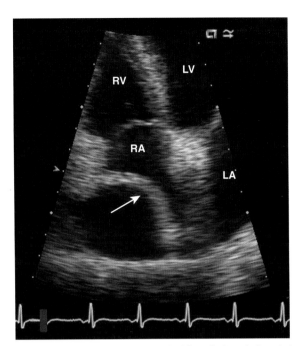

Figure 10–14. The RA free wall is examined frame by frame in the apical 4-chamber plane using zoom mode and a narrow sector. This end-systolic frame shows persistent systolic compression (or collapse) of the RA free wall consistent with tamponade physiology.

heart limits filling of the left heart, resulting in a lower forward stroke volume and blood pressure.

❏ If the patient has a low cardiac output or hypotension and a large pericardial effusion is present, further echocardiographic evaluation is not needed; prompt therapy is more appropriate.

Step 1: Look for right atrial systolic collapse

■ When intrapericardial pressure exceeds RA pressure, the RA free wall collapses in systole. (Figure 10–14)

■ RA free wall inversion for more than one third of systole is sensitive and specific for the diagnosis of tamponade physiology.

Key points

❏ Brief systolic inversion of the RA free wall may be seen without tamponade physiology.

❏ The RA free wall is best evaluated in the apical and subcostal 4-chamber views.

❏ Zoom mode provides optimal image resolution; a narrow 2D sector improves frame rate.

❏ Frame by frame analysis, to determine the number of frames with free wall inversion compared with the total frames in systole, improves the accuracy of this approach.

Step 2: Evaluate RV diastolic collapse

■ When intrapericardial pressure exceeds RV diastolic pressure, the RV free wall collapses in diastole. (Figure 10–15)

Key points

❏ Frame-by-frame analysis or use of an M-mode cursor through the RV free wall may be helpful for evaluation of the timing of RV free wall motion.

❏ RV diastolic collapse may be appreciated in parasternal long and short axis and in apical and subcostal 4-chamber views.

❏ RV diastolic collapse is less sensitive, but more specific, than brief RA systolic collapse for the diagnosis of pericardial tamponade.

❏ If the RV free wall is thickened due to hypertrophy or an infiltrative process, diastolic collapse may not occur even with elevated pericardial pressures.

Step 3: Examine for reciprocal respiratory changes in RV and LV volumes

■ An effusion with tamponade physiology results in a fixed total cardiac volume.

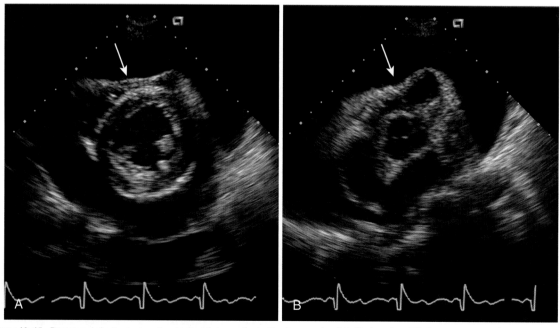

Figure 10–15. Parasternal short-axis views in mid-diastole in a patient with a large pericardial effusion, show RV diastolic collapse at the mid-ventricular (*A*) and RV outflow tract (*B*) levels. The RV chamber is very small, with a convex indentation of the RV free wall by the pericardial effusion.

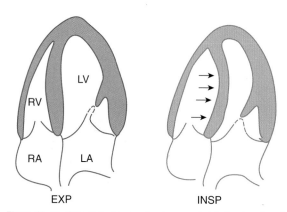

Figure 10–16. Schematic diagram showing an apical 4-chamber view at end-expiration (*EXP*) and during inspiration (*INSP*) with pericardial constriction. The increase in RV filling with inspiration results in a compensatory decrease in LV size, as the total cardiac volume is constrained by the thickened and adherent pericardium. This results in "septal shift" with inspiration.

- With a fixed total volume, the increase in right-sided filling with inspiration is matched by a reciprocal decrease in left-sided volumes.
- Conversely, with expiration there is a relative increase in left, compared with right, heart filling.

Key points

- ❏ The reciprocal changes in right- and left filling with respiration are best seen on 2D imaging in a 4-chamber view. (Figure 10–16)

- ❏ With inspiration, the ventricular septum shifts to the left, followed by a shift toward the right with expiration.
- ❏ An M-mode tracing of the septum from the parasternal window also may be helpful.

Step 4: Evaluate for reciprocal respiratory changes in RV and LV filling velocities

- Analogous to the changes in RV and LV volumes with respiration, the volume of inflow across the atrioventricular valves varies with respiration.
- With inspiration, there is an increase (>25%) in RV diastolic filling; with expiration, LV diastolic filling increases (by >25%). (Figure 10–17)

Key points

- ❏ The phase of respiration is recorded (using a respirometer) simultaneously with the ECG and Doppler velocity data.
- ❏ A slow sweep speed is used to include more than one respiratory cycle on the recording.
- ❏ The Doppler sample volume is positioned and a 2D image is recorded for several beats to ensure that the intercept angle between the Doppler beam and direction of inflow does not vary significantly with respiration. If there is a significant variation in intercept angle, observed differences in velocity with respiration may be an artifact due to assuming a constant angle in the Doppler equation.

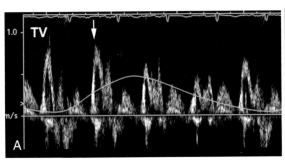
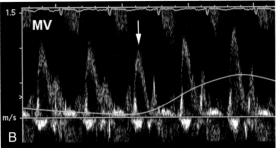

Figure 10–17. In this patient with a large pericardial effusion, ventricular inflow velocities across the tricuspid valve (*TV*) and mitral valve (*MV*) were recorded at a slow sweep speed simultaneously with a respirometer tracing. The cyan-colored respirometer tracing indicates inspiration as an upward deflection and expiration as a downward deflection. The TV tracing shows that the inflow velocity increases with inspiration with a peak velocity of only 0.29 m/s in expiration and 0.54 m/s with inspiration (an increase > 100%). There are reciprocal changes in transmitral flow, with the peak velocity decreasing from 0.82 m/s during expiration to 0.55 m/s on the first beat after inspiration.

- ❐ With tamponade physiology, RV diastolic filling increases and LV diastolic filling decreases on the first beat after inspiration.
- ❐ Evaluation of filling dynamics is challenging, so that an apparent lack of respiratory variation does not exclude the possibility of tamponade physiology.

Step 5: Determine if right atrial filling pressures are elevated

- ■ Elevated RA filling pressures are a sensitive, but not specific, sign of cardiac tamponade.
- ■ Echocardiographic evaluation of RA filling pressure is based on the size and respiratory variation of the inferior vena cava (IVC); a dilated IVC without respiratory variation and with dilated hepatic veins is called plethora of the IVC. (Figure 10–18)

Key points

- ❐ Images of the IVC are obtained from the subcostal view in spontaneously breathing patients.
- ❐ This method is not applicable in patients on positive pressure mechanical ventilation.
- ❐ There are many other causes for elevated RA pressures, other than tamponade physiology, so this finding is interpreted in the context of the other imaging findings.
- ❐ Tamponade may be present without plethora of the IVC if the patient is hypovolemic.

Step 6: Perform echo-guided pericardiocentesis if clinically indicated

- ■ Echocardiography may be used to guide the percutaneous pericardiocentesis procedure either to define the best approach to percutaneous drainage or to confirm the needle position in the pericardial space. (Figure 10–19)

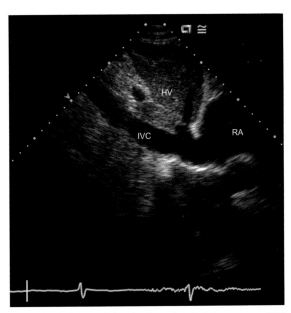

Figure 10–18. Subcostal view showing a dilated inferior vena cava (*IVC*) and hepatic vein in a patient with pericardial tamponade. With inspiration, there was no change in *IVC* diameter.

- ■ Echocardiography is used after pericardiocentesis to assess the amount of residual fluid. (Figure 10–20)

Key points

- ❐ Evaluation from parasternal, apical, and subcostal approaches demonstrates the depth and amount of pericardial fluid relative to the position of the transducer.
- ❐ Visualization of the tip of the needle is problematic because any segment of the needle passing through the 2D image plane may be mistaken for the tip 3D imaging may be helpful.

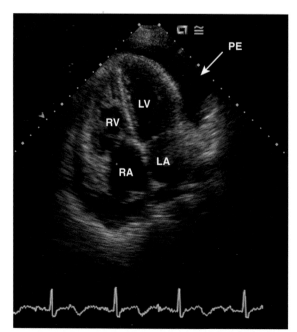

Figure 10–19. Apical 4-chamber view showing a large circumferential pericardial effusion, with relatively more fluid posterior and lateral to the LV, as is typical on echocardiography. Fluid is seen adjacent to the RA and a small amount of fluid is seen superior to the LA, in the oblique sinus of the pericardium that extends between the right and left pulmonary veins.

❑ The position of the needle is confirmed by injection of a small amount of agitated saline to produce a contrast effect.

Pericardial constriction

■ Pericardial constriction is the result of pericardial thickening and fibrosis with fusion of the parietal and visceral pericardium.
■ The thickened and rigid pericardium constricts the cardiac chambers, resulting in a limited total cardiac volume and a reduced cardiac output.

Key points

❑ Common causes of pericardial constriction include prior cardiac surgery or trauma, radiation therapy, and recurrent pericarditis.
❑ Like tamponade physiology, the fixed total cardiac volume with pericardial constriction results in reciprocal changes in right- and left-heart filling.
❑ Typically there is no significant pericardial effusion when constrictive pericarditis is present, although there are rare cases of effusive constrictive physiology.
❑ Clinically the differentiation of constrictive pericarditis (which is treated by pericardiotomy) and restrictive cardiomyopathy (which is treated medically) is problematic.

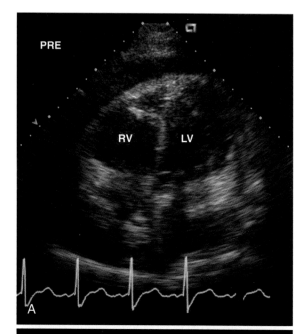

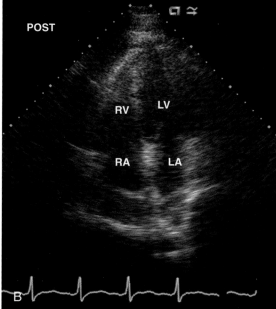

Figure 10–20. Echocardiographic monitoring of pericardiocentesis in the cardiac catheterization lab. At baseline (*PRE*), a foreshortened apical view shows a large pericardial effusion. After drainage of 1 L of fluid, repeat imaging shows a much smaller effusion at the apex, although some fluid persists adjacent to the RV and RA. Image quality is suboptimal because the patient is supine and removal of the fluid resulted in poorer acoustic access.

Step 1: Look for evidence of pericardial thickening

■ Pericardial thickening may be evident on 2D echocardiography as areas of increased echogenicity in the pericardial region. (Figure 10–21)

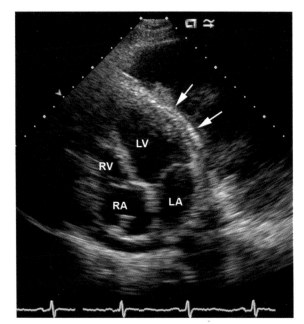

Figure 10–21. This long-axis views shows marked thickening of the pericardium posterior to the left ventricle in a patient later diagnosed with constrictive pericarditis. Pericardial thickening is differentiated from effusion by the echogenicity of the pericardial space.

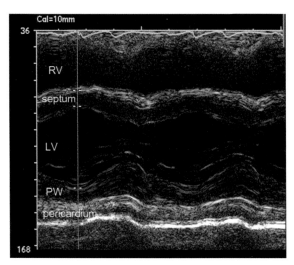

Figure 10–22. M-mode of pericardial thickening demonstrates a thick posterior pericardium that moves with the epicardium during the cardiac cycle.

- On M-mode tracings, pericardial thickening is evident as multiple dense parallel lines posterior to the LV endocardium that persist even with low gain settings. (Figure 10–22)

Key points

- ❏ Echocardiography is not sensitive for detection of pericardial thickening; cardiac computed tomographic (CT) or magnetic resonance

imaging (MRI) is preferred when measurement of pericardial thickness is needed.
- ❏ Pericardial thickening may be asymmetric so that a complete evaluation includes evaluation from parasternal, apical, and subcostal windows.

Step 2: Evaluate for anatomic evidence of constriction

- Typical findings in patients with pericardial constriction are enlarged atria (due to chronically elevated filling pressures), and small ventricles with normal systolic function.
- M-mode findings in constrictive pericarditis include reduced posterior motion of the LV posterior wall endocardium in diastole (<2 mm) and a brief rapid posterior motion of the ventricular septum in early diastole.

Key points

- ❏ There are no specific 2D imaging findings in patients with constrictive pericarditis.
- ❏ The diagnosis of constrictive pericarditis should be considered in the appropriate clinical setting (cardiac symptoms in a patient at risk of constrictive disease) if the echocardiogram does not show other causes for the patient's symptoms.
- ❏ Constrictive pericarditis most often is diagnosed in patients with unremarkable echocardiographic images.

Step 3: Perform Doppler studies to diagnose constriction

- Reciprocal respiratory changes in RV and LV diastolic filling, in the absence of a pericardial effusion, suggest the diagnosis of constrictive pericarditis. (Figure 10–23)
- Typically, pulmonary pressures are normal in patients with constrictive pericarditis but elevated (>60 mm Hg) in those with restrictive cardiomyopathy.

Key points

- ❏ With pericardial constriction, the normal myocardium allows rapid early diastolic filling of the chamber with normal relaxation and compliance. Once the chamber has reached the limit of total cardiac volume imposed by the rigid pericardium, ventricular filling abruptly halts.
- ❏ The ventricular inflow pattern shows a prominent early (E) filling velocity, a normal deceleration slope, and a very small atrial contribution to filling (due to elevated end-diastolic LV pressures).

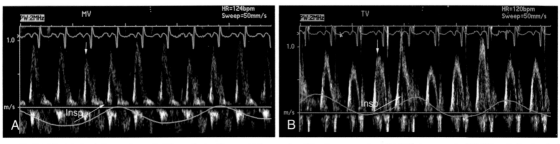

Figure 10-23. Ventricular inflow patterns in this patient with constrictive pericarditis show a marked (>25%) increase in RV filling during inspiration (*arrow*) with a reciprocal respiratory decrease (>25%) in LV diastolic filling.

TABLE 10-2 Comparison of Pericardial Tamponade, Constriction, and Restrictive Cardiomyopathy			
	Pericardial Tamponade	**Constrictive Pericarditis**	**Restrictive Cardiomyopathy**
Hemodynamics			
RA pressure	↑	↑	↑
RV/LV filling pressures	↑, RV = LV	↑, RV = LV	↑, LV > RV
Pulmonary artery pressures	Normal	Mild elevation (35-40 mm Hg systolic)	Moderate-severe elevation (≥60 mm Hg systolic)
RV diastolic pressure plateau		>1/3 peak RV pressure	>1/3 peak RV pressure
Radionuclide Diastolic Filling		Rapid early filling, impaired late filling	Impaired early filling
2D Echo	Moderate-large PE	Pericardial thickening without effusion	Left ventricular hypertrophy Normal systolic function
Doppler Echo	Reciprocal respiratory changes in RV and LV filling Inferior vena cava plethora	E > A on LV inflow Prominent *y* descent in hepatic vein Pulmonary venous flow = prominent *a* wave, reduced systolic phase Respiratory variation in IVRT and in *E* velocity	(1) Early in disease E < A on LV inflow (2) Late in disease E > A (3) Constant IVRT (4) Absence of significant respiratory variation
Other Diagnostic Tests	Therapeutic/diagnostic pericardiocentesis	CT or MRI for pericardial thickening	Endomyocardial biopsy

CT = computed tomography, IVRT = isovolumic relaxation time, LV = left ventricle, MRI = magnetic resonance imaging, PE = pericardial effusion.

❐ The RA inflow (hepatic vein) pattern shows a prominent atrial reversal, with prominent diastolic (and blunted systolic) ventricular filling.
❐ Pulmonary pressures are estimated based on the velocity in the tricuspid regurgitant jet and an estimate of RA pressure.

Step 4: Distinguish constrictive pericarditis from restrictive cardiomyopathy

■ Echocardiography alone often is inadequate to distinguish constrictive pericarditis from restrictive cardiomyopathy. (Table 10-2)

■ However, the possibility of these diagnoses often is first suggested by the echocardiographic findings.

Key points

❑ RA and LA filling pressures are increased in both conditions.

❑ RV and LV diastolic pressures are equal, even after volume loading, when constrictive pericarditis is present.

❑ Pulmonary systolic pressure typically is severely elevated with a restrictive cardiomyopathy.

❑ Severe biatrial enlargement is typical with restrictive cardiomyopathy.

❑ Early diastolic filling is rapid with constrictive pericarditis and is reduced with restrictive cardiomyopathy early in the disease course.

❑ However, with advanced restrictive physiology, ventricular compliance is reduced so that early diastolic filling may appear similar to the pattern seen with constrictive pericarditis.

❑ The LV myocardium is normal with constrictive pericarditis. With restrictive cardiomyopathy, LV wall thickness often is increased.

❑ Additional helpful studies are CT and/or MRI direct imaging of pericardial thickness, cardiac catheterization for simultaneous measurement of LV and RV diastolic pressures, and endomyocardial biopsy.

THE ECHO EXAM

Pericardial Effusion

Views
    Parasternal
    Apical
    Subcostal
Distinguish from pleural fluid
Size
    Small (<0.5 cm)
    Moderate (0.5-2.0 cm)
    Large (>2.0 cm)
Diffuse versus loculated
Evaluate for tamponade physiology if moderate or large
TEE if needed, especially in post-op pts

Pericardial Tamponade

CLINICAL FINDINGS

Low cardiac output
Elevated venous pressures
Pulsus paradoxus
Hypotension

2D ECHO

Moderate or large pericardial effusion
Right atrial systolic collapse (duration > ⅓ of systole)
Right ventricular diastolic collapse
Reciprocal respiratory changes in right and left
    ventricular volumes
Inferior vena cave plethora

DOPPLER

Respiratory variation in right and left ventricular
    diastolic filling
Increased right ventricular filling on first beat after
    inspiration
Decreased left ventricular filling on first beat after
    inspiration

Constrictive Pericarditis

M-MODE/2D

Pericardial thickening
Normal left ventricular size and systolic function
Left atrial enlargement
Flattened diastolic wall motion
Abrupt posterior motion of the ventricular septum in
    early diastole
Dilated inferior vena cava and hepatic veins

DOPPLER

Prominent *y* descent on hepatic vein or superior vena
    cava flow pattern
LV inflow shows prominent E velocity with a rapid early
    diastolic deceleration slope and a small or absent A
    velocity
Increase in LV IVRT by > 20% on first beat after
    inspiration
Respiratory variations in RV and LV diastolic filling
    (difference > 25%) with increased RV and decreased
    LV filling with inspiration
Tissue Doppler increased E'
Pulmonary venous flow shows prominent a wave and
    blunting of systolic phase

Left Ventricular Pseudo-Aneurysm

Abrupt transition from normal myocardium to
    aneurysm
Acute angle between myocardium and aneurysm
Narrow neck
Ratio of neck diameter to aneurysm diameter < 0.5
May be lined with thrombus

SELF-ASSESSMENT QUESTIONS

QUESTION 1

A 72-year-old woman presents with a 6-month history of progressive pedal edema and exertional dyspnea. Her medical history includes coronary disease and hypertension.

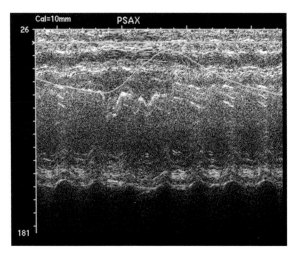

Figure 10–24.

The image provided (Figure 10–24) is most consistent with:

A. Cardiac tamponade
B. Primary pulmonary hypertension
C. Pericardial constriction
D. Dilated cardiomyopathy

QUESTION 2

A 55-year-old woman presents with a 3-month history of progressive pedal edema and exertional dyspnea. She has no significant past medical history.

Data from her transthoracic echocardiogram area is as follows:

LV end-diastolic volume	100 mL
LV posterior wall thickness	1.2 cm
LV ejection fraction	59%
LA indexed volume	45 mL/m^2
Mitral valve E wave velocity	1.7 m/s
Tissue Doppler E' velocity	0.05 m/s
IVC diameter	2.0 cm
Tricuspid regurgitant jet velocity	3.6 m/s

You conclude that the data are most consistent with:

A. Pericardial constriction
B. Dilated cardiomyopathy
C. Restrictive cardiomyopathy
D. Chronic obstructive pulmonary disease

QUESTION 3

A 54-year-old woman with acute myeloid leukemia presents with dyspnea.

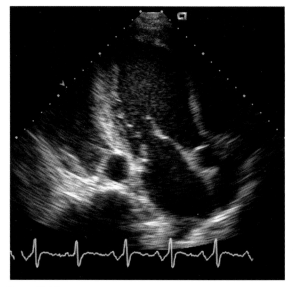

Figure 10–25.

Based on (Figure 10–25), the next best step in patient management is:

A. Pericardiocentesis
B. Thoracentesis
C. Ligation of the persistent left superior vena cava
D. Pericardial stripping

QUESTION 4

This 43-year-old man has a history of Hodgkin's lymphoma, initially diagnosed at age 18 years when he presented with fatigue and large pericardial and pleural effusions. At that time he was aggressively treated with chemotherapy and mantle radiation. He now presents with several months of progressive exertional dyspnea. This hepatic vein flow tracing is obtained (Figure 10–26).

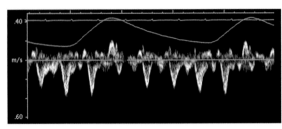

Figure 10–26.

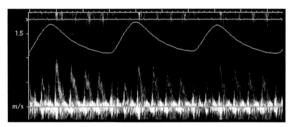

Figure 10–28.

The patient's current symptoms are most likely due to:

A. Prior chemotherapy
B. Recurrent pericardial effusion
C. Prior mantle field radiation
D. Recurrent pleural effusion

QUESTION 5

A 64-year-old female patient with end-stage renal disease presents with dyspnea and a blood pressure of 90/60 mm Hg. A TTE is ordered (Figure 10–27).

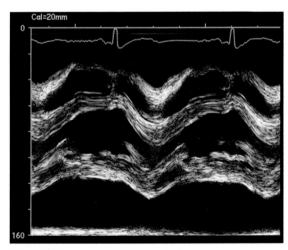

Figure 10–27.

Based on the image provided, what is your next step in the management of this patient?

A. Respirometer
B. Right heart catheterization
C. Cardiac CT
D. Pericardiocentesis

QUESTION 6

The following pulsed Doppler tracing was recorded across the mitral valve (Figure 10–28).

The most likely diagnosis for this patient is:

A. Normal respiratory variation
B. Pericardial constriction
C. Myocardial restriction
D. Chronic obstructive pulmonary disease

QUESTION 7

A 55-year-old woman with a history of viral cardiomyopathy with severe biventricular systolic dysfunction underwent placement of biventricular surgical ventricular assist devices. Cardiac output has decreased and you are asked to review an echocardiogram (Figure 10–29).

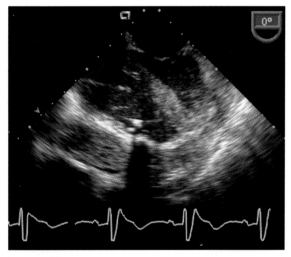

Figure 10–29.

Based on the image provided, the next best step in patient management is:

A. Reposition inflow cannula
B. Intravenous (IV) fluid administration
C. Hematoma evacuation
D. Cannula thrombus removal

QUESTION 8

A 78-year-old man presents with exertional dyspnea 6 years after coronary artery bypass grafting. Coronary angiography documents occlusion of one of his four bypass grafts. A TTE (Figure 10–30) is ordered and compared with a study he had done 5 years earlier.

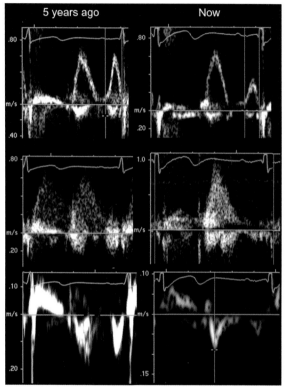

Figure 10–30.

Of the following options, what additional finding would most likely be present?

A. IVRT respiratory variation
B. Indexed LA volume 43 cm^3
C. LV dP/dt 800 mm Hg/s
D. IVC diameter 1.5 cm

QUESTION 9

A 58-year-old male with amyloidosis is undergoing evaluation for stem cell transplantation. TTE is performed (Figure 10–31).

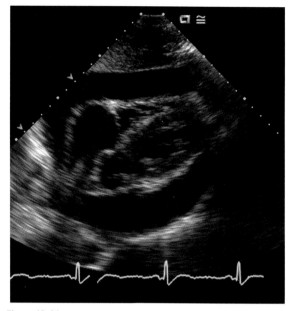

Figure 10–31.

Which of the following clinical conditions would most hinder further echocardiographic evaluation?

A. Pulmonary hypertension
B. Pleural effusion
C. Cardiac amyloidosis
D. Abdominal ascites

QUESTION 10

The following pulsed Doppler tracing was recorded across the tricuspid valve (Figure 10–32).

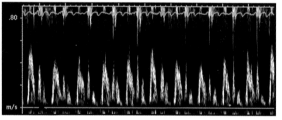

Figure 10–32.

The most likely diagnosis for this patient is:

A. Normal respiratory variation
B. Pericardial tamponade
C. Positive pressure ventilation
D. Pericardial constriction

ANSWERS

ANSWER 1: C

This is an M-mode tracing taken from the parasternal long-axis view. The RV is closer to the transducer and the interventricular septum is seen between the ventricles. Superimposed on the M-mode tracing is a tracing from a respirometer in green. During inspiration, the respirometer shows an upward deflection. Coincident with inspiration, there is septal shifting with a transient increase in RV size and a concordant decrease in LV size. The opposite occurs during expiration. Respiratory-dependent septal shifting is consistent with a fixed external obstruction to ventricular filling, as occurs in pericardial constriction. Pericardial constriction is typically a consequence of cyclic or chronic pericardial inflammation and is most commonly seen in inflammatory conditions or postcardiac surgical procedures. This patient is not in cardiac tamponade; there is no significant pericardial fluid between the right ventricular free wall and the transducer and fluid is not seen posterior to the heart. In primary pulmonary hypertension, the right ventricle is enlarged with flattened septal motion in systole and diastole due to RV pressure overload. With dilated cardiomyopathy the LV is enlarged with decreased systolic endocardial motion of the septum and posterior wall. In this case, the LV at end-diastole is normal at about 5 cm and the end-systolic dimension is 3.5 cm for a fractional shortening of 30%, which is normal.

ANSWER 2: C

This is a patient with restrictive cardiomyopathy. Patients with restrictive cardiomyopathy have relatively normal systolic function with significant diastolic dysfunction, often in the setting of increased LV wall thickness. This study shows decreased ventricular compliance and severely elevated LV filling pressure as reflected in the elevated E wave velocity of 1.7 m/s and a severely elevated E/E' of 34. The elevated LV filling pressure is also reflected in the severely elevated indexed LA volume (normal < 30 ml/m^2) and pulmonary hypertension, with only mildly increased central venous pressure. LV chamber size (indexed LV volume) is normal, with preserved systolic function and mild hypertrophy of the chamber walls, also characteristic of restrictive cardiomyopathy. For pericardial constriction, elevation in RV filling pressure is more pronounced than the increase in LV filling pressure, evidenced by dilation of the IVC, which is not seen in this case. Also, in constriction, myocardial tissue Doppler would be normal (normal E' velocity), with only mildly increased pulmonary pressures. This patient does not have a dilated cardiomyopathy; LV volume would be increased, with a decreased ejection fraction. Chronic obstructive pulmonary disease is not associated with LV diastolic dysfunction, and the severity of pulmonary hypertension is greater than expected for this diagnosis.

ANSWER 3: B

This patient has a large left-sided pleural effusion. The image presented is an apical long-axis view of the heart. The LV is closest to the transducer. Posterior to the heart, there is an echolucent space consistent with fluid. The circular structure is the descending thoracic aorta seen in cross section. Tracking posterior to the descending thoracic aorta is a large pleural effusion. A pleural and pericardial effusion can be differentiated by the tissue planes that bound the fluid collection. Fluid that tracks anterior to the descending aorta is pericardial. In this example, there is a trivial pericardial stripe seen just along the epicardial border, which is normal thickness. The descending aorta might be mistaken for a dilated coronary sinus, as seen in patients with a persistent left superior vena cava. However, the coronary sinus is not well seen on this image; it typically is closer to the atrioventricular groove and slightly superior to the descending aorta in this view. A persistent left superior vena cava is a normal variant and does not cause symptoms or require intervention. Pericardial stripping refers to surgical removal of a thickened pericardial when pericardial constriction is present.

ANSWER 4: C

This is a patient with pericardial constriction. The hepatic vein tracing shows the ECG, respirometer (inspiration is an upward deflection), and Doppler tracing, with care taken using 2D imaging to ensure that the Doppler angle did not change with respiration. The pulsed Doppler tracing from the hepatic vein shows a prominent RA filling curve in diastole with blunted filling in systole, typical of the "square root sign" of ventricular filling pressures with constriction. Filling increases on the first beat after inspiration and then declines dramatically (and in fact reverses on the first beat) with expiration. Late pericardial constriction is a relatively common complication in patients with Hodgkin's lymphoma who received mantle field (upper torso) radiation treatment in the 1980s and 1990s. Other late adverse effects of radiation therapy include diastolic ventricular dysfunction and accelerated valve calcification and coronary atherosclerosis. Pericardial constriction is less common with more contemporary treatments for Hodgkin's lymphoma, in which chemotherapy and more focused treatment fields are utilized.

Other respiratory-dependent changes in pericardial constriction that would be seen by echocardiography include reciprocal changes in Doppler inflows, increased on inspiration across the right valves and decreased on inspiration across the left valves, and an inspiratory increase in IVRT duration. Right heart catheterization would show equalization of intracardiac and pulmonary artery diastolic pressures. Anthracycline chemotherapy is cardiotoxic, and the potential cumulative effect of treatment is a dilated cardiomyopathy. In patients with severe ventricular dysfunction and volume overload, the IVC may be dilated, but anterograde flow in the hepatic vein would be normal. If there were significant concurrent tricuspid annular dilation and tricuspid regurgitation, hepatic vein systolic flow reversal might be seen but would not be dependent on the respiratory cycle. A pleural effusion would not affect RA Doppler inflow unless tamponade physiology was present.

ANSWER 5: D

This image shows an M-mode tracing taken from the parasternal short-axis view in a patient with a large pericardial effusion. There is a circumferential pericardial effusion, evidenced by an echolucent space between the transducer and the heart and a large echolucent space posterior to the heart, between the heart and pericardium, which is seen in the very far field. This patient has evidence of hemodynamic significance, with a small LV chamber size at the level of the mitral leaflet tips and a small RV chamber size (referenced to the side marks, the RV chamber size is approximately 1 cm in diameter in diastole). Additionally, there is late diastolic invagination of the RV free wall, a small posterior deflection, just at the onset of the QRS, which is also supportive of a hemodynamically significant effusion. With symptoms, hypotension and a large pericardial effusion, prompt pericardiocentesis is appropriate. Additional diagnostic information, such as intracardiac pressures or respiratory variation in tricuspid or mitral inflow, is not needed. Cardiac CT would also diagnose a pericardial effusion but is not needed with a diagnostic echocardiogram, and CT is less useful for determining the hemodynamic significance of an effusion. In a patient with suspected pericardial constriction, cardiac CT would aid in visualizing the pericardium and in measuring pericardial thickness.

ANSWER 6: B

This is a pulsed Doppler sample taken across the mitral valve in a patient with pericardial constriction. On the first beat after inspiration (upward deflection on green respirometer curve), there is a significant (>20%) decrease in the mitral E wave velocity and with expiration there is a higher mitral E wave velocity. These findings are consistent with impaired LV filling during inspiration and increased LV filling during expiration. The proposed mechanism for these changes is that the negative intrathoracic pressure with normal inspiration allows increased RV inflow. Because total heart volume is limited due to pericardial constriction, the increase in RV size results in a decrease in LV size and a reduction in LV filling with inspiration. The opposite changes occur during expiration, and these changes exceed the normal degree of variation in RV and LV inflow with respiration. These exaggerated reciprocal variations in respiratory flow are also seen in pericardial tamponade. With exaggerated respiratory effort, as can occur with chronic obstructive pulmonary disease, respiratory variation in inflow to the thinner-walled RV is commonly seen, but without external cardiac constraint, reciprocal changes in LV filling are not seen. In myocardial restriction, there is no external constraint on the heart and, although diastolic LV function is abnormal, reciprocal respiratory changes in ventricular filling are not seen.

ANSWER 7: C

This TEE 4-chamber view shows a large hematoma in the pericardial space, adjacent to the inflow cannula from the RV apex, identified by the bright echoes with dense distal shadowing. There is a 3-cm-thick echodense space around the heart with a thin pericardial stripe seen in the far field. The pericardial hematoma surrounds both ventricles and is the most likely cause of decreased cardiac output, either by compression of the inflow cannula or frank tamponade physiology. Thus, surgical evacuation of the hematoma was appropriate and resulted in marked clinical improvement in this patient. With an LV assist device, the LV chamber is usually small due to "unloading" by flow into the device. However, if the ventricular assist device flow rate is set too high, the LV chamber can collapse or the inflow cannula can abut the septum, resulting in impaired inflow into the device. In this case, the LV appears small and underfilled but the RV appears dilated, suggesting that a high flow rate is not the problem. Administration of IV fluid is unlikely to be helpful given the dilated RV seen on this image; total intravascular volume does not appear reduced. In the absence of a ventricular assist device, fluid administration partially alleviates tamponade physiology while awaiting pericardiocentesis; however, with a ventricular assist device, a further increase in RV diastolic pressure is unlikely to be helpful. The inflow cannula itself is not well seen and it would be difficult to diagnose an obstructive thrombus within the device on echocardiographic imaging due to image artifact from prosthetic material, although Doppler interrogation of cannula flow may be diagnostic, particularly if there is a change from a previous study.

ANSWER 8: A

This patient has Doppler evidence of pericardial constriction, likely a consequence of his prior bypass grafting surgery. In addition to the findings shown, respiratory variation in LV/RV inflow and the IVRT would be present. In pericardial constriction, myocardial function is normal, with normal LV relaxation and ventricular compliance, but diastolic filling of the ventricle is constrained externally by the rigid pericardium. The early component of diastolic filling, E wave, is normal, but the late atrial contribution, A wave velocity, is minimal because of elevated LV end-diastolic pressure. Therefore, the E/A ratio (*top*) is increased in this patient compared with his baseline study. On the pulmonary venous tracing (*middle*), higher LV filling pressure leads to blunting of the systolic component of LA filling compared with baseline. However, because myocardial function is normal, the E/E′ ratio remains in the normal range, with a baseline E/E′ of $0.65/1.1 = 6$ and a follow-up E/E′ of $0.65/0.08 = 8$, both of which are in the normal range and within measurement variability of each other. In constriction, the thickened pericardium encases the entire heart, and biventricular size is normal or only mildly increased; an indexed LA volume of 43 cm^3 is severely increased and would be more typical of restrictive cardiomyopathy. The LV *dP/dt* is normal (>1000 mm Hg/s) with pericardial constriction because LV systolic function is normal. Also, in constriction, return of blood is restricted, with severely increased central venous pressure, and the IVC would be dilated and plethoric, not normal caliber.

ANSWER 9: A

This subcostal 4-chamber view shows a large pericardial effusion. Both RV and LV chamber size are small and there is a large echolucent space anterior and posterior to the heart. The posterior fluid is seen between the posterior LV wall and the pericardium (seen in the very far field). Symptoms of a pericardial effusion typically include chest discomfort and dyspnea, but a slowly accumulating effusion may also be asymptomatic, as in this example. In a patient with a large pericardial effusion, cardiac tamponade is a clinical diagnosis based on evidence of hemodynamic compromise including tachycardia, hypotension, and a pulsus paradoxus. In addition, echo-Doppler findings suggesting tamponade physiology can be helpful in clinical decision making. Echocardiographic findings of hemodynamic significance include respiratory-dependent variation in ventricular inflow; with an increase in RV inflow on inspiration and a reciprocal decrease in LV inflow with inspiration. As a consequence, there are also concordant reciprocal changes in ventricular volumes with the respiratory cycle. Significant pulmonary hypertension increases intracavitary RV pressure, preventing RV compression, and thus may obscure classic echocardiographic features of tamponade. Cardiac amyloidosis is associated with restrictive LV filling on the transmitral Doppler tracing, with a high E/A ratio and low tissue myocardial velocity. However, amyloidosis does not cause respiratory-dependent variation in RV and LV filling and septal shifting is not present. Extracardiac fluid collections such as pleural effusion or abdominal ascites do not exert external circumferential pressure on the heart and therefore do not generate echocardiographic findings consistent with cardiac tamponade.

ANSWER 10: A

This is a pulsed Doppler sample taken across the tricuspid valve in a patient with a normal heart. Although a respirometer tracing is not shown, the degree of change in inflow velocity is within normal limits. With inspiration, negative intrathoracic pressure increases and there is an increase in RV inflow (tricuspid E wave velocity) up to 25% variation. With pericardial tamponade or constriction, reciprocal respiratory variation in ventricular inflow is greater than 25% between the first beat after inspiration and the first beat after expiration. Positive pressure ventilation eliminates the negative intrathoracic pressure of inspiration and normal respiratory variation in inflow is not seen.

11 Valvular Stenosis

AORTIC STENOSIS

STEP-BY-STEP APPROACH

Step 1: Determine the etiology of stenosis

based on: (Figure 11–1):
- Parasternal 2D images of the valve in long- and short-axis views
- Number of leaflets, mobility, thickness, and calcification
- Level of obstruction: valvular, subvalvular, or supravalvular

Key points

- Calcific changes usually start in the central part of the leaflets, resulting in a three-pointed star-shaped orifice.
- Rheumatic aortic valve disease affects the commissures and leaflet edges, with a triangular-shaped orifice, and is accompanied by rheumatic mitral valve changes.
- A bicuspid valve may appear trileaflet in diastole due to a raphe in one leaflet; the number of leaflets must be visualized when the valve is open in systole, taking care to identify each commissure, the points where the leaflets attach to the aortic wall.
- Subvalvular or supravalvular stenosis is distinguished from valvular stenosis based on the site of the increase in velocity and on the anatomy of the outflow tract.

Step 2: Evaluate severity of stenosis based on jet velocity, mean gradient, and valve area

Aortic jet velocity (Figure 11–2)

- CW Doppler gray-scale spectral recording of aortic jet velocity

Key points

- Use multiple acoustic windows (apical, suprasternal, right parasternal) with careful patient positioning and transducer angulation to avoid underestimation of velocity.

215

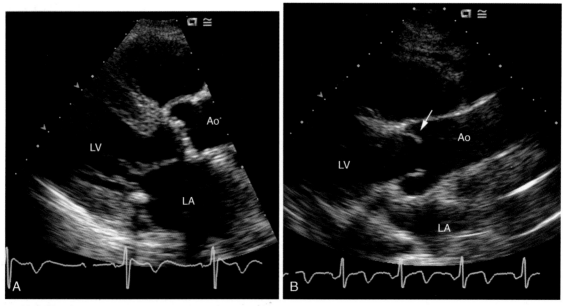

Figure 11–1. The etiology of aortic valve stenosis is evident on these two long views. *A,* With calcific valve disease, there is increased echogenicity of the leaflets, due to calcification and thickening, with reduced systolic opening of the leaflets. Short axis views may show a trileaflet or bicuspid valve, but the number of leaflets may be difficult to determine when significant calcification is present. *B,* In a patient with a congenitally bicuspid, non-calcified valve, the long-axis view shows thin leaflets with reduced systolic opening due to "doming" of the leaflets in systole (*arrow*), as seen by the curve at the tips of the leaflets.

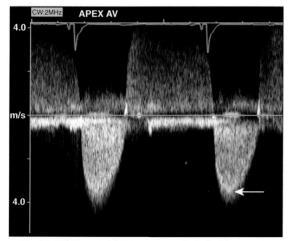

Figure 11–2. Aortic jet velocity is recorded using continuous wave (CW) Doppler. An optimal signal-to-noise ratio is obtained using a small dedicated transducer; the small footprint of this transducer also allows optimal positioning and angulation to align the ultrasound beam parallel to the direction of the stenotic jet. In this example, the scale has been adjusted to show both aortic stenosis and regurgitation. The aortic jet should show a denser signal around the edge and a smooth velocity curve. The difficulty in identifying the maximum velocity is seen in this example, with fuzzy linear signals at peak velocity that are due to the transit time effect. Maximum velocity is measured at the edge of the denser signal, as shown by the *arrow.*

❑ A dedicated small CW Doppler transducer provides the optimal signal-to-noise ratio and allows more precise angulation of the transducer.

❑ Decrease the gain, increase the wall filter, and adjust the baseline and scale to optimize identification of the maximum velocity.

❑ Use the gray-scale spectral displays because with some color displays the signal-to-noise ratio is poor and the edge of the spectral envelope may be blurred, leading to overestimation of velocity.

❑ A smooth velocity curve with a dense outer edge and clear maximum velocity should be recorded; fine linear echos at the peak of the curve are due to the transit time effect and are not included in measurements.

❑ Color Doppler is usually not helpful for jet direction because the jet is short with post-stenotic turbulence and because the elevational plane is not visualized.

Mean gradient

■ Transaortic pressure gradient (ΔP) is calculated from velocity (v) using the Bernoulli equation (Figure 11–3*)* as:

$$\Delta P = 4v^2$$

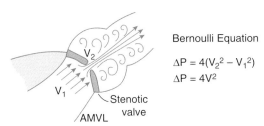

Bernoulli Equation

$$\Delta P = 4(V_2{}^2 - V_1{}^2)$$
$$\Delta P = 4V^2$$

Figure 11–3. This schematic diagram of the Bernoulli equation demonstrates aortic stenosis with laminar low velocity flow on the ventricular side of the valve, a small area of acceleration into the narrow orifice, and the high velocity jet of flow through the narrowed valve. The distal flow disturbance is shown by the *curved arrows*. The instantaneous pressure gradient (ΔP) across the valve is related to the proximal velocity (V_1) and jet velocity (V_2) as shown. Because the proximal velocity is much less than the jet velocity, and usually is less than 1 m/s, the simplified Bernoulli equitation uses only jet velocity in the equation.

Key points

Maximum gradient is calculated from maximum velocity: $\Delta P_{max} = 4v_{max}{}^2$

☐ When proximal velocity is greater than 1.0 m/s, it should be included in the Bernoulli equation, so that:

$$\Delta P = 4(v_{max}{}^2 - v_{proximal}{}^2)$$

☐ Mean gradient is calculated by tracing the velocity curve and averaging instantaneous gradients over the systolic ejection period. (Figure 11–4)
☐ Any underestimation of aortic velocity results in an even greater underestimation in gradients.

Continuity equation valve area *(Figure 11–5)*

■ Aortic valve area (AVA) is calculated as:

$$AVA = (CSA_{LVOT} \times VTI_{LVOT})/VTI_{AS\text{-}Jet}$$

■ The simplified continuity equation, which uses maximum velocities instead of velocity-time integrals (VTIs), also can be used:

$$AVA = (CSA_{LVOT} \times V_{LVOT})/V_{max}$$

Key points

☐ Outflow tract diameter is measured in the parasternal long-axis view in mid-systole using zoom mode and adjusting gain setting to optimize the blood–tissue interface. (Figure 11–6)
☐ Diameter (D) is measured immediately adjacent to the aortic leaflets from inner edge to inner edge. Calculate the circular cross-sectional area:

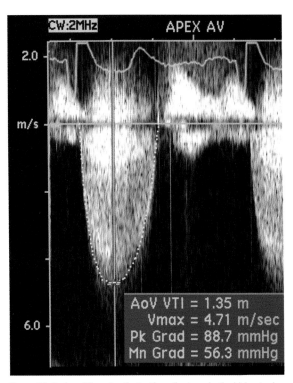

CW:2MHz   APEX AV

2.0

m/s

6.0

AoV VTI = 1.35 m
Vmax = 4.71 m/sec
Pk Grad = 88.7 mmHg
Mn Grad = 56.3 mmHg

Figure 11–4. In a different patient with aortic stenosis, the highest velocity aortic jet was obtained from an apical window. The baseline is moved and the scale is adjusted so that the stenotic signal fills the vertical range of the display. The horizontal axis or "sweep speed" is adjusted to 100 mm/s to allow accurate measurement. The Doppler curve is traced along the outer edge of the dark signal to obtain the velocity-time integral (VTI). The instantaneous pressure gradients over the systolic ejection period are averaged by the analysis package to provide the mean systolic gradient. Notice that the mean gradient is *not* calculated by using the mean velocity in the Bernoulli equation.

$$(CSA_{LVOT}) = 3.14(D/2)^2$$

☐ Outflow tract velocity is recorded with pulsed Doppler from the apical window with the sample volume positioned just apically from the flow acceleration into the valve. An aortic closing click on the spectral tracing indicates correct sample volume positioning.
☐ Move the baseline, adjust the velocity scale, and use an expanded time scale for accurate measurements (Figure 11–7).
☐ Trace the modal systolic velocity (VTI_{LVOT}) and measure peak velocity (V_{LVOT}).
☐ If outflow tract diameter cannot be accurately measured, calculate the ratio of outflow tract to aortic jet velocity:

$$Ratio = V_{LVOT}/V_{max}$$

☐ A ratio less than 0.25 indicates severe stenosis.

CONTINUITY EQUATION

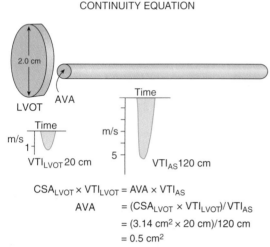

$$CSA_{LVOT} \times VTI_{LVOT} = AVA \times VTI_{AS}$$

$$AVA = (CSA_{LVOT} \times VTI_{LVOT})/VTI_{AS}$$
$$= (3.14 \text{ cm}^2 \times 20 \text{ cm})/120 \text{ cm}$$
$$= 0.5 \text{ cm}^2$$

Figure 11–5. The continuity equation is based on the principle that the volume of flow proximal to and in the narrowed valve must be equal. Flow for one cardiac cycle in the left ventricular outflow tract (LVOT) is shown as a cylinder with a diameter equal to LVOT diameter. Length is equal to the velocity-time integral (VTI) of LVOT flow (because the integral of velocity over time is distance, like traveling in a car). The flow through the orifice is shown as a cylinder with the cross-section equal to aortic valve area (AVA) and length equal to the VTI of the aortic stenosis (AS) jet. Because the volume of both cylinders is the same, the equation is solved for AVA as shown.

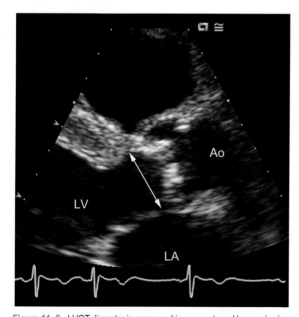

Figure 11–6. LVOT diameter is measured in a parasternal long-axis view in mid-systole from the inner edge of the septum to the inner edge of the anterior mitral leaflet, immediately adjacent to the aortic valve leaflets (*arrow*). A magnified image allows more accurate measurement, and typically several beats are measured to ensure a reproducible value. A typical outflow tract diameter is 2.2 to 2.6 cm in adult men and 2.0 to 2.4 cm in adult women. Outflow tract diameter in adults with aortic stenosis rarely changes over time, so the same value should be used when comparing sequential studies.

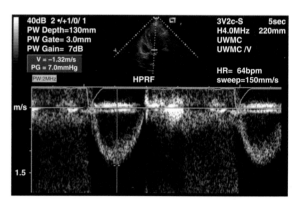

Figure 11–7. Although LVOT diameter is measured from the parasternal window, to provide axial resolution of the tissue–blood interfaces, with ultrasound imaging, LVOT velocity is recorded from the apical window to allow parallel alignment between the ultrasound beam and flow direction. Pulsed (or HPRF) Doppler is used to measure the velocity signal on the ventricular side of the aortic valve, in an anteriorly angulated 4-chamber view (as shown here) or in a long-axis view. The sample volume length or gate is adjusted to 2 to 3 mm and the sample volume is positioned as close to the valve as possible (often the closing click is seen), avoiding the small area of flow acceleration immediately adjacent to the stenotic orifice. The sample volume position should correspond to the site where LVOT diameter was measured. The velocity range and baseline are adjusted so the signal fits but fills the scale, using a fast (100–150 mm/s) horizontal axis scale. A smooth curve with a dense band of velocities ("envelope of flow") with a well-defined peak velocity should be seen. If there is spectral broadening at the peak, the sample volume position is moved slightly apically until a clear signal is obtained.

Step 3: Evaluate aortic regurgitation and ascending aorta (Figure 11–8)

- If regurgitation is significant (vena contracta ≥ 3 mm), evaluate as detailed in Chapter 12.
- Dilation of the ascending aorta may accompany aortic stenosis, particularly with a bicuspid valve.

Key points

- ❏ Most patients with aortic stenosis have some degree (usually mild) of regurgitation.
- ❏ With combined moderate stenosis and regurgitation, quantitation of both lesions is needed.
- ❏ The end-diastolic diameter of the aorta is measured at the sinuses, sinotubular junction, and mid-ascending aorta when aortic valve disease is present. (See Chapter 16)

Step 4: Evaluate the consequences of chronic pressure overload (Figure 11–9)

- Measure LV size and wall thickness and calculate ejection fraction as detailed in Chapter 6.
- Evaluate ventricular diastolic function as detailed in Chapter 7.
- Evaluate coexisting mitral regurgitation (if vena contracta ≥ 3 mm) as detailed in Chapter 12.
- Estimate pulmonary pressures as detailed in Chapter 6.

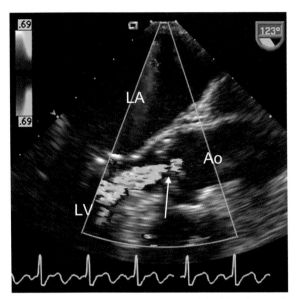

Figure 11–8. Aortic regurgitation is common in adults with aortic stenosis. Often evaluation based on vena contracta width (*arrow*) and the intensity of CW Doppler signal is adequate. This TEE long-axis view shows mild aortic regurgitation in a 48-year-old woman with severe calcific aortic stenosis related to prior radiation therapy.

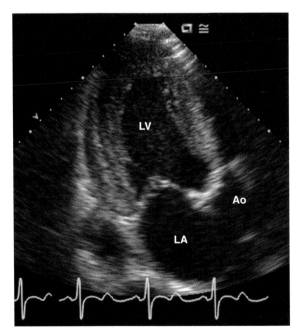

Figure 11–9. This apical long-axis view in a patient with severe aortic stenosis (note calcified valve) demonstrates a normal-size chamber with concentric hypertrophy, as expected with chronic pressure overload of the ventricle.

Key points

☐ Aortic stenosis typically results in concentric LV hypertrophy.

☐ Systolic function and ejection fraction remain normal in most patients but, occasionally, sys-

tolic dysfunction is identified in an asymptomatic patient.

☐ Diastolic dysfunction, usually impaired relaxation, is common.

☐ Pulmonary pressures may be elevated with longstanding severe aortic stenosis.

Step 5: Consider additional evaluation of aortic stenosis severity in selected cases

Key points

☐ The degree of valve calcification (mild, moderate, severe) is a simple, important parameter that is predictive of clinical outcome.

☐ The dimensionless ratio of outflow tract to aortic jet velocity provides a simple index of stenosis severity (normal, 1.0; mild, 0.5; severe, 0.25).

☐ Planimetry of valve area can be helpful in selected cases with excellent images, but caution is needed due to reverberations and shadowing from leaflet calcification. (Figure 11–10)

☐ Blood pressure should be recorded at the time of the velocity data acquisition; stenosis severity may be underestimated in hypertensive patients.

☐ With atrial fibrillation, several beats should be averaged for each measurement. (Figure 11–11)

☐ With low output aortic stenosis and a low LV ejection fraction, evaluation of hemodynamics at two different flow rates (e.g., at rest and with dobutamine) may be helpful.

MITRAL STENOSIS

STEP-BY-STEP APPROACH

Step 1: Evaluate mitral valve morphology (Figure 11–12)

■ Use long- and short-axis views of the mitral valve to demonstrate the typical findings of rheumatic valve disease:
  • Commissural fusion resulting in diastolic doming
  • Chordal shortening and fusion
■ Evaluate mitral valve leaflet mobility, thickening, calcification, and subvalvular disease using the morphology score (Table 11-1) or French classification. (Table 11-2)

Key points

☐ Rheumatic valve disease is the most common cause of mitral stenosis.

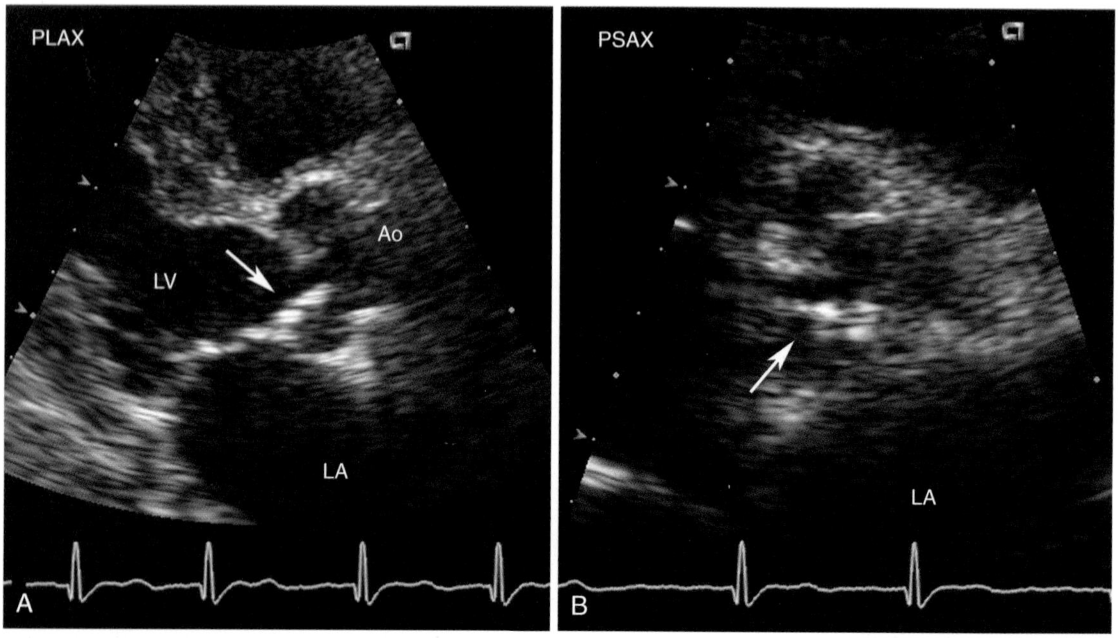

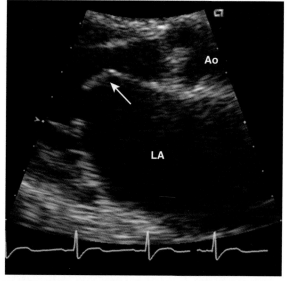

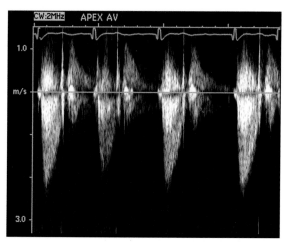

Figure 11–10. In the parasternal long-axis (PLAX) view, the calcified valve leaflet is seen (*arrow*). In the short-axis view of the valve, on TTE or TEE imaging, the apparent opening of the leaflets often can be visualized. Although planimetry of this apparent orifice may be helpful in selected cases, caution is needed to ensure the image plane is at the level of the orifice (consider where this short-axis plane is relative to the long-axis view in this patient), and that shadowing and reverberations from calcification do not obscure the leaflet edges.

Figure 11–11. When the cardiac rhythm is irregular, the velocity (and pressure gradient) across a stenotic valve varies with the length of the R-R interval because of an increased stroke volume with a longer diastolic filling period. This example shows the variation in aortic jet velocity (at a slow sweep speed to include multiple beats) in a patient in atrial fibrillation. Ideally, heart rate should be controlled before evaluation of stenosis severity is performed. Several beats are then averaged for each measurement. Signal quality in this example is suboptimal so additional efforts to improve patient and/or transducer positioning are needed.

Figure 11–12. In this parasternal long-axis view, the typical changes of rheumatic mitral stenosis are seen. There is diastolic doming (*arrow*) of the anterior mitral leaflet due to commisural fusion. The left atrium is enlarged but LV size is normal, as expected with mitral stenosis.

- ❏ Rarely, severe mitral annular calcification encroaches on the mitral orifice, but calcific stenosis is rarely severe.
- ❏ In addition to a numerical score, a narrative description of valve anatomy is helpful for deciding on the optimal intervention.

- ❏ The extent of commisural calcification and asymmetry of leaflet calcification should be noted.
- ❏ The subvalvular apparatus may be best seen on apical views (and may be poorly visualized on TEE).

TABLE 11-1   Mitral Valve Morphology* by 2D Echocardiography

Grade	Mobility	Subvalvular Thickening	Thickening	Calcification
1	Highly mobile valve with only leaflet tips restricted	Minimal thickening just below the mitral leaflets	Leaflets near normal in thickness (4-5 mm)	A single area of increased echo brightness
2	Leaflet mid and base portions have normal mobility	Thickening of chordal structures extending up to one-third of the chordal length	Mid-leaflets normal, considerable thickening of margins (5-8 mm)	Scattered areas of brightness confined to leaflet margins
3	Valve continues to move forward in diastole, mainly from the base	Thickening extending to the distal third of the chords	Thickening extending through the entire leaflet (5-8 mm)	Brightness extending into the mid-portion of the leaflets
4	No or minimal forward movement of the leaflets in diastole	Extensive thickening and shortening of all chordal structures extending down to the papillary muscles	Considerable thickening of all leaflet tissue (>8-10 mm)	Extensive brightness throughout much of the leaflet tissue

The total echocardiographic score is derived from an analysis of mitral leaflet mobility, valvar and subvalvar thickening, and calcification, graded from 0 to 4 according to the above criteria. This gives a total score of 0 to 16.
From Wilkins GT, Weyman AE, Abascal VM, et al.: Br Heart J 1988;60:299-308.

TABLE 11-2   The French Three-Group Grading of Mitral Valve Anatomy

Echocardiographic Group	Mitral Valve Anatomy
Group 1	Pliable noncalcified anterior mitral leaflet and mild subvalvular disease (i.e., thin chordae ≥10 mm long)
Group 2	Pliable noncalcified anterior mitral leaflet and severe subvalvular disease (i.e., thickened chordae <10 mm long)
Group 3	Calcification of mitral valve of any extent, as assessed by fluoroscopy, whatever the state of the subvalvular apparatus

From Iung B, Cormier B, Discimetiere P, et al.: J Am Coll Cardiol 1996;27:407-414.

Step 2: Evaluate the severity of mitral stenosis

2D planimetry of valve area (Figure 11–13)

■ Valve area is measured directly by tracing the orifice in a short-axis view at the leaflet tips.

Key points

❒ In a parasternal short-axis orientation, the image plane is slowly moved from the apex toward the base to identify the orifice of the funnel-shaped stenotic valve.

❒ The zoom mode is used to focus on the valve orifice, with the gain reduced to clearly show the tissue–blood interface.

❒ The inner border of the black–white interface is traced to obtain valve area.

❒ The orifice typically is a smooth, elliptical shape in patients with no prior procedures.

❒ After percutaneous or surgical valvotomy, the orifice is more irregular due to splitting of the fused commissures.

Mean gradient (Figure 11–14)

■ The Doppler velocity curve across the narrowed mitral orifice is recorded from the apical window.

■ Mean gradient is determined using the Bernoulli equation to average the instantaneous pressures gradients over the diastolic filling period.

Key points

❒ The mitral stenosis jet is directed toward the apex, so only minor adjustment of transducer position and angulation is needed to obtain a parallel angle between the Doppler beam and mitral jet; color flow Doppler can help with alignment.

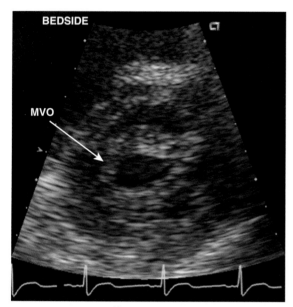

Figure 11–13. The rheumatic mitral valve orifice (*MVO*) is imaged in short axis, taking care to scan from apex toward base to identify the smallest area of the funnel-shaped stenotic orifice. The inner edge of the white–dark interface is traced to obtain valve area. The distance between the LV wall and the edge of the orifice reflects the degree of commisural fusion. These leaflets are uniformly echogenic, consistent with symmetric fibrosis and little calcification.

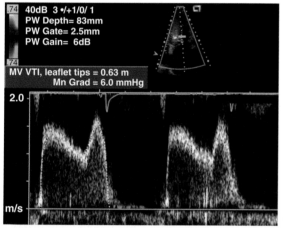

Figure 11–14. Measurement of the mean transmitral pressure gradient in a patient with mitral stenosis. The transmitral velocity is recorded with pulsed Doppler (including HPRF) or CW Doppler if needed to prevent signal aliasing, from an apical window with the baseline shifted and the velocity scale adjusted so that the Doppler velocity fits the vertical axis of the tracing. The time scale is set at 100 to 150 mm/s with the ECG included for timing. After a smooth Doppler curve with a narrow band along the outer edge and a clearly defined peak is obtained, the outer edge of the signal is traced. The analysis package averages the instantaneous gradients over the diastolic filling period. This patient is in sinus rhythm, which does not affect the accuracy of Doppler evaluation of stenosis severity.

☐ Transducer position and gain are adjusted to demonstrate a clear outer boundary of the velocity curve with a well-defined peak and a linear deceleration slope.

☐ The baseline is moved toward the edge of the display, the scale adjusted so the Doppler curve fits but fills the space, and gain and wall filters adjusted to decrease signal noise.

☐ Pulsed or high pulse repetition frequency (HPRF) Doppler may provide a more clearly defined velocity curve than CW Doppler.

☐ Movement of the heart with respiration may result in variation in the Doppler curve due to a variation in the intercept angle; if so, have the patient suspend respiration briefly during data recording.

Pressure half-time valve area (Figure 11–15)

■ The pressure half-time is calculated from the Doppler curve at the time interval between peak velocity and the peak velocity divided by 1.4.

■ The empiric constant 220 is divided by the pressure half-time ($T\frac{1}{2}$ in milliseconds) to estimate mitral valve area (MVA in cm^2):

$$MVA = 220/T\frac{1}{2}$$

Key points

☐ The peak velocity occurs at the onset of diastole with flow deceleration in mid-diastole.

☐ A clearly defined peak velocity is needed for an accurate pressure half-time measurement (Figure 11–16).

☐ The diastolic slope should be linear with a clearly defined edge; if a non-linear slope is obtained, the mid-diastolic segment of the curve should be used for the pressure half-time calculation (Figure 11–17).

☐ The pressure half-time may be inaccurate if left atrial or LV compliance is abnormal.

☐ If an atrial contraction is present, only the early diastolic portion of the curve is included in the pressure half-time calculation.

Continuity equation valve area

■ If further evaluation of mitral stenosis severity is needed, a continuity equation valve area can be calculated.

■ Transmitral stroke volume (SV) is divided by the velocity-time integral of the mitral stenosis jet (VTI_{MS}) to obtain mitral valve area:

$$MVA = SV/VTI_{MS}$$

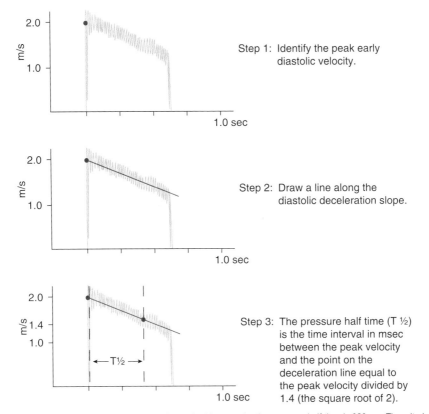

Step 1: Identify the peak early diastolic velocity.

Step 2: Draw a line along the diastolic deceleration slope.

Step 3: The pressure half time (T ½) is the time interval in msec between the peak velocity and the point on the deceleration line equal to the peak velocity divided by 1.4 (the square root of 2).

Figure 11–15. The mitral pressure half-time is calculated as shown. In this example, the pressure half-time is 320 ms. The mitral valve area is 220/320 = 0.7 cm², consistent with severe stenosis.

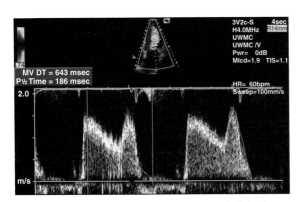

Figure 11–16. On the ultrasound system, the pressure half-time is measured by identifying the peak early diastolic velocity and then placing a line along the mid-diastolic deceleration slope. The quantitation software then calculates the time interval between the peak gradient and half the peak gradient. The empiric constant 220 is divided by the pressure half-time by to obtain valve area.

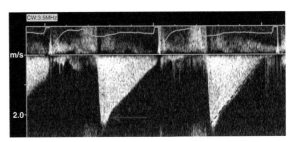

Figure 11–17. Transesophageal imaging in a 64-year-old woman with rheumatic mitral valve disease shows CW Doppler antegrade flow (away from the transducer) across the stenotic mitral valve. The initial diastolic slope (*arrow*) is steeper than the mid-diastolic slope. When there is an initial steep decline in velocity (often called a "ski-slope" pattern) with a flatter mid-diastolic slope, the pressure half-time is measured along the mid-diastolic portion of the curve, as shown on the second beat, extrapolating back to the onset of flow.

Step 3: Evaluate mitral regurgitation (Figure 11–18)

- If regurgitation is significant (vena contracta ≥ 3 mm), evaluate as detailed in Chapter 12.

Key points

- Most patients with rheumatic mitral stenosis have some degree of mitral regurgitation.

Key points

- Transmitral stroke volume is determined in the LV outflow tract (LVOT) or across the pulmonic valve.
- This approach is only accurate when there is no mitral regurgitation.

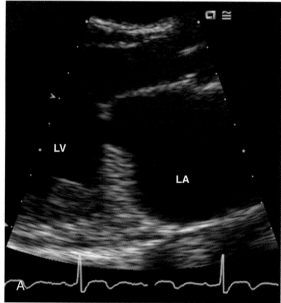

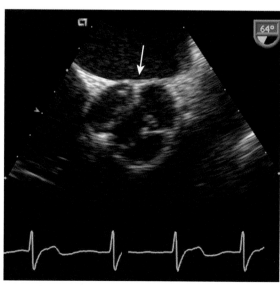

Figure 11–19. In the same patient as Figure 11–17, there is rheumatic involvement of the aortic valve with fusion (*arrow*) at all three commissures of the aortic valve and restricted leaflet opening. On transthoracic echo, her aortic jet velocity was 4.2 m/s with a functional valve area of 0.8 cm². She was scheduled for aortic valve replacement for severe symptomatic aortic stenosis; the purpose of the TEE was to decide if concurrent mitral valve replacement or repair was needed.

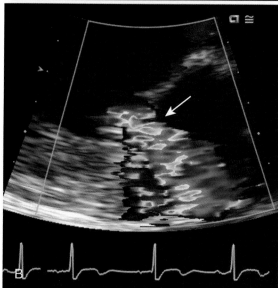

Figure 11–18. In this patient with mitral stenosis, the diastolic long-axis view shows typical diastolic doming due to commissural fusion (*A*). In systole, there is moderate-severe mitral regurgitation with a vena contracta (*arrow*) width of 1.0 cm (*B*).

Step 4: Examine aortic and tricuspid valves for rheumatic involvement

- When rheumatic mitral stenosis is present, careful evaluation of aortic and tricuspid valves is needed to detect rheumatic involvement (Figure 11–19).

Key points

- ❐ Rheumatic disease typically affects the mitral valve first, causing stenosis and/or regurgitation.
- ❐ The aortic valve is affected in about 35% of patients and the tricuspid valve in about 6% of patients with rheumatic mitral valve disease.
- ❐ The appearance of rheumatic disease affecting the aortic and tricuspid valves is similar to the mitral valve, with commissural fusion being the most consistent feature.

Step 5: Evaluate the consequences of mitral valve obstruction

- Measure LA size (Figure 11–20).
- Estimate pulmonary pressures as detailed in Chapter 6.
- Evaluate RV size and systolic function.

- ❐ With combined moderate stenosis and regurgitation, quantitation of both lesions is needed.
- ❐ The degree of mitral regurgitation may need to be evaluated by TEE because moderate or greater regurgitation is a contraindication to percutaneous valvotomy.

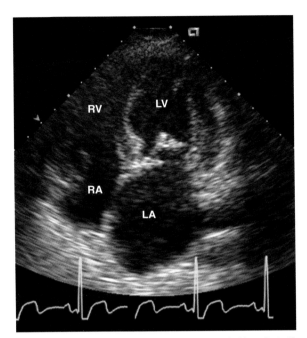

Figure 11–20. The marked degree of LA enlargement in this patient with rheumatic mitral stenosis is seen in an apical 4-chamber view. The LA area appears larger than the LV area in this diastolic frame.

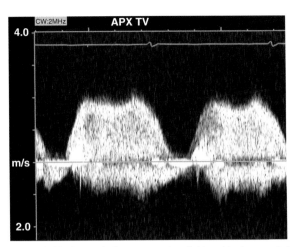

Figure 11–21. Antegrade flow across a stenotic tricuspid valve recorded with CW Doppler from an apical view. The velocity is markedly increased, with a mean gradient of 12 mm Hg, and the diastolic slope is very flat with a pressure half-time of 400 ms and a valve area of 0.6 cm².

Key points

▢ LA enlargement is usually present in patients with mitral stenosis and is related to the severity and chronicity of mitral valve obstruction.

▢ Pulmonary pressures are elevated passively due to the increased LA pressure. In addition, reactive pulmonary hypertension is seen with changes in the pulmonary vasculature that may persist after relief of mitral stenosis.

▢ RV enlargement and systolic dysfunction in patients with mitral stenosis may be due to pulmonary hypertension (pressure overload) or to rheumatic tricuspid regurgitation (volume overload).

TRICUSPID STENOSIS

■ Tricuspid stenosis is uncommon and usually is due to rheumatic tricuspid valve involvement in patients with mitral stenosis.

■ Evaluation of rheumatic tricuspid stenosis is similar to evaluation of mitral stenosis.

Key points

▢ Rheumatic tricuspid stenosis appears similar to mitral stenosis, with commisural fusion and diastolic bowing of the leaflets.

▢ Carcinoid disease can cause tricuspid stenosis with thickened, shortened leaflets.

▢ The antegrade tricuspid velocity curve, recorded from an RV inflow view or an apical approach, allows measurement of mean gradient and pressure half-time.

▢ Diastolic pressure gradients may be lower for the tricuspid, compared with mitral, stenosis (Figure 11–21).

▢ Planimetry of the stenotic tricuspid orifice rarely is possible with 2D imaging; three-dimensional (3D) imaging may be helpful in some cases.

PULMONIC STENOSIS (Figure 11–22)

■ The velocity across the pulmonic valve is recorded using pulsed or CW Doppler from a parasternal approach.

■ Maximum gradient is calculated using the Bernoulli equation.

■ Coexisting pulmonic regurgitation is evaluated by color and CW Doppler.

Key points

▢ Pulmonic stenosis usually is due to congenital heart disease and may be an isolated defect or a component of more complex congenital disease, such as Tetralogy of Fallot.

▢ Visualization of the pulmonic valve is challenging on both transthoracic and transesophageal imaging in adults; often Doppler data are used to infer valve pathology.

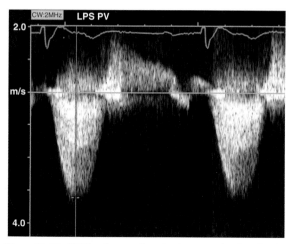

Figure 11–22. CW Doppler recording of pulmonary valve flow showing an antegrade velocity of 3.2 m/s, consistent with a maximum gradient of 41 mm Hg, or moderate pulmonic stenosis. Pulmonic regurgitation is seen above the baseline and appears to be moderate based on the relative density of retrograde versus antegrade flow. Pulmonary pressures are low, based on the low end-diastolic velocity of the regurgitant signal.

❑ Grading of stenosis severity is based on the maximum transvalvular pressure gradient (mild < 25 mm Hg; moderate 25–50 mm Hg; severe > 50 mm Hg).

❑ Pulmonic stenosis often is accompanied by significant pulmonic regurgitation, particularly if there has been a prior surgical or percutaneous procedure.

❑ Branch pulmonary artery stenosis may also be present and is difficult to evaluate by echocardiography, although evaluation of the proximal right and left pulmonary may be possible from a high parasternal short-axis view.

THE ECHO EXAM

Aortic Stenosis

Valve anatomy	Calcific Bicuspid (two leaflets in systole) Rheumatic
Stenosis severity	Jet velocity (V_{max}) Mean pressure gradient (ΔP_{mean}) LVOT/AS velocity ratio Aortic valve area (AVA)
Coexisting AR	Qualitative evaluation of severity
LV response	LV hypertrophy LV dimensions or volumes LV ejection fraction
Other findings	Pulmonary pressures Mitral regurgitation

AR, aortic regurgitation; AS, aortic stenosis; LVOT, left ventricular outflow tract.

EXAMPLE

An 82-year-old woman presents with dyspnea on exertion and is noted to have a 3/6 systolic murmur at the base, radiating to the carotids with a single S2 and a diminished carotid upstrokes.
Echocardiography shows a calcified aortic valve with:

Aortic jet velocity (V_{max})	4.2 m/s
Velocity time-integral (VTI_{AS})	68 cm
Mean gradient	45 mm Hg
LV outflow tract diameter ($LVOT_D$)	2.1 cm
LVOT velocity (V_{LVOT})	0.9 m/s

The *maximum jet velocity* of 4.2 m/s indicates severe stenosis, which is confirmed by calculation of maximum and mean pressure gradients.

Maximum pressure gradient is calculated from maximum aortic jet velocity (V_{max}) as:

$$\Delta P_{max} = 4\,(V_{max})^2 = 4\,(4.2)^2 = 71\,\text{mm Hg}$$

Mean pressure gradient is calculated by tracing the outer edge of the CW Doppler velocity curve, with the echo instrument calculating and then averaging instantaneous pressure gradients over the systolic ejection period. The simplified method for estimation of mean gradient is:

$$\Delta P = 2.4\,(V_{max})^2 = 2.4\,(4.2)^2 = 42\,\text{mm Hg}$$

In order to correct for transvalvular volume flow rate, the velocity ratio and valve area are calculated:
Velocity ratio is:

$$V_{LVOT}/V_{max} = 0.9/4.2 = 0.21\,\text{(dimensionless index)}$$

Aortic valve area is:

$$AVA = (CSA_{LVOT} \times VTI_{LVOT})/VTI_{AS\text{-}Jet}$$

Where cross-sectional area (CSA) of the LVOT is:

$$CSA_{LVOT} = \pi(LVOT_D/2)^2 = 3.14(2.1/2)^2 = 3.46\,\text{cm}^2$$

Thus:

$$AVA = (3.46\,\text{cm}^2 \times 14\,\text{cm})/68\,\text{cm} = 0.71\,\text{cm}^2$$

Simplified formula for valve area is:

$$AVA = (CSA_{LVOT} \times V_{LVOT})/V_{max}$$

Thus:

$$AVA = (3.46\,\text{cm}^2 \times 0.9\,\text{cm/s})/4.2\,\text{cm/s} = 0.74\,\text{cm}^2$$

This mean gradient (> 40 mm Hg), velocity ratio (<0.25), and valve area (<1.0 cm^2) are all consistent with severe stenosis.

Classification of Aortic Stenosis Severity

	Mild	Severe
Jet velocity (m/s)	<3.0	>4.0
Mean gradient (mm Hg)	<20	>40
Velocity ratio	>0.50	<0.25
Valve area (cm^2)	>1.5	<1.0

Quantitation of Aortic Stenosis Severity

Components	Modality	View	Recording	Measurements
LVOT diameter (LVOT$_D$)	2D	Parasternal long axis	Adjust depth, optimize endocardial definition, zoom mode	Inner edge to inner edge of LVOT, parallel and adjacent to aortic valve, mid-systole
LVOT flow V_{LVOT} VTI_{LVOT}	Pulsed Doppler	Apical 4-chamber (anteriorly angulated)	Sample volume 2–3 mm, envelope of flow with defined peak, start with sample volume at valve and move apically	Trace modal velocity of spectral velocity curve
AS-Jet V_{max} $VTI_{AS\text{-}Jet}$	CW Doppler	Apical, SSN, other	Examination from multiple windows, careful positioning, and transducer angulation to obtain highest velocity signal	Measure maximum velocities at edge of intense velocity signal $\Delta P_{max} = 4\,(V_{max})^2$
Continuity equation			$AVA\,(cm^2) = [\pi\,(LVOT_D/2)^2 \times VTI_{LVOT}]/VTI_{AS\text{-}Jet}$	
Simplified continuity equation			$AVA\,(cm^2) = [\pi\,(LVOT_D/2)^2 \times V_{LVOT}]/V_{AS\text{-}Jet}$	
Velocity ratio			Velocity ratio $= V_{LVOT}/V_{AS\text{-}Jet}$	

AS, aortic stenosis; CW, Continuous-wave; LVOT, left ventricular outflow tract; SSN, suprasternal notch; V_{LVOT}, LVOT velocity; V_{max}, maximum veiocity; VTI, velocity-time integral.

Mitral Stenosis

Valve anatomy	Valve thickness and mobility Calcification Commissural fusion Subvalvular involvement
Stenosis severity	2D valve area Mean pressure gradient Pressure half-time valve area
Left atrium	Size TEE for thrombus prevalvuloplasty
Coexisting MR	Qualitative evaluation of severity
Pulmonary vasculature	Pulmonary systolic pressure Right ventricular size and function
Other findings	Aortic valve involvement LV size and systolic function

2D, two-dimensional; MR, mitral regurgitation; TEE, transesophageal echocardiography.

EXAMPLE

A 26-year-old pregnant woman presents with dyspnea and is noted to have a diastolic murmur at the apex.

Echocardiography shows rheumatic mitral stenosis with:

MVA_{2D}	$0.8\ cm^2$
Mean ΔP	5 mm Hg
$T\frac{1}{2}$	260 ms
Mitral valve morphology score	
Leaflet thickness	2
Mobility	1
Calcification	1
Subvalvular	2
TOTAL	6
Tricuspid regurgitant jet velocity	3.1 m/s
Mitral regurgitation	Mild

Mean pressure gradient is calculated by tracing the outer edge of the CW Doppler velocity curve, with the echo instrument calculating and then averaging instantaneous pressure gradients over the systolic ejection period.

Doppler mitral valve area ($MVA_{Doppler}$) is calculated as:

$$MVA_{Doppler} = 220/T\tfrac{1}{2} = 220/260 = 0.85\ cm^2$$

The 2D mitral valve area and the pressure half-time valve area show reasonable agreement and both are consistent with severe mitral stenosis.

Pulmonary artery pressure (PAP) is:

$$PAP = 4(V_{TR})^2 + RAP = 4(3.1)^2 + 10\ mm\ Hg = 48\ mm\ Hg$$

Pulmonary pressure is moderately elevated consistent with a secondary response to severe mitral stenosis.

The mitral morphology score is low and only mild mitral regurgitation is present, indicating a high likelihood of immediate and long-term success with balloon mitral valvuloplasty. TEE is needed just before mitral valvuloplasty to evaluate for left atrial thrombus.

Classification of Mitral Stenosis Severity

	Mild	Severe
Mean gradient (mm Hg)	<5	>15
Pulmonary pressure (mm Hg)	<30	>60
Valve area (cm²)	>1.5	<1.0

Quantitation of Mitral Stenosis Severity

Parameter	Modality	View	Recording	Measurements
2D valve area	2D	Parasternal short axis	Scan from apex to base to identify minimal valve area	Planimetry of inner edge of dark–light interface
Mean gradient	HPRF Doppler	Apical 4-chamber or long axis	Align Doppler beam parallel to MS jet. Adjust angle to obtain smooth envelope, clear peak, and linear deceleration slope	Trace maximum velocity of spectral velocity curve
Pressure half-time	HPRF Doppler	Apical 4-chamber or long axis	Same as mean gradient. Adjust scale so velocity curve fills the screen. HPRF Doppler often has less noise than CW Doppler signal.	Place line from maximum velocity along mid-diastolic linear slope $MVA = 220/T\frac{1}{2}$

2D, two-dimensional; HPRF, high pulse repetition frequency; MS, mitral stenosis.

SELF-ASSESSMENT QUESTIONS

QUESTION 1

A 31-year-old man with a history of palpitations and a murmur is referred for echocardiography. The initial parasternal long-axis view is shown (Figure 11–23).

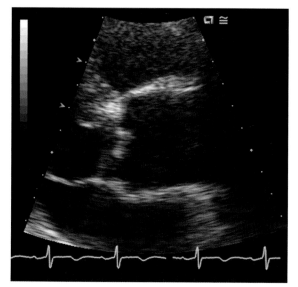

Figure 11–23.

The most likely diagnosis is:

A. Mitral valve prolapse
B. Subaortic stenosis
C. Bicuspid aortic valve
D. Ventricular septal defect
E. Calcific aortic stenosis

QUESTION 2

A 52-year-old male patient is referred for evaluation of exertional dyspnea. He has a history of congenital aortic stenosis and had undergone corrective surgery as a child. TTE demonstrates an ejection fraction (EF) of 68% without regional wall motion abnormalities. The aortic valve is heavily calcified with minimal systolic motion. These Doppler signals are obtained (Figure 11–24 A and B).

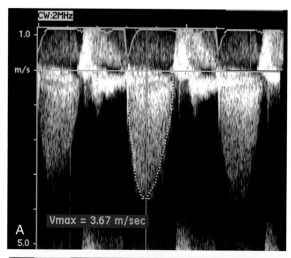

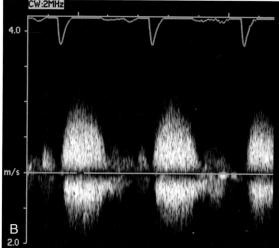

Figure 11–24 A and B.

The most appropriate next step in patient management is:

A. Transesophageal echocardiography
B. Dobutamine stress echocardiography
C. Coronary angiography
D. Repeat transthoracicl echocardiography

QUESTION 3

A 28-year-old woman who recently moved to the United States presents to establish care with a provider. A murmur is heard on examination and an echocardiogram is ordered (Figure 11–25).

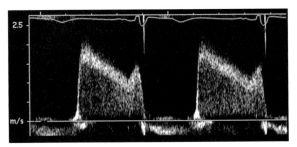

Figure 11–25.

The most likely diagnosis is:

A. Rheumatic valve disease
B. Tetralogy of Fallot
C. Bicuspid aortic valve
D. Myxomatous mitral valve disease
E. Ventricular septal defect

QUESTION 4

A 78-year-old woman presents with aortic stenosis. On physical examination her vital signs reveal a blood pressure of 144/80 mm Hg and heart rate of 56 bpm. On TTE, the aortic valve is severely calcified, with:

LV outflow tract diameter	2.4 cm
LV outflow tract peak velocity	0.9 m/s
LVOT velocity-time integral	12 cm
Aortic valve velocity	4.0 m/s
Aortic valve velocity-time integral	94 cm

Based on this data, do the following calculations:
Transaortic stroke volume _____
Cardiac output _____
Continuity equation aortic valve area
_____
Aortic velocity ratio _____
Overall, the degree of aortic stenosis is
_____

QUESTION 5

A 58-year-old woman is referred for echocardiography for new onset atrial fibrillation. She lives in a rural area and has not seen care providers regularly due to lack of insurance. The following image is obtained (Figure 11–26).

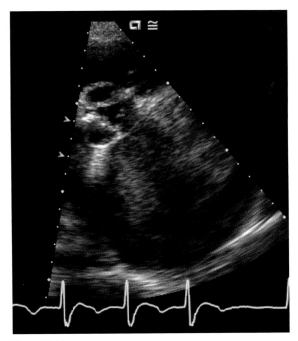

Figure 11–26.

The most likely cause of the abnormalities seen here is:

A. Endocarditis
B. Calcific valve disease
C. A systemic inflammatory disease
D. Rheumatic disease
E. Congenital bicuspid aortic valve

QUESTION 6

A 76-year-old man with coronary artery disease presents with exertional dyspnea. A recent angiogram shows chronic occlusion of his right coronary artery and no new coronary lesions. Echocardiography demonstrates a heavily calcified aortic valve, an EF of 40%, and regional wall motion abnormalities in the inferior wall and apex. The following data were obtained from a dobutamine stress echocardiogram at an infusion rate of 7.5 mcg/kg/m:

	Baseline	Dobutamine
Ejection fraction (%)	40	55
LVOT velocity (m/s)	0.7	0.8
Aortic maximum velocity (m/s)	3.5	4.2
Mean aortic gradient (mm Hg)	27	41
Aortic valve area (cm²)	0.8	0.8

These findings are most consistent with:

A. Lack contractile reserve
B. Severe aortic stenosis
C. Moderate aortic stenosis
D. Inadequate test

QUESTION 7

A 36-year-old woman with known rheumatic valve disease is referred for mitral valvotomy. Echocardiographic factors to consider in determining candidacy for percutaneous valvotomy include all of the following *except*:

A. Mitral valve leaflet thickening
B. Systolic anterior motion (SAM) of the chords
C. Mitral valve calcification
D. Mitral valve leaflet mobility
E. Chordal apparatus thickening

QUESTION 8

Doppler recordings recorded in a young woman with a systolic murmur and dyspnea are shown below (Figure 11–27). The diameter of the inferior vena cava (IVC) measured 1.8 cm with normal inspiratory collapse.

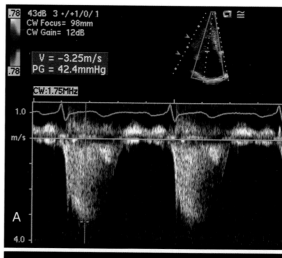

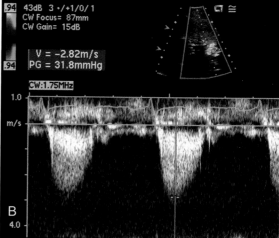

Figure 11–27.

Calculate the pulmonary arterial systolic pressure:
_____

QUESTION 9

A 36-year-old woman undergoing chronic dialysis therapy for end-stage renal disease presents for clinical follow-up. She denies cardiopulmonary symptoms, palpitations, or fever. Her exercise tolerance is unchanged from baseline. A TTE is ordered and the following image is obtained (Figure 11–28). The transmitral mean gradient is 3 mm Hg and there is mild mitral regurgitation.

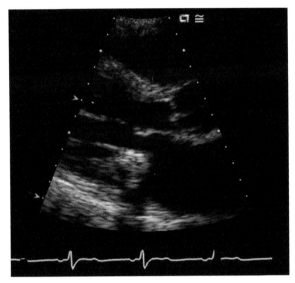

Figure 11–28.

These findings are most consistent with:

A. Rheumatic valve disease
B. Acute bacterial endocarditis
C. Mitral annular calcification
D. Left atrial myxoma
E. Persistent left superior vena cava

QUESTION 10

A 60-year-old woman with tricuspid valve stenosis is admitted to the hospital with dyspnea and pedal edema. The transtricuspid Doppler tracing is shown below (Figure 11–29).

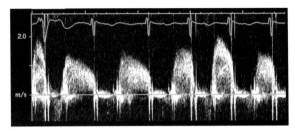

Figure 11–29.

In this case, the severity of stenosis is best assessed by measuring:

A. Average peak gradient, 3 cardiac cycles
B. Mean gradient, longest Doppler signal
C. Average mean gradient, 3 cardiac cycles
D. Peak late gradient, highest Doppler signal

QUESTION 11

An asymptomatic patient with rheumatic mitral stenosis is seen for routine follow-up. The diastolic flow curve shows an increased velocity and flat diastolic slope with a maximum velocity of 2.0 m/s.

The time interval between maximum velocity and various points on the diastolic flow curve are measured as follows:

1.8 m/s	190 msec
1.4 m/s	225 msec
1.0 m/s	250 msec
0.6 m/s	275 msec

Calculate the mitral valve area: _____

QUESTION 12

The following image (Figure 11–30) is consistent with:

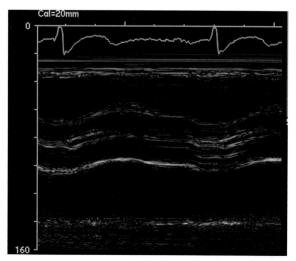

Figure 11–30.

A. Mitral stenosis
B. Aortic stenosis
C. Tricuspid stenosis
D. Pulmonic stenosis

ANSWERS

ANSWER 1: C

In this diastolic image (Figure 11–31) in a parasternal long-axis view, a bicuspid valve is evident by the anteriorly displaced aortic valve closure plane relative to the midpoint of the aortic root. The diagnosis of bicuspid aortic valve should be confirmed in systolic short-axis view (see below) showing the two leaflets and two commissures. In diastole, the aortic valve may appear trileaflet if there is a ridge of tissue, or raphe, where the leaflets would normally separate; this can be difficult to distinguish from a closed commissure on a diastolic image. In this patient, the anterior mitral valve leaflet appears normal and mitral prolapse would not be evident on a diastolic image in any case. There is no defect in the proximal ventricular septum to suggest a ventricular septal defect and there is no narrowing or membrane seen in the left ventricular outflow tract.

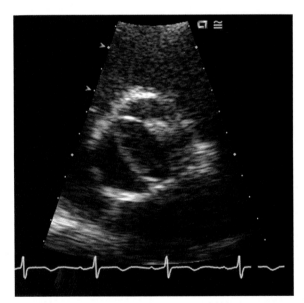

Figure 11–31.

ANSWER 2: D

The original ECG report describes normal systolic function and evidence of aortic stenosis, with a heavily calcified, immobile valve. However, the Doppler data are poor quality; the apparent maximum velocity does not fit with the rest of the clinical and imaging data. Thus, a repeat transthoracic study is recommended. TEE is helpful for visualization of valve anatomy and allows planimetry of valve area in some cases, but Doppler data for aortic stenosis on TEE are suboptimal because it is difficult to align the Doppler beam with the stenotic jet due to constraints of transducer position in the esophagus. Obviously, the noninvasive transthoracic data should be correctly recorded before proceeding to TEE. Dobutamine

stress echocardiography may be helpful to differentiate low-gradient severe aortic stenosis, but systolic function is preserved in this case. Coronary angiography might be appropriate if aortic stenosis is not severe, because coronary disease is an alternate explanation for his symptoms, but should be considered only after complete evaluation of the aortic valve.

For the repeat study, Doppler interrogation of the valve from multiple views with careful patient positioning and transducer angulation is needed to record the highest jet velocity. The first Doppler recording (Figure 11–24A) was taken from the apical window. A peak velocity of 3.7 m/s suggested only moderate-range stenosis in the setting of normal forward stroke volume but is a poor-quality signal without a clear Doppler envelope and a poorly defined peak velocity. The second Doppler recording (Figure 11–24B) (peak approximately 2.0 m/s) clearly underestimates the severity of stenosis and was not well aligned with the aortic jet (signal above and below the baseline). With the patient repositioned in a steep left lateral decubitus position, using an apical cutout in the exam table additional imaging provided velocity data from apical, suprasternal, high right parasternal, and subcostal views, with careful transducer angulation from each window. The apical CW Doppler signal (Figure 11–24C) was still suboptimal (4.0 m/s), but a higher velocity (>4.7 m/s) was obtained from a right parasternal window (Figure 11–24D) consistent with severe aortic stenosis.

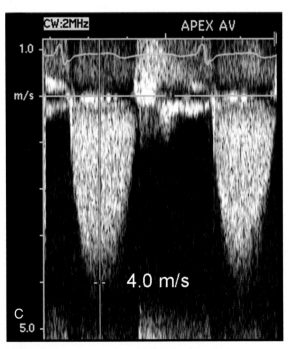

Figure 11–24 C.

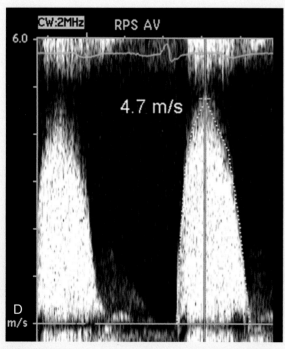

Figure 11–24 D.

ANSWER 4

The first step is to calculate the outflow tract cross-sectional area:

$$CSA_{LVOT} = \pi(LVOT_D/2)^2 = 3.14(2.4/2)^2 = 4.5 \text{ cm}^2$$

$$\text{Transaortic stroke volume (SV)} = CSA_{LVOT} \times VTI_{LVOT}$$
$$= 4.5 \text{ cm}^2 \times 12 \text{ cm} = 54 \text{ cm}^3 = 54 \text{ ml}$$

Cardiac output is:

$$SV \times \text{heart rate (56 bpm)} = 3024 \text{ mL} = 3.02 \text{ L/min}$$

The aortic jet is examined from both apical and high right parasternal windows with the highest jet velocity representing the most parallel intercept angle between the jet and ultrasound beam. The highest velocity signal is used to measure the VTI.

Continuity equation aortic valve area is:

$$AVA = SV/VTI_{AS\text{-Jet}} = 54 \text{ cm}^3/94 \text{ cm} = 0.6 \text{ cm}^2$$

The velocity ratio is:

$$V_{LVOT}/V_{max} = 0.9/4.0 = 0.23$$

These findings are all consistent with severe aortic stenosis, defined as an aortic velocity greater than 4.0 m/s and valve area less than 1.0 cm^2.

ANSWER 3: A

This is a transmitral Doppler tracing taken from an apical window with flow directed toward the transducer during diastole. The Doppler pattern is consistent with atrioventricular valve inflow with early filling (E wave) and late filling due to atrial contraction (A wave), and the markedly prolonged diastolic deceleration slope is consistent with obstruction of LV inflow at the valve level. The pressure half-time is 240 ms, consistent with a valve area of 220/240 or 0.9 cm^2 (try measuring it yourself on the image). Mitral stenosis is nearly uniformly caused by rheumatic valve disease and has wide geographic variation in prevalence and age at presentation. Mitral regurgitation due to myxomatous mitral valve disease and ventricular septal defect flow would both occur during systole. Regurgitation of a bicuspid aortic valve would occur during diastole but would not show evidence of atrial contraction. Also, peak end-diastolic velocity of an aortic regurgitant jet would be higher velocity than transmitral flow due to the higher transvalvular gradient between the aortic diastolic pressure and LV chamber. A common late complication of surgically treated Tetralogy of Fallot is pulmonic regurgitation. Similar to aortic regurgitation, pulmonic regurgitation would occur during diastole, but would not show evidence of atrial contraction, and the shape and magnitude of the velocity curve would reflect the pulmonary artery to RV diastolic pressure difference.

ANSWER 5: D

This parasternal short-axis image shows a trileaflet aortic valve with thickening along the leaflet edges and commisural fusion diagnostic for rheumatic aortic valve disease. The left atrium is severely enlarged and spontaneous contrast is seen, suggesting there also is severe mitral stenosis. Atrial fibrillation can be a presenting symptom with rheumatic valve disease. In the United States, many patients initially present at age 50 to 60 years, with about 80% of cases occurring in women. In immigrants from countries with a higher prevalence of rheumatic fever, valve disease presents at a younger age. Endocarditis results in valve vegetations, leaflet destruction, and abscess formation, not commisural fusion. Calcific aortic valve disease affects the body of the leaflet, not the leaflet edges or commissures. Systemic inflammatory diseases can affect the posterior aortic wall and aortic valve but typically cause aortic regurgitation, rather than stenosis, and would be unlikely to cause this degree of left atrial enlargement.

ANSWER 6: B

This patient has low output, low gradient aortic stenosis. The baseline data are either consistent with severe aortic stenosis in the setting of LV dysfunction or may be due to only moderate aortic stenosis with reduced leaflet opening secondary to the low transaortic flow rate. Dobutamine stress echocardiography is helpful in distinguishing between these diagnoses; with severe aortic stenosis, valve replacement is indicated, whereas with moderate stenosis, medical therapy is more appropriate. In this patient, there is a normal contractile response to dobutamine with an increase in stroke volume and an increase in ejection fraction from 40% to 55%. Despite the concurrent increase in both stroke volume and aortic jet velocity, the calculated aortic valve area remained the same at 0.8 cm^2, indicating that the aortic stenosis is severe and is the result of a "fixed" obstruction. The definition of severe aortic stenosis on dobutamine stress echocardiography is a valve area less than 1.0 cm^2 with an increase in stroke volume greater than 20% or an aortic velocity greater than 4.0 m/s at any flow rate. With a primary cardiomyopathy and moderate aortic stenosis, inadequate forward stroke volume to fully open the leaflets in systole may lead to smaller aortic valve orifice area calculations at rest. However, with dobutamine infusion, the increase in forward stroke volume results in greater leaflet opening and a larger valve area calculation. A lack of contractile reserve would lead to no change in cardiac output (ejection fraction) or stroke volume with dobutamine, not the situation in this case. The appropriate augmentation in cardiac output suggests this test was diagnostic (adequate).

ANSWER 7: B

Systolic anterior motion (SAM) of the chords is not a characteristic feature of mitral stenosis. SAM occurs with dynamic subaortic obstruction, as can occur with hypertrophic cardiomyopathy, often resulting in late systolic mitral regurgitation. SAM also can be seen with mitral valve prolapse and in some normal individuals, without associated outflow obstruction in either of these situations. Optimal results with percutaneous mitral valvotomy occur with fracturing of the fused commissures, allowing a larger orifice area. The features of mitral valve anatomy predictive of outcomes with percutaneous mitral valvotomy are described by a scoring system with four echocardiographic criteria: leaflet mobility, leaflet thickening, subvalvar (chordal) thickening, and mitral valve calcification. A score between 1 and 4 points is assigned to each criteria (more severe involvement = 4) and then summed. A score greater than 8 points is consistent with more leaflet thickening and calcification or more involvement of the subvalvular apparatus; these patients tend to have less optimal results because abnormal leaflet morphology remains after the procedure. Severe commisural calcification also is a poor prognostic sign because it increases the likelihood of a leaflet tear during the procedure, producing significant mitral regurgitation. Best results are seen in patients with a score less than 8 points and little commissural calcium.

ANSWER 8

Doppler signal A can be identified as the tricuspid regurgitant jet, taken from the apical 4-chamber view, based on a long ejection time with a Doppler signal that starts at the onset of the QRS signal. The peak velocity is elevated at 3.3 m/s, consistent with an RV–to–RA systolic pressure difference of 44 mm Hg. With a normal-caliber IVC and normal inspiratory collapse, right atrial pressure is about 5 mm Hg. Adding the estimated RA pressure to the RV–to–RA pressure difference, then, provides an estimated RV systolic pressure of 49 mm Hg. However, estimation of the pulmonary arterial systolic pressure from the tricuspid regurgitant jet assumes that there is no interceding pressure gradient between the pulmonary circulation and the RV. In this case, there is also pulmonic stenosis as shown in tracing B, recorded from the parasternal short-axis view. The pulmonic valve Doppler signal is differentiated from the tricuspid regurgitant signal by the relative delay in onset, accounted for by isovolumic contraction. The peak velocity of the pulmonic stenosis jet is 2.8 m/s, which corresponds to a pressure gradient of 32 mm Hg across the pulmonic valve, or between the RV and pulmonary artery in systole. This pressure gradient must be subtracted from the RV systolic pressure to obtain the estimated pulmonary systolic pressure ($49 - 32 = 17$ mm Hg), which is normal.

ANSWER 9: C

This parasternal long-axis image shows severe calcification of the posterior mitral valve annulus. There is a minimal transmitral pressure gradient without significant mitral regurgitation. Mitral annular calcification develops from progressive calcium deposition along and beneath the mitral valve annulus with relative sparing of the posterior mitral valve leaflet, appearing with an irregular, lumpy appearance. The mitral valve leaflets and chordae tendinae are generally not involved. In advanced cases of mitral annular calcification, there is encroachment on the mitral valve leaflets. There may be a mild inflow gradient or mild associated mitral regurgitation, but mitral annular calcification rarely requires surgery. Rheumatic mitral valve disease involves leaflet thickening and scarring along commissural lines with restriction of diastolic opening or "doming" of the anterior leaflet, which is not seen in this case. In addition, most of the calcific burden for rheumatic valve disease is seen at the leaflet tips rather than at the base of the valve or valve annulus. Bacterial endocarditis typically involves the atrial side of the leaflets and is associated with mitral regurgitation due to leaflet destruction or poor coaptation. A myxoma is a benign cardiac mass that typically originates from the atrial septum with an echodensity similar to tissue. A persistent left superior vena cava results in a dilated coronary sinus, which is seen as an echolucent area posterior to the mitral annulus in the long-axis view.

ANSWER 10: C

Tricuspid valve stenosis is nearly uniformly caused by rheumatic valve disease. The patient is in atrial fibrillation with variability in the R–to–R interval. With a shorter cardiac cycle, less time is spent in diastole, and diastolic LV filling is completed in a shorter interval. For these shorter cardiac cycles, the peak early inflow velocity is higher than in Doppler signals with a longer cardiac cycle duration. Because mean gradient averages the instantaneous gradients over the flow duration, the mean gradient will be higher on shorter cycle lengths and lower on long cycle lengths. In clinical practice, when significant variation in heart rate is present, any measurements of peak and mean gradients are averaged over several cardiac cycles. For mitral or tricuspid stenosis, mean gradients are more representative of stenosis severity than peak gradients.

ANSWER 11: 1.0 cm²

The pressure half-time (T $\frac{1}{2}$) is defined as the time required for the pressure gradient across an obstruction to decrease to half of its maximal value. Velocity is squared in the Bernoulli equation to calculate pressure gradient, so to calculate the velocity on the curve where the gradient is $\frac{1}{2}$ the maximum gradient, maximum velocity is divided by 1.4 (because 1.4 is the square root of 2). In this case, 2.0 m/s divided by 1.4 equals 1.4 m/s so the T $\frac{1}{2}$ is 225 ms. Then mitral valve area is calculated by the equation 220/T $\frac{1}{2}$, in this case 220/225 = 0.98 cm². Valve area calculations are only accurate to one decimal point so this calculation should be rounded up and reported at 1.0 cm², consistent with severe mitral stenosis.

ANSWER 12: B

This is an M-mode tracing through the aortic valve. Aortic valve motion is shown against time on the horizontal axis. The anterior and posterior aortic valve annulus is seen throughout the cardiac cycle with slight motion corresponding to systole and diastole. Within the annulus is a bright, calcified aortic valve best seen during diastole. During systole, there is little valve motion, consistent with aortic stenosis.

12 Valve Regurgitation

BASIC PRINCIPLES

Vena contracta (Figure 12–1)

- Narrowest width of the regurgitant jet, measured using color Doppler flow imaging

Key points

- ❐ Optimal color flow images show flow acceleration proximal to the regurgitant valve and distal jet expansion in the receiving chamber, with the vena contracta being the narrow neck between them.
- ❐ Vena contracta measurements are most accurate with:
    - The flow signal in the near field of the image (e.g., transthoracic parasternal long-axis views)
    - A narrow sector width to optimize frame rate
    - Zoom mode to increase image size
- ❐ Small differences in vena contracta width correspond to substantial changes in regurgitant severity grade so that if a precise and accurate measurement is not possible, other approaches should be used.

Proximal isovelocity surface area (PISA)

- Blood flow accelerates proximal to a regurgitant orifice.
- The aliasing velocity on color Doppler flow imaging provides visualization of a contour where all the blood cells have the same velocity (isovelocity). (Figure 12–2)
- The shape of this proximal isovelocity contour typically is a hemisphere so that the cross-sectional area (CSA) of this surface is $2\pi r^2$.
- Volume flow rate is cross-sectional area times velocity (in this case the aliasing velocity):

$$\text{Instantaneous flow rate}\,(\text{in cm}^3/\text{s}) = \text{CSA}\,(\text{cm}^2) \times V_{\text{aliasing}}\,(\text{cm/s})$$

239

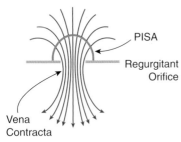

Figure 12–1. Schematic diagram showing the proximal jet geometry for valve regurgitation. Streamlines of blood flow are shown in red. Flow proximal to the regurgitant orifice increases in velocity as the flow stream narrows into the regurgitant orifice. A proximal isovelocity surface area PISA is represented by the blue line that connects points with the same velocity on each stream line. Multiple PISA are present proximal to the orifice, the PISA seen with color flow depends on the aliasing velocity of the color scale. The flow stream continues to narrow beyond the orifice with the narrowest point or vena contracta reflecting regurgitant severity.

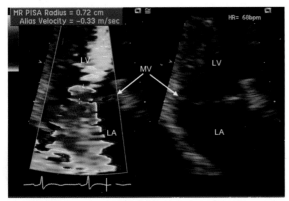

Figure 12–2. The proximal isovelocity surface area (PISA) is identified by the aliasing velocity (blue–red interface) proximal to the regurgitant valve seen in this zoomed image of the mitral valve in an apical 4-chamber view. The PISA is assumed to be hemispherical, although the image seen with color Doppler may be somewhat distorted, as in this example. The simultaneous 2D image on the right is helpful for identifying the valve plane.

Key points

❑ The PISA is best visualized from a window where the ultrasound beam is parallel to the flow direction, typically the apical long-axis or 4-chamber view.

❑ The aliasing velocity is decreased to 30 to 40 cm/s by shifting the Doppler baseline, which enhances PISA visualization.

❑ Both a narrow color sector and zoom mode are used for accurate measurement.

❑ PISA measures instantaneous flow rate (cm³/s). PISA must be integrated over the flow period to obtain flow volume (cm³ or mL).

❑ PISA may be inaccurate when the proximal flow field is not hemispherical, so this approach is more useful for central jets compared with eccentric jets.

❑ It is more difficult to visualize the PISA when regurgitation is mild, and it is more difficult to visualize a PISA for aortic, compared with mitral, regurgitation.

❑ Identification of the valve plane by two-dimensional (2D) imaging is critical because the PISA measurement is from the aliasing velocity to the valve orifice.

Regurgitant volume (Figure 12–3)

■ Regurgitant volume is the amount of blood that flows backward across the valve, measured in cm^3 or mL.

■ Regurgitant volume can be calculated by subtracting the stroke volume (SV) across a competent valve (forward SV) from the antegrade volume flow rate across the regurgitant valve (total SV):

$$\text{Regurgitant volume} = \text{Total SV} - \text{Forward SV}$$

■ Total SV also can be calculated by 2D echocardiographic measurement of LV stroke volume using the apical biplane approach.

Key points

❑ Transvalvular volume flow rate calculations are based on diameter measurements (using a circular cross-sectional area) and the velocity-time integral (VTI) of flow at that site:

$$SV = CSA \times VTI = \pi (D/2)^2 \times VTI$$

❑ Small errors in diameter measurement lead to large errors in calculated SV.

❑ The largest source of error is ensuring that diameter is measured at the same level as the VTI recording; this is particularly problematic for transmitral volume flow.

❑ When both aortic and mitral valves are regurgitant, pulmonic valve flow rate can be used for forward stroke volume.

❑ 2D LV volumes provide total SV when image planes and endocardial definition are adequate, but volumes may be underestimated if apical views are foreshortened.

Regurgitant orifice area

■ Conceptually, regurgitant orifice area (ROA) is the size of the defect in the closed valve that allows valve regurgitation.

■ The actual anatomy of the regurgitant orifice may be complex, sometimes with multiple sites of backflow across the valve.

■ The continuity equation applies to both antegrade and retrograde flow across a valve.

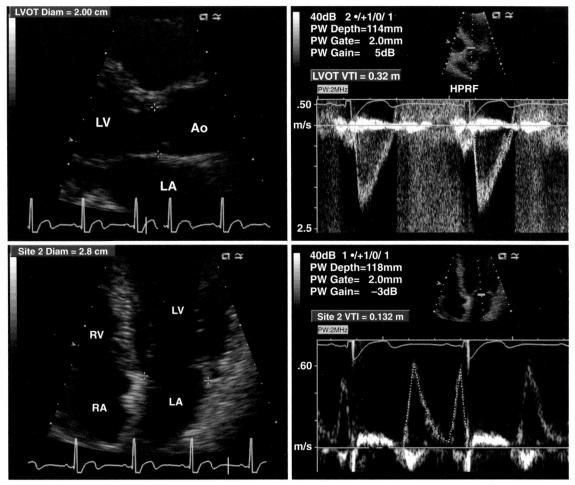

Figure 12–3. In this patient with aortic regurgitation, regurgitant volume is calculated as the difference between total stroke volume across the aortic valve and forward stroke volume across the mitral valve. The diameter (*D, left*) and velocity-time integral (*VTI, right*) for transaortic (*top*) and transmitral (*bottom*) flow are shown. Transaortic (total) stroke volume (TSV) is LVOT cross-sectional area (CSA = πr^2 = 3.14[2 cm/2]^2 = 3.14 cm^2) times the VTI (TSV = 3.14 cm^2 × 32 cm = 100 mL). Transmitral (forward) stroke volume (FSV) is π(3.1 cm/2)^2 × 13.2 cm = 64 mL. Then regurgitant stroke volume (RSV) is TSV − FSV or 100 mL − 64 mL = 36 mL. Regurgitant fraction is 36 mL/100 mL × 100% = 36%. These findings suggest moderate regurgitation.

- Thus, ROA can be calculated from regurgitant stroke volume and the VTI of the regurgitant jet (RJ) as:

$$\text{ROA}\left(\text{cm}^2\right) = \text{Regurgitant SV}\left(\text{cm}^3\right)/\text{VTI}_{\text{RJ}}\left(\text{cm}\right)$$

Key points

- ❏ ROA can be calculated using regurgitant SV calculated by any method.
- ❏ The continuous wave (CW) recording of the regurgitant jet is used to trace the VTI (Figure 12–4) to go with the regurgitant volume calculation from Figure 12–3.
- ❏ ROA also can be estimated using the PISA approach by dividing the PISA instantaneous volume flow rate by the maximum regurgitant jet velocity:

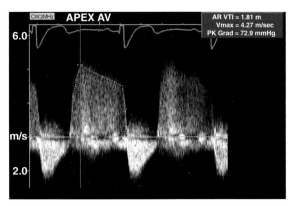

Figure 12–4. The velocity-time integral (VTI) of aortic regurgitant flow in the same patient shown in Figure 12–3 is used to calculate regurgitant orifice area (ROA) as the RSV/VTI = 36 cm^3/181 cm = 0.20 cm^2, again consistent with moderate regurgitation.

$$ROA\left(cm^{2}\right)=PISA\left(cm^{3}/s\right)/V_{RJ}\left(cm/s\right)$$

- ☐ The PISA estimated ROA reflects the instantaneous ROA only; thus, it is most useful for regurgitation that occurs equally throughout the flow period.
- ☐ In clinical practice, ROA should be calculated by more than one method, if possible, to ensure validity.

Distal flow reversals

- ■ The direction of blood flow distal to a regurgitant valve is reversed from normal when regurgitation is severe.
  - With severe mitral regurgitation, there is systolic flow reversal in the pulmonary veins.
  - With severe aortic regurgitation, there is holodiastolic flow reversal in the aorta. (Figure 12–5)
  - With severe tricuspid regurgitation, there is systolic flow reversal in the hepatic veins. (Figure 12–6)
- ■ This qualitative indicator is integrated with other findings in classifying overall regurgitant severity.

Key points

- ☐ These findings are more specific when flow reversal is more distal (e.g., abdominal compared with thoracic aorta for aortic regurgitation) and more severe (e.g., reversed versus blunted pulmonary vein systolic flow in mitral regurgitation).

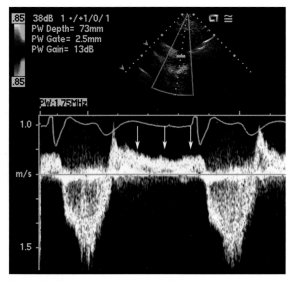

Figure 12–5. The Doppler flow signal in the descending thoracic aorta shows holodiastolic flow toward the transducer (reversal of flow, *arrows*) in this patient with moderate to severe aortic regurgitation. Holodiastolic flow reversal in the descending aorta also may be seen with other causes of diastolic flow exiting the proximal aorta, including a patent ductus arteriosus or a large arteriovenous fistula in an upper extremity.

- ☐ Flow reversal is sometimes seen even when regurgitation is not severe—for example, in hepatic and pulmonary veins in non-sinus rhythms, or in the descending aorta with a patent ductus arteriosus.
- ☐ Flow reversal is best detected with low wall filter settings, gain reduced to avoid channel crosstalk and with the scale adjusted to the velocity range of interest.
- ☐ Normal patterns of flow sometimes are mistaken for flow reversal.
  - In the descending aorta, early diastolic flow reversal is normal.
  - In the hepatic veins, the atrial reversal can be prominent and may appear to extend into early systole.

CW Doppler signal (Figure 12–7)

- ■ The shape of the CW Doppler signal reflects the instantaneous pressure differences between the two chambers.
- ■ The density of the CW Doppler signal, relative to antegrade flow, reflects the volume of regurgitant flow.

Key points

- ☐ The diastolic deceleration slope (or pressure half-time) of the aortic regurgitant signal is steeper (shorter) with more severe aortic regurgitation.
- ☐ A late systolic decline in velocity with mitral regurgitation reflects a rise in LA pressure, suggestive of a v-wave.
- ☐ Care is needed to ensure the Doppler recording is made with the ultrasound beam parallel to

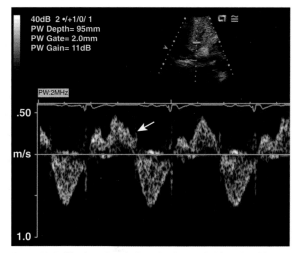

Figure 12–6. The hepatic vein flow signal, recorded from the subcostal window in the central hepatic vein shows flow toward the transducer in systole (*arrow*), also called systolic flow reversal, when severe tricuspid regurgitation is present.

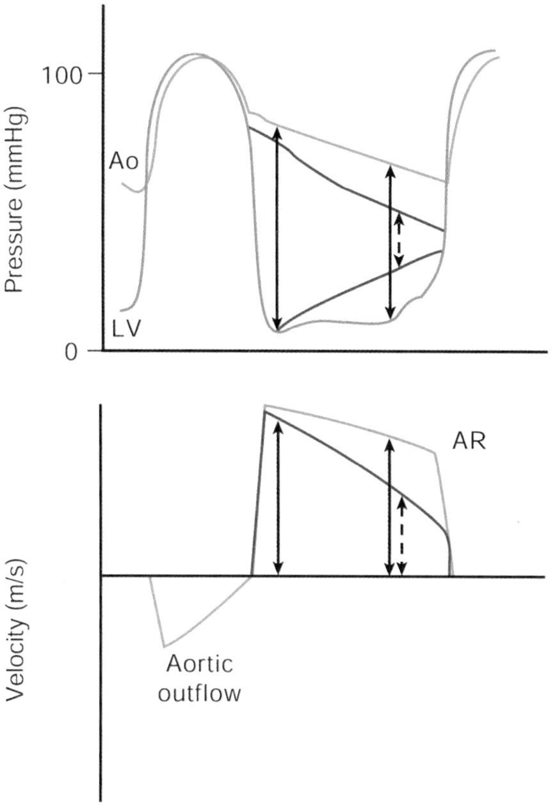

Figure 12–7. The shape of the CW Doppler velocity curve reflects the instantaneous pressure differences between the aorta and LV in diastole, with the relationship between LV and aortic (Ao) pressures (*top*) and Doppler velocities (*bottom*) shown for chronic (green) and acute (blue) aortic regurgitation.

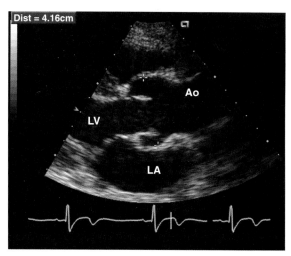

Figure 12–8. Parasternal long-axis view in a patient with aortic regurgitation showing dilated sinuses of Valsalva that may be the cause of valve dysfunction.

the direction of the regurgitant jet at the vena contracta.

❏ Optimal CW recordings of the regurgitant jets show a smooth velocity curve with a dense signal along the outer edge of the spectral signal.

❏ Recordings are enhanced using gray scale spectral analysis with the velocity scale adjusted to the range of interest, the wall filters increased to improve the signal-to-noise ratio, and gains lowered to avoid overestimation of velocities.

AORTIC REGURGITATION

Step-by-step approach

Step 1: Determine the etiology of regurgitation

■ Aortic regurgitation is due either to disease of the valve leaflets or abnormalities of the aortic root. (Figure 12–8)

■ Primary causes of aortic leaflet dysfunction include bicuspid valve, rheumatic disease, endocarditis, calcific disease, and some systemic diseases.

■ Aortic root enlargement resulting in aortic regurgitation may be due to Marfan syndrome, familial aortic aneurysm, hypertension, or aortic dissection.

Key points

❏ Long- and short-axis images of the aortic valve allow identification of a bicuspid aortic valve (two leaflets in systole), rheumatic disease (commissural fusion), vegetations, and calcific changes.

❏ Leaflet perforation or fenestration cannot be visualized but is inferred from the location of the regurgitant jet orifice identified by color Doppler.

❏ When aortic regurgitation is more than mild, the aorta should be measured at several sites as detailed in Chapter 16. The transducer is moved cephalad to visualize the ascending aorta.

❏ Marfan syndrome is characterized by loss of the normal acute angle at the sinotubular junction.

❏ Systemic inflammatory diseases associated with aortic regurgitation cause dilation of the aorta and thickening of the posterior aortic root extending onto the base of the anterior mitral leaflet.

Step 2: Determine the severity of regurgitation

■ Regurgitant severity is evaluated using a stepwise approach with integration of several types of data.

■ In addition to Doppler measures of regurgitant severity, the cause of regurgitation, and left ventricular (LV) size and systolic function are important parameters in clinical decision making.

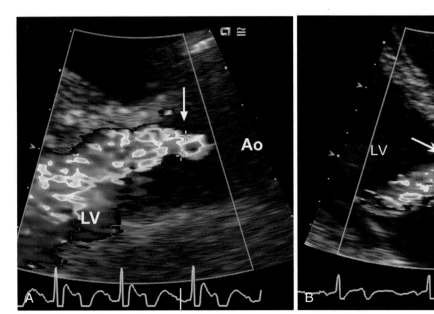

Figure 12–9. Examples of measuring vena contracta width with a centrally (*left*) and eccentrically (*right*) directed jet of aortic regurgitation. Vena contracta width in aortic regurgitation is best recorded in the parasternal long-axis view using zoom mode to focus on the aortic valve. The narrowest width of the regurgitant jet is measured, ideally with the proximal flow acceleration and distal jet expansion regions seen. Vena contract width is measured perpendicular to the jet direction; with an eccentrically directed jet, this measurement is not perpendicular to the LVOT.

Step 2A: Measurement of vena contracta width is the initial step in evaluation of aortic regurgitation (Figure 12–9)

Key points

- ❑ With aortic regurgitation, vena contracta usually is best measured in the parasternal long-axis view on transthoracic echocardiography (TTE) or the long-axis view at about 120 degrees rotation on transesophageal echocardiography (TEE).
- ❑ Vena contracta is measured as the smallest width of the jet, taking care with eccentric jets to avoid an oblique diameter measurement. (Figure 12–10)
- ❑ A vena contracta width less than 0.3 cm indicates mild regurgitation; a vena contracta width greater than 0.6 cm indicates severe regurgitation.
- ❑ Further evaluation is needed when vena contracta is 0.3 to 0.6 cm, when images of the vena contracta are suboptimal, or when further quantitation is needed for clinical decision making.

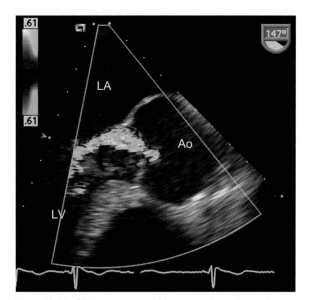

Figure 12–10. TEE long-axis view of the aortic valve in diastole in zoom mode showing a narrow eccentric jet of aortic regurgitation. The jet originates in the central part of the valve (note proximal acceleration region) but extends along the ventricular side of the non-coronary cusp and then down the anterior mitral valve leaflet. Vena contracta width is measured at the narrowest diameter of the jet; in this case, vena contracta width is almost perpendicular to the valve leaflet closure plane.

Step 2B: Evaluation of diastolic flow reversal in the descending aorta is a simple, reliable approach to evaluation of aortic regurgitant severity

Key points

- ❑ Holodiastolic flow reversal in the proximal abdominal aorta is highly specific for severe aortic regurgitation. (Figure 12–11)
- ❑ Holodiastolic flow reversal in the descending thoracic aorta is seen in some patients with moderate aortic regurgitation, as well as those with severe aortic regurgitation.
- ❑ Early diastolic flow reversal in the descending aorta is normal and should not be mistaken for aortic regurgitation.

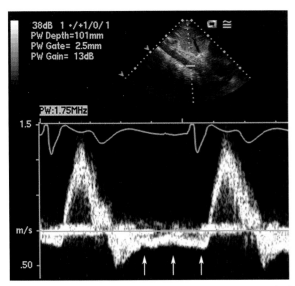

Figure 12–11. With severe aortic regurgitation, flow in the proximal abdominal aorta, recorded from the subcostal window, shows antegrade flow in systole with retrograde flow throughout diastole (*arrows*), reflecting severe backflow across the aortic valve.

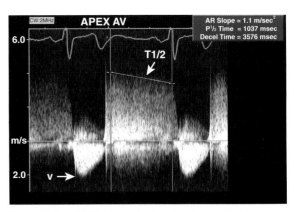

Figure 12–12. CW Doppler evaluation of aortic regurgitation provides information based on (1) the velocity of antegrade flow (*v*) reflecting both the volume of flow and coexisting valve stenosis, (2) the relative density of the regurgitant signal compared with the density of antegrade flow, and (3) the time course of the velocity signal. In this example, the diastolic slope is flat, with a pressure half-time greater than 1000 ms, and the signal is much less dense than antegrade flow; both these features are consistent with mild regurgitation.

☐ If holodiastolic aortic flow reversal is seen but there is no color Doppler evidence of severe aortic regurgitation, evaluate for a patent ductus arteriosus, which also causes aortic diastolic flow reversal due to flow from the aorta into the pulmonary artery.

Step 2C: CW Doppler evaluation of aortic regurgitation is a standard part of the evaluation (Figure 12–12)

Key points

☐ Aortic regurgitation usually is best recorded from an apical approach using CW Doppler because this window allows parallel alignment between the ultrasound beam and regurgitant jet.

☐ In cases with an eccentric posteriorly directed aortic regurgitant jet, the best intercept angle may be obtained from the parasternal window.

☐ On TEE a transgastric apical view may allow recording of the aortic regurgitant jet, but it may not be possible to obtain a parallel intercept angle using TEE.

☐ The density of the aortic regurgitant velocity signal compared with the density of the antegrade signal provides a qualitative measure of regurgitant severity. (Figure 12–13)

☐ In general, a steep diastolic deceleration slope (pressure half-time < 200 ms) is consistent with severe regurgitation, whereas a flat slope (>500 ms) indicates mild regurgitation. However, some patients with compensated

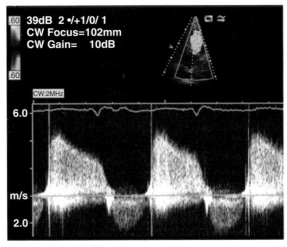

Figure 12–13. In this patient with severe aortic regurgitation, the CW Doppler signal in diastole is as (or more) dense as the antegrade flow signal in systole.

severe regurgitation have a long pressure half-time.

☐ Pressure half-time is measured using the same approach as measurement of pressure half-time in mitral stenosis. (See Chapter 11)

Step 2D: When further quantitation is needed, regurgitant volume and orifice area can be calculated

Key points

☐ The most common approach is to calculate total stroke volume across the aortic valve and then subtract forward stroke volume (calculated across the mitral or pulmonic valve) to determine regurgitant volume.

❏ Regurgitant orifice area is calculated by dividing regurgitant volume by the velocity-time integral (VTI) of the CW aortic regurgitation velocity curve.

❏ The proximal isovelocity surface area (PISA) often is difficult to visualize with aortic regurgitation.

❏ Methods to calculate regurgitant volume based on antegrade and retrograde flow in the descending aorta have been described but are not routinely used.

Step 3: Evaluate antegrade aortic flow and stenosis

■ Many patients with aortic regurgitation also have some degree of aortic stenosis.

■ However, antegrade aortic velocity is increased in patients with severe regurgitation because of the increased antegrade volume flow rate across the aortic valve in systole.

■ Thus, in addition to velocity and mean pressure gradient, aortic valve area should be calculated using the continuity equation as described in Chapter 11.

Step 4: Evaluate the consequences of chronic LV pressure and volume overload

■ The LV dilates in response to the chronic load imposed by aortic regurgitation with the extent of LV dilation reflecting the severity of regurgitation. (Figure 12–14)

■ Some patients develop irreversible LV dysfunction in the absence of symptoms so that the most important parameters to measure on echocardiography in patients with chronic severe aortic regurgitation are LV size and ejection fraction.

Key points

❏ LV end-diastolic and end-systolic dimensions, volumes, and ejection fraction are key measurements, with direct side-by-side comparison to previous examinations.

❏ Guidelines recommend M-mode ventricular dimension measurements because of better endocardial definition due to the high sampling rate of M-mode recordings.

❏ When the M-line cannot be aligned perpendicular to the long and short axes of the LV, 2D measurements can be used, taking care to optimally define the endocardium and to correctly measure the LV minor axis at end-diastole and end-systole.

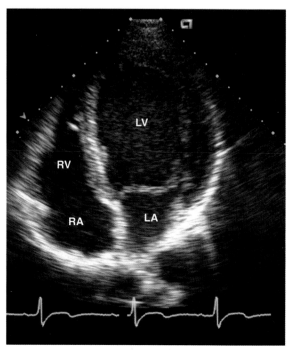

Figure 12–14. In this patient with severe aortic regurgitation, the apical 4-chamber view shows a dilated LV with increased sphericity (rounded shape of the LV apex).

❏ LV end-diastolic and end-systolic volumes and ejection fraction are measured using the 2D (or three-dimensional [3D]) apical biplane method.

❏ Indexing dimensions and volumes to body surface area is especially important in women and smaller patients.

❏ With severe aortic regurgitation, LV volumes are increased in direct proportion to the regurgitant volume; the stroke volume calculated using the biplane apical approach is the total stroke volume (forward SV plus regurgitant SV).

❏ The LV becomes more spherical in aortic regurgitation patients, so it is especially important to ensure that LV dimensions are measured at the same position on sequential examinations in each patient.

MITRAL REGURGITATION

Step-by-step approach

Step 1: Determine the etiology of regurgitation

■ Mitral regurgitation may be primary (due to abnormalities of the valve leaflets and chordae) or functional (secondary to LV dilation or dysfunction with normal leaflets).

- Primary causes of mitral leaflet and chordal dysfunction include myxomatous mitral valve disease (mitral valve prolapse), rheumatic disease, mitral annular calcification, and endocarditis. (Figure 12–15)
- LV dilation results in functional mitral regurgitation due to annular dilation and malalignment of the papillary muscles, resulting in tethering or "tenting" of the valve leaflets in systole.
- Ischemic mitral regurgitation may be due to papillary muscle dysfunction, regional dysfunction of the inferior-lateral wall, or diffuse LV dysfunction and dilation.
- Mitral regurgitation may be intermittent if reversible ischemia results in inadequate leaflet closure.

Key points

☐ Mitral valve anatomy is evaluated in multiple TTE views, including long-axis, short-axis, and 4-chamber image planes. If better definition of valve anatomy is needed for clinical decision making, TEE or 3D imaging may be helpful. (Figures 12–16 and 12–17)

☐ Imaging of the mitral valve allows identification of myomatous valve disease, rheumatic disease (commissural fusion), vegetations, and calcific changes.

☐ With myxomatous mitral valve disease, the degree of thickening, redundancy, and prolapse of each leaflet is described.

☐ The tip of a flail leaflet segment points toward the roof of the LA in systole; a severely prolapsing segment is curved so that the tip points toward the LV apex. (Figure 12–18)

☐ Restricted leaflet motion is characteristic of functional mitral regurgitation. The area defined by the tented leaflets and the annular plane at end-systole provides an index of the severity of restricted motion.

☐ 3D TEE is especially useful for evaluation of prolapse and chordal rupture in patients with myxomatous mitral valve disease.

Step 2: Determine the severity of regurgitation

- Regurgitant severity is evaluated using a stepwise approach with integration of several types of data.
- In addition to Doppler measures of regurgitant severity, the cause of regurgitation, LV size and systolic function, LA size, and pulmonary pressures are important parameters in clinical decision making.

Step 2A: Measurement of vena contracta width is the initial step in evaluation of mitral regurgitation (Figure 12–19)

Key points

☐ With mitral regurgitation, vena contracta usually is best measured in the parasternal

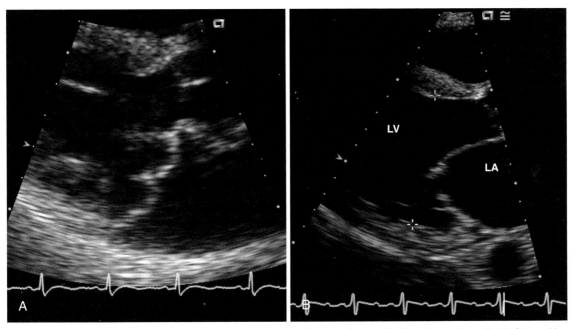

Figure 12–15. Examples of primary mitral regurgitation due to myxomatous mitral valve disease (*A*) with prolapse of both mitral leaflets on this end-systolic frame, and functional mitral regurgitation (*B*) due to leaflet tethering in a patient with a dilated cardiomyopathy.

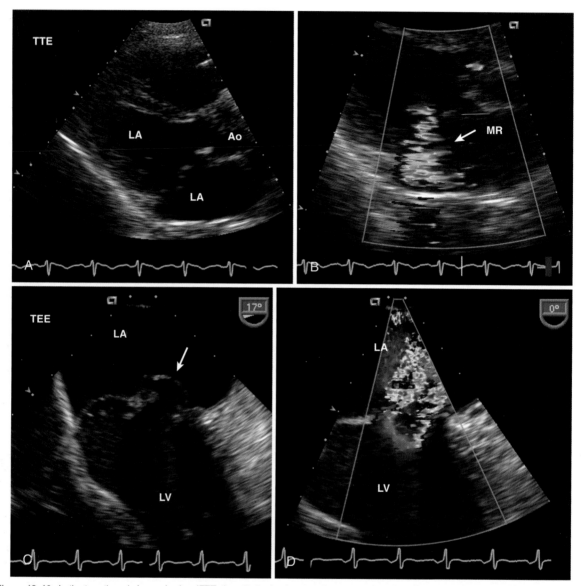

Figure 12–16. In the transthoracic long-axis view (*TTE*) the mitral valve is not well seen, although color Doppler shows a posteriorly directed mitral regurgitation (*MR*) jet. Transesophageal images (*TEE*) show severe prolapse of the posterior mitral leaflet (*arrow*) with severe mitral regurgitation with a wide vena contracta. The mitral leaflet curves into the left atrium (*LA*), but the tip of the leaflet points toward the LV apex, so these findings are consistent with severe prolapse, but not a flail segment, in this view.

long-axis view on TTE or the long-axis view at about 120 degrees rotation on TEE.

❏ Vena contracta is measured as the smallest width of the jet, taking care with eccentric jets to avoid an oblique diameter measurement. Both the proximal acceleration region and the distal jet expansion should be seen to ensure the narrowest segment of the jet is measured.

• A vena contracta width less than 0.3 cm indicates mild regurgitation; a vena contracta width of 0.7 cm indicates severe regurgitation.

• Further evaluation is needed when the vena contracta is between 0.3 and 0.7 cm, when images of the vena contracta are suboptimal, or when

further quantitation is needed for clinical decision making.

Step 2B: Evaluation of jet direction determines the next step in evaluation of mitral regurgitant severity

■ Central jets typically are seen with functional mitral regurgitation due to LV dilation.

■ Ischemic mitral regurgitation often results in an eccentric posteriorly directed jet.

■ Mitral valve prolapse often results in an eccentric regurgitant jet with the jet directed away from the affected leaflet. (Figure 12–20)

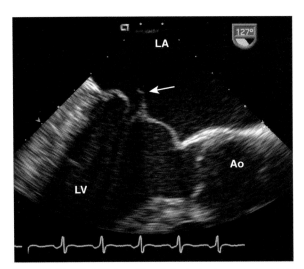

Figure 12–17. This TEE view of the mitral valve in a long-axis view shows the posterior mitral leaflet closure on the atrial side of the valve in systole. The tip of the central scallop of the posterior leaflet (*arrow*), seen in this view, points toward the roof of the *LA*, consistent with a flail leaflet segment.

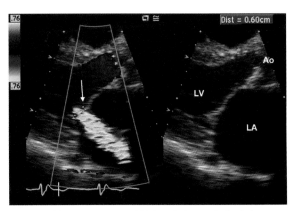

Figure 12–19. Vena contracta width for mitral regurgitation is best measured in a parasternal long-axis view using zoom mode to maximize the size of the image of the proximal jet geometry. The vena contracta is the narrow neck between the proximal acceleration on the ventricular side of the valve and jet expansion in the LA.

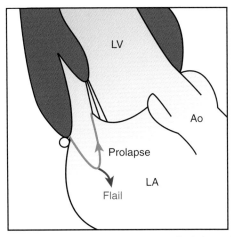

Figure 12–18. The term *prolapse* of the mitral leaflet indicates that the chordal connections of the leaflet to the papillary muscle are intact so that, regardless of the severity of prolapse, the tip of the leaflet still points toward the LV apex. With chordal rupture, the mitral leaflet segment becomes "flail" and the tip of the flail segment points toward the roof of the LA.

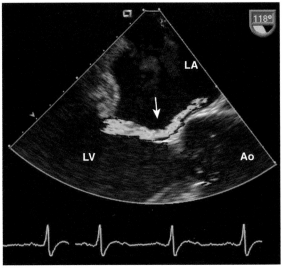

Figure 12–20. Color Doppler in a TEE long-axis view shows an eccentric anteriorly directed mitral regurgitant jet. With myxomatous mitral valve disease, the direction of the jet typically is opposite the affected leaflet. This anteriorly directed jet confirms that regurgitation is primarily due to involvement of the posterior valve leaflet.

❏ The duration of mitral regurgitation in systole can be visualized on frame-by-frame review of the cardiac cycle or can be inferred from the CW Doppler mitral regurgitation jet signal.

Step 2C: When clinically indicated, RV and ROA are calculated

Key points

❏ With late systolic mitral regurgitation or eccentric jets, total stroke volume is calculated across the mitral valve (SV_{MR}), and then forward stroke volume (calculated across the LV outflow tract [SV_{LVOT}] or pulmonic valve)

Key points

❏ With holosystolic regurgitation and a central jet, the PISA approach to quantitation of severity is appropriate; use of the PISA approach with late systolic mitral regurgitation or an eccentric jet is problematic.

❏ With an eccentric jet or late systolic mitral regurgitation, pulsed Doppler measurement of regurgitant volume and orifice area is appropriate.

is substracted to obtain regurgitant volume (Figure 12–21):

$$RV_{MR} = SV_{MR} - SV_{LVOT}$$

❏ The 2D biplane total LV stroke volume (SV_{2D}) can be used instead of transmitral flow to calculate regurgitant volume:

$$RV_{MR} = SV_{2D} - SV_{LVOT}$$

❏ Regurgitant orifice area is calculated by dividing regurgitant volume (RV) by the velocity time integral (VTI_{MR}) of the CW Doppler mitral regurgitation velocity curve during systole:

$$ROA = RV/VTI_{MR}$$

❏ The proximal isovelocity surface area approach provides instantaneous flow rate, which is divided by the peak mitral regurgitation velocity (V_{MR}) to estimate ROA:

$$ROA = (PISA \times V_{aliasing})/V_{MR}$$

❏ The regurgitant volume can be estimated using the PISA method by multiplying the ROA by the VTI of the mitral regurgitant jet:

$$RV = ROA \times VTI_{RJ}$$

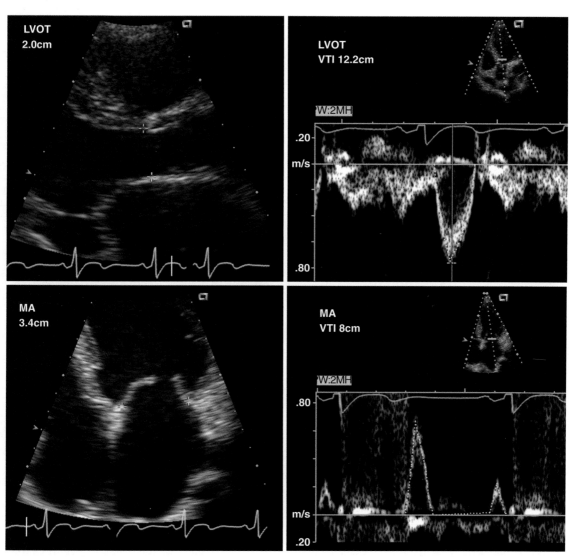

Figure 12–21. Calculation of regurgitant volume in a patient with mitral regurgitation (secondary to a dilated cardiomyopathy) is based on measurement of mitral (*bottom*) and aortic (*top*) annular diameter (*D, left*) and velocity-time integral (*VTI, right*). Total (transmitral) stroke volume (TSV) is the mitral annular cross-sectional area (CSA= πr^2 = 3.41[3.4 cm/2]^2 = 9.1 cm^2) multiplied by the VTI (TSV = 9.1 cm^2 × 8 cm = 73 mL). Transaortic (forward) stroke volume (FSV) is π(2.0 cm/2)^2 × 12.2 cm = 38 mL. Then regurgitant stroke volume (RSV) is TSV – FSV or 73 mL – 38 mL = 35 mL. Regurgitant fraction is 35 mL/78 mL × 100% = 45%. These findings suggest moderate regurgitation.

- The PISA images are optimized using an aliasing velocity of 30 to 40 cm/s. The radius (r) of the PISA is measured from the edge of the color corresponding to the aliasing velocity to the level of the closed leaflets in systole (Figure 12–22).
- Recording images for PISA measurement with and without color facilitates correct identification of the valve orifice plane.
- A quick estimate of ROA can be obtained by setting the aliasing velocity at close to 40 cm/s and assuming a mitral regurgitation maximum velocity of 5 m/s; then ROA is $r^2/2$.

Step 2D: Additional simple measures of regurgitant severity include pulmonary vein systolic flow reversal and the density of the CW Doppler signal

- Reversal or blunting of the normal pattern of pulmonary venous inflow into the LA in systole is seen in most patients with severe mitral regurgitation (Figure 12–23).
- The density of the CW Doppler mitral regurgitant curve, compared with the density of antegrade flow, indicates relative mitral regurgitant severity (Figure 12–24).

Key points

- The specific location of systolic flow reversal depends on jet direction, so that TEE imaging may be needed to evaluate all four pulmonary veins; the absence of systolic flow reversal on TTE does not exclude severe regurgitation.
- Systolic flow reversal may be present even when regurgitation is not severe in patients with atrial arrhythmias or other factors that affect normal atrial filling patterns.
- The CW Doppler mitral regurgitant jet usually is best recorded from an apical approach on TTE or a 4-chamber view on TEE because these windows allow parallel alignment between the ultrasound beam and regurgitant jet.
- In cases with an eccentric posteriorly directed regurgitant jet, the best intercept angle may be

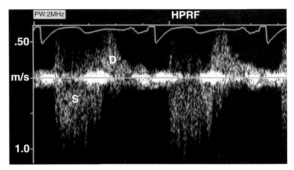

Figure 12–23. Pulmonary vein flow recorded on TTE from the apical 4-chamber view in the right superior pulmonary vein. Signal strength often is suboptimal, as in this example; even so, the flow into the LA in diastole (D) can be distinguished from the systolic (S) flow reversal due to severe mitral regurgitation.

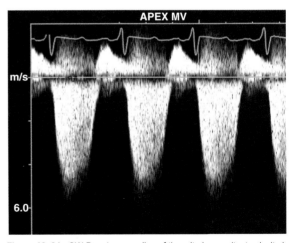

Figure 12–24. CW Doppler recording of the mitral regurgitant velocity is evaluated for (1) the velocity and deceleration curve of the antegrade flow in diastole, (2) the relative density of the retrograde flow compared with antegrade flow, and (3) the shape and timing of the regurgitant velocity curve. In this example, the antegrade flow is normal velocity (<1 m/s) with a steep deceleration curve indicating the absence of mitral stenosis. The regurgitant signal is almost as dense as antegrade flow and is holosystolic, consistent with severe regurgitation. In addition, the falloff in velocity in late systole, suggests that left atrial pressure is elevated in late systole, consistent with a v-wave and acute regurgitation.

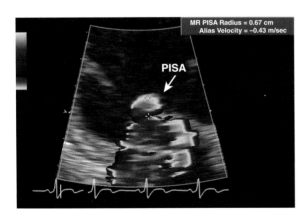

Figure 12–22. The proximal isovelocity surface area (*PISA*) is best visualized from the apical window, in a long-axis (as in this example) or 4-chamber view. Zoom mode is used to maximize the image size of the PISA, with a velocity scale without variance and with the baseline moved so that the aliasing velocity is about 40 cm/s. In this example, the instantaneous flow rate is calculated as the surface area of the PISA ($2\pi r^2 = 2 \times 3.14 \times [0.67 \text{ cm}]^2 = 2.8 \text{ cm}^2$ times the aliasing velocity of 43 cm/s, which equals 121 cm^3/s. If the mitral regurgitant maximum velocity is 5 m/s (500 cm/s), then regurgitant orifice area is (121 cm^3/s)/500 cm/s = 0.24 cm^2.

obtained from the parasternal window or occasionally from a suprasternal approach.

Step 3: Evaluate antegrade mitral flow and stenosis

- Patients with rheumatic mitral regurgitation often have some degree of mitral stenosis.
- All patients with severe mitral regurgitation have an elevated antegrade mitral velocity because of the increased antegrade volume flow rate across the mitral valve in diastole.
- Mitral stenosis is distinguished from a high volume flow rate by the mitral pressure half-time.

Step 4: Evaluate the consequences of chronic ventricular volume overload

- The LV dilates in response to the chronic load imposed by mitral regurgitation. However, the extent of LV dilation is much less than seen with aortic regurgitation because aortic regurgitation results in pressure and volume overload, whereas mitral regurgitation predominantly imposes a volume overload.
- The most important parameters to measure on echocardiography in patients with chronic severe mitral regurgitation are LV size and ejection fraction because some patients develop irreversible LV dysfunction in the absence of symptoms.

Key points

- ❏ LV end-diastole and end-systolic dimensions and volumes should be measured and compared side by side with previous examinations.
- ❏ Even a slight increase in systolic size is clinically significant because the threshold for intervention is close to the upper normal limit for LV size (> 40 mm).
- ❏ Guidelines recommend M-mode ventricular dimension measurements because of better endocardial definition due to the high sampling rate of M-mode recordings.
- ❏ When the M-line cannot be aligned perpendicular to the long and short axes of the LV, 2D measurements can be used, taking care to optimally define the endocardium and to correctly measure the LV minor axis at end-diastole and end-systole.
- ❏ LV end-diastolic and end-systolic volumes and ejection fraction are measured using the 2D (or 3D) apical biplane method.
- ❏ With severe mitral regurgitation, LV volumes are increased in direct proportion to the regurgitant volume; stroke volume calculated using the biplane apical approach is the total stroke volume (forward plus regurgitant).

- ❏ Ejection fraction measurement is accurate in patients with mitral regurgitation. Even a small decline in ejection fraction has important clinical implications for optimal timing of valve surgery, so precise measurement is essential.
- ❏ Measurement of LV *dP/dt* (rate of rise in pressure) from the mitral regurgitation jet is useful. (see Chapter 6)

Step 5: Evaluate other consequences of mitral regurgitation

- Left atrial enlargement is assessed as described in Chapter 2.
- Pulmonary systolic pressures are estimated as described in Chapter 6.
- RV size and systolic function are evaluated as described in Chapter 6.

PULMONIC REGURGITATION

Step-by-step approach

Step 1: Determine the etiology of regurgitation

- A small amount of pulmonic regurgitation is seen in most individuals. (Figure 12–25)
- Pathologic regurgitation most often is due to congenital heart disease, such as a repaired tetralogy of Fallot.

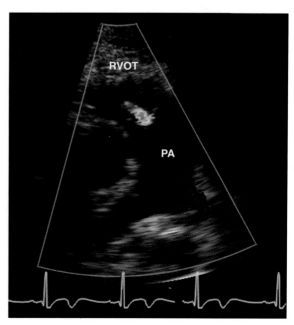

Figure 12–25. Color Doppler image of pulmonic regurgitation in a parasternal short-axis view in diastole. The vena contracta is narrow, reflecting mild regurgitation.

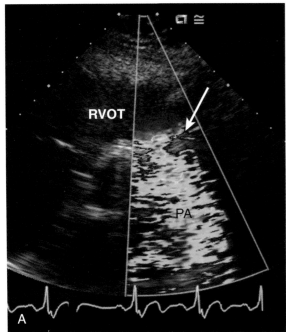

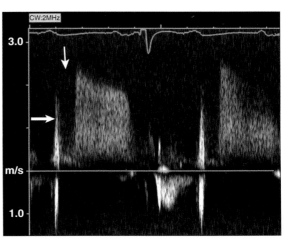

Figure 12–27. CW Doppler recording of pulmonic regurgitation. The signal is much less dense than antegrade flow, consistent with mild regurgitation. A prominent pulmonic closing click (*arrow*) is followed by an area of signal dropout, probably due to initial competence of the valve in early diastole, followed by the typical low-velocity diastolic curve of pulmonic regurgitation. The velocity-time course reflects the pulmonary artery–to–right ventricular pressure difference in diastole. Low-velocity flow is consistent with a small pressure gradient and thus normal pulmonary diastolic pressures.

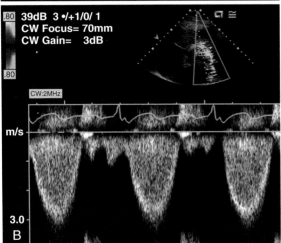

Figure 12–26. This patient with congenital pulmonic stenosis has thickened valve leaflets with a systolic increase in velocity at the leaflet level. CW Doppler shows moderate stenosis with a jet velocity of 3.2 m/s, but little regurgitation is detected.

■ The density and shape of the CW Doppler waveform are diagnostic. (Figure 12–27)
■ Further quantitation of pulmonic regurgitation is rarely needed.

Key points

❏ Pulmonic regurgitation is low velocity (if pulmonary diastolic pressure is normal), so the color Doppler display may show uniform laminar flow in diastole in the RV outflow tract. (Figure 12–28)
❏ The CW Doppler curve is especially helpful for detection of severe pulmonic regurgitation showing a dense signal with a steep deceleration slope that reaches the baseline at end-diastole. (Figure 12–29)

Step 3: Evaluate the consequences of right ventricular volume overload

■ Severe pulmonic regurgitation results in RV dilation and eventual systolic dysfunction.

Key points

❏ Evaluation of RV size and systolic function by echocardiography is largely based on qualitative evaluation of 2D images, using a scale of normal, mild, moderate, and severely abnormal.

Key points

❏ Imaging the pulmonic valve is difficult in adult patients.
❏ Thickened, deformed leaflets may be seen with congenital pulmonic valve disease. (Figure 12–26)

Step 2: Evaluate the severity of pulmonic regurgitation

■ Vena contracta width is helpful for evaluation of pulmonic regurgitation.

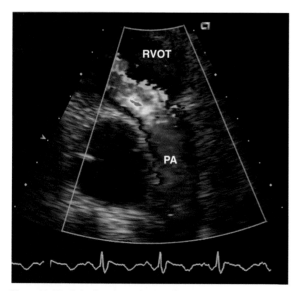

Figure 12–28. Color Doppler evaluation of the pulmonic valve in a parasternal short-axis view shows laminar flow filling the right ventricular outflow tract (*RVOT*) in diastole, consistent with severe pulmonic regurgitation. Because flow velocities are low, there is little variance, so that regurgitation may be missed on cine images but is evident on a frame-by-frame review.

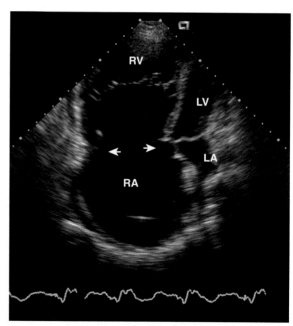

Figure 12–30. Apical 4-chamber view in a patient with Ebstein's anomaly of the tricuspid valve. The tricuspid valve leaflets are apically displaced so that the portion of the RV between the leaflets and the tricuspid annulus (*arrows*) has a right atrial pressure. Severe tricuspid regurgitation results in severe right atrial and RV enlargement. This patient has an intact atrial septum.

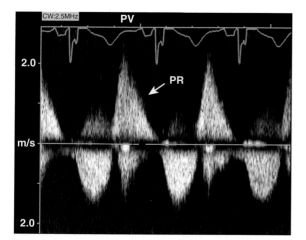

Figure 12–29. CW Doppler recording of pulmonary flow in a patient with severe pulmonic regurgitation (PR). The density of retrograde flow across the valve (above the baseline) is equal to the density of antegrade flow in systole. In addition, the end-diastolic velocity of the pulmonic regurgitation approaches zero, indicating equalization of diastolic pressures in the pulmonary artery and RV.

TRICUSPID REGURGITATION

Step-by-step approach

Step 1: Evaluate the etiology of tricuspid regurgitation

- Tricuspid regurgitation may be due to primary valve disease or may be secondary to annular dilation.
- Primary causes of tricuspid regurgitation include endocarditis, Ebstein's anomaly, rheumatic disease, carcinoid, and myxomatous disease.
- Secondary tricuspid regurgitation is seen with pulmonary hypertension of any cause, including mitral valve disease, pulmonary parenchymal disease, or primary pulmonary hypertension.

Key points

- ❑ Tricuspid valve vegetations are diagnosed on TTE or TEE.
- ❑ With Ebstein's anomaly there is apical displacement (insertion of tricuspid leaflet >10 mm apical from mitral valve leaflets) of one or more valve leaflets. (Figure 12–30)
- ❑ Carcinoid results in short, thick, and immobile valve leaflets.

- ❑ Sequential studies are helpful in distinguishing residual RV dilation or dysfunction after repair of tetralogy of Fallot from progressive postoperative changes.
- ❑ Cardiac magnetic resonance imaging allows quantitation of RV volumes and ejection fraction.

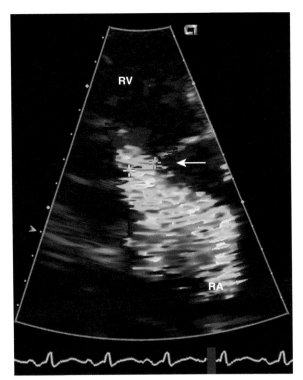

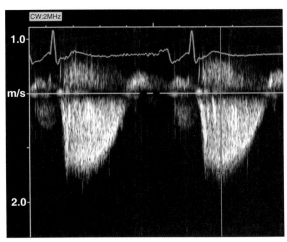

Figure 12–32. This CW Doppler recording shows severe tricuspid regurgitation with a dense systolic signal. The velocity is low because pulmonary pressures are normal and right atrial pressure is elevated due to severe tricuspid regurgitation.

Figure 12–31. The vena contracta of the tricuspid regurgitant jet is visualized in the RV inflow view from the parasternal window using the zoom mode to maximize resolution of the proximal jet geometry. The vena contract width of 4 mm is consistent with moderate regurgitation. Evaluation of the vena contracta is more accurate than visualization of the size of the flow disturbance in the right atrium (*RA*) for quantitation of tricuspid regurgitation.

❏ Rheumatic tricuspid disease occurs in 20% to 30% of patients with rheumatic mitral disease.

❏ The diagnosis of secondary tricuspid regurgitation is based on the presence of pulmonary hypertension and the absence of structural abnormalities of the leaflets.

Step 2: Evaluate the severity of tricuspid regurgitation

■ Vena contracta width is the key step in evaluation of tricuspid regurgitant severity.

■ Density of the CW Doppler velocity curve, relative to antegrade flow, is also helpful.

■ Systolic flow reversal in the hepatic veins is seen with severe tricuspid regurgitation.

Key points

❏ A vena contracta greater than 0.7 cm is specific for severe tricuspid regurgitation. (Figure 12–31)

❏ Vena contracta width is best measured in the parasternal short-axis or RV inflow view.

❏ A dense CW Doppler signal is seen with severe tricuspid regurgitation, but velocity reflects the RV–to–RA systolic pressure gradient, not regurgitant severity. (Figure 12–32)

❏ Evaluation of hepatic vein flow patterns is problematic unless sinus rhythm is present.

Step 3: Evaluate the consequences of right ventricular volume overload

■ Severe chronic tricuspid regurgitation is associated with RV enlargement.

■ RV systolic function may be normal or may be reduced with chronic tricuspid regurgitation.

■ RV size and systolic function are evaluated qualitatively as described in Chapter 6.

■ Right atrial size is increased with chronic tricuspid regurgitation.

THE ECHO EXAM

Aortic Regurgitation

Etiology	Valve abnormality Dilated aorta
Severity of regurgitation	Vena contracta width Descending aorta holosystolic flow reversal CW Doppler deceleration slope Calculation of RV, RF and ROA
Coexisting aortic stenosis	Aortic jet velocity
LV response	LV dimensions or volumes LV ejection fraction *dP/dt*
Other findings	Dilation of sinuses or ascending aorta Aortic coarctation (with bicuspid valve)

EXAMPLE

A 37-year-old man presents with an asymptomatic diastolic murmur. Echocardiography shows a bicuspid aortic valve with more than mild aortic regurgitation with:

Vena contracta width	5 mm
Descending aorta	Holodiastolic flow reversal in descending thoracic, but not proximal abdominal, aorta
CW Doppler	Aortic regurgitation (AR) signal less dense than antegrade flow $VTI_{AR} = 150$ cm
LVOT diameter ($LVOT_D$)	2.8 cm
VTI_{LVOT}	24 cm
Mitral annulus diameter	3.1 cm
VTI_{MA}	12 cm

The *vena contracta width* indicates more than mild aortic regurgitation, but this could be moderate or severe.

Holodiastolic flow reversal in the proximal abdominal aorta would be consistent with severe AR. Flow reversal in the descending thoracic aorta indicate at least moderate AR but is less specific for severe AR.

CW Doppler signal density indicates at least moderate AR, and a deceleration slope > 3 m/s^2 but < 5 m/s^2 is also consistent with moderate or severe aortic regurgitation.

Next, regurgitant volume (RV), regurgitant fraction (RF), and regurgitant orifice area (ROA) are calculated.

Using the LVOT and mitral annulus diameters (MA_D), the circular cross-sectional areas of flow are calculated:

$$CSA_{LVOT} = \pi (LVOT_D/2)^2 = 3.14(2.7/2)^2 = 6.2 \, cm^2$$

$$CSA_{MA} = \pi (MA_D/2)^2 = 3.14(3.1/2)^2 = 7.5 \, cm^2$$

Stroke volume across each valve (cm^3 = ml), then, is:

$$SV_{LVOT} = (CSA_{LVOT} \times VTI_{LVOT}) = 6.2 \, cm^2 \times 24 \, cm = 149 \, cm^3$$

$$SV_{MA} = (CSA_{MA} \times VTI_{MA}) = 7.5 \, cm^2 \times 12 \, cm = 91 \, cm^3$$

Regurgitant volume is calculated from transaortic flow (total stroke volume [TSV]) and transmitral flow (forward stroke volume [FSV]), as:

$$RV = TSV - FSV = 149 \, mL - 91 \, mL = 58 \, mL$$

Regurgitant fraction is:

$$RV = RSV/TSV \times 100\% = 58 \, mL/149 \, mL \times 100\% = 39\%$$

Regurgitant orifice area (ROA) is:

$$ROA = RSV/VTI_{AR} = 58 \, cm^3/204 \, cm = 0.28 \, cm^2$$

The RV, RF, and ROA all are consistent with moderate (but nearly severe) aortic regurgitation.

LVOT, left ventricular outflow tract; RSV, regurgitant stroke volume.

Quantitation of Aortic Regurgitation Severity

Parameter	Modality	View	Recording	Measurements and Calculations
Vena contracta width	Color flow imaging	Parasternal long axis	Angulate, decrease depth, narrow sector, zoom	Narrowest segment of regurgitant jet between proximal flow convergence and distal jet expansion
Descending aortic diastolic flow reversal	Pulsed Doppler	Subcostal and SSN	Sample volume 2-3 mm, decrease wall filters, adjust scale	Evidence for holodiastolic flow reversal
CW Doppler signal (intensity, slope, VTI)	CW Doppler	Apical	Careful positioning and transducer angulation to obtain clear signal	Compare signal intensity of retrograde to antegrade flow, measure slope along edge of dense signal
Volume flow at two sites (RV, RF, ROA)	2D and pulsed Doppler	Parasternal (2D) and apical	LVOT diameter and VTI Mitral annulus diameter and VTI	$TSV = SV_{LVOT} = (CSA_{LVOT} \times VTI_{LVOT})$ $FSV = SV_{MA} = (CSA_{MA} \times VTI_{MA})$ $RV = TSV - FSV$ $ROA = RSV/VTI_{AR}$

2D, two-dimensional; AR, aortic regurgitation; FSV, forward stroke volume; LVOT, left ventricular outflow tract ; MA, mitral annulus; RF, regurgitant fraction; RV, regurgitant volume; TSV, total stroke volume.

Quantitative Evaluation of Aortic Regurgitant Severity (ASE Guidelines)

Parameter	Mild	Moderate	Severe
Jet width/LVOT	<25%	25%-65%	>65%
Vena contracta (cm)	<0.3	0.3-0.6	>0.6
Pressure half-time (ms)	>500	200-500	<200
Regurgitant volume (mL/beat)	<30	30-60	>60
Regurgitant fraction (%)	<30	30-50	>50
Regurgitant orifice area (cm²)	<0.10	0.1-0.3	>0.30

ASE, American Society of Endocardiography; LVOT, left ventricular outflow tract.

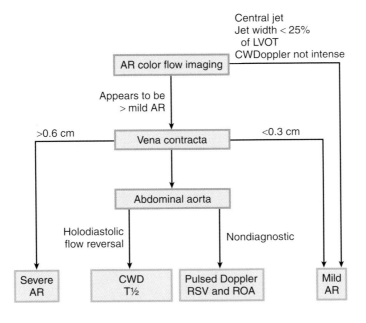

Mitral Regurgitation

Etiology	Primary valve disease Secondary (functional)
Severity of regurgitation	Vena contracta width Jet direction (central, eccentric) CW Doppler signal Calculation of regurgitant volume, regurgitant fraction, and regurgitant orifice area Central jet: PISA method Eccentric jet: volume flow at two sites Pulmonary vein flow reversal
LV response	LV dimensions or volumes LV ejection fraction *dP/dt*
Pulmonary vasculature	Pulmonary systolic pressure RV size and systolic function
Other findings	LA size

EXAMPLE

A 52-year-old man with a dilated cardiomyopathy presents with worsening heart failure symptoms. Echocardiography shows a dilated LV with an ejection fraction of 32% and a central jet of mitral regurgitation with:

Vena contracta width	8 mm
CW Doppler	MR signal as dense as antegrade flow with no evidence for a v-wave
dP/dt	840 mm Hg/s
Maximum MR velocity	4.6 m/s
VTI$_{MR}$	130 cm
PISA radius	1.2 cm
Aliasing velocity	30 cm/s
Right superior pulmonary vein	Systolic flow reversal

The vena contracta width indicates severe mitral regurgitation.

CW Doppler signal density indicates moderate to severe MR and the absence of a v-wave suggests a chronic disease process. The *dP/dt* is <1000 mmHg/s, consistent with decreased LV contractility.

Color flow indicates a central jet, so the proximal isovelocity surface area method can be used to quantitate regurgitant severity.

The PISA is calculated from the radius measurement as:

$$PISA = 2\pi r^2 = 2\pi(1.0\,cm)^2 = 6.3\,cm^2$$

The maximum instantaneous regurgitant flow rate (R_{FR}) is calculated from PISA and the aliasing velocity ($V_{aliasing}$) as:

$$R_{RF} = PISA \times V_{aliasing} = 6.3\,cm^2 \times 30\,cm/s = 189\,cm^3/s$$

Maximum regurgitant orifice area (instantaneous), then, is calculated from the R_{FR} and MR jet velocity (where 4.6 m/s = 460 cm/s):

$$ROA_{max} = R_{FR}/V_{MR} = (189\,cm^3/s)/460\,cm/s = 0.41\,cm^2$$

This ROA is consistent with severe mitral regurgitation. Regurgitant volume over the systolic flow period can be estimated as:

$$RV = ROA \times VTI_{MR} = 0.41\,cm^2 \times 130\,cm = 53\,cm^3 \text{ or mL}$$

This regurgitant volume is consistent with moderate mitral regurgitation.

If the jet is eccentric, quantitation should be performed using transaortic (forward) stroke volume and transmitral (total) stroke volume calculations, as illustrated for aortic regurgitation.

MR, mitral regurgitation; PISA, proximal isovelocity surface area; ROA, regurgitation orifice area; RV, regurgitant volume; V$_{MR}$, mitral regurgitation jet velocity; VTI$_{MR}$, mitral regurgitation velocity-time integral.

Quantitation of Mitral Regurgitation Severity

Parameter	Modality	View(s)	Recording	Measurements and Calculations
Vena contracta width	Color flow imaging	Parasternal long axis	Angulate, decrease depth, narrow sector, zoom	Narrowest segment of regurgitant jet between proximal flow convergence and distal jet expansion
Color flow imaging	Color flow imaging	Parasternal and apical	Narrow sector, decrease depth	Central vs. eccentric, anterior vs. posterior
CW Doppler signal	CW Doppler	Apical	Careful positioning, and transducer angulation to obtain clear signal	Compare signal intensity of retrograde to antegrade flow
PISA	Color flow imaging	A4C or apical long axis	Decrease depth, narrow sector, zoom, adjust aliasing velocity Adjust aliasing velocity so PISA is hemispherical, measure from aliasing boundary to orifice	$PISA = 2\pi r^2$ $R_{FR} = PISA \times V_{aliasing}$ $ROA_{max} = R_{FR}/V_{MR}$ $RV = ROA \times VTI_{MR}$
Volume flow at two sites	2D and pulsed Doppler	Parasternal (2D) and apical	LVOT diameter and VTI Mitral annulus diameter and VTI	$TSV = SV_{MA} = (CSA_{MA} \times VTI_{MA})$ $FSV = SV_{LVOT} = (CSA_{LVOT} \times VTI_{LVOT})$ $RV = TSV - FSV$ $ROA = RSV/VTI_{MR}$
2D LV total and Doppler LVOT forward SV	2D and pulsed Doppler	Parasternal (2D) and apical	LVOT diameter and VTI Apical biplane left ventricular volumes	$TSV = EDV - ESV$ (on 2D left ventricular volumes) $FSV = SV_{LVOT} = (CSA_{LVOT} \times VTI_{LVOT})$ $RV = TSV - FSV$ $ROA = RSV/VTI_{MR}$
Pulmonary vein flow	Pulsed Doppler	A4C on TTE, but TEE often needed	Pulmonary vein flow in all four veins	Qualitative, systolic flow reversal

2D, two-dimensional; A4C, apical 4-chamber view; CSA, cross-sectional area; EDV, end-diastolic volume; ESV, end-systolic volume; FSV, forward stroke volume; LVOT, left ventricular outflow tract; MA, mitral annulus; MR, mitral regurgitation; PISA, proximal isovelocity surface area; R_{FR}, regurgitant flow rate; ROA, regurgitant orifice area; RSV, regurgitant stroke volume; RV, regurgitant volume; SV, stroke volume; TEE, transesophageal echocardiography; TSV, total stroke volume; TTE, transthoracic echocardiography; VTI, velocity-time integral.

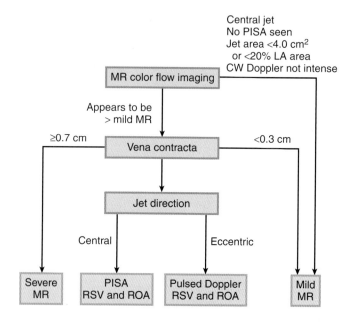

Quantitative Evaluation of Mitral Regurgitant Severity (ASE Guidelines)

Mitral Regurgitation	Mild	Moderate	Severe
Jet area (cm²)	<4 cm² or <20% left atrial area	20%-40%	>40% left atrial area
Vena contracta (cm)	<0.3	0.3-0.7	>0.7
Regurgitant volume (mL)	<30	30-60	>60
Regurgitant fraction (%)	<30	30-50	>50
Regurgitant orifice area (cm²)	<0.20	0.2-0.4	>0.40

ASE, American Society of Echocardiography.

SELF-ASSESSMENT QUESTIONS

QUESTION 1

This Doppler signal (Figure 12–33) was recorded on a TTE.

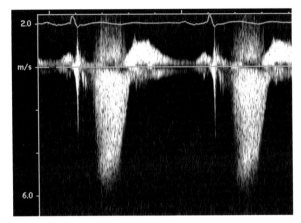

Figure 12–33.

The most likely diagnosis is:

A. Bicuspid aortic valve
B. Mechanical prosthetic valve
C. Hypertrophic cardiomyopathy
D. Mitral valve prolapse

QUESTION 2

A TTE was requested in a 50-year-old woman with decreased exercise tolerance. Initial image quality with fundamental imaging was not optimal; therefore, harmonic imaging was utilized. The results of the study are listed:

Left ventricle:	LV end-diastolic dimension 4.8 cm, ejection fraction 68%
Aortic valve:	Trileaflet with mild regurgitation; maximum antegrade velocity 1.5 m/s
Mitral valve:	Mildly thickened with mild regurgitation
Pulmonic valve:	Full leaflet excursion with mild regurgitation
Tricuspid valve:	Mild regurgitation; maximum regurgitant velocity 2.1 m/s

The most abnormal finding on this study is:

A. Aortic valve function
B. Mitral valve function
C. Pulmonic valve function
D. Tricuspid valve function

QUESTION 3

A 41-year-old man with a history of surgically repaired complex congenital heart disease presents with progressive exertional dyspnea. On physical examination, his blood pressure is 110/74 mm Hg; pulse is 40 bpm. Cardiac auscultation reveals a murmur. There is no clubbing or cyanosis. The following Doppler flow (Figure 12–34) is recorded on a transthoracic study.

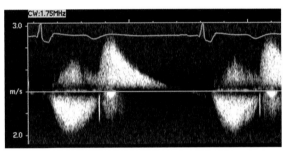

Figure 12–34.

The best next step in patient management is:

A. Cleft mitral valve repair
B. Repair of ventricular septal defect patch leak
C. Pulmonic valve replacement
D. Stenting of pulmonary artery branch stenosis

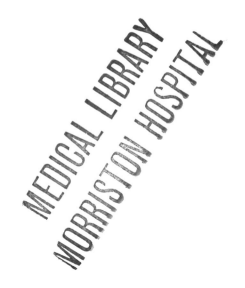

MEDICAL LIBRARY MORRISTON HOSPITAL

QUESTION 4

This Doppler image (Figure 12–35) was recorded in a 62-year-old man with chronic mitral valve disease and decreased exercise tolerance. Calculate the regurgitant orifice area, regurgitant fraction, and regurgitant volume:

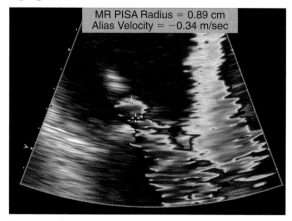

> MR PISA Radius = 0.89 cm
> Alias Velocity = −0.34 m/sec

Figure 12–35.

Antegrade transmitral VTI	18.6 cm
Mitral annulus diameter	3.2 cm
Mitral regurgitant maximum velocity	4.7 m/s
Mitral regurgitant VTI	158 cm

Regurgitant orifice area _____
Regurgitant volume _____
Regurgitant fraction _____

QUESTION 5

Which of the following measures is *least* consistent with severe mitral regurgitation?

    A. Mitral E-wave velocity 2.5 m/s
    B. Mitral vena contracta 0.8 cm
    C. Maximum regurgitant velocity 5.2 m/s
    D. Regurgitant orifice area 0.5 cm^2

QUESTION 6

A 40-year-old man, asymptomatic with a known bicuspid aortic valve, undergoes routine TTE, and the following data are obtained.

LV end-diastolic dimension	7.1 cm
LV ejection fraction	48%
Tricuspid regurgitation jet velocity	3.3 m/s
Aortic sinus diameter	4.2 cm
Aortic jet vena contracta	0.8 cm

The most compelling finding to recommend cardiac surgery, based on these data, is:

    A. Vena contracta
    B. LV function
    C. Pulmonary pressure
    D. Ascending aorta size
    E. Pressure half-time $(T\frac{1}{2})$

QUESTION 7

In a patient with myxomatous mitral valve disease, which of the following echocardiographic findings is *most* consistent with a partial flail posterior leaflet?

    A. Vena contracta 0.4 cm
    B. Pulmonary vein systolic flow reversal
    C. Mitral regurgitation *dP/dt* 780 mm Hg/s
    D. Anteriorly directed jet

QUESTION 8

Echocardiography in a 55-year-old patient with coronary artery disease shows an ejection fraction of 30%, thinning and akinesis of his inferior wall, and significant mitral regurgitation. The PISA radius measures 1.2 cm. Which of the following is *not* needed to calculate the regurgitant volume?

    A. Mitral regurgitant peak velocity (V_{MR})
    B. Mitral valve inflow velocity time integral (VTI_{MV})
    C. Mitral regurgitant aliasing velocity ($V_{aliasing}$)
    D. Mitral regurgitant velocity time integral (VTI_{MR})

QUESTION 9

In an acutely ill patient admitted to the intensive care unit, a murmur is heard on physical examination, and a TTE is performed (Figure 12–36).

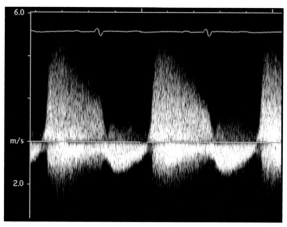

Figure 12–36.

The most likely diagnosis is:

A. Severe mitral regurgitation
B. Severe tricuspid regurgitation
C. Severe aortic regurgitation
D. Severe pulmonic regurgitation

QUESTION 10

Echocardiographic data are recorded in a patient with a diastolic murmur (Figure 12–37).

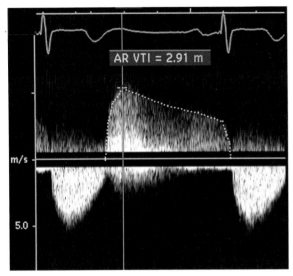

Figure 12–37.

Mitral valve inflow VTI	15.0 cm
LV outflow tract VTI	29.0 cm
LV outflow tract diameter	2.4 cm

Given these data, calculate the following for this patient:

Aortic regurgitant volume _____
Aortic regurgitant fraction _____
Aortic regurgitant orifice area _____

QUESTION 11

For each of the three Doppler flows shown (Figure 12–38) indicate the most likely diagnosis using the following choices:

A. Aortic regurgitation
B. Mitral regurgitation
C. Pulmonic regurgitation
D. Tricuspid regurgitation

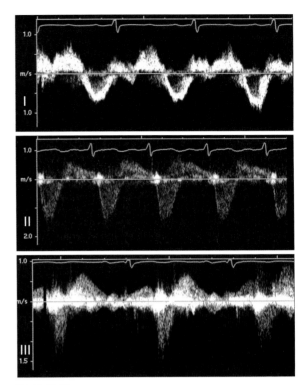

Figure 12–38.

QUESTION 12

This M-mode tracing (Figure 12–39) is most consistent with:

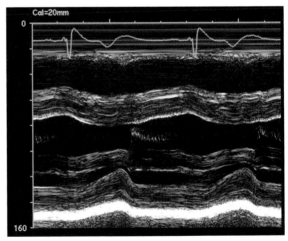

Figure 12–39.

A. Aortic regurgitation
B. Hypertrophic cardiomyopathy
C. Dilated cardiomyopathy
D. Mitral valve prolapse
E. Mitral stenosis

ANSWERS

ANSWER 1: D

This is a CW Doppler signal of the mitral valve taken from the apical view. The LV inflow pattern shows the early diastolic E-wave filling and the late diastolic atrial A wave, corresponding to atrial contraction. During systole, flow is directed away from the transducer. There is absence of flow in early systole, with abrupt onset of flow in mid- to late systole. This is characteristic of mitral valve prolapse where the valve is competent earlier in systole, until buckling and prolapse of the mitral valve into the left atrium leads to poor leaflet coaptation and mitral regurgitation. The color M-mode tracing below (Figure 12–40) shows mitral regurgitation coinciding with prolapse of the posterior mitral valve leaflet.

Aortic stenosis due to a bicuspid aortic valve would show an ejection curve throughout systole and probably would show aortic regurgitation in diastole. A dynamic LV outflow gradient due to hypertrophic cardiomyopathy does peak in late systole, but flow starts with LV ejection with an upward curving or "dagger-shaped" waveform, indicative of progressive systolic obstruction rather than the abrupt late-systolic flow onset characteristic of mitral valve prolapse. A mechanical aortic or mitral prosthetic valve Doppler signal would show a bright mechanical click corresponding to opening and closing of the valve occluders. Shadowing of the left atrium by a prosthetic mitral valve will hinder evaluation of prosthetic regurgitation, but if prosthetic regurgitation is present, occasionally a faint holosystolic regurgitation Doppler signal can be seen during systole.

ANSWER 2: A

Aortic regurgitation, even trace or mild severity, is only seen in approximately 5% of patients with a normal heart. Mild aortic regurgitation of a trileaflet aortic valve commonly indicates leaflet thickening, as can occur with aortic sclerosis, or mild aortic root dilation. In contrast, with improved imaging techniques, physiologic regurgitation of the atrioventricular valves (tricuspid and mitral) and the pulmonic valve can be seen in up to 80% of patients with normal hearts and is usually of no clinical significance. With improved image quality, most echocardiogram studies are now performed using harmonic imaging, rather than fundamental imaging, which often makes thin structures such as the mitral valve leaflets appear mildly thickened.

ANSWER 3: C

This is a CW Doppler tracing across the pulmonic valve in a patient with surgically repaired tetralogy of Fallot. Surgical repair of tetralogy of Fallot includes closure of the ventricular septal defect with a synthetic patch and relief of the RV outflow tract obstruction. The level of RV outflow obstruction may be subvalvular or valvular, so the surgical repair may include resection of obstructive muscle and enlargement of the RV outflow tract with an infundibular patch, often with a concurrent surgical pulmonic valvotomy. Although this procedure relieves stenosis, it often creates some degree of regurgitation so that the most common late complication of surgically repaired tetralogy of Fallot is progressive pulmonic valve regurgitation. Color Doppler imaging often

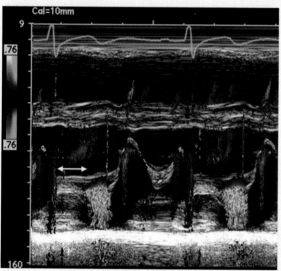

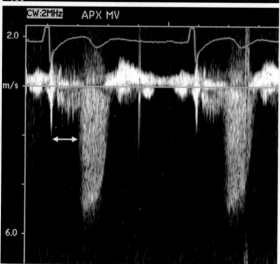

Figure 12–40.

underestimates the severity of pulmonic regurgitation because the unobstructed forward and reverse flow appears uniform in color, without a "flow disturbance." Pulsed or CW Doppler recordings are diagnostic with a dense diastolic regurgitant signal, comparable to the intensity of anterograde flow, with the flow curve reaching the baseline in mid-systole due to rapid equalization of pressure in the pulmonary artery and right ventricle, as in this case. In a symptomatic patient or one with progressive RV dilation and systolic dysfunction, pulmonic valve replacement is indicated.

A mitral regurgitant velocity curve would show a much higher velocity (at least 4.5 m/s) due to the LV–to–LA pressure gradient in systole. Similarly, flow across a small ventricular septal defect shows a high velocity systolic velocity curve, reflecting the difference between LV and RV pressure, with lower velocity diastolic flow if LV diastolic pressure exceeds RV diastolic pressure. If a large ventricular septal defect with Eisenmenger physiology were present, there would be bidirectional flow across the defect; however, the patient would be cyanotic on physical examination. Pulmonary artery branch stenosis would show a higher-velocity systolic flow and no diastolic flow reversal.

ANSWER 4

Regurgitant orifice area	0.36 cm^2
Regurgitant volume	57 mL
Regurgitant fraction	38%

The first step in this calculation is to measure the proximal isovelocity surface area (PISA). This is the surface area of the 3D hemisphere on the LV side of the valve where the velocity is the same everywhere on the surface (e.g., isovelocity), defined by the color aliasing velocity. The radius of the hemisphere from the aliasing velocity to the valve plane is 0.89 cm. The surface area of a hemisphere is $2\pi r_{hemisphere}^2$. Thus:

$$PISA = 2\pi r^2 = 2(3.14)(0.89)^2 = 4.97 \text{ cm}^2$$

The regurgitant orifice area is calculated based on the continuity principle that the volume of blood flow through the PISA and through the regurgitant orifice are equal and that volume flow rate equals the cross-sectional area of flow times the velocity at that site. Thus, for a single point in the cardiac cycle:

$$PISA \times V_{aliasing} = ROA \times V_{MR}$$

The ROA (at that point in the cardiac cycle), then, is calculated as:

$$ROA = PISA \times (V_{aliasing}/V_{MR}) = 4.97 \text{cm}^2 \times (0.34/4.7)$$
$$= 0.36 \text{ cm}^2$$

Regurgitant volume is the volume of blood that goes backward through the valve with each cardiac cycle. Regurgitant volume is calculated as the product of the velocity time integral of the regurgitant jet and the regurgitant orifice area:

$$RV = ROA \times VTI_{MR} = 0.36 \text{ cm}^2 \times 158 \text{ cm}$$
$$= 57 \text{ cm}^3 \text{ or } 57 \text{ mL}$$

The regurgitant fraction is the fraction of transmitral flow that is regurgitant relative to the total amount of flow pumped by the heart across the valve. Total antegrade flow (total stroke volume) across the mitral valve is calculated as the product of the velocity time integral of antegrade flow and the area of the mitral valve annulus:

$$Total SV = \pi r_{MVA}^2 \times VTI_{MV} = 3.14(3.2 \text{ cm}/2)^2 \times 18.6 \text{ cm}$$
$$= 149 \text{ cm}^3 \text{ or } 149 \text{ mL}$$

Then,

$$RF = RV/Total SV \times 100\% = 57 \text{ mL}/149 \text{ mL} \times 100\%$$
$$= 38\%$$

These calculations are all consistent with moderate mitral regurgitation.

ANSWER 5: C

The maximum mitral regurgitant jet velocity reflects the LV–to–LA pressure gradient and is not a useful measure of regurgitant severity. Although with severe acute regurgitation, the increased LA pressure and decreased systolic blood pressure (and decreased LV pressure) may result in a lower maximum regurgitant velocity, with chronic regurgitation, velocity primarily reflects systolic blood pressure. The increased regurgitant volume of severe mitral regurgitation results in an increased antegrade transmitral stroke volume and the mitral opening pressure (the LA–to–LV pressure difference in early diastole) is increased; both these factors results in a high antegrade mitral flow velocity (with a steep deceleration slope) when severe mitral regurgitation is present. The transmitral E wave is typically increased over 1.5 m/s. The vena contracta is the narrowest diameter of the regurgitant jet at the valve plane, usually measured in the long-axis view of the valve. A wider vena contracta implies a larger regurgitant orifice area and more severe regurgitation. A vena contracta width greater than 0.7 cm is consistent with severe regurgitation. The regurgitant orifice area is a measure of the "hole" through which blood is regurgitant. A regurgitant orifice area larger than 0.4 cm^2 is consistent with severe mitral regurgitation.

ANSWER 6: B

Patients with symptomatic, severe valvular regurgitation should be referred for surgical intervention. In asymptomatic patients, evidence of the progressive effect of the regurgitant volume load with either LV dilation or a decline in systolic function is the primary criteria to prompt earlier surgical intervention. Because a small subset of patients do not develop cardiopulmonary symptoms despite LV dilation or a decline in function, periodic imaging in asymptomatic patients is indicated once regurgitation is diagnosed. Current guidelines recommend valve surgery in asymptomatic patients with severe aortic regurgitation and an end-diastolic dimension of 75 mm or more, an end-systolic dimension of 55 mm or more, or an ejection fraction less than 50%. Surgery is recommended in this case based on the decreased ejection fraction.

A tricuspid regurgitation jet velocity of 3.3 m/s suggests that the RV systolic pressure is at least 44 mmHg over RA pressure, supporting at least moderate pulmonary hypertension. However, pulmonary hypertension is not a primary indication for aortic valve replacement. The pressure half-time $(T\frac{1}{2})$ is the time interval between the peak transvalvular pressure gradient and half the initial gradient. For the aortic regurgitant jet, a pressure half-time of less than 200 ms indicates rapid equalization of pressures between the aorta and LV, consistent with severe regurgitation. However, with chronic disease, the pressure half-time may be normal despite severe regurgitation. The vena contracta of 0.8 cm confirms that this patient has severe aortic regurgitation, which by itself is not an indication for valve surgery in the absence of symptoms. A subset of bicuspid aortic valve patients have associated dilation of the aortic root, and current guidelines recommend root replacement when aortic diameter exceeds 5.0 cm. If the patient is already undergoing valve replacement for stenosis or regurgitation, root replacement should be considered at a diameter of 4.5 cm.

ANSWER 7: D

A partial flail leaflet leads to failure of leaflet coaptation. With posterior mitral leaflet prolapse, the tip of the posterior leaflet prolapses into the left atrium. During systole, the flail tip is more cephalad and the regurgitant jet enters the left atrium eccentrically across the back of the anterior leaflet, directed anteriorly as seen in the apical 4-chamber view (Figure 12–41) in this patient.

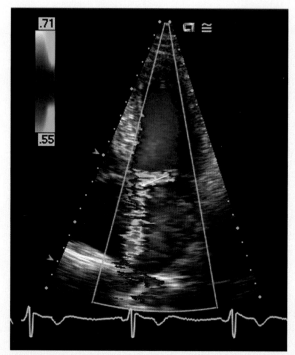

Figure 12–41.

Entrainment of the regurgitant jet along the wall of the atrium may make the jet appear smaller. A vena contracta of 0.4 is consistent with only moderate regurgitation; a partial flail leaflet is typically associated with severe regurgitation. Pulmonary vein systolic flow reversal is consistent with severe regurgitation but does not help in determining the specific leaflet involved unless systolic flow reversal is present in some, but not all, pulmonary veins. In patients with LV systolic dysfunction, the poorly functioning LV does not generate a transmitral gradient rapidly and the initial slope of the mitral regurgitant jet decreases to below 1000 mmHg/sec. With myxomatous mitral valve disease and regurgitation, LV systolic function usually is normal.

ANSWER 8: B

The PISA area is measured as $2\pi r_{hemisphere}^{2}$. Calculation of the regurgitant orifice area utilizes the continuity principle where $PISA \times V_{aliasing} = ROA \times V_{MR}$. The equation is rearranged and regurgitant orifice area is calculated as $ROA = PISA \times (V_{aliasing}/V_{MR})$. The regurgitant volume is the volume of blood that is regurgitant through the valve with each cardiac cycle and is the product of the velocity time integral of the regurgitant jet and the cross-sectional area at the point of regurgitation, or regurgitant volume = ROA $\times VTI_{MR}$. The mitral valve inflow velocity-time integral (VTI_{MV}) is not needed to calculate the regurgitant volume. VTI_{MV} is needed to calculate the regurgitant fraction, or the fraction of transmitral flow that is regurgitant relative to total anterograde flow. Total anterograde flow across the mitral valve is the product of the VTI_{MV} and the cross-sectional area at the mitral valve annulus. The regurgitant fraction, then, is:

Regurgitant Fraction = Regurgitant Volume/Total Flow

ANSWER 9: C

This is a CW Doppler signal showing flow away from the transducer in systole with a shape that might be antegrade flow in a great vessel (aorta or pulmonary artery) or might be regurgitant flow across an atrioventricular (mitral or tricuspid valve). However, the maximum velocity is less than 2 m/s, which excludes mitral regurgitation, and the short duration of the systolic signal suggests that tricuspid regurgitation is unlikely. The antegrade ejection velocity might be transaortic flow or transpulmonic flow. However, the diastolic signal has an initial diastolic velocity of 4 m/s, indicating a 64 mm Hg gradient between the great vessel and ventricle. Although this might be pulmonic regurgitation if severe pulmonary hypertension were present, the timing is more consistent with aortic regurgitation. These data were recorded in a patient with acute severe aortic regurgitation. The end-diastolic velocity of the regurgitation jet, about 2 m/s, indicates the end-diastolic gradient between the aorta and LV is only 16 mm Hg, consistent with a low aortic and high LV diastolic pressure in this acutely ill patient. In addition, the diastolic regurgitant signal is as dense as antegrade systolic flow consistent with severe aortic regurgitation. The steep diastolic deceleration slope indicates rapid equalization of pressure between the aorta and LV during diastole, consistent with acute, rather than chronic, regurgitation.

ANSWER 10

Regurgitant volume	25 mL
Regurgitant fraction	19%
Regurgitant orifice area	0.09 cm²

In this patient with aortic regurgitation, the stroke volume across the aortic valve is the sum of anterograde flow and regurgitant flow or total stroke volume. Assuming a competent mitral valve, the anterograde flow across the mitral valve (SV_{MV}) equals forward stroke volume. To calculate the volume flow rate (stroke volume) at each valve, the area and velocity time integral at each site are needed. Stroke volumes are calculated by multiplying cross-sectional area and velocity time integral at that site. Thus:

$$SV_{MV} = CSA_{MV} \times VTI_{MV\ INFLOW} = \pi(D/2)^2 \times$$
$$VTI_{MV\ INFLOW} = 3.14(3.0/2)^2 \times 15\ cm = 106\ cm^3$$

$$SV_{LVOT} = CSA_{LVOT} \times VTI_{LVOT} = \pi(D/2)^2 \times VTI_{LVOT} =$$
$$3.14(2.4/2)^2 \times 29\ cm = 131\ cm^3$$

Regurgitant volume (RV_{AR}) is the difference between SV_{LVOT} and SV_{MV}:

$$RV_{AR} = SV_{LVOT} - SV_{MV} = 131\ cm^3 - 106\ cm^3 =$$
$$25\ cm^3\ or\ 25\ mL$$

The regurgitant fraction is the proportion of regurgitant volume compared with the total transaortic flow:

$$RF = RV_{AR}/SV_{LVOT} = 25\ mL/131\ mL = 19\%$$

The ROA is then calculated by dividing regurgitant stroke volume by the VTI_{AR}.

$$ROA = RV_{AR}/VTI_{AR} = 25\ cm^3/291\ cm = 0.09\ cm^2$$

An ROA less than 0.1 cm², a regurgitant volume of 25 mL, and a regurgitant fraction of 19% are all consistent with mild aortic regurgitation. These data are congruent with the visual impression from the CW Doppler signal with a faint diastolic regurgitant signal compared with antegrade flow.

ANSWER 11: ID, IIA, IIIB

1. This is a pulsed Doppler sample taken from the hepatic vein in a patient with severe tricuspid regurgitation. The image is acquired from the subcostal view with flow from the hepatic vein to the IVC directed antegrade, away from the transducer. The venous flow pattern is evident with a brief flow curve toward the transducer after atrial contraction and atrial filling during diastole. Peak flow velocities in the hepatic vein are low, and the scale is set with a maximum velocity of 0.6 m/s. With severe tricuspid regurgitation, there is systolic flow reversal in the hepatic vein, shown as flow in systole directed toward the transducer following the QRS complex instead of the normal pattern of RA filling in systole, as well as diastole. Pulmonary vein flow also shows a venous flow pattern, but diastolic filling would be directed toward the transducer from the transthoracic approach.

2. This is a pulsed Doppler recording taken from the descending thoracic aorta in a patient with severe aortic regurgitation. The antegrade flow in systole at 1.3 m/s with an ejection type curve that identifies this as a great artery. This is unlikely to be the pulmonary artery because the velocity peaks in early systole and is shorter in duration and higher in velocity than typical pulmonary artery flow. The holodiastolic (extends continuously from the beginning to end of diastole) flow reversal seen as flow directed toward the transducer during diastole is consistent with moderate to severe aortic regurgitation.

3. This is a pulsed Doppler sample of the pulmonary vein flow in a patient with severe mitral

regurgitation due to mitral valve prolapse. Diastolic LV filling with flow directed toward the transducer is seen, identifying this as pulmonary venous inflow. In systole, early systolic flow toward the transducer is seen, consistent with normal LV filling. However, in late systole flow is reversed (directed away from the transducer), suggesting late systolic mitral regurgitation.

ANSWER 12: A

This is an M-mode tracing from the parasternal long-axis view. The mitral valve is seen in the mid-portion of the left ventricle. During diastole, the mitral valve is open and the anterior mitral valve leaflet shows a rapid fluttering motion. This motion is the result of the aortic regurgitant jet impinging on the thin flexible anterior mitral leaflet. Regurgitation is likely only mild because the E-point septal separation is normal and there is no LV dilation. Other findings on the M-mode tracing are concentric LV hypertrophy (thick walls with a small chamber) and marked posterior pericardial thickening. With hypertrophic cardiomyopathy, asymmetric thickening of the septum compared with the posterior wall is seen, and if there is obstruction, systolic anterior motion of the mitral leaflets is present. Left ventricular chamber size is normal, not consistent with a dilated cardiomyopathy; in addition, the separation between the mitral E point and the septum is increased with LV dilation and systolic dysfunction. With mitral valve prolapse, the mitral leaflets are thickened and there is late systolic buckling of the mitral valve leaflet posteriorly on the M-mode tracing. If mitral stenosis were present, leaflet thickening with a reduced diastolic opening and a flat diastolic leaflet slope would be seen.

Prosthetic Valves

BASIC PRINCIPLES

- Evaluation of prosthetic valves by echocardiography is based on the same principles as evaluation of native valve disease.
- Fluid dynamics (and Doppler flows) depend on the specific valve type and size. (Figure 13–1)
- Dysfunction of mechanical valves usually is due to valve thrombosis resulting in systemic embolism, incomplete closure (regurgitation), or inadequate opening (stenosis).
- Dysfunction of tissue valves usually is due to leaflet degeneration (regurgitation) or calcification (stenosis).
- All prosthetic valves are at risk of endocarditis, which often primarily affects the annular ring rather than the valve leaflets.

Key points

- ❐ There are several types of tissue valves, which can be classified as stented, stentless, or combined valve-root prostheses (including homograft valves).

- ❐ A stented tissue valve is recognized by the three valve struts; a stentless tissue valve may be indistinguishable from a normal native valve.
- ❐ Transcatheter aortic valve implantation can be performed either from the femoral artery retrograde across the valve or from the left ventricular (LV) apex antegrade across the valve.
- ❐ Transcatheter valves consist of a tissue valve mounted in an expandable stent. Once deployed, the echocardiographic appearance is similar to a stentless tissue valve. (Figure 13–2)
- ❐ The most common mechanical valve now implanted is a bileaflet design with two semicircular disks that open to form a central slit-like orifice and two larger lateral openings.
- ❐ Other types of mechanical valves include single disk valves that "tilt" to open, either on a central strut or with hinges in the annular ring. Ball-cage valves may still be seen in some patients.
- ❐ On echocardiography, mechanical valves result in ultrasound reverberations and shadowing that limit direct visualization of valve function.

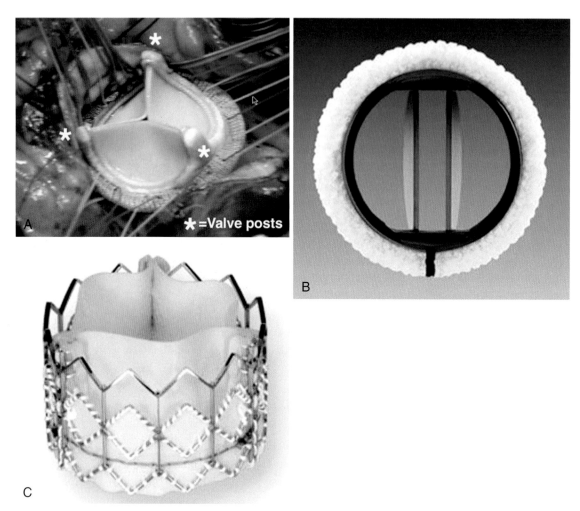

Figure 13–1. Examples of a (*A*) bioprosthetic aortic valve at the time of surgical implantation; (*B*) bileaflet mechanical valve; and (*C*) transcatheter bioprosthetic valve. *A, From Oxom D, Otto C: Atlas of Intraoperative Echocardiography, 2007, Philadelphia: Elsevier. B, Courtesy St Jude Medical, Inc. St Paul, MN. C, Courtesy Edwards SAPIEN Investigational Transcatheter Heart Valve. Available at www.edwards.com/products/transcathetervalves/sapienthv.htm.*

STEP-BY-STEP APPROACH

Step 1: Review the clinical and operative data

- Information on the operative procedure is reviewed before the echocardiographic examination.
- The valve type and size, obtained from the medical record or the patient's valve ID card, are included on the echocardiographic report.
- Blood pressure and heart rate at the time of the echocardiogram are recorded.

Key points

- ❑ Information in the operative report helps guide the echocardiographic image acquisition and improves the final interpretation.

- ❑ With aortic valve surgery, key features are valve replacement versus resuspension, concurrent replacement of the aortic root either above the sinotubular junction or including the sinuses of Valsalva, and surgical coronary reimplantation (with aortic root surgery).
- ❑ With mitral valve surgery, key features are valve repair or replacement, preservation of the mitral leaflets and chords with valve replacement, amputation of the LA appendage, and whether a concurrent atrial ablation (e.g., maze) procedure was done.
- ❑ The valve type and size determine the expected hemodynamics and are important for distinguishing normal prosthetic Doppler data from prosthetic valve stenosis or regurgitation.
- ❑ On early postoperative studies, unexpected findings are discussed directly with the surgeon

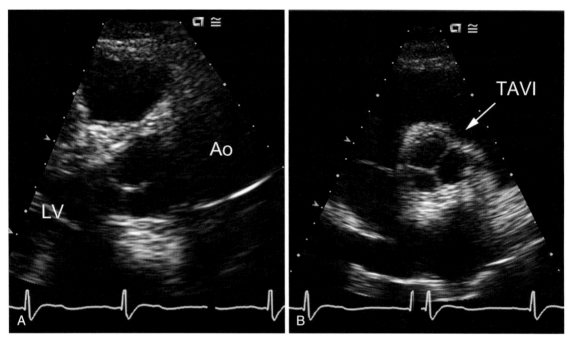

Figure 13–2. Transcatheter aortic valve seen in a parasternal long-axis (*A*) and short-axis (*B*) views with a trileaflet tissue valve similar in appearance to a native aortic valve. Increased paravalvular echogenicity represents the native calcified valve that is pushed aside by the stent of the transcatheter valve.

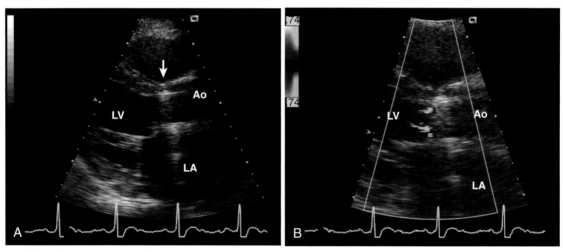

Figure 13–3. *A*, Parasternal long-axis view of a mechanical aortic valve showing the reverberations along the ultrasound beam path (*arrow*), with (*B*) color Doppler showing the normal small eccentric aortic regurgitant jets with a bileaflet valve.

to correlate with observations during the surgical procedure.

Step 2: Obtain images of the prosthetic valve

- Prosthetic aortic valves are imaged in parasternal long- and short-axis views. (Figure 13–3)

- Prosthetic mitral valves are imaged in parasternal long and short axis and in apical 4-chamber and long-axis views. (Figure 13–4)
- Transesophageal echocardiography (TEE) imaging is needed to evaluate the LA side of mechanical mitral prosthetic valves, due to shadowing from the transthoracic approach, when valve dysfunction is suspected. (Figure 13–5)

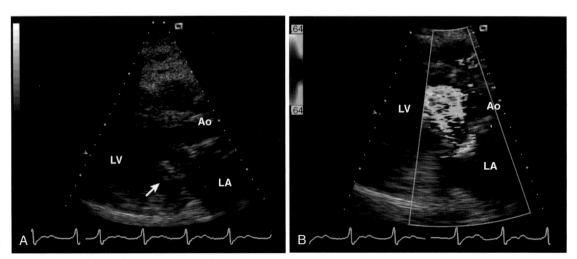

Figure 13–4. *A,* Parasternal long-axis view of a stented tissue mitral valve prosthesis with the typical appearance of the struts (*arrow*) protruding into the LV, with (*B*) color Doppler showing the inflow stream directed toward the ventricular septum.

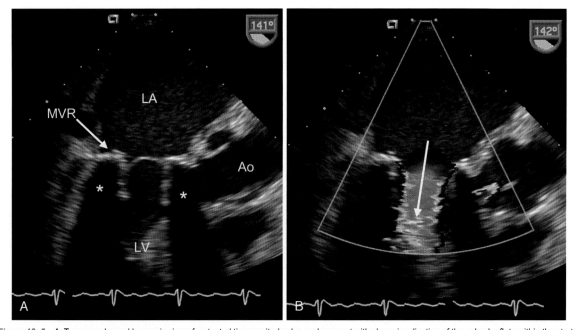

Figure 13–5. *A,* Transesophageal long-axis view of a stented tissue mitral valve replacement with clear visualization of the valve leaflets within the struts. With the transducer on the atrial side of the valve, the acoustic shadow and reverberations obscure the LV (*asterisks*) but not the LA side of the valve, resulting in improved detection of prosthetic valve dysfunction. *B,* Color Doppler shows the inflow stream filling the valve ring, directed toward the ventricular septum.

■ TEE also often provides better images of the posterior aspect of aortic valve prostheses.

Key points

❑ Transthoracic imaging of mechanical valves is limited by reverberations and shadowing. Even so, the leaflets and annular region may be adequately evaluated by this approach for most baseline or follow-up studies in clinically stable patients.

❑ Tissue valves have a trileaflet structure similar to a native aortic valve. Mitral tissue valves are stented to provide support for the leaflets, with the leaflets well seen in both parasternal and apical views.

❑ With aortic tissue valves, support is provided either by stents, by attachment directly to the aortic wall (stentless valves), or by implanting an intact valve and root (sometimes called a "mini-root" approach). The aortic tissue prosthesis is well seen in long- and short-axis views.

□ When prosthetic valve dysfunction is suspected on clinical grounds or based on TTE findings, both TTE and TEE are recommended.

Step 3: Record prosthetic valve Doppler data

- Antegrade velocities across the prosthetic valve are recorded with pulsed and CW Doppler.
- Prosthetic valve regurgitation is evaluated using CW and color Doppler.

Key points

□ Both tissue and mechanical valves are inherently stenotic compared with normal native valves.
□ The normal antegrade velocity and pressure gradient depends on the specific valve type, valve size, heart rate, and cardiac output. (Table 13-1)
□ Ideally, Doppler data are compared with the patient's own baseline postoperative examination, done when the patient had fully recovered from surgery and was clinically stable.

□ If a baseline examination is not available, recorded data are compared with published data for that valve type and size
□ A small amount of regurgitation is normal with most prosthetic valves.

Step 3A: Evaluate for prosthetic valve stenosis

- Maximum and mean gradients are calculated with the Bernoulli equation from transvalvular velocities. (Figure 13–6)
- Continuity equation valve area can be calculated for aortic valve prostheses. (Figure 13–7)
- The mitral pressure half-time for prosthetic valves is measured in the mitral position. (Figure 13–8)

Key points

□ LV outflow tract diameter is measured from the 2D images for calculation of valve area. The valve size may differ from the subaortic anatomy and so cannot be substituted for this diameter measurement.

TABLE 13-1   Normal Reference Values of Effective Orifice Areas for the Prosthetic Valves

	No. of Patients,* %	19	21	23	25	27	29
STENTED BIOPROSTHETIC VALVES							
Medtronic Intact	129 (10.2)	0.85	1.02	1.27	1.40	1.66	2.04
Medtronic Mosaic	390 (30.8)	1.20	1.22	1.38	1.65	1.80	2.00
Hancock II	53 (4.2)	...	1.18	1.33	1.46	1.55	1.60
Carpentier-Edwards Perimount	59 (4.7)	1.10	1.30	1.50	1.80	1.80	...
St. Jude Medical X-cell	21 (1.7)	...	...	...	...	...	...
STENTLESS BIOPROSTHETIC VALVES							
Medtronic freestyle	368 (29.1)	1.15	1.35	1.48	2.00	2.32	...
St. Jude Medical Toronto SPV	60 (4.7)	...	1.30	1.50	1.70	2.00	2.50
MECHANICAL VALVES							
St. Jude Medical Standard	151 (11.9)	1.04	1.38	1.52	2.08	2.65	3.23
St. Jude Medical Regent	13 (1.0)	1.50	2.00	2.40	2.50	3.60	4.80
MCRI On-X	18 (1.4)	1.50	1.70	2.00	2.40	3.20	3.20
Carbomedics	3 (0.2)	1.00	1.54	1.63	1.98	2.41	2.63

From Blais et al: Circulation 108:983, 2003.

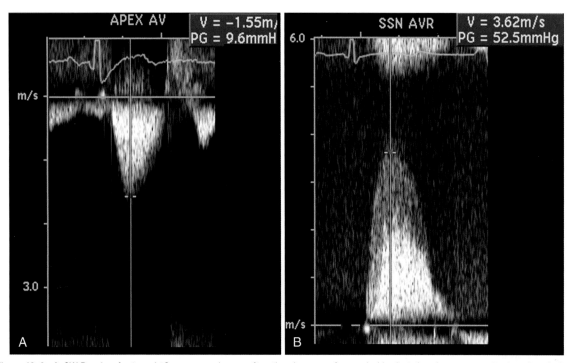

Figure 13–6. *A*, CW Doppler of antegrade flow across a homograft aortic valve soon after surgical implantation shows a normal antegrade velocity of 1.6 m/s. *B*, CW Doppler 10 years after implantation in this 32-year-old man now shows a velocity of 3.6 m/s in association with leaflet calcification, consistent with moderate prosthetic valve stenosis.

$$SV_{LVOT} = SV_{AVR}$$
$$CSA_{LVOT} \times VTI_{LVOT} = EOA \times VTI_{AVR}$$
$$EOA = (CSA_{LVOT} \times VTI_{LVOT})/VTI_{AVR}$$

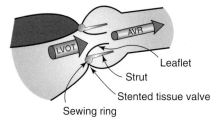

Figure 13–7. Schematic drawing of the continuity equation with a stented tissue aortic valve replacement (*AVR*). Stroke volume (*SV*) proximal to the valve in the LV outflow tract (*LVOT*) equals SV through the aortic valve replacement. SV at each site is equal to the cross-sectional area of flow (*CSA*) times the velocity-time integral (*VTI*) of flow at that site. LVOT flow is measured with pulsed Doppler from an apical approach. CSA$_{LVOT}$ is calculated as a circle from a mid-systolic LVOT diameter measurement, and the VTI of flow through the valve prosthesis is measured with CW Doppler, usually from the apical approach. This equation then is solved for the aortic prosthetic effective orifice area (*EOA*).

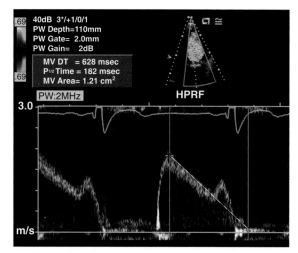

Figure 13–8. High pulse repetition frequency Doppler recording of antegrade flow across a tissue mitral prosthesis is consistent with mild stenosis, with a pressure half-time of 182 ms and estimated functional valve area of 1.2 cm^2.

❏ When measurement of outflow tract diameter is difficult, the ratio of the velocity proximal to the valve and in the orifice is used as a measure of stenosis severity.

❏ With bileaflet mechanical valves, the small central orifice often results in high velocities due to local acceleration, which should not be mistaken for prosthetic valve stenosis.

❏ The mitral pressure half-time is used to calculate valve area, as for native mitral stenosis. Often the pressure half-time itself is reported.

❏ "Patient–prosthesis mismatch" describes a normally functioning prosthetic valve that has a valve area inadequate for the patient's body size. (Figure 13–9)

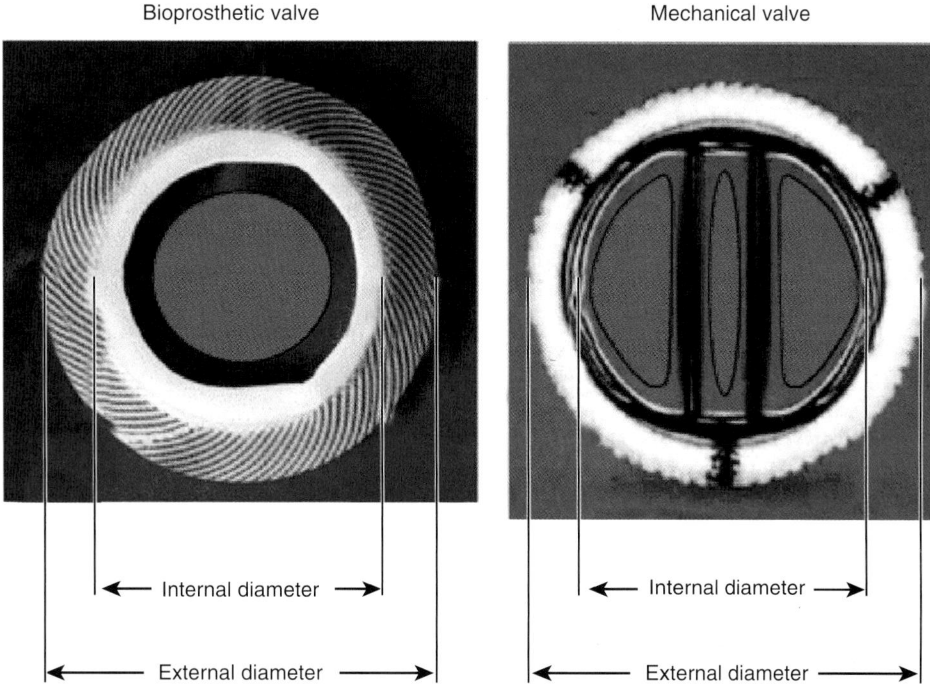

Bioprosthetic valve

Mechanical valve

←— Internal diameter —→

←— Internal diameter —→

←——— External diameter ———→

←——— External diameter ———→

Figure 13–9. View of a bioprosthesis and a bileaflet mechanical valve with the leaflets in a fully open position. The area highlighted in pink is the effective orifice area. Patient–prosthesis mismatch is present when the effective orifice area is smaller than needed to maintain a normal cardiac output at rest and with exercise without an excessive increase in transvalvular pressure gradient. *From Pibarot P, Dumesnil JG: Prosthesis-patient mismatch: definition, clinical impact, and prevention. Heart 2006;92(8):1022-1029.*

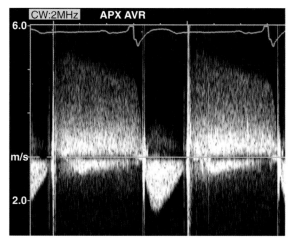

CW:2MHz   APX AVR

6.0

m/s

2.0

Figure 13–10. Prosthetic aortic valve regurgitation recorded with CW Doppler from an apical approach shows prominent valve clicks. The diastolic aortic regurgitant signal is much less dense than the antegrade systolic signal, consistent with mild regurgitation.

Step 3B: Evaluate for prosthetic valve regurgitation

- Prosthetic valve regurgitation is evaluated using CW and color Doppler (Figure 13–10).
- Evaluation of prosthetic mitral regurgitation requires TEE; transthoracic imaging is nondiagnostic due to shadowing and reverberation by the valve prostheses.
- A small amount of prosthetic regurgitation is normal; moderate to severe prosthetic regurgitation or any degree of paraprosthetic regurgitation is pathologic.

Key points

- Prosthetic regurgitation often is first detected with CW Doppler due to the high signal-to-noise ratio, excellent tissue penetration, and wide beam geometry of CW Doppler (Figure 13–11).
- Normal prosthetic regurgitation has a weak CW Doppler signal and typically is brief in duration.
- A dense regurgitant CW Doppler signal is an indication for further evaluation (Figure 13–12).
- Normal prosthetic regurgitation on color Doppler is spatially localized adjacent to the valve, has a small vena contracta and jet area, is through the prosthesis (not paravalvular), and is brief in duration.
- The exact pattern of normal prosthetic regurgitation depends on the valve type—for example, central with bioprosthetic valves, two eccentric jets with bileaflet mechanical valves.

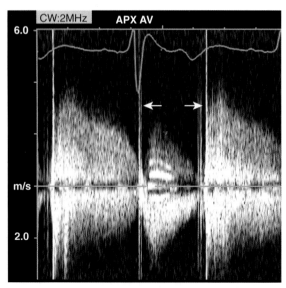

Figure 13–11. Transthoracic apical CW Doppler of an aortic valve prosthesis. Prominent linear signals due to valve opening and closing are seen (*arrows*). The dense bands in systole are a common artifact, but the moderately dense signal of aortic regurgitation is consistent with at least moderate regurgitation. The signal is seen on both sides of the baseline suggesting a nonparallel intercept angle, likely due to an eccentric jet direction.

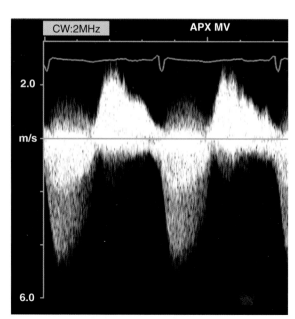

Figure 13–12. Transthoracic apical CW Doppler after mitral valve repair. The antegrade flow velocity is increased to over 2 m/s and a systolic signal is present. The systolic signal is consistent with mitral regurgitation (not LV outflow) based on the timing of flow. The density of the signal suggests that more than trivial regurgitation is present. TEE is needed for further evaluation to avoid shadowing by the annular ring.

❐ Pathologic prosthetic valve regurgitation on color Doppler often is paravalvular, has a larger vena contracta and jet area, and lasts longer during the cardiac cycle.

❐ Significant prosthetic regurgitation, especially of the mitral valve, may not be detectable on transthoracic imaging.

Step 4: Evaluate left ventricular geometry and function

■ After valve surgery, LV dilation and hypertrophy typically regress, but many patients have persistent abnormalities.

■ Systolic ventricular dysfunction often improves after valve surgery, but diastolic dysfunction may be evident for many years.

■ LV geometry and systolic and diastolic function are evaluated in patients with prior heart valve surgery as detailed in Chapters 6 and 7.

Key points

❐ After aortic valve replacement for aortic stenosis, LV hypertrophy regresses and systolic function improves, but diastolic dysfunction may be chronic.

❐ After valve replacement for aortic or mitral regurgitation, LV dilation and systolic dysfunction improve in most patients, but a subset have irreversible LV dilation and systolic dysfunction.

❐ In patients with isolated mitral stenosis, LV size and systolic function usually are normal both before and after valve surgery.

❐ Comparison of the early postoperative study with the preoperative exam helps distinguish residual ventricular abnormalities from new ventricular dysfunction.

Step 5: Measure pulmonary pressures and evaluate right heart function

■ There is an immediate decrease in pulmonary pressures after valve surgery that is directly related to the fall in LA pressure (e.g., the passive component of pulmonary hypertension).

■ The late decrease in pulmonary pressures is variable and depends on the extent of irreversible changes in the pulmonary vasculature.

■ Pulmonary pressures and right heart function are evaluated in patients with prior heart valve surgery as detailed in Chapters 6 and 7.

Key points

❐ Measurement of pulmonary pressures on the early postoperative study serves as the baseline for subsequent studies.

After mitral valve surgery, recurrent pulmonary hypertension might be due to prosthetic regurgitation, which otherwise might be missed on TTE.

RV systolic function usually improves when pulmonary pressures decline after valve surgery.

SPECIFIC VALVE TYPES

Aortic valves

Bioprosthetic aortic valves

■ Tissue aortic valve have three thin leaflets, similar to a native aortic valve.

■ With stented tissue valves, the three stents are seen in both long- and short-axis views.

■ The flow profile and hemodynamics are similar to a native valve with only a small degree of central regurgitation.

Key points

Aortic tissue valves are well visualized in long- and short-axis views both on transthoracic imaging from a parasternal window and on TEE from a high esophageal window.

Both TTE and TEE may be needed for complete evaluation when endocarditis is suspected because each approach visualizes the part of the valve that is obscured by the ring shadow from the other approach.

Antegrade flow across the valve is recorded from the apical window using CW Doppler. Alignment with flow is usually not optimal on a TEE study.

Valve regurgitation is evaluated by color Doppler in the short- and long-axis views of the valve, with measurement of vena contracta, as described in Chapter 12 for native valves, when possible (Figure 13–13).

Valve regurgitation also is evaluated with CW Doppler from the apical view, with the velocity scale, gain, and filters adjusted to demonstrate the regurgitant flow signal (Figure 13–14).

Transcatheter aortic valve implantation

■ TEE often is used for correct positioning of a transcatheter valve at the time of implantation.

■ The echocardiographic appearance of an aortic prosthesis implanted by the transcatheter approach is similar to a stentless tissue valve.

Key points

Aortic annulus diameter measured in the long-axis view at the aortic cusp insertion in mid-

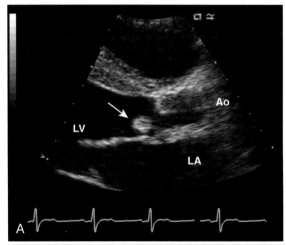

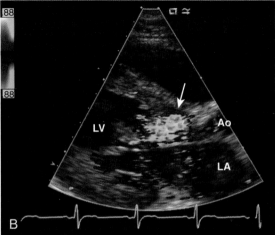

Figure 13–13. This bioprosthetic aortic valve has a flail leaflet (*arrow*) with color Doppler showing regurgitation that fills the LV outflow tract in diastole, consistent with severe regurgitation.

systole is used to choose the correct valve size for implantation.

TEE aortic annulus measurement is recommended when transthoracic views are suboptimal.

The normal antegrade velocity across a transcatheter implanted aortic valve is lower than for most bioprosthetic valves, typically about 2 m/s.

Mild paravalvular regurgitation often is present after transcatheter aortic valve implantation due to irregularities in the contact between the valve stent and the compressed, calcified native valve.

Valved conduits or valve resuspension

■ The native aortic valve may be sutured inside a tube graft replacement of the aortic root (called valve resuspension or the David procedure). (Figure 13–15)

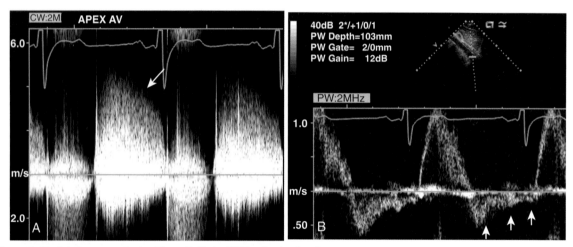

Figure 13–14. *A*, In the same patient as Figure 13–13, the CW Doppler signal confirms severe regurgitation with an equal signal density for antegrade systolic and retrograde diastolic aortic flow. *B*, Pulsed Doppler recording in the proximal abdominal aorta shows holodiastolic flow reversal, again consistent with severe aortic regurgitation.

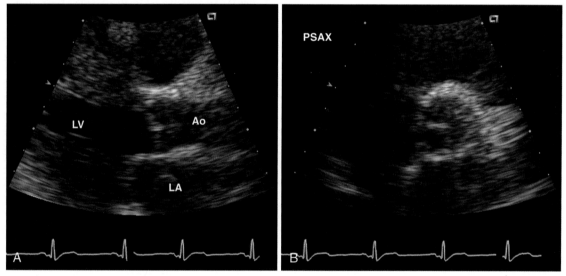

Figure 13–15. The native aortic valve has been resuspended within an aortic tube graft replacement, resulting in normal-appearing leaflets in long- and short-axis views, with increased echogenicity of the aortic walls.

- A combined tissue aortic valve with an attached segment of aorta (either a homograft or hetero-graft) may be used when endocarditis is present or there is involvement of the aorta.
- When aortic root replacement includes the sinuses of Valsalva, the right and left coronary ostium are reimplanted into the prosthetic aorta. (Figure 13–16)

Key points

- ❑ The structure and dimensions of the aorta at each level (annulus, sinuses, sinotubular junction, and mid-ascending aorta) are measured in patients who have undergone aortic valve surgery.
- ❑ The coronary reimplantation sites are best seen on TEE imaging (Figure 13–17). Postoperative echocardiographic findings may include para-aortic edema, hematoma, or surgical material. Review of the images with the surgical team is helpful in distinguishing expected postoperative findings from infection or bleeding. (Figure 13–18)
- ❑ With valve resuspension or any other sub-coronary stentless valve implantation, the height and symmetry of the commissures affects valve function, so these valves are imaged

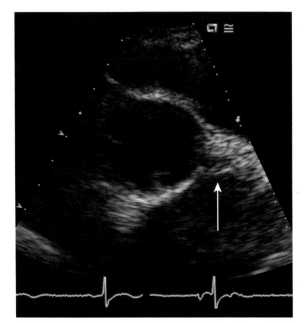

Figure 13–16. Transthoracic short-axis view just superior to the aortic valve, showing the reimplanted left main coronary artery (*arrow*) in a 32-year-old man with Marfan syndrome and root replacement.

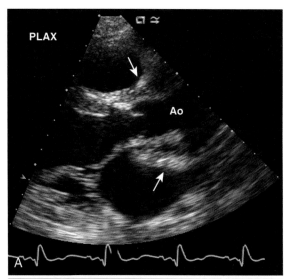

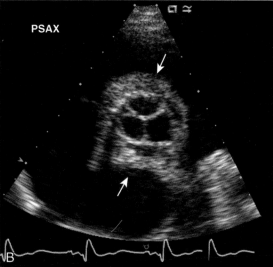

Figure 13–18. Replacement of the ascending aorta and resuspension of the aortic valve complicated by periaortic postoperative hematoma and tissue edema (*arrows*), seen in parasternal long-axis and short-axis views.

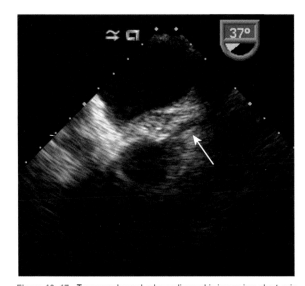

Figure 13–17. Transesophageal echocardiographic image in a short-axis view of the aorta just superior to the aortic valve showing the reimplanted left main coronary (*arrow*) after valve resuspension surgery.

using a higher-frequency transducer and zoom mode.

Mechanical aortic valve

■ Both stenosis and regurgitation of a mechanical valve in the aortic position can be evaluated on transthoracic imaging.

■ TEE is needed when the indication for echocardiography is bacteremia, fever, or embolic events.

■ A mechanical valve may be used in a composite aortic root and valve replacement, with coronary reimplantation (the Bentall or modified Bentall procedure).

Key points

❏ An aortic mechanical prosthesis is best imaged in long- and short-axis views from the parasternal transthoracic or high esophageal windows. (Figure 13–19)

❏ Infection typically involves the paravalvular region so imaging includes evaluation of the

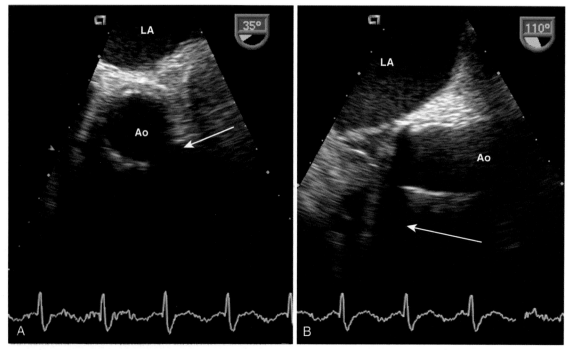

Figure 13–19. TEE short-axis (*A*) and long-axis (*B*) images of a mechanical aortic valve. In short axis, the circular sewing ring with minor irregularity at the suture sites is seen. The posterior aspect of the sewing ring shadows the anterior aspect (*arrow*). Similarly, in the long-axis view, the valve itself casts shadows and reverberations (*arrow*) that obscure the LV outflow tract and anterior aspect of the valve. Evaluation of an aortic valve prosthesis typically requires both TTE and TEE imaging.

aortic wall thickness, identification of the coronary ostium and visualization of the paravalvular region.

❐ Antegrade velocity is recorded using CW Doppler from the apical window. Prominent valve opening and closing clicks often are seen.

❐ A high antegrade velocity (and small calculated valve area) for a bileaflet valve in the aortic position may be due either to normal valve function (with a high velocity in the central slit-like orifice), patient prosthesis mismatch, or valve stenosis. These conditions are differentiated based on clinical information, other echocardiographic findings, and, in some cases, other diagnostic evaluation such as computed tomographic imaging or fluoroscopy of valve motion. (Figure 13–20)

❐ Prosthetic aortic valve regurgitation is evaluated with color Doppler in short- and long-axis views of the valve (TTE or TEE) with identification of jet origin (valvular or paravalvular) and vena contracta width.

❐ Normal regurgitation of a bileaflet mechanical valve typically consists of two or more eccentric small jets that originate at the closure points of the valve occluders with the sewing ring.

❐ CW Doppler is used to evaluate prosthetic aortic regurgitation based on the density and time course of the diastolic regurgitant signal.

❐ Diastolic flow reversal in the descending aorta, as with native valve regurgitation, is also useful for evaluation of prosthetic aortic regurgitation.

Mitral valves

Mitral valve repair

■ The most common mitral valve repair involves resection of a segment of the posterior leaflet, with a suture line in the mid-segment of the posterior leaflet and placement of an annuloplasty ring. (Figure 13–21)

■ Other procedures used for mitral valve repair include transfer of a segment of the anterior leaflet to the posterior leaflet, use of artificial chords, suturing of the anterior and posterior leaflets together in their midsegments (Alfieri repair), and a variety of other techniques.

■ Percutaneous approaches to mitral valve repair in development include deployment of a device in the coronary sinus to mimic an annuloplasty ring and a clip or suture to mimic an Alfieri-type repair.

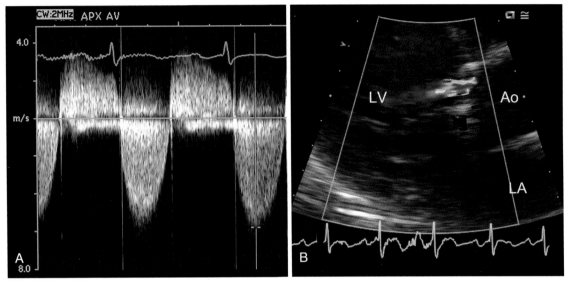

Figure 13–20. In this patient who was noncompliant with anticoagulation, severe stenosis of the mechanical aortic valve prosthesis is present due to valve thrombosis with (*A*) an antegrade velocity of 5.2 m/s and (*B*) mild regurgitation.

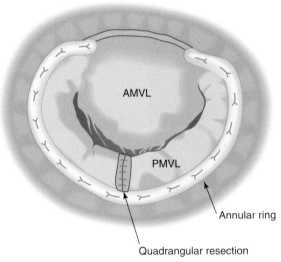

Figure 13–21. View of the mitral valve from the LA side after valve repair, showing the suture in the posterior leaflet at the site of resection of the prolapse segment and the annuloplasty ring. *From Stewart WJ, Griffin BP: Intraoperative Echo in Mitral Valve Repair In Otto CM: The Practice of Clinical Echocardiography, ed 3. Philadelphia, Elsevier, 2007.*

Key points

❏ Knowledge of details of the repair procedure is helpful for interpreting the echocardiographic findings.

❏ The mitral annuloplasty ring causes shadows and reverberations that may obscure mitral regurgitation from the transthoracic approach; TEE is indicated when regurgitation is suspected. (Figure 13–22)

❏ Mitral valve repair may be associated with a mild degree of functional stenosis, which is evaluated based on mean pressure gradient and pressure half-time valve area, as for a native valve.

❏ With a successful repair, there is no more than trace to mild (1+) residual mitral regurgitation.

❏ Recurrent mitral regurgitation after valve repair is evaluated as for a native valve.

❏ An infrequent complication of mitral valve repair is subaortic obstruction due to systolic anterior motion of the mitral leaflets. This complication is related to the size and rigidity of the annuloplasty ring.

Bioprosthetic mitral valves

■ Bioprosthetic mitral valves are stented with the stents typically oriented slightly toward the ventricular septum.

■ Imaging and Doppler evaluation of a bioprosthetic mitral valve are similar to evaluation of a native valve.

■ Shadowing and reverberations from the sewing ring and stents decrease the accuracy of TTE for evaluation of valve dysfunction; TEE is more accurate when a prosthetic mitral valve is present. (Figure 13–23)

Key points

❏ With a prosthetic mitral valve, inflow into the LV is directed toward the ventricular septum, the opposite of the normal diastolic vortex in the LV.

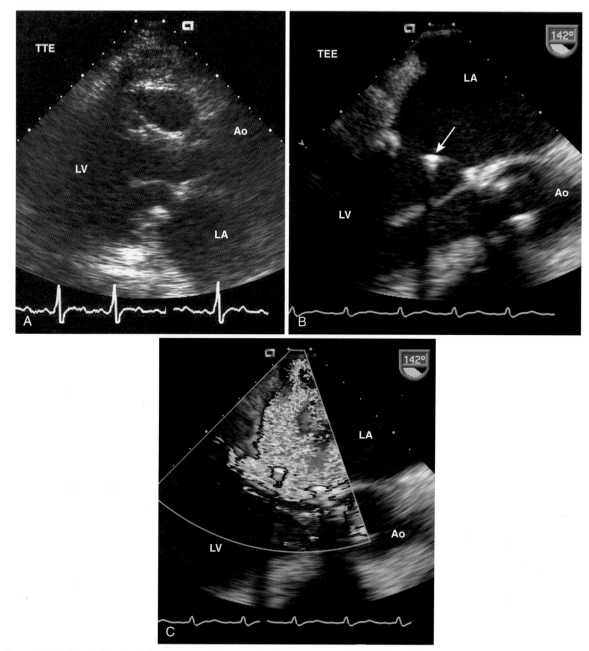

Figure 13–22. *A,* TTE after mitral valve repair may have limited image quality, and shadowing by the valve ring may obscure Doppler evaluation of regurgitation. *B,* TEE offers better image quality and the shadows from the annuloplasty ring now are projected toward the LV. Note the abnormal position of the annuloplasty ring on the TEE view. *C,* Color Doppler confirmed severe mitral regurgitation, which was not evident on transthoracic imaging.

❏ Recording of antegrade flows and calculation of pressure gradient and valve area are no different than for a native mitral valve.

❏ Although the apical window usually provides a parallel alignment for Doppler recordings, in some cases, the mitral inflow can be recorded from a parasternal window, depending on the orientation of the valve inflow stream.

❏ Prosthetic regurgitation is evaluated with CW and color Doppler, as for a native valve, but TEE is considered when valve dysfunction is suspected because significant regurgitation may not be detected from the transthoracic approach.

❏ A small amount of central regurgitation is normal for a bioprosthetic valve.

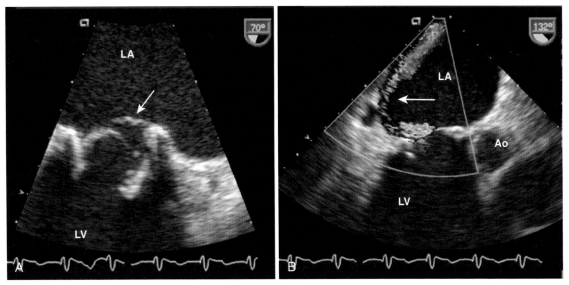

Figure 13–23. A stented bioprosthetic mitral valve with a flail leaflet and an eccentric jet of severe mitral regurgitation, seen on transesophageal but not transthoracic imaging.

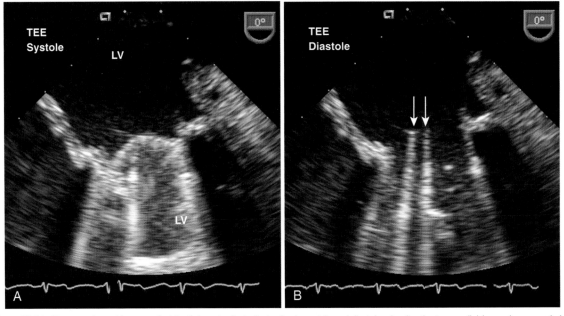

Figure 13–24. Transesophageal images of a bileaflet mechanical mitral valve in systole and diastole, showing the two parallel (*arrows*) open occluders in diastole.

Mechanical mitral valves

- The valve occluders are best seen from the apical transthoracic or high esophageal window, using zoom mode to focus on the mitral valve. (Figure 13–24)
- Antegrade flow across the valve is recorded from the apical window, using pulsed or CW Doppler, depending on the maximum transvalvular velocity.

- Evaluation for regurgitation requires TEE because the LA is shadowed by the prosthesis itself, both from the parasternal and apical windows.

Key points

- Adjustments in the rotation of the image plane from the standard views may be needed to show both leaflets, from both the transthoracic and transesophageal approach.

❏ CW Doppler is especially important for detection of mechanical mitral valve regurgitation because the broad CW beam may detect a regurgitant signal that is obscured by shadowing on color Doppler flow imaging. (Figure 13–25)

❏ Other clues that suggest mitral prosthetic regurgitation on TTE include a high antegrade velocity across the mitral valve and recurrent (or persistent) pulmonary hypertension.

❏ TEE provides superior imaging of the posterior aspects of the prosthetic mitral valve and is more accurate than TTE for diagnosis of prosthetic regurgitation.

❏ Clear definition of the leaflets and annular ring allows visualization of the normal regurgitant jets that originate at the closure plane of the occluders with the sewing ring.

❏ Paravalvular regurgitation originates outside the sewing ring, often has an identifiable proximal isovelocity surface area on the ventricular side of the valve, and typically has a very eccentric jet direction in the LA. (Figure 13–26)

❏ Pulmonary venous flow patterns in patients with mechanical mitral valves are affected by atrial rhythm, atrial mechanical function, and mitral valve hemodynamics, as well as by the presence of mitral regurgitation.

❏ Paravalvular regurgitation may be clinically important regardless of hemodynamic severity because it may be a sign of infection or may be a cause of hemolytic anemia.

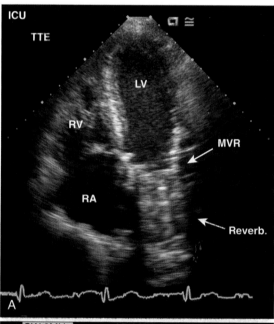

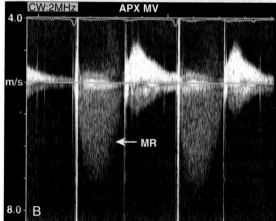

Figure 13–25. *A,* On TTE, the mechanical mitral valve results in reverberations and shadows obscuring the LA in the apical 4-chamber view. *B,* However, with CW Doppler, a systolic signal (*arrow*) consistent with mitral regurgitation is detected.

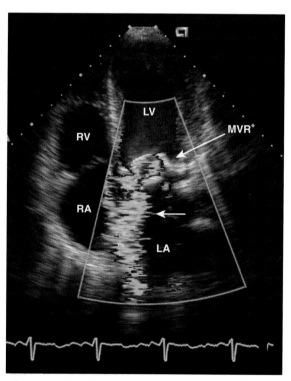

Figure 13–26. Transthoracic apical 4-chamber view in a patient with a tissue mitral prosthesis and paravalvular regurgitation shows a very eccentric jet (*arrows*) that hugs the atrial septum and was missed on initial parasternal images.

Tricuspid valve prostheses and rings

- Tricuspid valve replacement is uncommon, but either a stented bioprosthetic or a mechanical valve is used. (Figure 13–27)
- In patients undergoing mitral valve surgery, a tricuspid annuloplasty ring often is placed if severe tricuspid regurgitation is present or if there is annular dilation with moderate regurgitation.
- Evaluation of a prosthetic tricuspid valve is similar to evaluation of a mitral valve replacement.

Key points

- ❏ Tricuspid valve prostheses often can be fully evaluated on TTE because the valve is close to the chest wall and because the RA can be evaluated from the parasternal window, without shadowing by the valve prosthesis.
- ❏ TEE imaging is helpful when transthoracic images are non-diagnostic.
- ❏ Antegrade flows are recorded using pulsed or CW Doppler from the apical window for calculation of pressure gradients and pressure half-time valve area.
- ❏ Prosthetic tricuspid regurgitation is evaluated by standard approaches using CW and color Doppler.

Pulmonic valve replacements

- Most pulmonic valve replacements are seen in patients with congenital heart disease.
- Pulmonic valve substitutes include homografts; bioprosthetic valves, either in a conduit or isolated; and transcatheter valve implantation.
- Transcatheter pulmonic valves are typically placed in patients with a prior surgically implanted conduit. The transcatheter valve is analogous to a trileaflet tissue bioprosthesis mounted in an expandable stent.
- Mechanical valves are occasionally used in the pulmonic position.

Key points

- ❏ Visualization of prosthetic pulmonic valves from either transthoracic or TEE approaches often is limited in adults. Alternate diagnostic procedures, such as cardiac magnetic resonance imaging or cardiac catheterization and angiography, often are needed.
- ❏ Antegrade velocity is recorded with pulsed or CW Doppler in the parasternal short axis or RV outflow view. (Figure 13–28)
- ❏ Pulsed and color Doppler are used to document the level of obstruction. Many of these patients

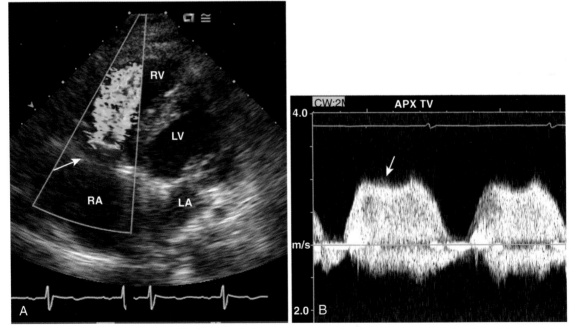

Figure 13–27. Apical view of a tissue tricuspid valve with color Doppler showing proximal acceleration (*arrow*) and a stenotic jet inflow signal. CW Doppler shows a high velocity and long pressure half-time, consistent with severe prosthetic stenosis.

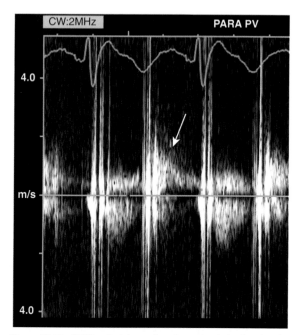

Figure 13–28. CW Doppler interrogation of a mechanical pulmonic valve replacement with the transducer in a high parasternal position. The scale has been set with a wide velocity range to examine both for stenosis and regurgitation. In this case, the antegrade velocity is only mildly increased, prominent valve clicks are present, and there is a diastolic signal (*arrow*) most consistent with tricuspid inflow (note timing relative to antegrade pulmonary flow).

also have subvalvular or supravalvular pulmonic stenosis. Stenosis also can occur at the distal anastomosis site of the conduit or in the branch pulmonary arteries.

❑ Severe prosthetic regurgitation is seen as to-and-fro flow on color Doppler; because the pressure difference is low, there may be little evidence of a flow disturbance.

❑ On CW Doppler, severe prosthetic pulmonic regurgitation is seen as a diastolic signal with a density equal to antegrade flow and a steep slope, often reaching the baseline before the end of diastole. (See Figure 17–28)

THE ECHO EXAM

Prosthetic Valves

TRANSTHORACIC EXAMINATION		TRANSESOPHAGEAL EXAMINATION	
Imaging	Valve leaflet thickness and motion LV size, wall thickness, and systolic function	*Imaging*	Valve leaflet thickness and motion Examine atrial side of mitral prostheses LV size, wall thickness, and systolic function
Doppler	Antegrade prosthetic valve velocity Evaluate for stenosis Search carefully for regurgitation Pulmonary artery pressures	*Doppler*	Antegrade prosthetic valve velocity Evaluate for stenosis Search carefully for regurgitation Pulmonary artery pressures

Transthoracic Doppler Evaluation of Prosthetic Valves

Components	Modality	View	Recording	Measurements
Antegrade flow velocity	Pulsed or CW Doppler	Apical	Antegrade transmitral or transaortic velocity	Peak velocity (compare to normal values for valve type and size)
Measures of valve stenosis	Pulsed and CW Doppler	Apical	Careful positioning to obtain highest velocity signal	Mean gradient Aortic valves: ratio of LVOT to aortic velocity Mitral valve: pressure half-time
Valve regurgitation	Color imaging and CW Doppler	Parasternal, apical, SSN	Jet origin, direction, and size on color CW Doppler of each valve Pulmonary vein flow Descending aorta flow	Vena contracta width Intensity of CW Doppler signal Pulmonary vein systolic flow reversal (MR) Descending aorta flow reversal (AR)
Pulmonary pressures	CW Doppler	RV inflow and apical	TR jet velocity IVC size and variation	Calculate PAP as $4v^2$ of TR jet plus estimated RA pressure.

AR, atrial regurgitation; CW, continuous wave; IVC, inferior vena cava; LVOT, left ventricular outflow tract; MR, mitral regurgitation; PAP, pulmonary artery pressure; TR, tricuspid regurgitation; SSN, suprasternal notch.

ECHOCARDIOGRAPHIC SIGNS OF PROSTHETIC VALVE DYSFUNCTION

Increased antegrade velocity across the valve
Decreased valve area (continuity equation or T ½)
Increased regurgitation on color flow
Increased intensity of CW Doppler regurgitant signal
Progressive chamber dilation
Persistent LV hypertrophy
Recurrent pulmonary hypertension

Transesophageal Evaluation of Prosthetic Valves

Components	Modality	View	Recording	Limitations
Valve Imaging	2D echo	High esophageal	Mitral valve in high esophageal 4-chamber view Aortic valve in high esophageal long- and short-axis views	Aortic valve prosthesis may shadow anterior segments of the aortic valve. With both aortic and mitral prostheses, the aortic shadow may obscure the mitral prosthesis.
Antegrade flow velocity	Pulsed or CW Doppler	High esophageal or transgastric apical	Antegrade transmitral or transaortic velocity	Alignment of Doppler beam with transaortic valve flow may be problematic; compare with TTE data.
Measures of valve stenosis	Pulsed and CW Doppler	High esophageal or transgastric apical	Careful positioning to obtain highest velocity signal	Mean gradient Aortic valves: ratio of LVOT to aortic velocity (alignment may be suboptimal) Mitral valve: pressure half-time
Valve regurgitation	Color imaging and CW Doppler	High esophageal with rotational scan	Document origin of jet and proximal flow acceleration, and jet size and direction	Measure vena contracta, record pulmonary venous flow pattern, search carefully for eccentric jets.
Pulmonary pressures	CW Doppler	RV inflow and apical	TR jet velocity IVC size and variation	Calculate PAP as 4v² of TR jet plus estimated RA pressure. May be difficult to align Doppler beam parallel to TR jet; correlate with TTE data.

2D, two-dimensional; CW, continuous wave; IVC, inferior vena cava; LVOT, left ventricular outflow tract; PAP, pulmonary artery pressure; TR, tricuspid regurgitation; TTE, transthoracic echocardiography.

EXAMPLE

A 62-year-old man with a mechanical mitral valve replacement 2 years ago for myxomatous mitral valve disease presents with increasing heart failure symptoms and a systolic murmur. He is in chronic atrial fibrillation. Transthoracic echocardiography shows:

LA anterior-posterior dimension	5.7 cm
LV dimensions (systole/diastole)	6.2/3.8 cm
Ejection fraction	56%
Transmitral E velocity	1.8 m/s
Mitral pressure half-time	100 ms
TR jet velocity	3.2 m/s
IVC size and variation	Normal

Color flow imaging shows ghosting and reverberations in the LA region, but no definite regurgitant jet can be identified. CW Doppler shows a mitral regurgitant signal that is incomplete in duration and not as dense as antegrade flow.

This transthoracic study is difficult to interpret without a previous study for comparison. The LA and LV dilation and the borderline ejection fraction may be residual from before the valve surgery or could represent progressive changes after valve replacement. Pulmonary artery pressure (PAP) is moderately elevated at:

$$PAP = 4(V_{TR})^2 + RAP = 4(3.2)^2 + 10 = 41 + 10 = 51 \text{ mm Hg}$$

Again, pulmonary hypertension may be residual or recurrent after valve surgery, but the presence of pulmonary hypertension suggests the possibility of significant prosthetic mitral regurgitation.

Although a clear regurgitant jet is not demonstrated due to shadowing and reverberations from the valve prosthesis, the high antegrade flow velocity with a short pressure half-time and detection of regurgitation with CW Doppler indicate that further evaluation is needed.

Transesophageal echocardiography (TEE) demonstrates a paravalvular mitral regurgitant jet with a proximal acceleration region seen at the lateral aspect of the annulus, a vena contracta width of 7 mm, and an eccentric jet directed along the posterior-lateral LA wall. The left pulmonary veins show definite systolic flow reversal; the right pulmonary veins show blunting of the normal systolic flow pattern. These findings are consistent with severe paraprosthetic regurgitation.

On TEE imaging, the LV was not well visualized due to shadowing and reverberations from the mitral prosthesis; although transgastric short-axis views were obtained, ejection fraction could not be calculated. The maximum tricuspid regurgitation jet obtained on TEE was 2.9 m/s. Because a higher jet was obtained on transthoracic imaging, the TEE jet most likely underestimates pulmonary pressures.

In summary, this patient has severe paraprosthetic mitral regurgitation with LA and LV dilation, moderate pulmonary hypertension, and a borderline ejection fraction. As is typical with prosthetic valves, the combination of transthoracic and TEE was needed for diagnosis.

QUESTION 1

For each of the following four images, the valve shown is a:

A. Bileaflet mechanical valve
B. Mechanical valve, unknown type
C. Stented bioprosthetic valve
D. Stentless bioprosthetic valve
E. Normal native valve

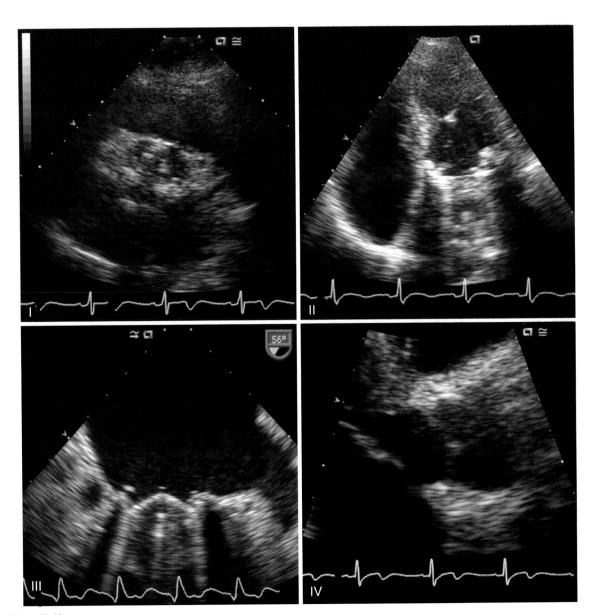

Figure 13–29.

QUESTION 2

This 44-year-old man presented for evaluation of atypical chest pain. He had undergone aortic valve replacement for aortic regurgitation 8 years ago with placement of a 27 mm stented bioprosthetic valve. A postoperative echocardiogram demonstrated an aortic velocity of 2.4 m/s, mean transaortic gradient of 19 mm Hg, and valve area of 1.5 cm^2. Data from the current study are shown in Figure 13–30. Measure the aortic valve velocity and calculate the maximum transaortic gradient and valve area.

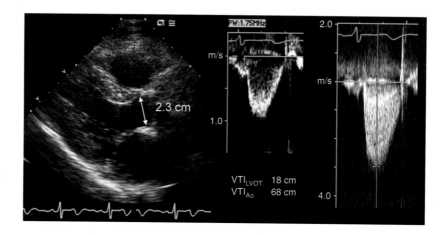

Figure 13–30.

QUESTION 3

A 43-year-old woman with aortic valve replacement 20 years ago for congenital aortic stenosis presents for routine follow-up. She is asymptomatic and physically active with no exercise limitation, but no previous echocardiograms are available. A systolic murmur is noted on examination and the echocardiogram shows the following Doppler data:

The best next step in patient management is:

A. Exercise treadmill testing
B. Transesophageal echocardiography
C. Calculate continuity equation valve area
D. Chest computed tomographic imaging
E. LV strain rate imaging

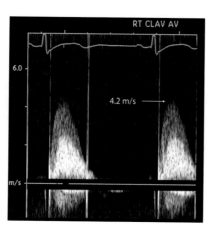

Figure 13–31.

QUESTION 4

This 88-year-old woman presented with worsening heart failure and hemoptysis. She had undergone bio-prosthetic mitral valve replacement 12 years ago for severe mitral stenosis with an early postoperative baseline echocardiogram that showed normal LV and RV size and function, normal prosthetic valve function, and a pulmonary systolic pressure of 40 mm Hg. On exam now she has a blood pressure of 100/70 mm Hg, heart rate of 74 bpm with an irregular pulse, jugular venous pressure of 20 cm H_2O, distant heart sounds, and bilateral pulmonary rales. The following Doppler tracings were recorded on the current study.

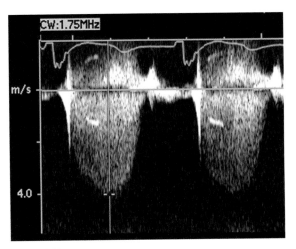

Figure 13–32.

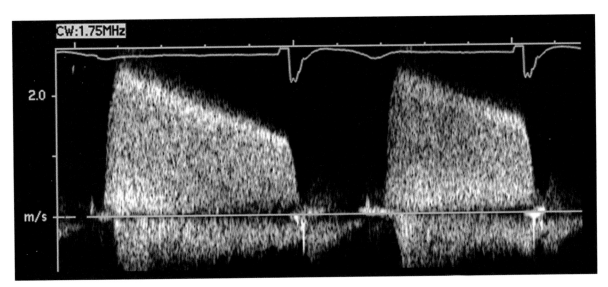

Figure 13–33.

The most likely cause of her current symptoms is:

A. Pulmonary embolus
B. LV systolic dysfunction
C. Severe mitral regurgitation
D. Rheumatic aortic valve disease
E. Mitral stenosis

QUESTION 5

Using the data shown for Question 4, calculate the following:

Pulmonary systolic pressure: _____
Mitral valve area: _____

QUESTION 6

In the patient with this echocardiographic image, which of the following clinical findings is most likely present?

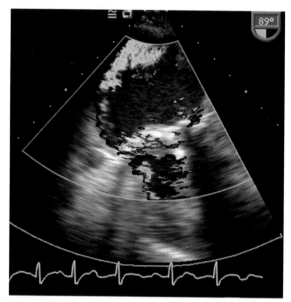

Figure 13–34.

A. Elevated reticulocyte count
B. Diastolic murmur
C. Wide pulse pressure
D. S4 gallop
E. Thrombocytopenia

QUESTION 7

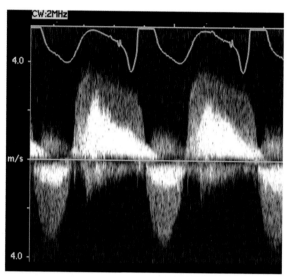

Figure 13–35.

This Doppler tracing obtained in a patient with prior valve surgery is consistent with all of the following except:

A. Aortic stenosis
B. Aortic regurgitation
C. Mitral stenosis
D. Mitral regurgitation

QUESTION 8

A 71-year-old woman presented for a second opinion regarding possible aortic patient–prosthesis mismatch. She had undergone a 19 mm pericardial bioprosthetic aortic valve replacement 2 years ago but continued to have symptoms of atypical chest pain.

On exam, she is an older anxious woman with a blood pressure of 120/80 mm Hg, pulse of 72 bpm, body surface area of 1.9 cm^2, and an aortic ejection murmur but no evidence of heart failure. Echocardiography shows a normal-appearing prosthetic valve with the following Doppler data.

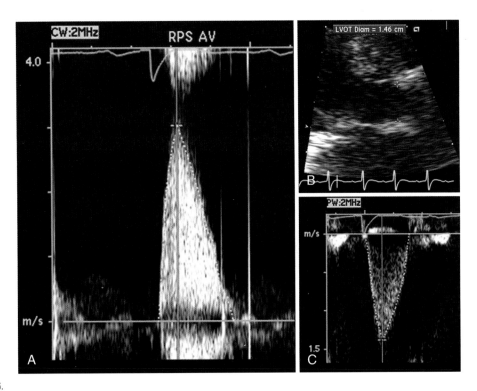

Figure 13–36.

The most likely diagnosis in this patient is:

A. No prosthetic valve dysfunction
B. Prosthetic valve stenosis
C. Prosthetic valve regurgitation
D. Patient–prosthesis mismatch

QUESTION 9

Match each of the following diagnostic issues with the most useful imaging modality:
1. Prosthetic aortic valve function
2. Prosthetic mitral valve function
3. Aortic graft pseudoaneurysm
4. Aneurysm of the aortic-mitral intervalvular fibrosa
5. Aortic valve paravalvular abscess
6. Bioprosthetic tricuspid valve vegetation
7. LV function with a mechanical mitral valve

A. Transthoracic 2D imaging
B. Transthoracic Doppler
C. TEE 2D imaging
D. TEE Doppler
E. Chest computed tomographic imaging

QUESTION 10

This echocardiographic image was obtained on the postoperative baseline study after bioprosthetic mitral valve replacement.

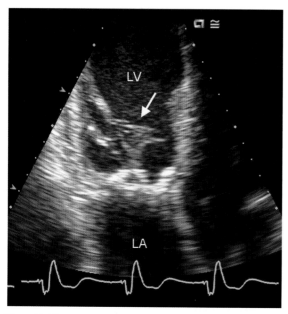

Figure 13–37.

What is the most likely diagnosis for the structure indicated by the arrow?

A. Vegetation
B. Valve strut
C. Mitral valve
D. Ruptured papillary muscle
E. LV thrombus

QUESTION 11

This 75-year-old man underwent surgical aortic valve repair 10 years ago for endocarditis resulting in prolapse of the noncoronary cusp. He has done well postoperatively and has been followed annually with echocardiograms showing mild to moderate residual aortic regurgitation. He now presents with a cough, fatigue, and a low-grade fever. On exam his blood pressure is 158/40 mm Hg, pulse is 113 bpm, and irregular and bibasilar rales are present. This Doppler flow tracing was recorded.

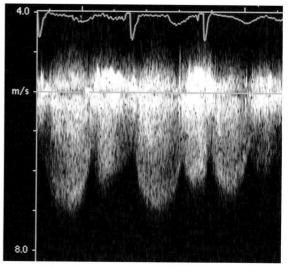

Figure 13–38.

The most likely new diagnosis in this patient is:

A. Acute mitral regurgitation
B. Aortic to LA fistula
C. Severe pulmonary hypertension
D. Severe aortic stenosis
E. Patent ductus arteriosus

ANSWERS

ANSWER 1

A. Stented bioprosthetic valve: This is a zoomed image of an aortic valve prosthesis in the parasternal short-axis view in an 82-year-old woman who underwent valve replacement for severe aortic stenosis 4 years ago. The three struts of the valve are seen at the perimeter of the valve with thin leaflets between the struts, consistent with the typical appearance of a bioprosthetic stented aortic valve.

B. Mechanical valve, unknown type: This apical 4-chamber view shows a mechanical mitral valve with extensive reverberations and shadowing distal to the valve, obscuring the LA in an 85-year-old woman who had undergone valve surgery 10 years ago. The exact valve type cannot be discerned on this still-frame image, but it is most likely a "low profile" valve (bileaflet or single tilting disk) rather than a ball-and-cage valve, which protrudes further into the LV cavity.

C. Bileaflet mechanical valve: This TEE image recorded in the 2-chamber plane (note the image plane rotation angle and the LA appendage) shows the typical appearance of a bileaflet mechanical valve. The disks are closed in systole, forming a "tent-shaped" closure within the sewing ring. Distal to the valve the LV is obscured by shadowing from the sewing ring and reverberations from the valve disks. The small dense echo on the atrial side of the medial aspect of the sewing ring most likely is a valve suture.

D. Stentless bioprosthetic valve: This zoomed parasternal long-axis diastolic image of the aortic valve might be mistaken for a normal native valve, given the thin normal appearance of the aortic valve leaflets. However, there is increased echodensity in the paravalvular region, both anteriorly and posteriorly, consistent with the extra tissue of a stentless bioprosthetic valve. This image emphasizes the importance of complete and correct clinical information for interpretation of echocardiographic data, as this patient was known to have a stentless aortic bioprosthesis.

ANSWER 2

Aortic velocity	3.0 m/s
Maximum gradient	36 mm Hg
Aortic valve area	1.1 cm^2

The aortic velocity shown is about 3.0 m/s, corresponding to a maximum transaortic pressure gradient of $4(3)^2$ or 36 mm Hg. Calculation of mean gradient requires averaging the instantaneous pressure gradients over the systolic ejection period, so this maximum gradient cannot be compared directly with the baseline postoperative mean gradient. However, aortic velocity has increased from 2.4 to 3.0 m/s, suggesting possible early prosthetic valve stenosis. This is a central flow orifice valve with anatomy similar to a native aortic valve, so continuity equation valve area can be calculated. The measured LV outflow tract diameter ($LVOT_D$), not the implanted valve size, should be used in the valve area calculation. Thus, in this example, LV outflow tract cross-sectional area (CSA_{LVOT}) is:

$$CSA_{LVOT} = \pi r^2 = 3.14(2.3/2)^2 = 4.15 \text{ cm}^2$$

Aortic valve area (AVA), then, is:

$$AVA = CSA_{LVOT} \times VTI_{LVOT}/VTI_{Ao}$$
$$= 4.15 \text{ cm}^2 \times (18 \text{ cm}/68 \text{ cm}) = 1.1 \text{ cm}^2$$

For a quicker valve area calculation, maximum LV outflow tract and aortic velocities can be substituted for velocity-time integrals:

$$AVA = CSA_{LVOT} \times V_{LVOT}/V_{Ao}$$
$$= 4.15 \text{ cm}^2 \times (0.8 \text{ m/s}/3.0 \text{ m/s}) = 1.1 \text{ cm}^2$$

These findings suggest there has been a decrease in functional aortic valve area compared with the early postoperative study, which is consistent with early calcific degeneration of a 10-year-old bioprosthetic valve in a young patient. However, this degree of stenosis is unlikely to account for symptoms of chest pain so that evaluation for other causes is appropriate.

ANSWER 3: D

This is a Doppler recording of transaortic flow based on the presence of prominent valve opening and closing clicks, an ejection type velocity curve, and the timing of flow relative to the QRS signal. The triangular shape of the signal suggests normal valve function because stenotic valves usually have a more rounded systolic curve with a late peaking maximum velocity. However, the velocity of 4.3 m/s is much greater than expected for this valve type. This high velocity most likely is due to low acceleration in the central slit-like orifice of the bileaflet valve, with pressure recovery distally resulting in only a modest valve gradient. The denser signal within the aortic curve supports this possibility and likely is the flow velocity through the larger lateral valve orifice. However, the possibility of valve thrombosis or pannus formation limited disk excursion must be excluded by direct visualization of leaflet motion. Simple fluoroscopy can be used to evaluate mechanical disk motion, with careful adjustment of imaging angle to visualize the leaflets. However, chest computed tomographic imaging is preferable because it allows direct visualization of both leaflet motion and the subvalvular region. Computed tomographic imaging showed normal valve function in this patient (Figure 13–31b).

Exercise treadmill testing can be helpful to clarify symptom status with native or prosthetic valve stenosis but is not needed in this asymptomatic patient. TEE might provide better images of the posterior aspects of the prosthetic valve, but shadowing and reverberations would now obscure the anterior valve structures, making it difficult to exclude prosthetic valve stenosis. The continuity equation valve area will be falsely reduced if the apparent aortic velocity is recorded from the small central flow orifice. LV strain rate imaging allows detection of early LV dysfunction when aortic valve disease is present but would not be helpful for evaluation of valve function in this patient.

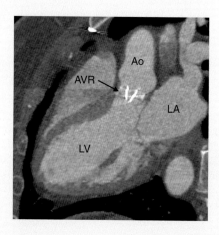

ANSWER 4: E

These Doppler recordings show a high velocity tricuspid regurgitant jet, consistent with pulmonary hypertension, and a transmitral flow signal consistent with an elevated transmitral gradient and small valve area. The tricuspid regurgitant signal is identified based on systolic flow with a long flow period relative to the QRS and with the typical rapid, followed by slow, rate of rise in velocity with a late peaking curve. The transmitral flow curve is in diastole with a typical passive flow pattern of an early diastolic peak and linear fall off in velocity throughout diastole. Atrial fibrillation is present with no discernable A-velocity. The slow diastolic decline in velocity is consistent with mitral stenosis.

Pulmonary embolus might be associated with pulmonary hypertension, but transmitral flow would be normal. LV systolic dysfunction would result in a reduced dP/dt on the mitral regurgitant velocity signal, which is not shown here. Severe mitral

regurgitation would result in an increased antegrade transmitral velocity, but the diastolic slope would be steep. Rheumatic aortic valve disease is present in about a third of patients with rheumatic valve disease, and the mitral stenosis signal appears similar in shape to aortic regurgitation. However, diastolic velocities are lower across the mitral valve compared with the aortic valve; with a diastolic blood pressure of 70 mm Hg, the initial diastolic velocity for aortic regurgitation would be about 4 m/s.

ANSWER 5

Pulmonary systolic pressure	79 mm Hg
Mitral valve area	0.6 cm²

The tricuspid regurgitant velocity is 4.0 m/s, reflecting a RV-to-RA systolic pressure difference of 64 mm Hg. Images of the inferior vena cava are not provided to estimate RA pressure; the central venous pressure was estimated to be about 20 cm H₂O (or 15 mm Hg) based on physical examination of the neck veins. The conversion factor for units of pressure is 1.36 cm H₂O for each mm Hg. Thus, adding RA pressure to the RV–RA pressure difference, the estimated pulmonary systolic pressure is 79 mm Hg.

With this bioprosthetic valve, mitral valve area is calculated from the mitral pressure half-time $(T\frac{1}{2})$, as for native mitral valve stenosis. On the first beat, the peak transmitral velocity is 2.3 m/s, corresponding to an instantaneous pressure gradient of 21 mm Hg. The $T\frac{1}{2}$ is measured on the time axis from this point to the point on the diastolic deceleration slope where the pressure drop is half the initial gradient. A pressure gradient of 11 mm Hg corresponds to a velocity of 1.66 m/s. Finding this point on the Doppler signal, drawing a vertical line to the time axis, and then measuring the time interval from peak velocity to this point, provides a $T\frac{1}{2}$ of 370 ms. Mitral valve area is $220/T\frac{1}{2}$ or 0.6 cm². These findings are consistent with severe prosthetic mitral stenosis. Although tissue valve durability usually is longer in older patients, at surgery the bioprosthetic valve was severely calcified with restricted leaflet motion.

ANSWER 6: A

This is a TEE 2-chamber view of a patient with a mechanical mitral valve prosthesis showing an eccentric paravalvular mitral regurgitant jet. Paravalvular mitral regurgitation can cause hemolysis resulting in an elevated reticulocyte count. Most often, hemolysis is well tolerated and the patient is able to maintain a relatively normal red blood cell count, although sometimes vitamin and iron supplementation is needed. Rarely is surgical or percutaneous intervention needed to close the paravalvular leak unless there also is a large volume of regurgitant flow. This patient likely has a systolic (not diastolic murmur). A wide pulse pressure is typical for aortic, not mitral, regurgitation. An S4 gallop will not be present because the electrocardiogram shows atrial fibrillation. The platelet count should be normal, although blood clotting likely is abnormal due to warfarin anticoagulation for a mechanical valve and atrial fibrillation.

ANSWER 7: D

This CW Doppler tracing shows a systolic ejection velocity below the baseline (recorded from the apex) with a maximum velocity about 3 m/s consistent with mild aortic stenosis or with a prosthetic aortic valve. In diastole, mild aortic regurgitation is seen with a signal that starts with aortic valve closure and extends to aortic valve opening, with a maximum early diastolic velocity about 3.5 m/s and passive diastolic deceleration with a flat slope. Overlapping with the aortic regurgitant signal is a denser diastolic signal that has a time delay between aortic closure and onset of flow, consistent with the isovolumic relaxation period, indicating that this is transmitral flow. The peak velocity over 2 m/s and slightly prolonged deceleration slope suggest mild mitral stenosis or a prosthetic mitral valve, as was the case in this patient. There should be a time interval between the end of transmitral flow and aortic ejection, but this finding is obscured by a poor signal-to-noise ratio. There is no atrial contribution to LV diastolic filling because this is a ventricular paced rhythm (see electrocardiogram) and the atrial rhythm likely is atrial fibrillation. This tracing does not show evidence of mitral regurgitation; a different Doppler beam angle is needed for better evaluation of mitral valve function.

ANSWER 8: D

The Doppler data show an aortic velocity of 3.0 m/s with an LV outflow tract diameter of only 1.5 cm and an LV outflow tract velocity of 1.4 m/s. The circular LV outflow tract cross-sectional area (CSA) is 1.77 cm^2. Aortic valve area calculated with the continuity equation is:

$$AVA = CSA_{LVOT} \times V_{LVOT}/V_{Ao}$$
$$= 1.77 \text{ cm}^2 \times (1.4 \text{ m/s}/3.0 \text{ m/s}) = 0.8 \text{ cm}^2$$

When indexed for body size,

$$\text{Indexed AVA} = 0.8 \text{ cm}^2/1.9 \text{ m}^2 = 0.42 \text{ cm}^2/\text{m}^2$$

These data are consistent with severe patient–prosthesis mismatch, defined as a prosthetic aortic valve indexed area less than 0.65 cm^2/m^2. The reason for patient–prosthesis mismatch in this patient is the very small LV outflow tract. Ideally, patient–prosthesis mismatch is avoided by calculating the expected valve

area divided by body size before valve implantation; if the expected valve area is too small, an alternate valve choice or an aortic root enlarging procedure can be considered. Once patient prosthesis mismatch is present, decision making is more difficult because correction would require another surgical procedure. Both short- and long-term outcomes are worse when patient–prosthesis mismatch is present, but the increase in late mortality is seen only in patients younger than age 70, patients with a body mass index less than 30 kg/m^2, and those with LV systolic dysfunction (ejection fraction < 50%). This patient is older than age 70, she has normal LV function, and it is not clear that her symptoms are related to her valve size. Her body mass index is 27 kg/m^2, so she may benefit from weight reduction. In addition, her transvalvular mean gradient is only 14 mm Hg and the LV outflow to aortic velocity ratio is only 1.4/3.0 = 0.47, neither of which support a significant hemodynamic effect from the small valve prosthesis. Thus, although she meets the definition for patient–prosthesis mismatch, there is no evidence for significant stenosis or regurgitation. In any case, this patient has declined further interventions and continues to do well with medical therapy.

ANSWER 9: 1B, 2D, 3E, 4C, 5A, 6A, 7A

Evaluation of a patient with suspected prosthetic valve dysfunction often requires both transthoracic and TEE imaging. Transthoracic imaging is optimal for measurement of LV volumes and ejection fraction because the LV often is foreshortened on TEE and may be shadowed by the mitral or aortic valve prosthesis. Transthoracic imaging usually is preferred for a bioprosthetic tricuspid valve because this valve is anterior in the chest and thus well seen from this approach. However, TEE imaging may be needed if transthoracic images are suboptimal. Transthoracic Doppler is the best approach for evaluation of prosthetic aortic valve function because the Doppler beam can be aligned from an apical window parallel with transvalvular flow and aortic regurgitation can be evaluated in both parasternal and apical views. In contrast, on TEE, alignment of the Doppler beam with transaortic flow is problematic and evaluation of regurgitation is limited by shadowing of the LV outflow tract by the prosthetic valve.

In patients with a prosthetic mitral valve, the LA side of the prosthesis is shadowed on transthoracic imaging so that TEE is recommended whenever prosthetic mitral regurgitation is suspected. Similarly, TEE is much more sensitive than transthoracic imaging for detection of a prosthetic paravalvular abscess because it allows imaging of the LA side of the aortic and mitral valve prostheses. Of course, an anteriorly located aortic paravalvular abscess may be seen on transthoracic imaging, but absence of an anterior abscess does not exclude posterior annular infection. With involvement of structures outside the narrow window provided by echocardiographic imaging, such as an aortic root pseudoaneurysm, wide field imaging modalities, such as chest computed tomography, are recommended.

ANSWER 10: C

This image shows the native mitral valve chords and part of the mitral leaflet, which were retained at the time of mitral valve replacement. Maintenance of mitral annular–papillary muscle continuity helps prevent loss of LV systolic contractile function with surgical mitral valve replacement. Typically the prosthetic valve is inserted centrally and the posterior leaflets and chords are left connected to the papillary muscle behind the prosthetic valve sewing ring. The anterior leaflet may be partially retained or may be resected, leaving freely mobile chordal remnants. A mitral vegetation would be more likely on the LA side of the valve; infection of the sewing ring with annular abscess formation instead of a typical vegetation is common with a prosthetic valve. Valve struts are more uniform in appearance and do not protrude this far into the LV cavity. A ruptured papillary muscle results in a disrupted muscle head moving freely in the LV, attached to the mitral valve; normal attachments of the chords to the papillary muscle can be seen on this image. An LV thrombus usually occurs in an area of regional dysfunction, often the apex, and is adherent to the LV myocardium.

ANSWER 11: A

This Doppler tracing shows a diastolic signal with a peak velocity and diastolic slope (see first beat) consistent with known aortic regurgitation. The diastolic flow is directed away from the transducer, so the probe position likely is parasternal with a posteriorly directed aortic regurgitant jet. In systole there is an ejection-type (rapid rise and fall with curved waveform) signal with a peak velocity about 5.5 m/s. This is most consistent with mitral regurgitation, given a systolic blood pressure of 158 mm Hg; even with an LA pressure of 20 mm Hg, the Bernoulli equation indicates that velocity should be at least 6 m/s if the intercept angle between the jet and ultrasound beam was parallel. In this example, a nonparallel intercept angle is likely with the transducer in a parasternal position. The relatively rapid fall-off in velocity in late systole suggests acute regurgitation with an elevated LA pressure. This patient had a mitral valve vegetation with an adjacent leaflet perforation, and blood cultures were positive for alpha-hemolytic *Streptococcus*.

With an aortic-to-LA fistula, high velocity continuous flow in systole and diastole would be seen reflecting the high aortic-to-LV pressure difference. The typical valve-type velocity curves would not be seen. Pulmonary hypertension cannot be diagnosed from these data; a tricuspid regurgitant jet would be longer in duration and overlap with aortic regurgitation at the onset and end of flow. If the systolic signal were due to aortic stenosis, a slight time interval before and after aortic regurgitation would be seen corresponding to the isovolumic relaxation and contraction periods. A patent ductus arteriosus would show continuous flow in the pulmonary artery with a lower velocity, reflecting the pressure difference from the descending aorta to the pulmonary artery, and the distinct valve-type curves would not be seen.

Endocarditis

BASIC PRINCIPLES

- Echocardiographic evaluation for endocarditis uses an integrated approach with transthoracic (TTE) and transesophageal (TEE) echocardiography, depending on the clinical setting and the initial echocardiographic findings.
- The modified Duke criteria for infective endocarditis are the current clinical standard.
- The primary goals of the echocardiographic examination in a patient with suspected or known endocarditis are to:
  - Detect and describe valvular vegetations
  - Quantitate degree of valve dysfunction
  - Identify paravalvular abscess or other complications
  - Evaluate hemodynamics effects of valve dysfunction on ventricular size and function and on pulmonary pressures *and*
  - Provide prognostic data on clinical course and need for surgical intervention

Key points

- Definite endocarditis is present when blood cultures are positive and diagnostic findings are present on echocardiography; these are called "major criteria" for the diagnosis of endocarditis.
- Diagnostic echocardiographic findings for endocarditis are:
  - Typical vegetation on a valve or prosthetic material
  - Paravalvular abscess
  - New prosthetic valve dehiscence *or*
  - New valvular regurgitation
- In the absence of the major criteria (blood cultures and echocardiographic findings), the minor criteria for diagnosis of endocarditis are:
  - Predisposing heart condition or IV drug use
  - Fever
  - Vascular phenomenon (arterial emboli, mycotic aneurysm, conjunctival hemorrhage, etc.)
  - Immunologic phenomenon (glomerulonephritis, rheumatoid factor, etc.) *and*
  - Other microbiologic evidence
- Definite endocarditis is based on the presence of two major *or* one major plus three minor *or* all five minor criteria. Possible endocarditis is based on one major plus one minor *or* three minor criteria.

STEP-BY-STEP APPROACH

Step 1: Review the clinical data

- Key clinical data in the patient undergoing echocardiography for suspected endocarditis are:
  - Blood culture results
  - History of underlying cardiac disease or intravenous drug use
  - Other evidence of endocarditis (fever, embolic events, PR interval prolongation
  - Any contraindication to TEE
- The clinical data help focus the echocardiographic examination so that particular attention is directed toward:
  - Detection of right-sided vegetations in patients with a history of intravenous drug use
  - Comparison of the current study with previous examinations in patients with underlying valve pathology
  - Additional imaging, often with TEE, of prosthetic valves and pacer leads

Key points

- ❏ The sensitivity of echocardiography for detection of valve vegetations depends as much on the diligence of the exam as on image quality; therefore, a pretest estimate of the likelihood of disease is helpful to the sonographer.
- ❏ Review of previous imaging studies before performing the exam allows quick recognition of new abnormalities.
- ❏ Clinical data are critical for interpretation of echocardiographic data. The echo appearance of a cardiac tumor, thrombus, and infected vegetation are similar—the final diagnosis is based on integration of echocardiographic and clinical data.
- ❏ Clinical data determine the urgency and most appropriate initial diagnostic modality as well as the need for any subsequent studies.

Step 2: Choose transthoracic and/or transesophageal echocardiography (Table 14-1)

- Most centers perform TTE first in patients with suspected endocarditis.
- Transthoracic imaging is followed by TEE if transthoracic images are nondiagnostic, if a prosthetic valve is present, or if the patient has a high risk of endocarditis.
- TEE is an appropriate initial diagnostic approach in patients with a prosthetic valve or other intracardiac devices (such as pacer leads).

- In a patient with suspected or known endocarditis, TEE is recommended if clinical data suggest paravalvular abscess.

Key points

- ❏ TEE is more sensitive for detection of valve vegetations compared with transthoracic imaging (a sensitivity of about 90% vs. about 70%). (Figure 14–1)
- ❏ TEE is more sensitive for detection of paravalvular abscess compared with transthoracic imaging (sensitivity greater than 90% vs. about 50%).
- ❏ TEE is the preferred approach in patients with prosthetic valves or other intracardiac devices (such as pacer leads) for detection of vegetations and evaluation of valve dysfunction. (Figure 14–2)
- ❏ Transthoracic imaging provides more reliable measurements of LV size and ejection fraction, because images of the LV are often oblique or foreshortened on TEE views.
- ❏ Transthoracic imaging provides more accurate Doppler evaluation of stenotic valves and estimation of pulmonary pressures because TEE often results in nonparallel intercept angle between the Doppler beam and high-velocity jet.
- ❏ When TEE is contraindicated but endocarditis is suspected on clinical grounds, a repeat transthoracic study in 5 to 10 days has additive value, with the prevalence of diagnostic findings increasing from 20% on the initial study to 40% on the repeat examination.

Step 3: Examine valve anatomy to detect valvular vegetations

- Valvular vegetations on echocardiography are seen as an abnormal, irregular mass attached to the valve apparatus. (Figure 14–3)
- Valvular vegetations typically are attached to the upstream side of the valve leaflet (e.g., atrial side of the mitral or tricuspid valve, LV side of aortic valve). (Figure 14–4)
- Motion of a vegetation typically is chaotic, with a spatial range in excess of normal valve excursion and a temporal pattern of rapid oscillations. (Figure 14–5)

Key points

- ❏ In addition to standard views of each valve, the image plane is slowly moved from side to side (or in a rotational sweep on TEE) because vegetations often are seen only in oblique views.

TABLE 14-1 ACC/AHA 2006 Recommendations for Echocardiography in Infective Endocarditis		
	Transthoracic Echo (TTE)	**Transesophageal Echo (TEE)**
Suspected Endocarditis		
1. Detection of valvular vegetations (with or without positive blood cultures)	Recommended	
2. Known valve disease with positive blood cultures and nondiagnostic TTE		Recommended
3. Persistent staphylococcal bacteremia without a known source		Reasonable
4. Nosocomial staphylococcal bacteremia		May be considered
5. Intracardiac device (pacer or defibrillator)	Recommended	Recommended if TTE nondiagnostic
Known Endocarditis		
1. Evaluation of valve hemodynamics	Recommended	Recommended if TTE nondiagnostic
2. Detect and assess complications (abscess, perforation, shunt)	Recommended	Recommended
3. Reassessment of valve function in high-risk patients (e.g., virulent organism, clinical deterioration, persistent or recurrent fever, new murmur, persistent bacteremia)	Recommended	
Prosthetic Valve Endocarditis		
1. Diagnosis and complications	TEE is preferred approach	Recommended
2. Patient with a prosthetic valve and a persistent fever without bacteremia or a new murmur.	Reasonable	
3. Reevaluation of prosthetic valve endocarditis during antibiotic therapy in the absence of clinical deterioration.	May be considered	
Peri-operative Management		
1. Preoperative evaluation in patients with known infective endocarditis		Recommended
2. Intraoperative TEE in patients undergoing valve surgery for infective endocarditis		Recommended

Derived from Bonow RO, Carabello BA, Chatterjee K, de LA, Jr., Faxon DP, Freed MD, et al. ACC/AHA 2006 guidelines for the management of patients with valvular heart disease: a report of the American College of Cardiology/American Heart Association Task Force on Practice Guidelines (writing Committee to Revise the 1998 guidelines for the management of patients with valvular heart disease) developed in collaboration with the Society of Cardiovascular Anesthesiologists endorsed by the Society for Cardiovascular Angiography and Interventions and the Society of Thoracic Surgeons. J Am Coll Cardiol 2006 Aug 1;48(3):e1-148.

Recommended = Class I, Reasonable = Class IIa, May be considered = Class IIb.

- ❐ Zoom mode, a narrow sector, high transducer frequency, and harmonic imaging are used to enhance details of valve anatomy (Figure 14–6).
- ❐ An M-mode recording through suspected vegetation seen on 2D imaging helps distinguish

vegetation from an artifact or valve tissue, based on the pattern and speed of motion of the structure.
- ❐ Vegetations may be missed on TTE; transesophageal imaging has a higher sensitivity for

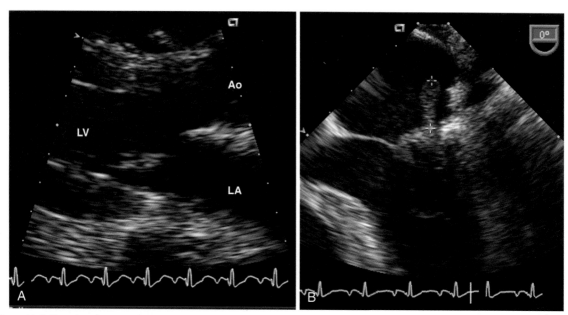

Figure 14–1. Transthoracic (*A*) and TEE (*B*) views of the mitral valve in a patient with bacteremia. The large mobile mitral valve vegetation is easily seen on the TEE images but was barely visible on the transthoracic study. This typical vegetation is attached to the upstream side of the valve (atrial side of mitral valve), is not as echodense as the valve tissue, is irregular in shape, and has a chaotic pattern of motion that is separate from the normal motion of the valve tissue.

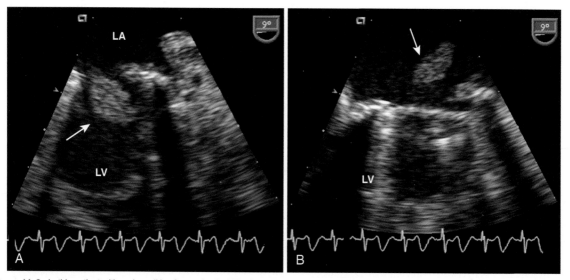

Figure 14–2. In this patient with endocarditis of a mechanical bileaflet mitral valve, the transthoracic study did not show valve vegetations due to shadowing and reverberations by the prosthesis. These TEE images show a large irregular mass, consistent with a vegetation, attached to the valve that prolapses into the LV in diastole (*A*) and the LA in systole (*B*).

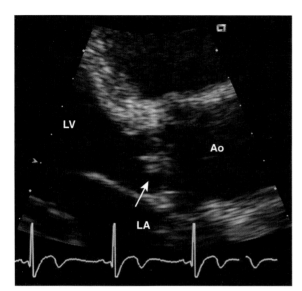

Figure 14–3. Small linear mobile echo densities on the ventricular side of the aortic valve in diastole may be a vegetation or a normal variant called Lambl's excrescences, small fibrous strands attached near the tip of each valve cusp that are more prevalent with age. This patient had positive blood cultures and associated aortic regurgitation, with a clinical course consistent with endocarditis.

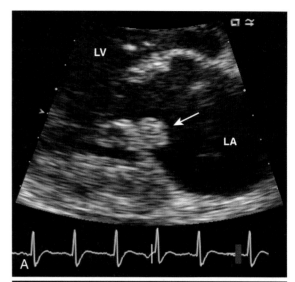

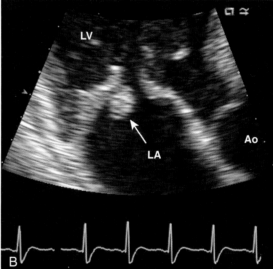

Figure 14–4. Parasternal (A) and apical (B) long-axis zoomed images of the mitral valve show an echodensity on the atrial side of the posterior leaflet, consistent with a vegetation.

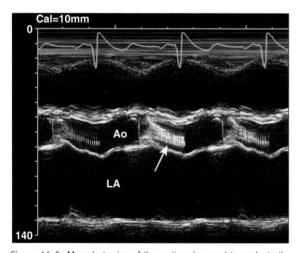

Figure 14–5. M-mode tracing of the aortic valve used to evaluate the motion of a small linear echodensity in a patient referred for possible endocarditis. The M-mode shows fine oscillations of the mass in diastole, suggesting a vegetation rather than nonspecific leaflet thickening.

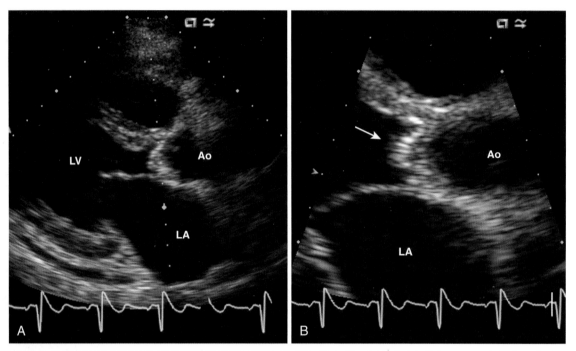

Figure 14–6. This long-axis view at a standard depth (*A*) shows a thickened prolapsing aortic valve in diastole. Using zoom mode (*B*) the valve is seen in more detail with real-time images showing independent rapid oscillating motion of the prolapsing tissue, suggestive of a vegetation.

detection of vegetation due to improved image quality.

❑ Other valve masses may be mistaken for an infected vegetation, including (Figure 14–7):

- Papillary fibroelastoma
- Partial flail mitral leaflet or chord
- Non-bacterial thrombotic endocarditis
- Valve thrombus (especially with prosthetic valves)
- Normal valve variants (such as Lambl's excrescence)
- Ultrasound artifacts

❑ Valvular vegetations tend to decrease in size and increase in echogenicity with effective therapy. However, some vegetations may still be present years after active infection.

Step 4: Evaluate valve dysfunction due to endocarditis

■ Vegetations are associated with distortion of valve anatomy and destruction of valve tissue, typically resulting in valve regurgitation. (Figure 14–8)

■ The presence and severity of valve dysfunction are evaluated no differently than in a patient with valve disease of any cause. (see Chapters 12 and 13)

■ Valve regurgitation in a patient with endocarditis often is acute, rather than chronic, in duration.

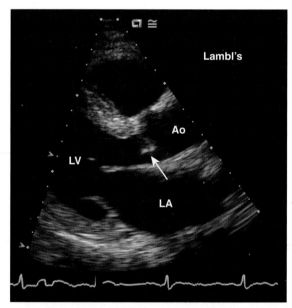

Figure 14–7. Example of a Lambl's excrescence on the aortic valve in diastole. A Lambl's excrescence can be difficult to distinguish from a vegetation but often is smaller, more linear and echodense, is not associated with valve dysfunction, and does not change in size or appearance on sequential studies.

Key points

❑ Vegetations may impede complete valve closure, resulting in regurgitation at the coaptation plane with either native or prosthetic valves.

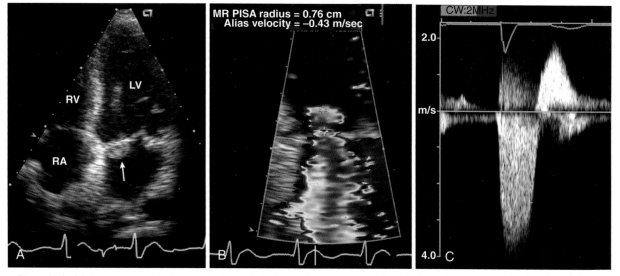

Figure 14–8. A large mass is seen on the LA side of the mitral valve consistent with a vegetation (*A*). Although the mass is distant from the coaptation point, color Doppler shows significant regurgitation, which is quantitated with standard approaches, including the proximal isovelocity surface area method (*B*) and the CW Doppler signal (*C*).

- ❏ Valve destruction results in regurgitation due to leaflet perforation or deformity of the leaflet edge.
- ❏ Regurgitation of prosthetic valves often is paravalvular due to infection in the annulus with valve dehiscence. (Figure 14–9)
- ❏ About 10% of patients with endocarditis do not have significant valve regurgitation due to the location of the vegetation at the leaflet base, which does not impair valve function.
- ❏ Rarely, a large vegetation causes stenosis due to obstruction of the native or prosthetic valve orifice by the vegetation mass.
- ❏ Prosthetic valve stenosis can result from a small, infected vegetation or thrombus impinging on normal disk excursion.

Step 5: Evaluate for the possibility of a paravalvular abscess or fistula

- ■ A paravalvular abscess is present in 20% to 60% of native aortic valve endocarditis cases and in about 15% of mitral valve infections. (Figure 14–10)
- ■ Paravalvular infection occurs in more than 60% of prosthetic valve endocarditis cases.
- ■ On echocardiography, a paravalvular abscess may be echolucent or echodense.
- ■ A paravalvular aortic abscess often communicates with the aortic lumen, appearing as an aneurysm of the sinus of Valsalva. (Figure 14–11)
- ■ Rupture of paravalvular infection into adjacent chambers results in an infected fistula. (Figure 14–12)

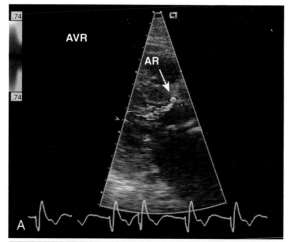

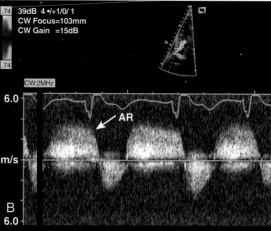

Figure 14–9. An eccentric jet of aortic regurgitation that originates anterior to the valve sewing ring is seen in a parasternal long-axis view (*A*). CW Doppler recorded from the apical window shows a similar density of antegrade and retrograde aortic flow, suggesting significant regurgitation may be present.

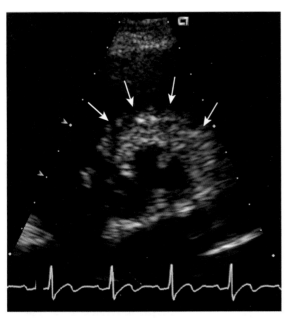

Figure 14–10. A paravalvular abscess can be difficult to detect on transthoracic imaging. In this parasternal short-axis view, there is increased echogenicity in the para-aortic region that may be due to abscess formation.

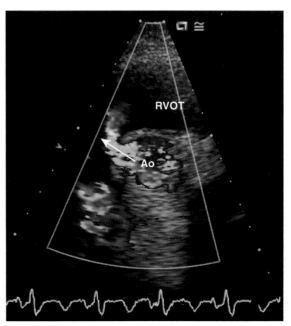

Figure 14–12. Infection of an aortic valve prosthesis resulting in a fistula from the aorta to the RV outflow tract seen on TTE in a parasternal short-axis view. The appearance is similar to a ventricular septal defect, but Doppler interrogation showed both diastolic and systolic flow more consistent with flow from the aorta into the RV.

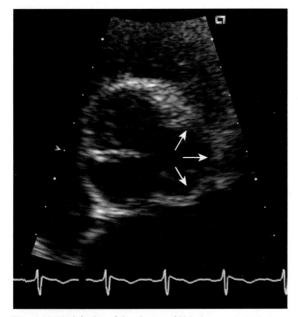

Figure 14–11. Infection of the sinuses of Valsalva can present as an asymmetric dilation of the sinus, as seen with the left coronary sinus of Valsalva in this image. Comparison with previous images and TEE imaging both are helpful in distinguishing an infected sinus from a benign congenital dilation of the sinus.

Key points

☐ TEE is indicated when a paravalvular abscess is suspected because the sensitivity of transthoracic imaging is low.

☐ Aortic paravalvular infection often is recognized based on distortion of the normal contours of the sinuses of Valsalva.

☐ Paravalvular aortic infection may extend into the base of the anterior mitral leaflet, resulting in mitral leaflet perforation. (Figure 14–13)

☐ An aortic paravalvular abscess may rupture into the LV (resulting in severe aortic regurgitation) or into the LA, RA, or RV outflow tract (resulting in a fistula).

☐ With prosthetic aortic valves, infection may result in an aneurysm of the aortic-mitral intervalvular fibrosa (a space between the aortic and mitral valve that communicates with the LV). (Figure 14–14)

☐ A mitral paravalvular abscess may extend into the pericardium, resulting in purulent pericarditis.

Step 6: Measure the hemodynamic consequences of valve dysfunction

■ Valve dysfunction due to endocarditis may result in ventricular dilation and dysfunction or in pulmonary hypertension.

■ Because regurgitation often is acute, evidence of chronic volume overload may be absent even when regurgitation is severe.

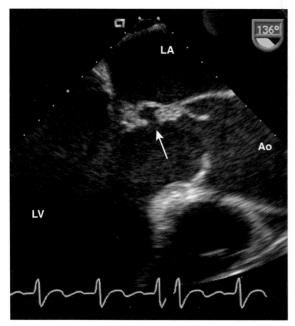

Figure 14–13. In this patient with aortic valve endocarditis, infection has extended into the base of the adjacent anterior mitral leaflet with thickening and a small perforation.

Key points

☐ Evaluation of the patient with endocarditis includes measurement of LV dimensions, volumes, and ejection fraction as detailed in Chapter 6.

☐ Pulmonary systolic pressure is estimated as described in Chapter 6.

☐ Early (mid-diastolic) closure of the mitral valve may be seen on M-mode when acute severe aortic regurgitation is present due to the rapid rise in diastolic LV pressure.

☐ The time course of the CW Doppler recording of valve regurgitation may show evidence of hemodynamic decompensation:

• A rapid decline in velocity in late systole with mitral (or tricuspid) regurgitation suggests a left (or right) atrial v wave.

• A steep diastolic deceleration slope with aortic regurgitation suggests acute regurgitation with an elevated LV end-diastolic pressure. (Figure 14–15)

☐ LV systolic function may be impaired, without LV dilation, with acute severe aortic regurgitation due to endocarditis, possibly due to the effects of systemic infection, combined with a shift to the steep segment of the LV pressure volume curve.

Step 7: Look for other complications of endocarditis

■ More than one cardiac valve may be affected, due either to primary infection at more than one site

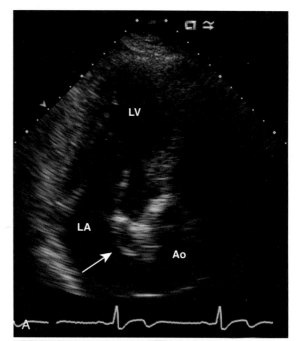

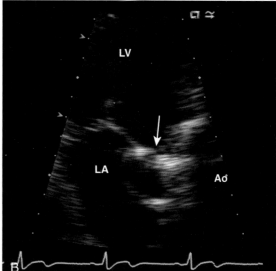

Figure 14–14. In the apical long-axis view (A), a curved pulsatile echo-free space (arrow) is seen between the posterior aortic root and LA. Using zoom mode (B), the narrow neck where this aneurysm of the aortic mitral intervalvular fibrosa communicates with the LV is seen (arrow).

or by direct extension of infection to adjacent structures.

■ Septic coronary artery emboli, resulting in myocardial infarction, occur in 10% of patients.

■ Endocarditis may occur at intracardiac sites other than valve leaflets, including a mitral or tricuspid valve chord, a Chiari network or Eustachian valve, or the RA wall in a region abraded by the tip of a central catheter.

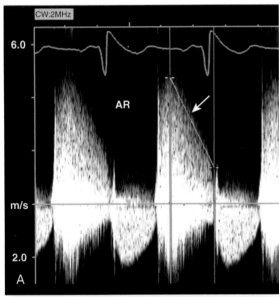

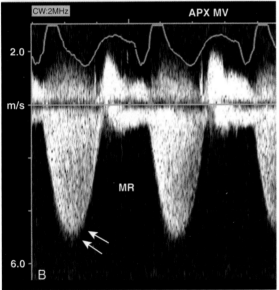

Figure 14–15. Regurgitation due to endocarditis often has an acute onset. Acute aortic regurgitation (A) shows a dense signal with a steep deceleration slope due to rapid equalization of aortic and LV pressures in diastole. With acute mitral regurgitation (B), an early fall-off from peak velocity is due to an increased LA systolic pressure and v wave.

■ A pericardial effusion may be present, either as a nonspecific sign of systemic infection or due to direct extension of infection.

Key points

❏ Once a vegetation has been detected on one valve, careful evaluation for infection of other valves is needed.

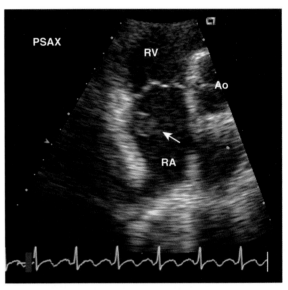

Figure 14–16. A rounded mass is seen in the RA attached to the free wall, near the distal tip of a central venous line, in this zoomed parasternal short-axis view. This might be a thrombus or an infected vegetation, depending on blood culture results and clinical evidence of infection.

❏ The presence of a regional wall motion abnormality in a patient with endocarditis is consistent with a coronary embolus from a valve vegetation.
❏ Intracardiac sites subject to injury, such as the RA wall in a patient with a central catheter or the tricuspid valve in a patient with an indwelling right heart catheter, should be carefully examined for evidence of infection. (Figure 14–16)

SPECIAL SITUATIONS

Right-sided endocarditis

■ Only 6% to 13% of febrile intravenous drug users have endocarditis.
■ In intravenous drug users, infection affects the right side of the heart (predominantly the tricuspid valve) in 75% of cases. (Figure 14–17)
■ Most cases of right-sided endocarditis in drug users are due to *Staphylococcus aureus*, and persistent infection or abscess formation requiring surgery occurs in less than 25% of cases.
■ Pulmonary emboli due to right heart vegetations may result in elevated pulmonary pressures.
■ Left-sided involvement occurs in 25% to 35% of endocarditis cases in patients with a history of intravenous drug use.

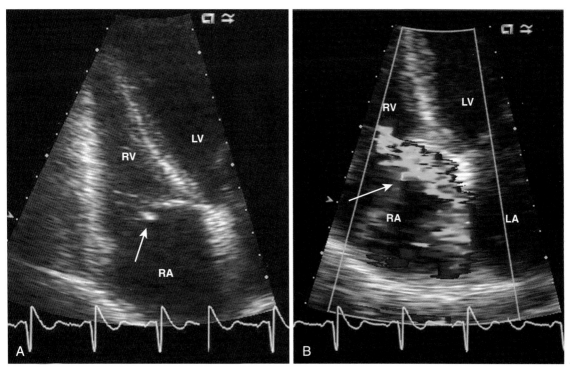

Figure 14–17. In an intravenous drug user with positive blood cultures for *S. aureus,* this apical 4-chamber view with angulation toward the right heart shows a small mobile echodensity on the atrial side of the tricuspid valve (*A*). Color flow (*B*) shows an eccentric jet of moderate tricuspid regurgitation.

- TTE is adequate for evaluation of tricuspid valve endocarditis, but TEE may be needed to exclude left heart involvement.

Prosthetic valves

- Blood cultures should be drawn before any antibiotic therapy in febrile patients with a prosthetic heart valve.
- TEE is indicated in all patients with a prosthetic heart valve and positive blood cultures.
- TEE should be considered in patients with a prosthetic heart valve and suspected endocarditis because transthoracic imaging is inadequate to exclude prosthetic valve infection.
- More than 50% of patients with prosthetic valve endocarditis require surgical intervention.

Pacer/defibrillator leads

- Blood cultures should be drawn before any antibiotic therapy in febrile patients with an intracardiac device.
- If pacer/defibrillator leads are not optimally seen by transthoracic imaging, TEE should be performed.
- Vegetations on the pacer wire are detected in less than 25% of cases on transthoracic imaging but

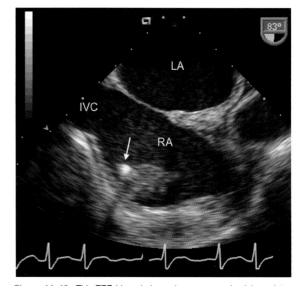

Figure 14–18. This TEE bicaval views shows a pacer lead (*arrow*) traversing the RA chamber with an attached echogenic mass that showed independent mobility. The appearance is consistent with vegetation or a thrombus.

are seen in more than 90% on TEE when infection is present. (Figure 14–18)
- The differential diagnosis of a mobile mass on a pacer lead includes thrombus. Thrombus and vegetation cannot be distinguished by echocardiography.

Staphylococcus aureus bacteremia

- TEE is reasonable in patients with persistently positive blood cultures for *S. aureus*, even if the transthoracic study is negative.
- Chronic indwelling central venous catheters may be a source of thrombus or infection. TEE allows imaging of the catheter tip in the RA in the 90-degree longitudinal view.
- A mobile mass attached to the catheter tip is consistent with thrombus or vegetation.
- Thrombus or infection also may involve the adjacent RA wall.

THE ECHO EXAM

Endocarditis
Duke Criteria (Short Version)

Definite Endocarditis	2 major *or* 1 major + 3 minor *or* 5 minor criteria
Major Criteria	Bacteremia with a typical organism Echo evidence of endocarditis
Minor Criteria	Predisposing condition Fever Vascular phenomenon Immunologic phenomenon Other microbiologic evidence

Echocardiographic Approach

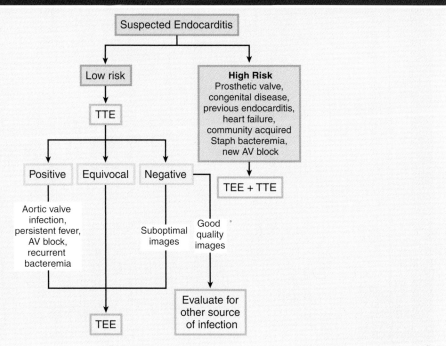

Diagnostic Echo Findings in Endocarditis

	Definition	Exam Points	Diagnostic Value	Limitations
Valvular vegetations	Mass attached to leaflet with independent motion	Use multiple acoustic windows and image planes. Angle between standard views. Use a high-frequency transducer and zoom mode.	Vegetations have high specificity for diagnosis of endocarditis. TEE is more sensitive than TTE for detection of vegetations.	Noninfective masses, healed vegetations, and artifacts may be mistaken for a vegetation.
Leaflet destruction	New or worsening valve regurgitation	Use standard Doppler approaches for detection and quantitation of valve dysfunction. With perforation, the regurgitation jet is from the midportion of leaflet, distant is from expected zones of leaflet coaptation	Valve dysfunction in association with a vegetation is diagnostic for endocarditis.	Other causes of valve dysfunction must be considered. With prosthetic mitral valve, TEE is essential when endocarditis is suspected.
Abscess	Infected area adjacent to valve, usually in the aortic or mitral annulus	Use multiple acoustic windows and image planes. Angle between standard views. Use zoom mode.	TEE is much more sensitive than TTE for detection of paravalvular abscess.	Cardiac abscesses may be echolucent or echodense.
Aneurysm or pseudoaneurysm	Localized dilation of a valve leaflet, aortic sinus or aortic-mitral intervalvular fibrosa (aneurysm), or a contained rupture (pseudoaneurysm)	Look for an abnormal contour of valve leaflets, aortic sinuses, or a space between the base on the anterior mitral leaflet and aortic root. Examine the para-aortic region for excess echodensity. Use color Doppler to examine flow in these regions.	Echo findings of aneurysm or pseudoaneurysm are accurate and can be used for clinical decision making.	TEE often is needed for accurate diagnosis.
Fistula	Abnormal communication between cardiac chambers or great vessels	An aortic paravalvular abscess can rupture into the LA, RA, or RV outflow tract.	Color Doppler detection of abnormal flow combined with pulsed and CW Doppler to define flow hemodynamics is diagnostic for a fistula.	The full extent of tissue destruction is difficult to assess with imaging approaches.
Prosthetic valve dehiscence	Detachment (partial) of the prosthetic valve from the annular tissue	Look for excess motion ("rocking") of the prosthetic valve (>20 degrees).	Valve dehiscence usually is accompanied by severe paravalvular regurgitation.	Valve "rocking" is diagnostic but rarely seen.

CW, continuous wave; LA, left atrium; RA, right atrium; TEE, transesophageal echocardiography; TTE, transthoracic echocardiography.

EXAMPLE

A 28-year-old man with a known bicuspid aortic valve presents with a 2-week history of fevers and fatigue. Physical examination shows a blood pressure of 120/40 mm Hg and a harsh diastolic murmur at the left sternal border. Blood cultures (three sets) are positive for *Streptococcus viridans*. With a predisposing factor, fevers, and positive blood cultures with a typical organism, the pretest likelihood of endocarditis is very high (>90%).

Transthoracic echocardiography (TTE) shows a bicuspid aortic valve with a mass on the ventricular side of the leaflets with independent motion. LV size and systolic function are normal. Color flow Doppler shows aortic regurgitation with an eccentric jet and a vena contracta width of 7 mm, CW Doppler shows a dense signal with a deceleration slope of 120 ms, and there is holodiastolic flow reversal in the proximal abdominal aorta.

The TTE findings are diagnostic for endocarditis, so that this patient now has two major Duke criteria and a diagnosis of *definite endocarditis*. With his bicuspid aortic valve, there may have been some degree of underlying aortic regurgitation. However, the normal LV size and the steep deceleration slope of the CW aortic regurgitant jet are consistent with superimposed *acute* aortic regurgitation. Aortic regurgitation is *severe* as evidenced by a wide vena contracta and holodiastolic flow reversal in the aorta.

The following day, a prolonged PR interval (first-degree atrioventricular block) is noted on the echocardiogram and transesophageal echocardiography (TEE) is performed. The TEE shows an echolucent area in the aortic annulus region consistent with abscess and the patient is referred for prompt surgical intervention.

SELF-ASSESSMENT QUESTIONS

QUESTION 1

Echocardiography is requested in a 32-year-old man with no prior medical problems, who presented with a 2-week history of fevers and fatigue and was found to have blood cultures positive for *Staphylococcus aureus*. Evaluation for the cause of bacteria has been unrevealing. Physical examination is remarkable only for a temperature of 38.5° C and a systolic murmur.

Which of these additional echocardiographic findings would then meet the Duke criteria for definite endocarditis?

 A. Mitral valve prolapse
 B. Mild mitral regurgitation
 C. Bicuspid aortic valve
 D. Pulmonic regurgitation
 E. None of the above

QUESTION 2

Echocardiography is requested in a 28-year-old woman with a known mitral valve prolapse, fevers, and blood cultures positive for *Streptococcus viridans*. Physical examination demonstrates a mid-systolic click and late systolic murmur at the apex, radiating to the axilla, consistent with mitral valve prolapse. There is no evidence of heart failure on exam. Echocardiography shows mitral valve prolapse with mild to moderate late-systolic mitral regurgitation.

The most appropriate next step is:

 A. Transesophageal echocardiogram
 B. Compare with previous echocardiograms
 C. Reassurance with watchful waiting
 D. 2-week course of IV antibiotics
 E. Repeat echo in 2 weeks

QUESTION 3

Echocardiography was requested in this 36-year-old man with a 1-week history of fever and a new murmur. He has no history of cardiac dysfunction, denies intravenous drug use, and is taking no medications.

Physical exam shows an ill-appearing man with a temperature of 38.5° C, a blood pressure of 95/61 mm Hg, and a pulse of 110 bpm. Laboratory data and blood cultures are pending.

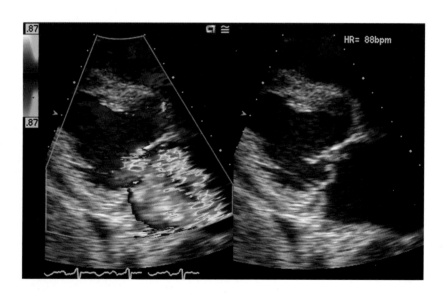

Figure 14–19.

List five abnormal findings evident on this image:

1. _____
2. _____
3. _____
4. _____
5. _____

QUESTION 4

A 62-year-old man is admitted to the intensive care unit with hypotension and pulmonary edema. After endotracheal intubation and stabilization, a bedside echocardiogram is performed. This tracing is recorded from an apical window.

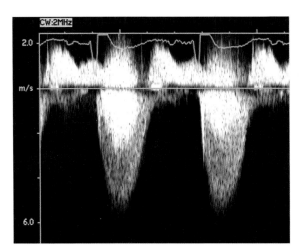

Figure 14–20.

The most likely diagnosis is:

A. Moderate mitral stenosis
B. Severe aortic stenosis
C. Ventricular septal rupture
D. Severe pulmonary hypertensions
E. Acute mitral regurgitation

QUESTION 5

A 24-year-old woman presents for evaluation of a murmur. She has a history of aortic valve endocarditis complicated by an aortic annular abscess for which she underwent homograft aortic valve replacement 3 months ago.

The findings in this parasternal short-axis view (Figure 14–21) and the CW Doppler recording of the flow disturbance is most consistent with:

A. Aortic regurgitation
B. Ventricular septal defect
C. Aorta to LA fistula
D. Perforated anterior mitral leaflet
E. Aortic annular abscess

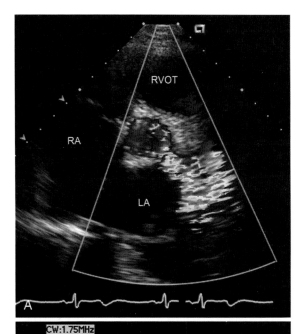

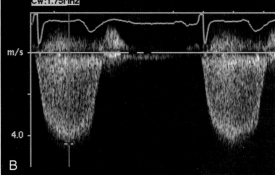

Figure 14–21.

QUESTION 6

A 67-year-old man in the intensive care unit with pneumonia and respiratory failure is referred for echocardiography for possible endocarditis, in the setting of fevers and positive blood cultures. A still-frame long-axis view of the mitral valve is shown (Figure 14–22).

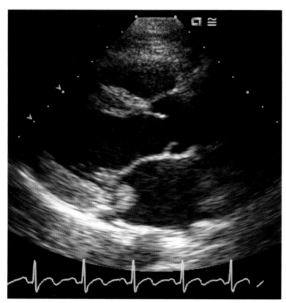

Figure 14–22.

What feature of this mitral valve abnormality would most reliably distinguish a vegetation from mitral valve prolapse?

- A. Diffuse leaflet thickening
- B. Systolic prolapse into the LA
- C. Independent mobility
- D. Involvement of both leaflets
- E. Severity of mitral regurgitation

QUESTION 7

TTE was requested in a 69-year-old man with end-stage liver disease and a fever. He has no history of cardiac disease and blood cultures are negative. An echocardiogram is obtained (Figure 14–23).

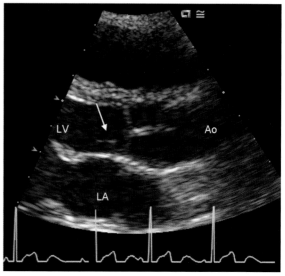

Figure 14–23.

The most likely diagnosis is:

- A. Bacterial endocarditis
- B. Lambl's excrescence
- C. Papillary fibroelastoma
- D. Nonbacterial thrombotic endocarditis
- E. Ultrasound artifact

QUESTION 8

A 61-year-old man with a history of multiple myeloma presents with a 2-week history of increasing lower extremity edema and is noted to have a new systolic murmur on examination. The following images are obtained (Figure 14–24).

The best next step for quantitation of regurgitant severity is:

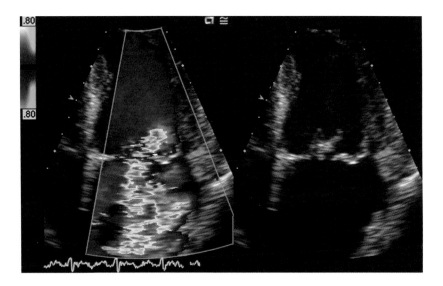

Figure 14–24.

A. Transesophageal echocardiography
B. Increase Nyquist limit to 1.2 m/s
C. Increase color Doppler gain
D. Widen color Doppler sector scan
E. Move color Doppler velocity baseline

QUESTION 9

In a 61-year-old man (same patient as question 8) with new onset mitral regurgitation and probable endocarditis, the following data were obtained.

Calculate:

Regurgitant orifice area _____

Regurgitant volume _____

Overall regurgitation severity _____

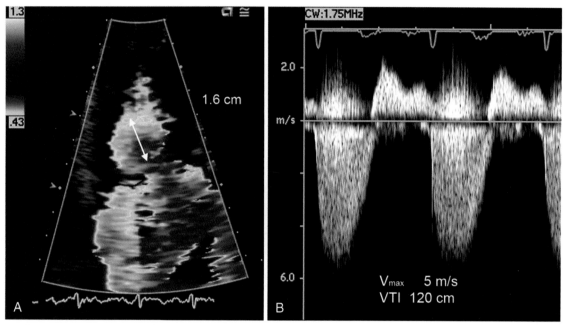

Figure 14–25.

ANSWERS

ANSWER 1: E

This patient has one major criteria (typical blood cultures for endocarditis) and one minor criteria (fever) and thus only meets the Duke criteria for *possible* endocarditis before the echocardiogram is requested. The major criteria for endocarditis on echocardiography are a definite valvular vegetation, paravalvular abscess, prosthetic valve dehiscence, or new valvular regurgitation. This patient does not have any of these findings; mild mitral and pulmonic regurgitation are seen in most normal adults and are not considered diagnostic for new valve regurgitation. Mitral valve prolapse and bicuspid aortic valve are anatomic conditions that predispose to endocarditis and are considered only a minor criteria for the diagnosis. The diagnosis of definite endocarditis requires two major or one major plus three minor criteria; in this example there are at most one major plus two minor criteria.

ANSWER 2: A

In the American College of Cardiology/American Heart Association (ACC/AHA) 2006 recommendations for echocardiography in infective endocarditis, TEE is recommended in patients with known valvular heart disease, positive blood cultures, and a nondiagnostic transthoracic study. Thus, TEE imaging is recommended in this patient because the likelihood of endocarditis is high and the TEE has a higher sensitivity than TTE for detection of a valvular vegetation. Although comparison with previous echocardiograms is appropriate, TEE should be performed even if there is no obvious change on side-by-side comparison of images. Reassurance with watchful waiting is not appropriate because this patient most likely has endocarditis. Antibiotics should be started immediately but the duration of therapy should be longer than 2 weeks if endocarditis is present. Repeat echocardiography in 2 weeks is most helpful in following treatment of endocarditis to ensure vegetation size is stable or decreasing with effective therapy. In some lower risk patients, it may be reasonable to defer TEE and repeat a TTE in several days when endocarditis is a possibility but this approach would not be appropriate in this higher-risk patient.

ANSWER 3

These color and 2D long-axis images show:

LA enlargement
LV enlargement
Posterior mitral leaflet prolapse

A vegetation on the anterior mitral valve leaflet, near the coaptation point
Anteriorly directed mitral regurgitation

The clinical presentation is consistent with bacterial endocarditis, and if his blood cultures are positive, the finding of a valvular vegetation on echocardiography is diagnostic based on the Duke criteria. In addition, it is likely that this patient has worsening of undiagnosed chronic mitral regurgitation due to mitral valve prolapse to explain the LA and LV enlargement, which are atypical for acute valve regurgitation.

ANSWER 4: E

This high-velocity systolic signal directed away from the apex might be due to aortic stenosis, mitral regurgitation, tricuspid regurgitation (if severe pulmonary hypertension is present), or a ventricular septal defect. All of these are possible with this clinical presentation; for example, this patient could have a post–myocardial infarction ventricular septal defect or papillary muscle rupture. This signal can be identified as mitral regurgitation based on the timing relative to the QRS (starts early) and associated diastolic flow signal. In diastole, an LV filling curve is seen with an E and A wave, with velocities typical of left (not right) heart filling. The systolic signal begins and ends exactly at the end and beginning of the diastolic flow signal, confirming this is mitral regurgitation, not aortic stenosis, which would have slight gaps in the onset and offset of flow due to isovolumic contraction and relaxation. In fact, the denser aortic signal can be seen "underneath" the mitral regurgitant signal on the first beat. The shape of the velocity curve is suggestive of *acute* regurgitation, with a rapid decline in velocity in late systole, instead of the more rounded waveform of chronic regurgitation. With acute regurgitation, the rise in LV pressure (or v wave) as the regurgitant flow fills the small noncompliant chamber results in a smaller pressure difference (and lower velocity) between the LV and LA. Endocarditis can present as pulmonary edema or cardiogenic shock if there is valve destruction with severe regurgitation, as in this example. Echocardiography reliability identifies the valve dysfunction and may demonstrate the cause of regurgitation—for example, vegetations consistent with endocarditis or a wall motion abnormality and papillary muscle rupture consistent with myocardial infarction. In addition to stabilizing the patient, blood cultures should be obtained when new severe regurgitation is present. Mitral stenosis can present acutely if there is a concurrent medical issue (such as infection or anemia) with increased cardiac demand, but Doppler would show the typical *diastolic* flow signal. A high-velocity tricuspid regurgitant jet due to pulmonary hypertension is longer in duration than mitral regurgitation and the associated flow in diastole is lower-velocity tricuspid, not mitral, inflow. It can be challenging to separate a ventricular septal defect signal from mitral regurgitation, but duration typically is longer and the mitral inflow signal is usually not seen in diastole. Instead, low-velocity left to right flow across the septal defect may be seen in diastole along with the high velocity systolic jet.

ANSWER 5: D

These findings are consistent with a perforated anterior mitral leaflet. The color Doppler image demonstrates a flow disturbance entering the LA from either the aorta or the LV outflow tract; it is difficult to be certain of the position of this image plane relative to the aortic valve in the short-axis plane. The corresponding long-axis view showed the flow disturbance originating at the base of the anterior mitral leaflet. Review of the operative report showed that the aortic homograft was trimmed to retain a segment of the anterior mitral leaflet base, which was used to repair the native mitral valve. The perforation is between the homograft and native leaflet tissue. The CW Doppler is diagnostic showing a high-velocity systolic waveform consistent with mitral regurgitation. Although the Doppler signal for a ventricular septal defect might be similar, there usually is a low-velocity diastolic component because of the slight diastolic pressure difference between the ventricles, and the color flow image is not consistent with a ventricular septal defect. An aortic to LA fistula would exhibit high-velocity systolic *and diastolic* flow due to the higher aortic, relative to LA, diastolic pressure. An aortic annular abscess may have areas of flow, but the CW Doppler velocity is low and the color signal is localized to the area adjacent to the valve. Aortic regurgitation is a likely complication of endocarditis but, of course, is a diastolic flow signal from the aorta into the LV.

ANSWER 6: C

The typical finding with either mitral valve prolapse or a mitral valve vegetation is an echogenic mass (leaflet or vegetation) that prolapses into the LA in systole. Diffuse leaflet thickening is a nonspecific finding that often is present with mitral prolapse; however, a vegetation cannot be excluded if the valve is abnormal. The most useful distinguishing feature of a vegetation is rapid chaotic motion that is independent of the motion of the mitral valve leaflet. This may be demonstrated by 2D imaging, but M-mode can be helpful to demonstrate the irregular motion,

separate from leaflet motion. Distinguishing a ruptured chord from a vegetation is problematic as both show independent mobility, although a ruptured chord usually is thinner and shorter than a vegetation and the tip points toward the roof of the LA. Both mitral valve prolapse and endocarditis may involve one or both leaflets; the severity of mitral regurgitation will depend on the extent of mitral prolapse or the degree of tissue destruction with endocarditis and thus does not distinguish between these processes.

ANSWER 7: B

A faint linear echodensity is seen in the LV outflow tract with a normal aortic valve and normal-size LV and LA. This appearance is most consistent with a Lambl's excrescence—a small filamentous structure, more often seen on the ventricular side of the valve—which is a normal variant with an increasing prevalence with age. Endocarditis typically results in larger vegetations on the downstream side of the valve (LV side of aortic valve) in association with leaflet tissue destruction resulting in valve regurgitation. A papillary fibroelastoma is a benign tumor attached to the valve leaflet that appears as a mobile mass; although typically an incidental finding, a larger papillary fibroelastoma can be associated with thrombosis and adverse clinical events. Nonbacterial thrombotic endocarditis typically appears as a globular mass (or masses) attached to the upstream side (aortic side of aortic valve) in patients with systemic inflammatory disorders. These vegetations tend to be multiple, sessile masses on the leaflets. This might be an ultrasound artifact given the smooth linear appearance, but there is no obvious structure between the mass and transducer that might cause a reverberation artifact at this location.

ANSWER 8: E

These images show an abnormal mitral valve with irregular thickening and incomplete leaflet coaptation. Although a definite valvular vegetation is not seen, these changes are concerning for tissue destruction; endocarditis is a strong possibility given these findings, especially if the murmur is new. Mitral regurgitation severity can be quantitated in this view from measurement of the proximal isovelocity surface area (PISA). The first step is to change the aliasing velocity (Nyquist limit) to about 0.3 to 0.4 m/s, which can be done by decreasing the Nyquist limit directly, but preferably is done by moving the color Doppler baseline down so that aliasing of flow away from the transducer occurs at a lower velocity. This provides a larger (more easily measured) and more hemispheral shape of the PISA. TEE is helpful when transthoracic images are suboptimal but is not needed for quantitation with excellent images, as in this case. The Nyquist limit is determined by the color sector depth and can only be decreased, not increased. Widening the color sector might show more of the LA but would decrease frame rate and would not be helpful in imaging proximal jet geometry.

ANSWER 9

Regurgitation orifice area: 1.38 cm^2
Regurgitant volume 166 ml
Overall regurgitant severity: Severe

The color Doppler image has been optimized for measurement of the PISA, with the color scale showing no variance and with the baseline moved so that the aliasing velocity for flow away from the transducer is 0.43 m/s, which then is the velocity at the color change that defines the PISA. The radius of the PISA (from color change to valve plane) is 1.6 cm. The surface area of the PISA is

$$2\pi r^2 = 2(3.14)(1.6 \text{ cm})^2 = 16 \text{ cm}^2$$

The instantaneous regurgitant orifice area (ROA) is this surface area multiplied by the aliasing velocity and then divided by the maximum mitral regurgitant jet velocity (units of m/s are converted to cm/s to match the units of the PISA measurement in cm^2):

$$ROA = (16 \text{ cm}^2 \times 43 \text{ cm/s})/500 \text{ cm/s} = 1.38 \text{ cm}^2$$

Regurgitant volume is calculated by multiplying the ROA by the mitral regurgitant velocity-time integral (VTI), in this case,

$$1.38 \text{ cm}^2 \times 120 \text{ cm} = 166 \text{ cm}^3 \text{ or } 166 \text{ mL}$$

This is very severe mitral regurgitation, with severe defined as a ROA ≥ 0.4 cm^2 and a regurgitant volume of 60 mL or greater.

Cardiac Masses and Potential Cardiac Source of Embolus

BASIC PRINCIPLES

STEP-BY-STEP APPROACH
    Left Atrial Thrombi
    Left Ventricular Thrombi
    Right Heart Thrombi
    Nonprimary Cardiac Tumors
    Primary Cardiac Tumors

    Vegetations
    Benign Valve-Associated Lesions
    Patent Foramen Ovale
    Evaluation for Cardiac Source of Embolus

THE ECHO EXAM

SELF-ASSESSMENT QUESTIONS

BASIC PRINCIPLES

■ The first step in evaluation of a cardiac mass on echocardiography is to determine if the findings are due to an ultrasound artifact or an actual anatomic finding. (Figure 15–1)

■ A prominent normal cardiac structure of a normal anatomic variant may be mistaken for an abnormal mass.

■ Ultrasound has limited utility for determination of tissue type; diagnosis of a cardiac mass is based on location, attachment, appearance, and any associated abnormalities.

Key points

❑ Image quality for evaluation of a cardiac mass is optimized by using:
  • Highest transducer frequency with adequate tissue penetration
  • Acoustic access adjacent to the structure of interest (e.g., transthoracic apical for ventricular thrombi versus transesophageal [TEE] for atrial thrombi)
  • Visualization of the motion of the mass with the cardiac cycle
  • Use of a narrow sector and zoom mode once a mass is identified
  • Careful gain and processing adjustments (excessive or inadequate gain can obscure a mass)
  • Off-axis views from standard image planes

❑ A detailed knowledge of cardiac anatomy and normal variants allows recognition of structures that may mimic a cardiac mass.

❑ Echocardiography cannot identify the etiology of a cardiac mass based on appearance. A differential diagnosis for the echocardiographic finding is based on the location, appearance, size, mobility, physiologic effects, and other findings associated with the mass.

❑ Clinical data and other echocardiographic findings often provide clues about the identity of a cardiac mass (e.g., a left atrial mass in a patient with severe rheumatic mitral stenosis likely is an atrial thrombus).

STEP-BY-STEP APPROACH

Left atrial thrombi

■ Left atrial thrombi most often form in the atrial appendage, particularly in patients with atrial fibrillation. (Figure 15–2)

■ Thrombi may be seen in the body of the LA with severe stasis of blood flow (e.g., with mitral stenosis).

■ TEE is required to exclude LA thrombi when clinically indicated.

Key points

❑ TTE is not sensitive for the diagnosis of LA thrombi due to the distance between the transducer and LA (limiting image quality at that depth) and the small size and location in the atrial appendage of most thrombi.

❒ The LA appendage may be visualized on trans- thoracic imaging in a parasternal short-axis view or in an apical two-chamber view, but image quality often is limited.

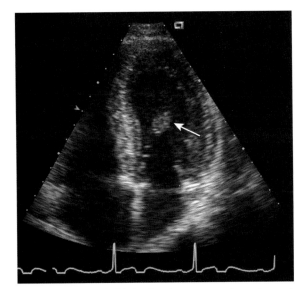

Figure 15–1. In this apical 4-chamber view, an apparent mass is seen in the LV chamber. Given the relationship of this mass to the anterior mitral leaflet, this most likely is a normal papillary muscle tip, seen in a oblique view. This diagnosis can be confirmed by scanning posteriorly to show its connection to the lateral LV wall.

❒ TEE images of the LA appendage are obtained from a high esophageal position. Evaluation includes:

- Use of a high transducer frequency (typically 7 MHz)
- A narrow image sector and zoom mode
- Visualization in at least two orthogonal views, typically in views rotated to 0 degrees and 60 degrees
- Pulsed Doppler recording of atrial appendage flow with the sample volume about 1 cm from the junction of the atrial appendage with the LA chamber

❒ The normal Doppler velocity with atrial con- traction is more than 0.4 m/s; lower velocities in sinus rhythm suggest contractile dysfunction.

❒ The LA appendage has normal trabeculations that are distinguished from thrombus by their continuity with and echogenicity similar to the appendage wall, as well as their lack of indepen- dent mobility. (Figure 15–3)

❒ Reverberation artifact from the ridge between the left upper pulmonary vein and LA append- age may hinder definitive exclusion of an appendage thrombus.

Left ventricular thrombi

■ LV thrombus formation occurs in regions of blood flow stasis or low-velocity flow.

■ LV thrombi most often form in an akinetic or dyskinetic apex after myocardial infarction. (Figure 15–4)

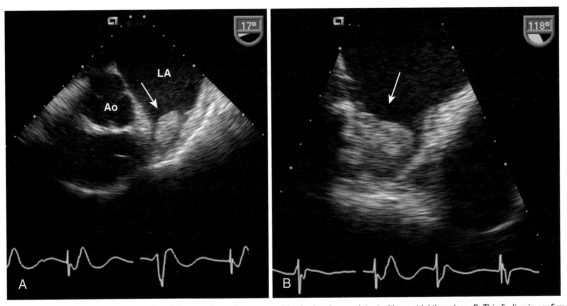

Figure 15–2. A, Transesophageal view of the LA appendage shows an ovoid echodensity consistent with an atrial thrombus. B, This finding is confirmed in an orthogonal view at 118 degree rotation using a magnified image.

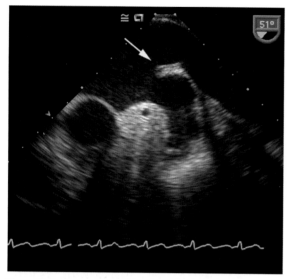

Figure 15–3. Transesophageal imaging of the LA appendage at about 50 degrees using a 7 MHz transducer frequency. The normal ridge between the LA appendage and left superior pulmonary vein is well seen (*arrow*). The LA appendage was imaged in several planes to evaluate for possible thrombus. The small circular echolucent structure seen between the LV outflow tract and LA is a cross section of the circumflex coronary artery.

■ LV thrombi also are seen in patients with severely reduced LV systolic dysfunction.

Key points

❑ TTE from the apical window is the optimal approach to detection of LV thrombi, with a sensitivity of 92% to 95% and a specificity of 86% to 88%.
❑ Detection of LV apical thrombi is enhanced by:
  • A steep left lateral decubitus patient position on a stretcher with an apical cutout
  • Use of a high transducer frequency (typically 5-7 MHz)
  • Standard and oblique image planes of the apex, especially medial angulation from a lateral transducer position
  • A shallow depth setting
❑ Myocardial trabeculations are differentiated from thrombi by their linear shape with an echodensity similar to and attachment to the myocardium. (Figure 15–5)
❑ Left echo contrast is helpful is identifying thrombus when image quality is suboptimal.
❑ Transesophageal imaging is not sensitive for diagnosis of LV apical thrombi because the apex is in the far field of the image and the true apex may not be included in the image plane.

Right heart thrombi

■ RA thrombi may be seen in patients with central lines that abrade the RA wall.
■ Thrombi also may form on permanent pacer leads in the RA or RV.
■ Peripheral venous thrombi may embolize to the right heart and become entangled in the tricuspid valve chords or a RA Chiari network. (Figure 15–6)

Key points

❑ Normal echogenic structures in the RA that may be mistaken for a thrombus include:
  • Eustachian valve or Chiari network. (Figure 15–7) *and*
  • Crista terminalis. (Figure 15–8)
❑ Eustachian valves and Chiari networks are thin filamentous structures that extend from the region of the inferior vena cava toward the superior vena cava. The bright mobile echos of a Chiari network may look similar to echo contrast in the RA.
❑ The RA and RV are examined in parasternal short-axis and RV inflow views, in the apical 4-chamber view, and from the subcostal window.
❑ Transesophageal imaging provides improved visualization of the right heart when thrombi are suspected.

Nonprimary cardiac tumors

■ Nonprimary cardiac tumors are 20 times more common than primary cardiac tumors.
■ Nonprimary tumors can involve the heart by:
  • Direct extension
  • Metastatic spread of disease
  • Production of biologically active substances
  • Side effects related to treatment of the primary tumor
■ Nonprimary cardiac tumors most often involve the pericardium but also may invade the myocardium. They rarely appear as intracardiac masses. (Figure 15–9)

Key points

❑ The most common nonprimary cardiac tumors, in order of frequency, are:
  • Lung
  • Lymphoma
  • Breast
  • Leukemia
  • Stomach
  • Melanoma
  • Liver
  • Colon

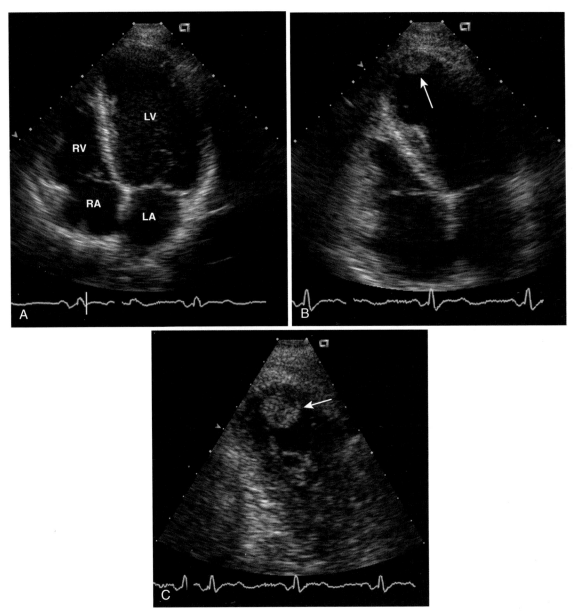

Figure 15–4. *A,* In the standard apical 4-chamber view in the patient with a dilated cardiomyopathy, there is no evidence for thrombus formation in the akinetic apex, despite using harmonic imaging and a 4 MHz transducer frequency. *B,* However, with a slight decrease in depth, increase in gain, adjustment of focal depth, and posterior angulation of the image plane, a protruding apical thrombus now is evident. *C,* The apical thrombus is best seen at a shallower image depth with further posterior angulation of the image plane.

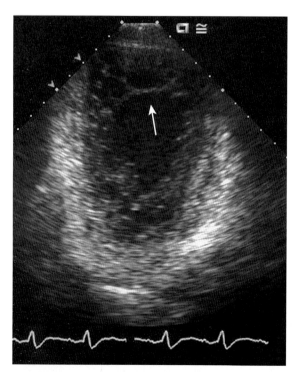

Figure 15–5. An echodensity was seen in the LV apex. The transducer frequency was increased to 4 MHz, the focal depth decreased, and the transducer moved medially and angulated laterally from the apical position for further evaluation. The linear echo traversing the apex is consistent with prominent trabeculation, not thrombus, because it connects with myocardium at both ends.

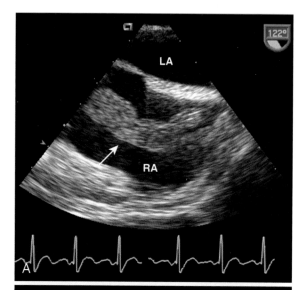

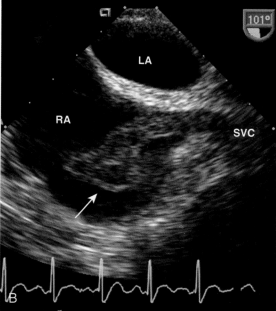

Figure 15–6. *A*, In this TEE long-axis view of the RA, a large, echogenic, tubular, mobile mass is seen in the RA. *B*, Slight medial turning of the TEE probe demonstrates that the mass originates from the region of the superior vena cava. By imaging in multiple planes, the attachment of this mass to a chronic indwelling catheter was demonstrated. The location, clinical setting, and appearance of the mass are most consistent with thrombus.

- ❐ All these tumors may involve the pericardium by direct extension (breast, lung) or by metastatic spread, presenting with a pericardial effusion, sometimes with tamponade physiology. (Figure 15–10)
- ❐ Renal cell carcinoma may extend up the inferior vena cava into the RA and may be removed surgically "en bloc" with the primary tumor.
- ❐ Carcinoid heart disease is characterized by thickening and shortening of the right heart valve leaflets, resulting in pulmonic and tricuspid regurgitation.
- ❐ Some chemotherapy affects myocardial function, so periodic monitoring of ejection fraction by echocardiography often is recommended.
- ❐ Radiation therapy that included cardiac structures in the treatment field may have very late (20 years or greater) adverse cardiac effects, including valve disease, accelerated coronary atherosclerosis, pericardial constriction, and myocardial fibrosis.
- ❐ TTE in standard views usually is adequate for evaluation of nonprimary cardiac tumors, but

TEE provides improved image quality when needed.

Primary cardiac tumors

- ■ Primary cardiac tumors in adults usually are histologically benign.

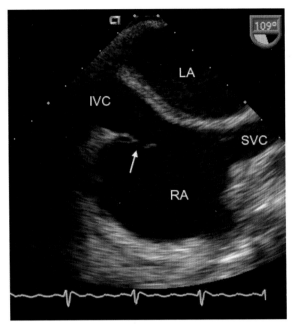

Figure 15–7. In this TEE bicaval view, a linear mobile echo originating from the junction of the inferior vena cava (*IVC*) and right atrium (*RA*) is seen, consistent with a normal Eustachian valve. In some patients this embryologic remnant is more extensive, forming a network of filamentous strands extending from the region of the inferior to the superior vena cava (*SVC*). This finding, called a Chiari network, may appear on TTE imaging as bright mobile echos with chaotic motion in the RA often best appreciated in parasternal short axis, RV inflow and subcostal 4-chamber views.

- Benign cardiac tumors result in adverse clinical outcomes due to:
  - Obstruction of blood flow *and*
  - Embolization
- Primary cardiac tumors most often present on echocardiography as an intracardiac mass.

Key points

- ☐ The most common primary cardiac tumors in adults, in order of frequency, are:
  - Myxoma (Figure 15–11)
  - Pericardial cyst
  - Lipoma
  - Papillary fibroelastoma (Figure 15–12)
  - Angiosarcoma (malignant)
  - Rhabdomyosarcoma (malignant)
- ☐ Myxomas most often are seen in the LA (75% of cases), attached by a narrow stalk to the center of the interatrial septum. Myxomas less often are seen in the RA, LV, and RV.
- ☐ A pericardial cyst is a single or multilobed sac lined by mesothelium that communicates with the pericardial space. Pericardial cysts are rare but, when present, most often are seen adjacent to the RA.

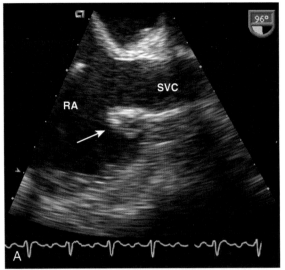

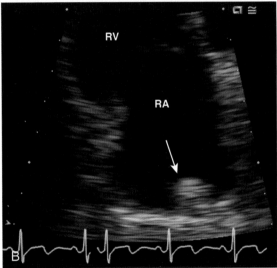

Figure 15–8. This TEE long-axis image (*A*) of the superior vena cava (*SVC*) and right atrium (*RA*) demonstrates the crista terminalis (*arrow*), the ridge at the junction of the trabeculated and smooth segments of the RA wall. The crista terminalis often is seen in the transthoracic apical 4-chamber view (*B*) as a slight bump on the superior aspect of the RA wall.

- ☐ Papillary fibroelastomas typically are small masses attached to the downstream side of a cardiac valve. The appearance is similar to a vegetation (except that vegetations usually are on the upstream side of the valve) but blood cultures are negative and clinical signs of endocarditis are absent.
- ☐ Lipomatous hypertrophy of the interatrial septum is common, with a typical appearance of sparing of the fossa ovalis. If in doubt, computed tomographic imaging confirms adipose tissue.
- ☐ Malignant primary cardiac tumors are rare, usually seen as an intracardiac mass.

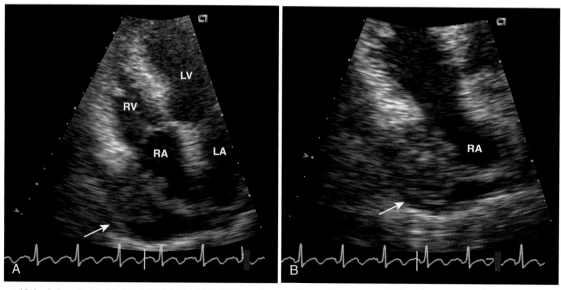

Figure 15–9. *A,* An apical 4-chamber view shows an inhomogeneous mass either attached to or invading the RA free wall. *B,* A magnified view shows the anatomy in more detail but does not provide a tissue diagnosis. This mass clearly is not an artifact, thrombus, vegetation, or normal variant. A benign primary cardiac tumor is unlikely because the appearance is atypical for a myxoma or fibroma, given the apparent involvement of the atrial wall. Thus, this most likely is a metastatic tumor of the heart or, less likely, a primary cardiac malignancy.

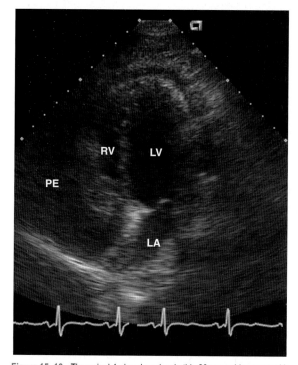

Figure 15–10. The apical 4-chamber view in this 29-year-old woman with non-Hodgkin's lymphoma shows a large pericardial effusion (*PE*) that compresses the RV. The RA is nearly obliterated and could only be identified with color flow imaging. Cardiac tumors may present with an effusion, without a mass.

❏ The goals of echocardiography in patients with a cardiac tumor are:
  • Define the location and extent of tumor involvement
  • Evaluate obstruction or regurgitation due to the tumor
  • Evaluate any associated pericardial effusion and signs of tamponade
❏ Often both transthoracic and transesophageal imaging are needed to fully evaluate a cardiac tumor. Masses located in the LA may be missed on transthoracic imaging. (Figure 15–13)

Vegetations

■ Vegetations are infected or noninfected masses of platelets and fibrin debris, typically attached to a valve leaflet.
■ The vegetations of nonbacterial thrombotic endocarditis (NBTE) are small and attached to the downstream (compared with upstream with infective vegetations) side of the valve. (Figure 15–14)
■ Infective vegetations are discussed in Chapter 14.

Key points

❏ The most critical step in evaluation of a patient with an intracardiac mass, especially a valve vegetation, is to obtain blood cultures for possible infective endocarditis.
❏ Like infective endocarditis, nonbacterial thrombotic endocarditis is diagnosed based on a

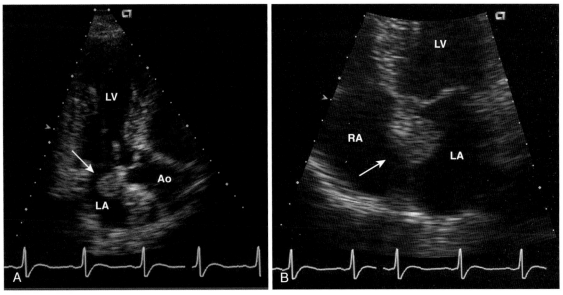

Figure 15–11. The location and smooth contour of this LA mass, seen in an apical long axis view (A) and a 4-chamber view (B), is consistent with an atrial myxoma.

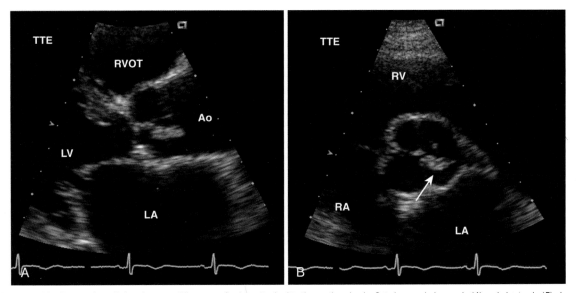

Figure 15–12. On transthoracic imaging, a mobile mass of echos attached to the aortic valve leaflets is seen in long axis (A) and short axis (B) views. This patient had no clinical evidence of infective endocarditis and no evidence for a systemic inflammatory disease, so the most likely diagnosis is a papillary fibroelastoma.

combination of clinical and echocardiographic findings.

- ❑ TEE is more accurate for diagnosis of nonbacterial valve vegetations compared with transthoracic imaging.
- ❑ Valve involvement by noninfected vegetations is seen in patients with systemic inflammatory diseases (i.e., systemic lupus erythematosus) and some malignancies.

Benign valve-associated lesions

- ■ Nodules of Arantius are small nodules at the central coaptation points of the semilunar valves.
- ■ Lambl's excrescences are thin, mobile, linear echodensities seen on the downstream side of a valve, most commonly the aortic valve.
- ■ Calcification of the posterior mitral annulus is common in the elderly.

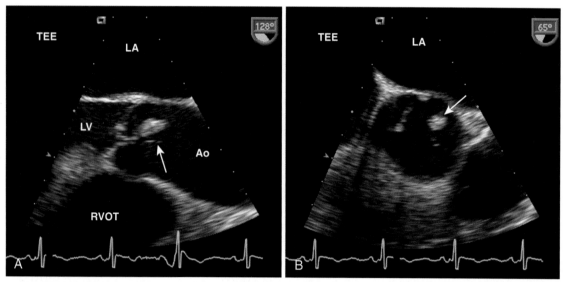

Figure 15–13. In the same patient as Figure 15–12, TEE imaging in long-(A) and short-(B) axis views of the aortic valve appear similar to the transthoracic views, although image quality is improved due to use of a 7 MHz TEE transducer.

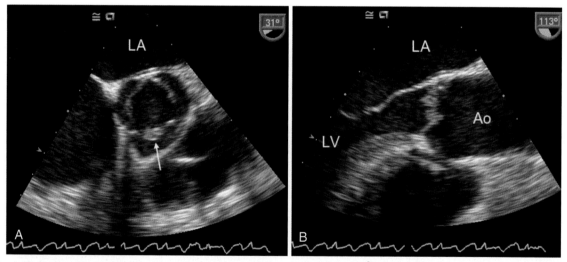

Figure 15–14. A small mass (arrow) is seen on the right coronary cusp of the aortic valve on this TEE short-axis image (A) with the long-axis view (B) showing small masses at the leaflet base and at the leaflet tip. These masses showed independent motion in real time suggestive of vegetations. The patient had no clinical signs of endocarditis and blood cultures were negative, so these findings may be due to nonbacterial thrombotic endocarditis.

Key points

- ❏ Nodules of Arantius typically are more prominent with age on the aortic side of the valve.
- ❏ Lambl's excrescences also are more common in older patients, are most often seen in the LV outflow tract, and may be mistaken for a vegetation. They less often are seen on the LA side of the mitral valve.
- ❏ Caseous calcification of the mitral annulus is a rare variant of mitral annular calcification, appearing as a smooth, round periannular mass with a central echolucent zone by echocardiography.

Patent foramen ovale

- ■ A small communication (patent foramen ovale) between the RA and LA is present in 20% to 30% of adults.
- ■ In some patients, a patent foramen ovale is associated with a contour abnormality of the septum with bulging from the midline more than 15 mm (atrial septal aneurysm). (Figure 15–15)

- There is a higher prevalence of patent foramen ovale in patients with a cryptogenic stroke.

Key points

- Shunting at the atrial level is sometimes seen with color Doppler but often requires a saline

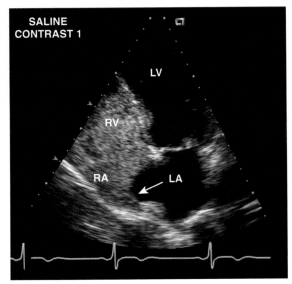

Figure 15–15. An atrial septal aneurysm is seen in this apical 4-chamber view with saline contrast used to opacify the right heart. The atrial septum deviates from left to right in the region of the fossa ovalis with a radius of more than 15 mm at the maximum curvature point.

contrast injection for detection. (Figures 15–16 and 15–17)

- A patent foramen ovale allows blood flow from RA to LA when RA pressure exceeds LA pressure. In some patients, shunting occurs at rest; in others, a right to left shunt is seen only after Valsalva maneuver to transiently increase RA pressure.
- Appearance of echo contrast in the LA within three beats of right heart opacification is consistent with a patent foramen ovale. Later appearance of contrast (after three to five cycles) may be due to transpulmonary passage.
- Longer digital clip lengths, which include entry of contrast into the right heart and at least five beats after RA opacification, are needed for evaluation of a saline contrast study. Review of videotaped images may be needed to include an adequate number of cardiac cycles with each injection.
- At least two saline contrast injections are needed, one at rest and one with Valsalva maneuver. However, accuracy is optimized with a total of four contrast injections, two at rest and two with Valsalva.
- TEE is more sensitive than transthoracic imaging for detection of a patent foramen ovale. (Figure 15–18)
- In patients with chronically elevated RA pressures (such as severe pulmonary hypertension

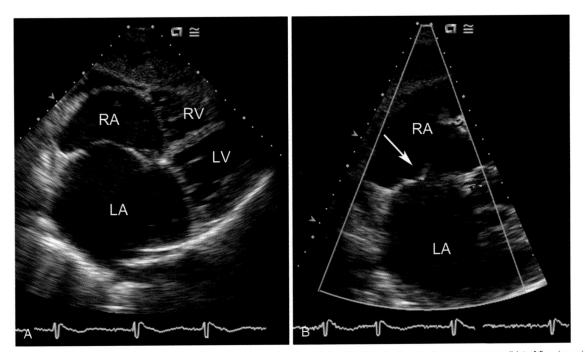

Figure 15–16. A, In a subcostal 4-chamber view the atrial septum bulges towards the RA. B, Color Doppler demonstrates a small jet of flow (arrow) from left to right across the interatrial septum consistent with a patent foramen ovale.

with right heart failure), persistent right to left shunting may result in arterial oxygen desaturation.

❑ Echocardiography (transesophageal or intra-cardiac) can be used to guide percutaneous closure of a patent foramen ovale. (Figure 15–19)

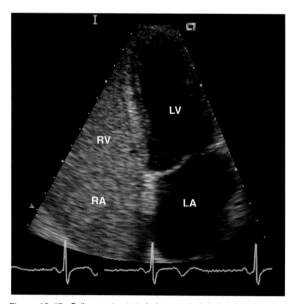

Figure 15–17. Saline contrast study in an apical 4-chamber view in a patient with a systemic embolic event shows no evidence for contrast in the left heart either at rest or with Valsalva maneuver, indicating the absence of a patent foramen ovale.

EVALUATION FOR CARDIAC SOURCE OF EMBOLUS

■ Echocardiography requested to evaluate for a cardiac source of embolus should include a saline contrast study for detection of patent foramen ovale.

■ A careful examination for cardiac thrombi, tumors, valvular vegetations, and aortic atheroma, often with TEE, is needed when a cardiac source of embolus is suspected.

Key points

❑ If atrial fibrillation is present, an LA thrombus is a likely cause of clinical events, even if not detected on TEE.

❑ Embolic events in patients with mechanical prosthetic valves must be presumed to be related to the prosthetic valve, regardless of echocardiographic findings.

❑ Aortic atheroma, detected on TEE, are associated with an increased prevalence of embolic events.

❑ TEE to evaluate for a cardiac source of embolus is recommended in patients with:

• Abrupt occlusion of a major peripheral or visceral artery

• Cerebrovascular emboli events in patients younger than age 45 years

• Cerebrovascular events without other evident causes in patients of any age

• Whenever clinical management would be altered based on the echocardiographic findings

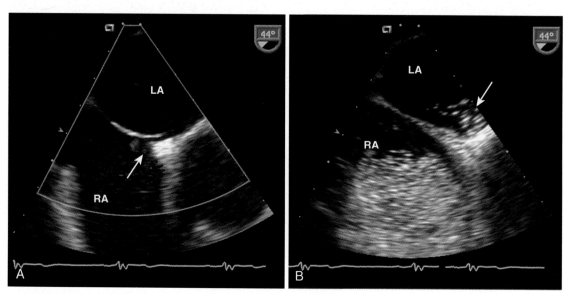

Figure 15–18. *A,* TEE in a patient with a cryptogenic stroke shows the typical "flap valve" appearance of a patent foramen ovale with color Doppler demonstrating a narrow red flow signal in the slitlike orifice. *B,* With peripheral injection of saline contrast, there is prompt appearance of microbubbles in the LA *(arrows)* on the first cardiac cycle, consistent with passage across a patent foramen ovale.

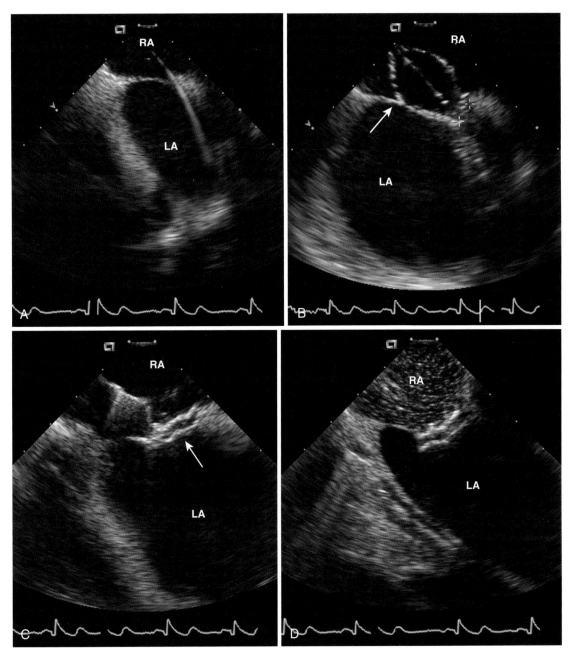

Figure 15–19. Intracardiac echocardiographic (ICE) guidance of percutaneous closure of a patent foramen ovale. The transducer tip (top of the sector) is in the RA, with the septum in the mid-field and LA in the far field of the images. *A,* The guiding catheter has been passed through the patent foramen ovale. *B,* A sizing balloon is inflated to measure the defect size. *C,* The closure device is in position but still attached to the catheter seen in the RA. *D,* The guiding catheter has been removed and contrast injected into the right heart. The parallel linear echos of the closure device are seen positioned on the atrial septum with no evidence for residual shunting.

Cardiac Massess and Sources Embolus
Structures That May Be Mistaken for an Abnormal Cardiac Mass

Left atrium	Dilated coronary sinus (persistent left superior vena cava) Raphe between left superior pulmonary vein and left atrial appendage Atrial suture line after cardiac transplant Beam-width artifact from calcified aortic valve, aortic valve prosthesis, or other echogenic target adjacent to the atrium Interatrial septal aneurysm
Right atrium	Crista terminalis Chiari network (Eustachian valve remnants) Lipomatous hypertrophy of the interatrial septum Trabeculation of right atrial appendage Atrial suture line after cardiac transplant Pacer wire, Swan-Ganz catheter, or central venous line
Left ventricle	Papillary muscles Left ventricular web (aberrant chordae) Prominent apical trabeculations Prominent mitral annular calcification
Right ventricle	Moderator band Papillary muscles Swan-Ganz catheter or pacer wire
Aortic valve	Nodules of Arantius Lambl's excrescences Base of valve leaflet seen en face in diastole
Mitral valve	Redundant chordae Myxomatous mitral valve tissue
Pulmonary artery	Left atrial appendage (just caudal to pulmonary artery)
Pericardium	Epicardial adipose tissue Fibrinous debris in a chronic organized pericardial effusion

Distinguishing Characteristics of Intracardiac Masses

Characteristic	Thrombus	Tumor	Vegetation
Location	LA (especially when enlarged or associated with mitral valve disease) LV (in setting of reduced systolic function or segmental wall abnormalities)	LA (myxoma) Myocardium Pericardium Valves	Usually valvular Occasionally on ventricular wall or Chiari network
Appearance	Usually discrete and somewhat spherical in shape or laminated against left ventricular apex or left atrial wall	Various: may be circumscribed or may be irregular	Irregular shape, attached to the proximal (upstream) side of the valve with motion independent from the valve
Associated findings	Underlying etiology usually evident Left ventricular systolic dysfunction or segmental wall motion abnormalities (exception: eosinophilic heart disease) Mitral valve disease with left atrial enlargement	Intracardiac obstruction depending on site of tumor Clinically: fevers, systemic signs of endocarditis, positive blood cultures	Valvular regurgitation usually present

LA, left atrium; LV, left ventricle.

QUESTION 1

What is the most likely diagnosis for the mass (*arrow*) seen in this echocardiographic image?

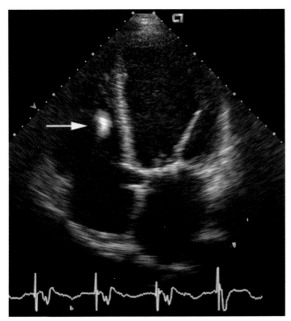

Figure 15–20.

A. Central venous catheter
B. Pacer lead
C. Moderator
D. Apical thrombus

QUESTION 2

Doppler data were recorded during an elective TEE in an outpatient.

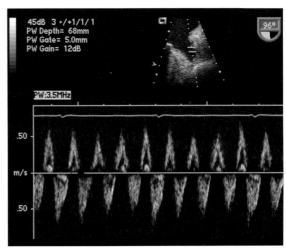

Figure 15–21.

This Doppler recording is most consistent with:

A. Normal sinus rhythm
B. Atrial fibrillation
C. Atrial flutter
D. Ventricular tachycardia
E. Ventricular fibrillation

QUESTION 3

On transthoracic imaging requested to evaluate for intracardiac thrombus, the following image was obtained.

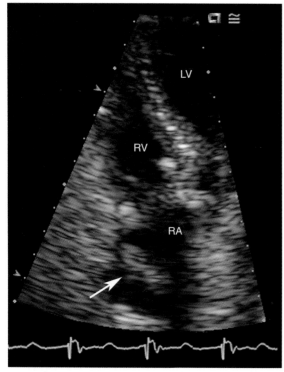

Figure 15–22.

The most likely explanation for the echo-density indicated by the arrow is:

A. Acoustic shadowing
B. Pacer lead
C. Normal structure
D. Electronic interference
E. Adipose tissue

QUESTION 4

This M-mode tracing was obtained in a patient referred for evaluation of an embolic stroke.

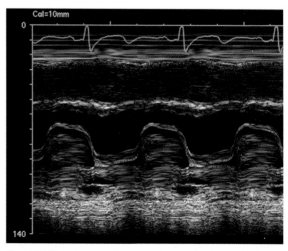

Figure 15–23.

This finding is most consistent with:

A. Normal
B. Mitral stenosis
C. Aortic stenosis
D. Atrial septal aneurysm
E. Atrial myxoma

QUESTION 5

What is the most likely diagnosis for the structure indicated by the *arrow?*

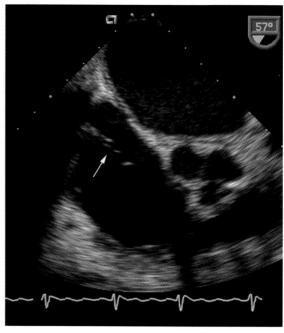

Figure 15–24.

A. Artifact
B. Atrial septal aneurysm
C. Central venous catheter
D. Chiari network
E. Crista terminalis

QUESTION 6

Echocardiography was requested in this 72-year-old man to evaluate for cardiac source of embolus. During the examination, discontinuity in the posterior LA wall was noted (*arrow*).

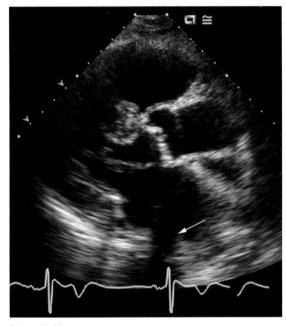

Figure 15–25.

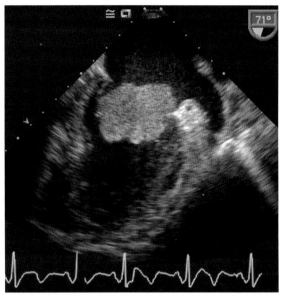

Figure 15–26.

The most likely cause of his symptoms is:

A. Pulmonary embolus
B. LV dysfunction
C. Atrial fibrillation
D. Mitral valve obstruction
E. Endocarditis

QUESTION 8

TEE was requested before elective cardioversion in this patient with atrial fibrillation and a prosthetic mitral valve.

The most likely cause of this echo appearance is:

A. Acoustic shadowing
B. Atrial myxoma
C. Mitral valve prosthesis
D. Annular abscess
E. Descending thoracic aorta

QUESTION 7

A 32-year-old man presented with exertional dyspnea and had this echocardiographic finding.

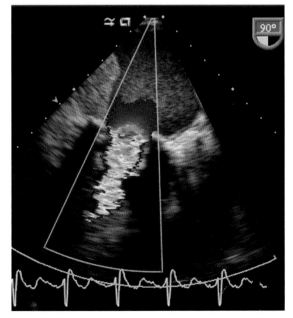

Figure 15–27.

Based on this image, the most appropriate next step is:

A. Obtain further views to evaluate the LA appendage
B. Cancel planned cardioversion
C. Proceed with cardioversion followed by full-dose anticoagulation treatment
D. Administer anticoagulation for 24 hours before cardioversion
E. Perform urgent repeat mitral valve replacement

QUESTION 9

TEE was requested to evaluate for potential cardiac sources of embolus in a 73-year-old woman with a transient ischemic event.
Figure 15–28

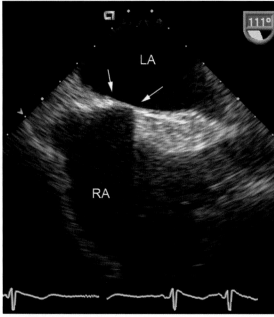

Figure 15–28.

This finding is diagnostic of:

A. Atrial septal aneurysm
B. Patent foramen ovale
C. Atrial myxoma
D. Lipomatous hypertrophy
E. Atrial septal occluder device

QUESTION 10

A 44-year-old man presents with confusion and difficulty in word finding to the neurology service. A stroke is diagnosed and echocardiography is requested to evaluate for an intracardiac shunt. Resting images demonstrate normal biventricular chamber size and function. There are no significant valvular abnormalities. Incidental note is made of a Eustachian valve and atrial septal aneurysm. The indexed LA volume is 41 mL/m^2. Agitated saline contrast was injected in the right antecubital vein at rest and again with Valsalva maneuver. On careful review of these two cine loops, the rest image showed no shunt. On the post-Valsalva loop, following opacification of the RA, the atrial septal aneurysm is seen bowing to the left and three microbubbles were seen in the left heart after four cardiac cycles. These data are most consistent with:

A. Transpulmonary contrast
B. Patent foramen ovale (PFO)
C. Nondiagnostic study

ANSWER 1: B

This bright dense "mass" seen in the RV most likely is a pacer lead seen in cross section. This diagnosis can be confirmed by reviewing the clinical history (or asking the patient) and by imaging in other views to demonstrate the length of the pacer lead as it traverses the RA and RV with the tip in the RV apex. A central venous catheter should be in the superior vena cava or RA; in the rare event that a central catheter extends into the RV, the echodensity of the plastic catheter is less than the metallic pacer leads and often two parallel echos are seen with a catheter. A pulmonary artery catheter usually is seen in the RV outflow tract rather than the mid–RV chamber, and the presence of a pulmonary artery catheter is obvious during image acquisition because these patients are in the intensive care unit and the catheter is visible externally. The moderator band is a normal muscle band closer to the RV apex, extending from the free wall to septum, with an echodensity similar to the rest of the myocardium. Ventricular thrombi are unusual in the RV but, when present, have an echodensity similar to myocardium and occur in regions of myocardial dysfunction. Peripheral venous thrombi may embolize to the heart and lodge in the RV or tricuspid valve apparatus, with a tubular shape reflecting formation in a peripheral vein.

ANSWER 2: C

This Doppler signal was recorded in the LA appendage, seen in the two-dimensional image in the 90 degree view, with the Doppler sample volume about 1 cm into the appendage. Regular flow in and out of the atrial appendage at a rate about 300 bpm is seen with a velocity about 0.5 m/s in both directions. This is consistent with atrial flutter with typical atrial (and appendage) contractions at a rate of 300 bpm. Normal sinus rhythm results in flow out of the atrial appendage following the P wave on the electrocardiogram with a single velocity peak of at least 0.4 ms/s with each cardiac cycle. Atrial fibrillation results in rapid, irregular, low-velocity flow waves from the atrial appendage. Ventricular tachycardia and ventricular fibrillation affect the contraction of the LV, not the LA, and usually are associated with hemodynamic compromise.

ANSWER 3: C

The differential diagnosis of this echodensity in the region of the RA includes an RA mass (tumor or thrombus) or a prosthetic device (central line or pacer lead), but this location and shape is most consistent with the normal RA wall, with a small amount of pericardial fluid around the atrium. A central line or pacer lead would be more echodense with a linear appearance and were excluded in this patient by clinical history. A saline contrast study showed contrast filling the normal RA cavity but not the pericardial space, confirming that is the normal RA free wall.

Acoustic shadowing results in loss of the reflected signal, not an echodensity. Electronic interference appears as a geometric pattern across the entire image. Adipose tissue may be seen in the atrioventricular groove or in the interatrial septum (lipomatous hypertrophy but both those locations are distant from the location of this echodensity. Cardiac magnetic resonance imaging or TEE would be helpful if the diagnosis remained unclear.

ANSWER 4: E

This is an M-mode tracing of the mitral valve, with the structures seen, from anterior to posterior, including the RV, septum, mitral valve, and posterior LV wall. An aortic valve M-mode would show the parallel walls of the aorta anterior to the LA. An atrial septal aneurysm is not usually seen well by M-mode given the orientation of the atrial septum relative to the chest wall. The diastolic slope of the anterior leaflet is flat, as is seen with mitral stenosis, but leaflet excursion and E-point septal separation are normal. In addition, there are multiple parallel echos moving with the mitral valve, seen filling the space between the anterior and posterior leaflets in diastole. This finding is consistent with a mass, most likely an LA myxoma (*arrow*) prolapsing in the mitral orifice in diastole, as confirmed on two-dimensional imaging.

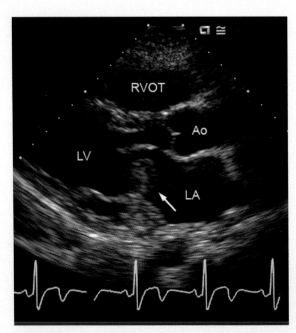

Figure 15-29.

ANSWER 5: D

This is a TEE short-axis view of the LA, atrial septum, and RA, with the aortic valve seen in an oblique image plane. The arrow points to a linear irregular echodensity that originates near the inferior vena cava and extends into the RA, most consistent with a Chiari network, which is a normal variant consisting of a thin tissue network extending from the inferior vena cava across the RA to the superior vena cava. The term *Eustachian valve* is used when the membrane at the inferior vena cava junction is very localized and *Chiari network* is used when it extends (often with fenestrations) from the inferior vena cava to the superior vena cava. On TTE imaging, often only bright mobile echos, similar to the appearance of contrast microbubbles, are seen, but on TEE imaging the structure itself can be identified. An artifact is unlikely because there are no structures closer to the transducer likely to cause reverberations. The atrial septum appears normal with a thin fossa ovalis and no evidence for an atrial septal aneurysm. Central venous catheters usually enter the RA from the superior vena cava and have a smoother appearance, with two parallel echos reflecting the hollow catheter structure. The crista terminalis is a ridge of atrial tissue seen at the superior aspect of the RA in a 4-chamber view.

ANSWER 6: A

This parasternal long-axis view shows acoustic shadowing from a heavily calcific aortic valve resulting in apparent discontinuity in the posterior LA wall. An atrial myxoma appears as a mass in the LA; although calcification can be seen with a myxoma, a mass would be evident. A prosthetic mitral valve also causes acoustic shadowing, but the location would be directly posterior to the mitral valve, and this image shows a native mitral valve with only mild annular calcification (with another small acoustic shadow). An annular abscess due to endocarditis is located in the annular region and often is echodense, rather than echolucent. The descending thoracic aorta is immediately posterior to the LA in this view (not well seen in this example) but would not cause an apparent discontinuity in the atrial wall.

ANSWER 7: D

This TEE 2-chamber view shows a large mass attached to the mitral valve, which prolapses into the mitral orifice in diastole, resulting in obstruction to LV inflow, which is the most likely cause of his symptoms. This mass is most likely an LA myxoma given the location, size, nonhomogenous appearance, and slightly irregular borders. Vegetations due to endocarditis typically are smaller and associated with valve destruction; a vegetation large enough to obstruct flow is rare except with fungal infections. Atrial fibrillation is not present because P waves are seen on the electrocardiogram. Pulmonary emboli are difficult to visualize by echocardiography because the distal pulmonary vessels are not well seen, although thrombus-in-transit may occasionally be identified in the right heart. Ventricular function cannot be evaluated on this still-frame image but is expected to be normal with a small chamber due to impaired diastolic filling.

ANSWER 8: B

This TEE 2-chamber view shows an enlarged LA with marked spontaneous contrast and a large mural LA thrombus. Thus, the elective cardioversion should be cancelled due to the high risk of an embolic event. Cardioversion followed by anticoagulation is appropriate only if there is no thrombus visualized. When a thrombus is present, several weeks or months of anticoagulation are appropriate before re-evaluation for resolution of thrombus. Additional views to visualize the atrial appendage are not needed because a definite thrombus has already been identified. In fact, the LA appendage was removed at the time of mitral valve replacement in this patient which explains why an atrial appendage is not seen in this view. Review of the operative report before TEE is recommended to ascertain if the mitral valve procedure included atrial appendage ligation or removal. The color Doppler signal with a relatively narrow antegrade jet across the valve is suggestive of prosthetic valve stenosis, but additional Doppler hemodynamic data are needed to confirm this diagnosis.

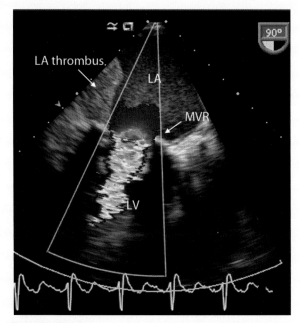

Figure 15–30.

ANSWER 9: D

In this TEE bicaval view of the LA and RA, the atrial septum appears intact with a normal thin fossa ovalis (between *arrows*) but with marked thickening and increased echodensity of the rest of the septum, diagnostic for lipomatous hypertrophy of the interatrial septum. This benign normal variant is commonly seen, with prevalence increasing with age and body mass index. Although the fossa ovalis appears relatively thin, it is normal thickness and is not deviated toward either side. The definition of an atrial septal aneurysm is deviation by 1.5 cm or more, which this image does not demonstrate. A patent foramen ovale may or may not be present, but diagnosis requires color Doppler and a saline contrast injection. If a secundum or primum atrial septal defect were present, the right heart chambers would be enlarged and there would be a discontinuity in the atrial septum. With a sinus venosus atrial septal defect, the septum might appear intact in this view but the right heart would still be enlarged. An atrial septal occluder device results in prominent echodensities on both sides of the fossa ovalis, in a shape consistent with the specific device implanted.

ANSWER 10: C

This is a nondiagnostic study for several reasons: only two contrast injections were performed, the patient may not have performed an adequate Valsalva maneuver due to confusion, and contrast was seen in the left heart four cardiac cycles after appearance in the RA. These borderline results should prompt further evaluation due to the clinical presentation of stroke in a patient younger than age 45 years and because there is

an increased likelihood of a patent foramen ovale in patients with an atrial septal aneurysm.

The most common use of agitated saline contrast echocardiography is for detection of an intracardiac shunt at the atrial level, either due to a patent foramen ovale or atrial septal defect. Even though flow is predominantly from left to right, there is a small amount of right to left flow due to the similar and low pressures in the RA and LA. Thus, when agitated saline contrast is injected into the venous system, some contrast passes from right to left across the septum and is seen in the LA within three cardiac cycles of appearance in the RA. An image plane (usually a transthoracic 4-chamber view or a TEE bicaval view) that shows both the RA, LA and interatrial septum is recorded with capture of several beats to ensure that the appearance of contrast in the RA and several following beats are recorded. An adequate contrast study fully opacifies the RA. Digital processing may occasionally introduce image artifacts; therefore, review of videotaped images, if available, is also performed. Under normal respiration there usually is no interatrial shunt even when a patent foramen ovale is present because RA pressure is lower than LA pressure except very briefly during isovolumic contraction and in early ventricular diastole. However, with induced increases in RA pressure, as occurs transiently with Valsalva maneuver or cough, right to left shunting can be seen.

Most saline microbubbles that enter the pulmonary microcirculation become fragmented and are absorbed before entering the pulmonary veins and draining into the LA; however, a few microbubbles may pass through the pulmonary bed, particularly if there are pulmonary arteriovenous communications, and these (often smaller) microbubbles are seen in the left heart five or more cycles after appearance in the RA.

In addition to technical factors, there are several other causes of a nondiagnostic saline contrast study. If LA pressure is elevated, as suggested in this case with increased LA volume, then less right to left interatrial shunting would occur; in some cases a "negative contrast" effect is seen as the unopacified blood from the LA enters the contrast-filled RA. A prominent Eustachian valve may lead to a falsely negative study as it directs superior vena caval flow toward the tricuspid valve, reducing the amount of contrast delivered to the atrial septum. Additionally, a nondiagnostic study may also occur if Valsalva effort and timing are not optimal; this is common when contrast studies are done during conscious sedation for a TEE, resulting in an inadequate transient increase in RA pressure. Last, to reduce the likelihood of a nondiagnostic study, multiple contrast injections are often required. In this case, only one injection at rest and one with Valsalva was performed. Ideally, at least two injections at rest and two with Valsalva (a total of four) are performed.

16 Echocardiographic Evaluation of the Great Vessels

BASIC PRINCIPLES

- A systematic approach is need for echocardiographic evaluation of the great vessels.
- Transesophageal imaging is more sensitive than transthoracic imaging for detection of aortic aneurysm and dissection.
- Wider field of view tomographic imaging techniques, including chest computed tomography or cardiac magnetic resonance imaging, provide optimal evaluation of the great vessels.

Key points

☐ Many segments of the aorta and pulmonary artery can be visualized on transthoracic imaging, but:
  - Evaluation of branch pulmonary arteries and the branching of systemic arteries from the aorta often is not possible.

- Ultrasound imaging artifacts must be distinguished from an intraluminal dissection flap.
☐ The term *aortic root* includes the aortic annulus, sinuses of Valsalva, sinotubular junction, and ascending aorta.
☐ When the echocardiogram is nondiagnostic or equivocal, additional imaging techniques should be recommended, based on the clinical signs and symptoms.

STEP-BY-STEP APPROACH

Transthoracic echocardiography

- Examination of the aorta is based on visualization of several segments from different acoustic windows.
- The sequence suggested here follows the sequence of a standard transthoracic study; other exam sequences may be appropriate with an acute clinical presentation.

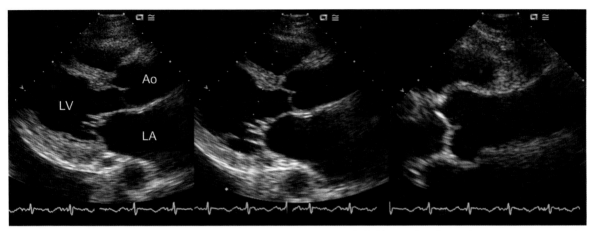

Figure 16–1. Standard parasternal long-axis view showing the proximal ascending aorta (*left*). The transducer is moved up an interspace to visualize additional segments of the ascending aorta (*center*), and then the image is zoomed to improve resolution of the aortic sinuses, sinotubular junction, and ascending aorta for accurate measurements (*right*).

Step 1: Record blood pressure and ensure the patient is medically stable

■ Aortic disease often presents as a medical/surgical emergency; appropriately trained health care providers should be available during the study.
■ Blood pressure is recorded at the beginning of the study because findings may change with altered loading conditions.

Key points

❐ When time is of the essence, limited imaging and Doppler data should be focused on the specific clinical question.
❐ It may be appropriate to proceed directly to TEE when aortic dissection is suspected; the echocardiographer should consult with the referring provider to ensure that the most appropriate test is performed in a timely manner.

Step 2: Assess the aortic root from the parasternal window

■ The aortic root is seen in the standard and high parasternal long-axis view. (Figures 16–1 and 16–2)
■ Diameter measurements are reported at end-diastole for the aortic annulus, sinuses of Valsalva, and sinotubular junction and in the mid-ascending aorta. (Figure 16–3)
■ Color Doppler allows detection of aortic regurgitation and evaluation of the flow pattern in the ascending aorta.

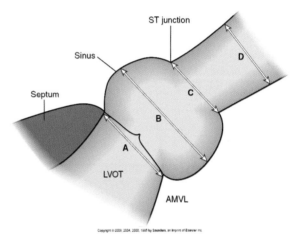

Figure 16–2. In addition to standard measurement at the annulus and sinuses of Valsalva, the sinotubular junction and mid-ascending aorta are measured when the aorta is dilated as shown in this schematic illustration.

Key points

❐ After recording the standard parasternal long axis view of the aortic root, the transducer is moved up one or more interspaces to visualize as much of the ascending aorta as possible.
❐ The sinotubular junction is defined as the top of the sinuses of Valsalva and is recognized by the acute angle at the transition from the curved sinuses to the tubular ascending aorta.
❐ Aortic dimensions are measured on two-dimensional images from the inner white–black

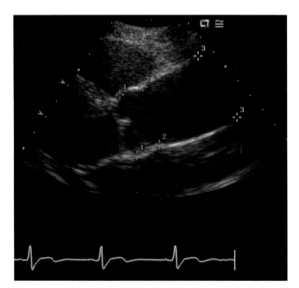

Figure 16–3. Example of measurements at the sinuses (*1*), sinotubular junction (*2*), and mid-ascending aorta (*3*) in a patient with mild aortic dilation. By convention, echo measurements are made at end-diastole from the inner white-black border of the anterior wall to the black–white border of the posterior aortic wall. Care is needed to ensure that the image plane is centered in the aorta and that measurements are perpendicular to the long axis of the vessel. An off-center image plane with underestimate aortic size; conversely, oblique measurements will overestimate aortic size.

border to the inner black–white border of the aortic lumen.

❏ Comparison of measurements on serial studies or by different modalities should be made at the same time point in the cardiac cycle.

❏ In comparing measurements from different modalities (computed tomography and magnetic resonance imaging), both imaging physics differ and measurement norms may vary, leading to apparent discrepancies.

Step 3: Assess the descending thoracic aorta from the parasternal and apical windows

■ The mid-portion of the descending thoracic aorta can be visualized from the parasternal long axis view, posterior to the left atrium (LA), by rotating the image plane clockwise to obtain a longitudinal view of the aorta. (Figure 16–4)

■ The descending thoracic aorta also can be imaged from the apical two-chamber view by lateral angulation of the image plane. (Figure 16–5)

■ Color Doppler is helpful in distinguishing image artifacts from an intraluminal flap in these views.

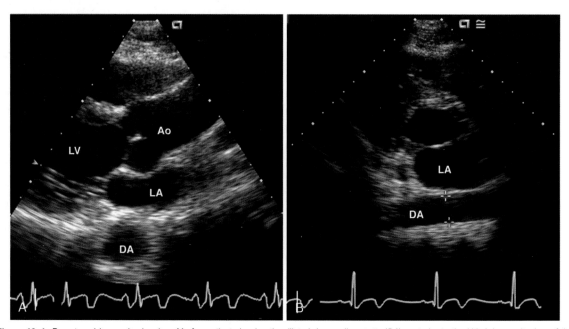

Figure 16–4. Parasternal long axis view in a Marfan patient showing the dilated descending aorta (*DA*) posterior to the LV. A long-axis view of the descending thoracic aorta can be obtained by rotating the transducer clockwise into a parasternal short-axis plane.

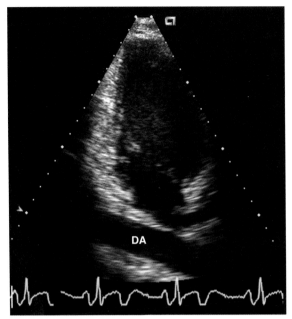

Figure 16–5. Another segment of the descending thoracic aorta is imaged in the same patient as Figure 16–4 from the apical 2-chamber view with lateral angulation of the image plane.

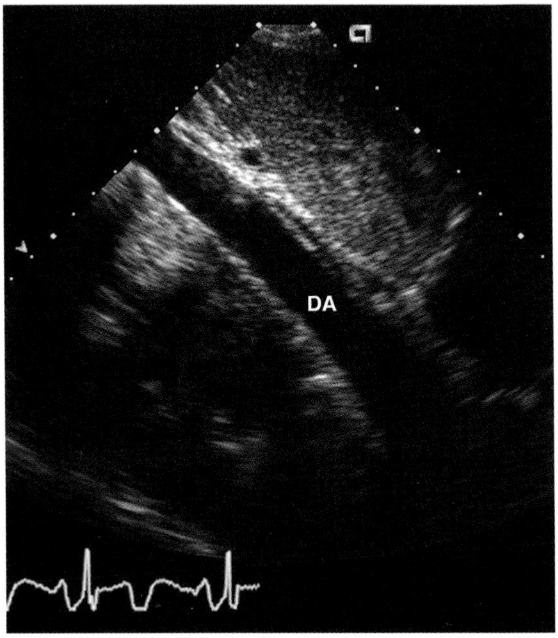

Figure 16–6. The proximal abdominal aorta seen from the subcostal window.

Key points

- ❏ Dilation of the descending aorta and dissection flaps can be identified in these views when image quality is adequate.
- ❏ Only some segments of the descending thoracic aorta are visualized so that significant pathology may be missed.
- ❏ The aorta is in the far field of the image in these views, limiting evaluation for aortic atheroma.
- ❏ In patients with a large left pleural effusion, the descending aorta can be imaged from the posterior chest wall, using the pleural effusion as an acoustic window.

Step 4: Assess the proximal abdominal aorta from the subcostal window

- ■ The proximal abdominal aorta is seen in the subcostal view by medial angulation from the inferior vena cava image plane. (Figure 16–6)
- ■ Holodiastolic flow reversal is seen in the proximal abdominal aorta in patients with severe aortic valve regurgitation. (See Figure 12–5)

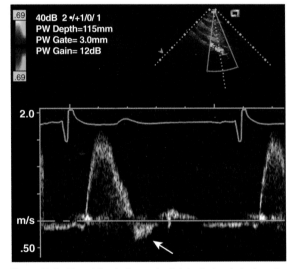

Figure 16–7. Normal flow in the proximal abdominal aorta is characterized by antegrade flow in systole, brief early diastolic reversal (arrow), low-velocity forward flow in mid-diastole, and then a slight flow reversal at end-diastole.

Key points

- ❏ Diameter of the proximal abdominal aorta is routinely measured in patients with aortic disease, such as Marfan syndrome.
- ❏ With a normal pattern of flow, antegrade systolic flow is followed by early diastolic flow reversal due to coronary blood flow, mid-diastolic low-velocity antegrade flow, and a very brief late diastolic flow signal due to elastic recoil of the aorta. (Figure 16–7)
- ❏ In order to detect the holodiastolic flow reversal seen with severe aortic regurgitation, the filters are adjusted to show low-velocity flow.

☐ Holodiastolic flow reversal also is seen with other aortic diastolic flow abnormalities, such as a patent ductus arteriosus, surgical systemic-to-pulmonary shunt (e.g., Blalock-Taussig shunt) or aorto-pulmonary window, or other large arteriovenous communication, such as an upper extremity dialysis fistula in patients with end-stage renal disease.

Step 5: Assess the aortic arch and proximal descending thoracic aorta from the suprasternal notch window

■ The aortic arch is visualized in long- and short-axis views from the suprasternal notch window. (Figure 16–8)
■ Pulsed Doppler recordings of flow in the proximal descending aorta show holodiastolic flow reversal when moderate to severe aortic regurgitation is present (Figure 16–9). The normal flow pattern is shown in Figure 16–10.

Key points

☐ The aortic arch is measured in its mid-section, where the ultrasound beam is perpendicular to the aortic walls.
☐ The descending aorta appears to "taper," even when normal, due to the oblique plane of the ultrasound image compared with the curvature of the aorta.
☐ The distance from the aortic valve that holodiastolic flow reversal persists, correlates with regurgitant severity. Thus, reversal in the proximal descending aorta is seen with moderate regurgitation, but reversal in the abdominal aorta indicates severe regurgitation.
☐ The right pulmonary artery is seen in cross section, under the arch, in the long-axis view of the aortic arch.
☐ A longitudinal view of the left pulmonary artery can be obtained by leftward rotation and angulation of the image plane.

Step 6: Decide if TEE or other imaging procedures are needed

■ Echocardiographic interpretation should first describe the imaging and Doppler findings, along with a differential diagnosis for these findings. The level of confidence in any diagnosis should be indicated.
■ Second, the interpretation should indicate any areas of uncertainly and, in conjunction with the referring physician, suggest additional diagnostic procedures.

Key points

☐ Complete evaluation of the aorta may require additional imaging procedures, including:
  • Transesophageal echocardiography
  • Chest computed tomography

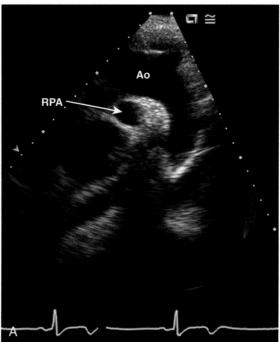

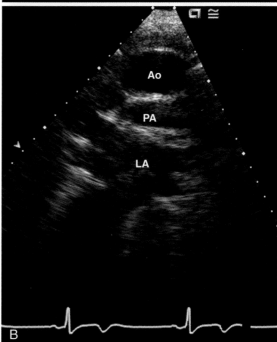

Figure 16–8. The long-axis view of the aortic arch (*A*) shows segments of the ascending and descending thoracic aorta, the arch, and the origins of the head and neck vessels. The right pulmonary artery is seen under the curve of the arch. In the short-axis view of the arch (*B*), the LA and pulmonary veins are seen inferior to the right pulmonary artery.

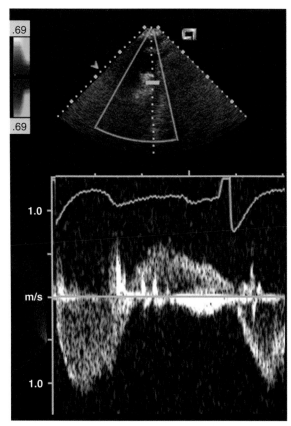

Figure 16–9. In a patient with severe aortic regurgitation, holodiastolic flow is seen in the descending thoracic aorta. The diastolic flow signal is above the baseline from the end of ejection up to the start of the next ejection period.

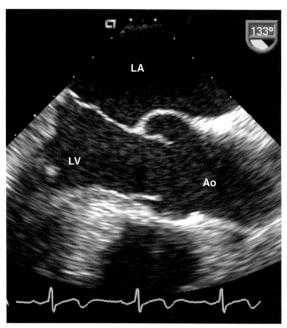

Figure 16–11. A long-axis view of the ascending aorta is obtained by TEE at about 120 to 140 degrees rotation with the probe withdrawn in the esophagus to see the ascending aorta.

- Cardiac magnetic resonance (CMR) imaging
- Cardiac catheterization with aortography
- ❑ Selection of the most appropriate diagnostic modality depends on several clinical factors, including the differential diagnosis, acuity of symptoms, concurrent diseases, and local expertise in imaging.

Transesophageal echocardiography

Step 1: Image the aortic root from a high esophageal position

- ■ Long-axis views of the ascending aorta provide excellent image quality for detection of aortic dilation or dissection.
- ■ Short-axis images provide confirmation of findings and are helpful in distinguishing artifact from intraluminal abnormalities.
- ■ Color Doppler evaluation of the flow pattern in the aortic root helps identify dissection flaps.

Key points

- ❑ The long-axis view typically is obtained at 120 degrees rotation, but there is individual variability, so the image plane should be adjusted to show the aortic root in a long-axis orientation. (Figure 16–11)
- ❑ From the long-axis view, the transducer is moved up in the esophagus to image as much of the ascending aorta as possible.

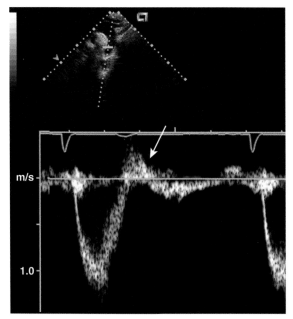

Figure 16–10. Normal flow in the descending thoracic aorta shows early diastolic flow reversal (corresponding to diastolic coronary blood flow), low-velocity forward flow in mid-diastole, and slight reversal at end-diastole. This patient had no aortic regurgitation.

- ❏ Slow medial and lateral turning of the image plane from the long-axis view may identify abnormalities not seen in the centered long-axis view.
- ❏ The short-axis view is used to provide an orthogonal image plane. The short-axis view should be recorded from the aortic valve level to as high as possible in the ascending aorta. (Figure 16–12)
- ❏ Color Doppler in long- and short-axis views may show flow in two lumens when a dissection is present.
- ❏ The mid- and distal ascending aorta may be better seen by decreasing the rotation to about 100 degrees and slightly withdrawing the probe.
- ❏ The distal ascending aorta just proximal to the arch is often not well seen due to the interposed air column (trachea) between the esophagus and aorta.
- ❏ Imaging artifacts commonly seen in the ascending aorta often include linear reverberations from the aorta itself or adjacent structures. Artifacts are distinguished from anatomic abnormalities by examination in at least two imaging planes; their location, appearance, and pattern of motion relative to the aortic wall; and correlation with color Doppler flow patterns.

Step 2: Evaluate aortic valve anatomy and function

- ■ The presence of aortic valve disease prompts careful evaluation for associated disease of the aortic root.

TABLE 16-1 Upper Limits of Normal Aortic Dimensions in Adults

	Men	Women	Indexed for BSA (Men and Women)
Aortic annulus	3.1 cm	2.6 cm	1.6 cm/m²
Sinus of Valsalva	4.0 cm	3.6 cm	2.1 cm/m²
Sinotubular junction	3.6 cm	3.2 cm	1.9 cm/m²

Data from Roman MJ et al: Am J Cardiol 1989;64:507-512.

TABLE 16-2 Equations for Calculation of Expected Aortic Sinus Dimension Based on Body Size

Patient Age	Expected Sinus Dimension (cm)
<20 years	1.02 + 0.98 (BSA)
20-39 years	0.97 + 1.12 (BSA)
40 years or older	1.92 + 0.74 (BSA)

BSA, body surface area data from Roman MJ et al: Am J Cardiol 1989;64:507-512.

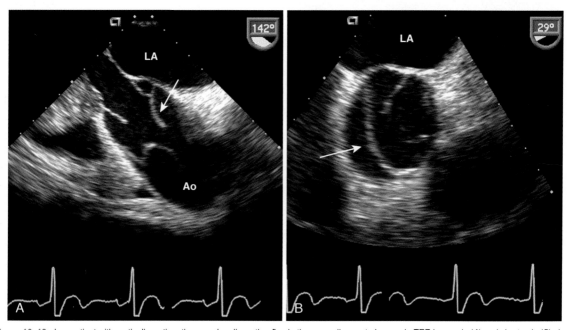

Figure 16–12. In a patient with aortic dissection, the complex dissection flap in the ascending aorta is seen in TEE long-axis (*A*) and short-axis (*B*) views of the ascending aorta.

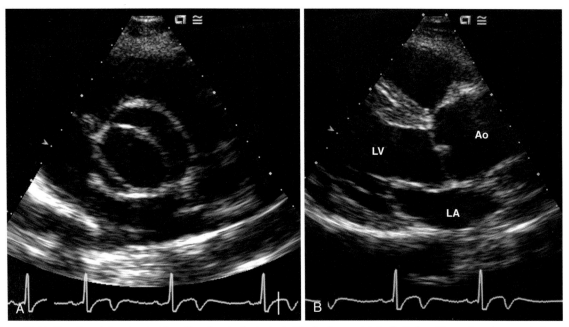

Figure 16–13. Transthoracic imaging of a bicuspid aortic valve in short-axis (*A*) often is associated with dilation of the aortic root as seen in the corresponding long-axis view (*B*).

■ Conversely, aortic root disease may result in aortic valve regurgitation.

Key points

❏ The risk of aortic dilation and dissection is higher in patients with a congenitally bicuspid or unicuspid valve, compared with those with a trileaflet valve. (Figure 16–13)

❏ Aortic disease may result in aortic regurgitation either due to dilation of the aortic root and central noncoaptation of the leaflets or due to extension of a dissection flap into the valve, resulting in a flail leaflet.

❏ Aortic valve anatomy and function is evaluated with 2D imaging and color Doppler in a long-axis view at about 120 degrees rotation and in the short-axis view, at about 30 degrees rotation.

❏ Additional scanning medially and laterally from the long-axis view and superiorly and inferiorly from the short-axis view also is helpful.

Step 3: Examine the descending thoracic aorta

■ The descending thoracic aorta is well visualized on TEE by turning the image plane posteriorly.
■ The short-axis view is recorded with the transducer slowly withdrawn from the transgastric level to the high esophagus. (Figure 16–14)

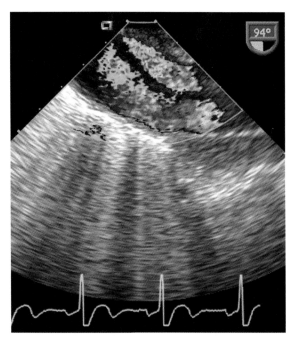

Figure 16–14. TEE imaging of the descending thoracic aorta in a longitudinal view in a patient with aortic dissection, obtained by turning the transducer toward the patient's back and then rotating the image plane by about 90 degrees.

■ The aortic arch is visualized from the high TEE position by turning the image plane medially with inferior angulation.

Key points

❑ Long-axis views of the descending aorta supplement short-axis views and are helpful for evaluation of any abnormal findings. However, the long axis view alone may miss abnormalities that are located medial and lateral to the image plane.

❑ Color flow provides visualization of flow in the true and false lumens when dissection is present.

❑ Color flow also is helpful in distinguishing image artifacts from dissection flaps and atheroma.

❑ When the aorta is tortuous, care is needed to distinguish intraluminal abnormalities from an oblique image plane.

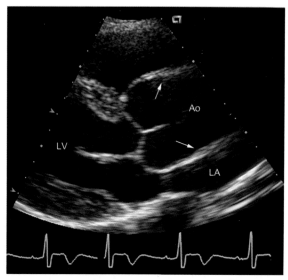

Figure 16–15. In patients with Marfan syndrome, the normal acute angle between the curved sinuses and tubular ascending aorta at the sinotubular junction is attenuated (*arrows*), resulting in a "water balloon" appearance of the aorta.

SPECIAL CONSIDERATIONS

Chronic aortic dilation

■ There are many causes of aortic dilation, including:
  • Hypertension
  • Atherosclerosis
  • Familial aortic aneurysm
  • Marfan syndrome and other connective tissue disorders
  • Aortic dilation associated with congenital unicuspid and bicuspid aortic valves
  • Inflammatory diseases of the aorta including tertiary syphilis, giant cell arteritis, and Takayasu's arteritis
  • Systemic inflammatory diseases including ankylosing spondylitis

■ Echocardiography provides accurate measurement of the aortic root and often provides anatomic clues about the cause of disease.

Key points

❑ Hypertensive aortic dilation usually is mild and accompanied by LV hypertrophy, aortic valve sclerosis, and mitral annular calcification.

❑ Marfan syndrome is characterized by loss of the normal acute angle at the sinotubular junction. Early in the disease, this finding may be subtle; late in the disease the aortic root appears globular with no discernible sinotubular junction. (Figure 16–15)

❑ Aortic dilation associated with congenital valve abnormalities is independent of valve hemodynamics.

❑ Aortic dilation due to an inflammatory process usually is characterized by increased thickness of the aortic walls.

❑ In ankylosing spondylitis, the increase in aortic wall thickness extends into the base of the anterior mitral valve leaflet, with the appearance of a subaortic "bump" in a long-axis view.

❑ Takayasu's arteritis typically involves the aortic arch and branches, resulting in areas of stenosis and dilation, but the descending aorta also may be involved.

Aortic dissection

Step 1: Use the basic approach for evaluation of the aorta to identify the dissection flap

■ The characteristics of a dissection flap (Figure 16–16) are:
  • A thin, linear, mobile intraluminal echo
  • Motion independent of the aortic walls
  • Separation of the lumen into two channels

■ Sites where there is communication between the true and false lumens may be identified with color Doppler.

■ An ascending aortic dissection usually requires surgical intervention, so it is especially important to determine if a dissection flap is present in the ascending aorta.

■ TEE is more sensitive than transthoracic imaging for detection of aortic dissection and should be the initial echo procedure when this diagnosis is suspected.

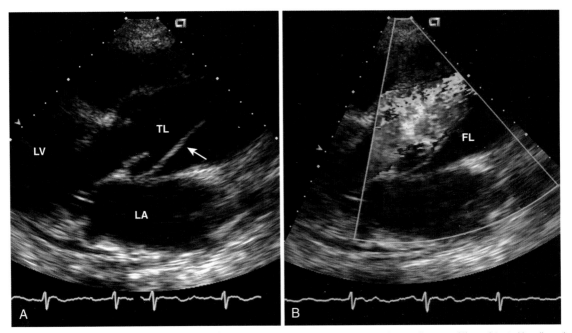

Figure 16–16. Transthoracic parasternal long-axis view showing a linear echo in the lumen of a dilated ascending aorta (*A*) consistent with a dissection flap (*arrow*) separating the true lumen (*TL*) from the false lumen (*FL*). In real time, this linear echo showed motion separate from the motion of the aortic wall and was seen in multiple image planes. Color Doppler (*B*) shows flow only in the true lumen.

Key points

❐ Imaging artifacts may be mistaken for a dissection flap. Approaches to avoiding a false positive diagnosis include imaging the flap in more than one imaging plane, demonstrating flow in two separate lumens, and demonstrating the three key characteristics of a dissection flap.

❐ There may be more than one entry site from the true into the false lumen and multiple exit sites may be detected distally.

❐ The false lumen may be thrombosed. In this situation the flap does not move and the false lumen is filled with an irregular echodensity, consistent with thrombus.

❐ Localized dissection into the aortic wall may result in a crescent-shaped intramural hematoma, without a dissection flap. (Figure 16–17)

❐ Outcomes with intramural hematoma and dissection are similar.

❐ Extraluminal, periaortic hematoma in association with aortic dissection is a poor prognostic marker.

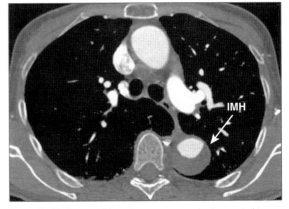

Figure 16–17. Intramural hematoma seen on a chest computed tomography scan in the descending thoracic aorta. These findings can be seen on TEE but may be difficult to distinguish from atheromatous or extra-aortic disease.

Step 2: Look for complications of aortic dissection

■ Complications of aortic dissection include:
 • Pericardial effusion
 • Aortic regurgitation

 • Extension of the dissection flap into a coronary artery
 • Involvement of arteries that arise from the aorta
■ Echocardiography may detect the central complications of aortic dissection, but evaluation of branch vessels typically requires other imaging techniques.

Key points

☐ Pericardial effusion may be due to rupture of the dissection into the pericardial space. Because the effusion is acute, tamponade physiology may be present with only a small effusion.

☐ Aortic regurgitation may be due to aortic dilation with central noncoaptation of the leaflets or due to a flail leaflet from extension of the dissection flap into the valve. (Figure 16–18)

☐ Extension of a dissection flap into the coronary artery may be visualized on TTE or TEE imaging in some cases. More often, the key finding is a regional wall motion abnormality due to ischemia in the myocardium supplied by the dissected vessel.

☐ The proximal segments of the left carotid and subclavian and right brachiocephalic artery may be seen by echocardiography in some cases. However, accurate evaluation of these vessels and more distal arteries (renal, mesenteric, etc.) requires other imaging approaches.

Sinus of Valsalva aneurysm

■ Congenital sinus of Valsalva aneurysms are irregularly shaped, thin-walled outpouchings of the sinus.

■ Rupture into adjacent chambers results in a fistula from the aorta into the RV, RA, or LA, depending on which sinus is affected.

■ Acquired sinus of Valsalva aneurysms usually are due to endocarditis and typically have a rounded symmetric shape. (Figure 16–19)

Key points

☐ Rupture of a right coronary sinus aneurysm is into the RV, left coronary sinus into the LA, and noncoronary sinus into the RA.

☐ Flow in the fistula from the aorta is continuous with high-velocity flow in both systole and diastole, reflecting the systolic and diastolic pressure differences between the aortas and receiving chamber.

☐ Acquired aneurysms due to infection may extend below the aortic valve, into the base of the septum. Imaging in long-axis views helps determine the level and extent of involvement.

Aortic pseudoaneurysms

■ An aortic pseudoaneurysm is a contained aortic rupture. (Figure 16–20)

■ Pseudoaneurysms may occur after aortic surgery due to dehiscence at the proximal or distal anastomosis or at a coronary reimplantation site.

Key points

☐ A pseudoaneurysm is detected as an echolucent space adjacent to the aorta. The pseudoaneurysm may be echodense if hematoma is present.

☐ A pseudoaneurysm should be suspected when a para-aortic mass is found in a patient with recent or remote surgery on the ascending aorta.

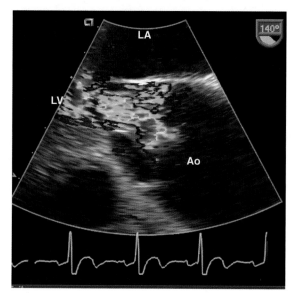

Figure 16–18. An aortic dissection can result in severe aortic regurgitation, as seen in this TEE long-axis view, due to extension of the dissection flap into the aortic valve leaflet.

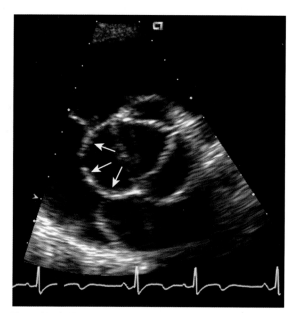

Figure 16–19. This short-axis view of the aortic valve shows the valve leaflets open to a triangular shape in systole. There is asymmetric dilation of the sinuses of Valsalva, most prominently involving the noncoronary sinus (*arrows*), consistent with a sinus of Valsalva aneurysm.

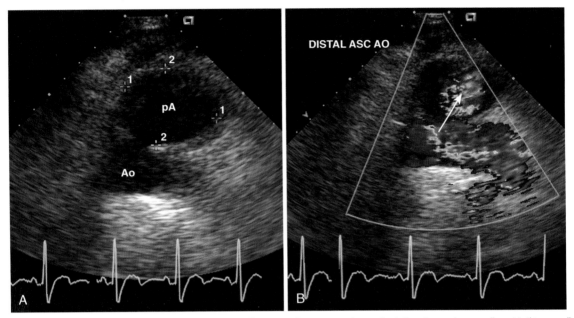

Figure 16–20. In a patient with a Dacron tube graft replacement of the ascending aorta, an abnormal echolucent space is seen adjacent to the ascending aorta, near the distal anastomosis site. The 3.5 by 4.5 cm diameter (measurements 1 and 2 shown) space appears lined by thrombus (A). Color Doppler demonstrates flow from the aorta into this space, consistent with a contained aortic rupture or pseudoaneurysm (pA).

❐ Although often initially diagnosed by echocardiography, evaluation of the size and origin of the pseudoaneurysm often requires a wide field of view imaging approach, such as cardiac magnetic resonance imaging or computed tomography.

Atherosclerotic aortic disease

■ Aortic atheromas may be detected on TEE imaging of the ascending and descending thoracic aorta and are a marker of coronary disease. (Figure 16–21)

■ Atheroma that protrude into the aortic lumen and atheroma associated with mobile thrombus are associated with an increased risk of embolic events.

Key points

❐ Atheroma is identified as irregular focal areas of thickening of the aortic wall, with or without associated calcification.

❐ Images of the aortic arch are limited, even with TEE, but atheroma may be detected from a high esophageal position in some cases.

Persistent left superior vena cava

■ A persistent left superior vena cava is a normal variant in which left upper extremity venous return enters the RA via the coronary sinus.

Key points

❐ A dilated coronary sinus is seen in cross section, posterior to the left atrium, in long-axis views, and in long axis with posterior angulation from a 4-chamber view.

❐ The persistent left superior vena cava may be directly visualized in some cases; Doppler flow shows low-velocity antegrade systolic and diastolic flow.

❐ A persistent left superior vena cava can be confirmed with saline contrast injection into the left upper extremity venous system, where saline contrast opacifies the coronary sinus prior to entering the right atrium.

Pulmonary artery

Clinical concerns

■ Isolated abnormalities of the pulmonary artery are rare; most pulmonary artery disease is associated with congenital heart disease. (Figure 16–22)

■ Idiopathic dilation of the pulmonary artery is an uncommon abnormality in which a dilated pulmonary artery is seen in the absence of other congenital lesions.

■ Thrombus in the pulmonary artery may be seen on transesophageal or transthoracic imaging in some cases, but echocardiography is not an accurate approach to diagnosis of pulmonary embolism.

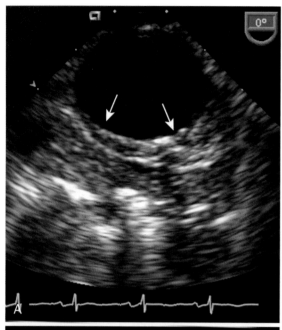

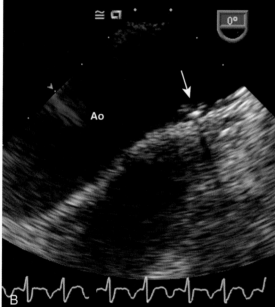

Figure 16–21. The descending thoracic aorta was evaluated in sequential short-axis images (*A*) as the transducer was withdrawn in the esophagus. From a high esophageal position, the image plane was turned medially and angulated inferiorly to show the aortic arch and ascending aorta (*B*). The irregular thickening of the aortic wall with an area of calcification (with shadowing) is consistent with an aortic atheroma.

Key points

- ❑ Abnormalities of the pulmonary artery associated with other congenital heart disease include pulmonary artery dilation and branch pulmonary artery stenosis.
- ❑ Pulmonary artery dissection is rare.

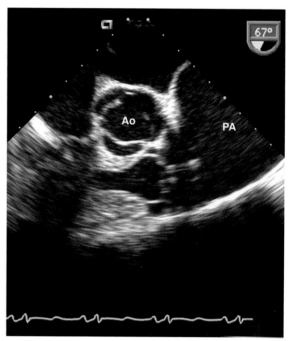

Figure 16–22. Severe dilation of the pulmonary artery seen on TEE in a patient with congenital heart disease.

Basic echocardiographic approach

- ■ The pulmonary artery is visualized in the transthoracic short-axis view by angulation superiorly to demonstrate the bifurcation of the main pulmonary artery. (see Figure 16–23)
- ■ Images also can be obtained in the transthoracic RV outflow view.
- ■ TEE imaging of the pulmonary artery is challenging and requires high esophageal views.
- ■ Color, pulsed, and continuous wave (CW) Doppler allow detection of pulmonic regurgitation and abnormal pulmonary artery flow patterns.

Key points

- ❑ In adults, visualization of the lateral wall of the pulmonary artery is difficult due to limitation of the acoustic window by the adjacent lung.
- ❑ Pulmonary artery diameter measurements are mainly helpful in adults with congenital heart disease, and may be better made by other imaging techniques.
- ❑ A small amount of pulmonic regurgitation is normal and is characterized by a narrow jet on color Doppler and a low-intensity, low-velocity spectral Doppler signal.
- ❑ With pulmonary hypertension, the pulmonic regurgitant velocity is increased, reflecting the

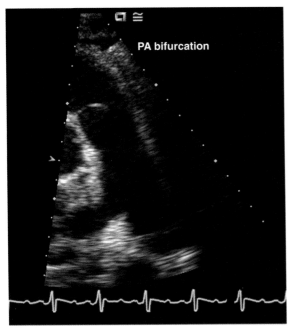

Figure 16–23. In the short axis view of the aortic valve, the pulmonary artery is seen. Often the lateral wall is difficult to delineate in adults.

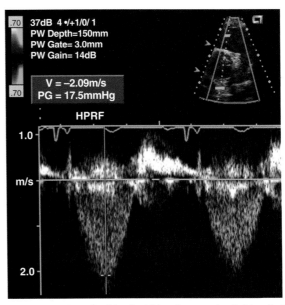

Figure 16–24. Stenosis of the distal right pulmonary artery in this patient with a repaired tetralogy of Fallot is demonstrated using high pulse repetition frequency Doppler to localize the origin of the high velocity jet.

elevation of pulmonary diastolic pressure, and there is a shortened time-to-peak velocity and mid-systolic deceleration in the antegrade flow signal.

❏ With branch pulmonary artery stenosis, a high-velocity signal may be detected with spectral Doppler, even when image quality is suboptimal. (see Figure 16–24)

❏ With a patent ductus arteriosus, the diastolic flow from the descending aorta into the pulmonary artery is seen with color and spectral Doppler.

❏ Full evaluation of the main pulmonary artery and branches in patients with congenital heart disease usually requires cardiac magnetic resonance or computed tomographic imaging.

THE ECHO EXAM

Disease of the Great Vessels
Examination of the Aorta

Aortic Segment	Modality	View	Recording	Limitations
Aortic root	TTE	Parasternal long axis	Images of sinuses of Valsalva, aortic annulus and sinotubular junction	Shadowing of posterior aortic root.
	TEE	High esophageal long axis	Standard long-axis plane by rotating to about 120-130 degrees	
Ascending	TTE	Parasternal long axis	Move transducer superiorly to image sinotubular junction and ascending aorta	Only limited segments visualized, variable between patients.
	TTE Doppler	Apical	LV outflow tract and ascending aorta flow recorded with pulsed or CW Doppler from an anteriorly angulated 4-chamber view	Velocity underestimation if the angle between the Doppler beam and flow is not parallel.
	TEE	High esophageal long axis	From long-axis view, move transducer superiorly and adjust rotation as needed to image ascending aorta	The distal ascending aorta may not be visualized.
Arch	TTE	Suprasternal	Long- and short-axis views of aortic arch	Descending aorta appears to taper as it leaves the image plane
	TEE	High esophageal	From the short-axis view of the initial segment of the descending thoracic aorta, turn the probe toward the patient's right side and angulate inferiorly	View not obtained in all patients. The aortic segment at the junction of the ascending aorta and arch may not be visualized.
Descending thoracic	TTE	Parastenal and modified apical views	Rotate from long-axis view to image thoracic aorta in long axis posterior to LV. From apical 2-chamber view, use lateral angulation and counterclockwise rotation to image aorta	Depth of thoracic aorta on TTE limits image qualtiy. TEE usually needed for diagnosis.
	TTE Doppler	Suprasternal	Descending aorta flow recorded with pulsed Doppler from SSN view	Low wall filters needed to evaluate for holodiastolic flow reversal.
Proximal abdominal	TTE	Subcostal	Long axis of proximal abdominal aorta	Only the proximal segment is visualized.
	TTE Doppler	Transgastric	Proximal abdominal aorta flow recorded with pulsed Doppler	Low wall filters needed to evaluate for holodiastolic flow reversal.
	TEE	Transgastric	From the transgastric position, portions of the abdominal aorta may be seen posteriorly.	Does not allow evaluation of entire abdominal aorta.

CW, continuous wave; LV, left ventricle; SSN, suprasternal notch; TEE, transesophageal echocardiogrpahy; TTE, transthoracic echocardiography.

AORTIC DISSECTION

Dissection flap
  In aortic lumen
  Independent motion
  True and false lumen
  Entry sites
  Thrombosis of false lumen
Intramural hematoma
Indirect findings
  Aortic dilation
  Aortic regurgitation
  Coronary ostial involvement
  Pericardial effusion

COMPLICATIONS OF THORACIC AORTIC DISSECTION

Aortic valve regurgitation
  Due to aortic root dilation
  Due to leaflet flail
Coronary artery occlusion due to dissection at the
  orifice
  Ventricular fibrillation
  Acute myocardial infarction
Distal vessel obstruction or occlusion
  Carotid (stroke)
  Subclavian (upper limb ischemia)
Aortic rupture
Into the pericardium:
  Pericardial effusion
Into the mediastinum:
  Pericardial tamponade
Into the pleural space:
  Pleural effusion
  Exsanguination

SINUS OF VALSALVA ANEURYSM

Congenital
  Complex shape
  Protrusion into right ventricular outflow tract
  Fenestrations
Acquired
  Infection or inflammation
  Symmetric shape
  Communication with aorta
  Potential for rupture

AORTIC ATHEROMA

Complex (≥4 mm or mobile)
Associated with:
  Coronary artery disease
  Cerebroembolic events

SELF-ASSESSMENT QUESTIONS

QUESTION 1

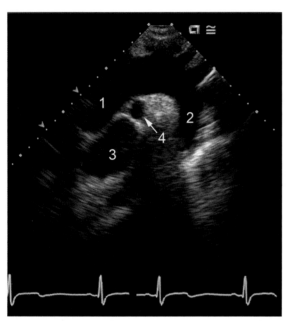

Figure 16–25.

Identify the structures numbered 1 to 5 by matching with the following list:

A. Descending aorta
B. Ascending aorta
C. Left ventricle
D. Left atrium
E. Right pulmonary artery
F. Left pulmonary artery
G. Brachiocephalic vein
H. Azygous vein

QUESTION 2

What is the structure indicated by the asterisk?

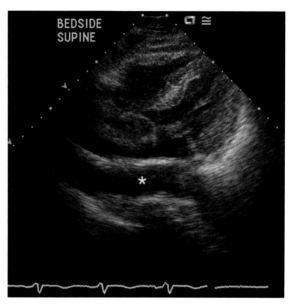

Figure 16–26.

How would you confirm this diagnosis?

QUESTION 3

This image was obtained in a 48-year-old man with an acute onset of chest pain.

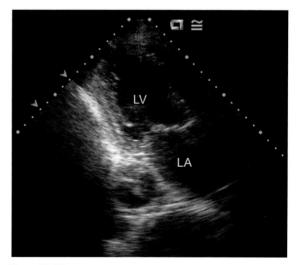

Figure 16–27.

The most likely diagnosis is:

A. Pulmonary embolism
B. Acute myocardial infarction
C. Mediastinal hematoma
D. Aortic dissection
E. Costochondritis

QUESTION 4

Echocardiography is requested in a 26-year-old man with atypical chest pain and no history of cardiac dysfunction. The following image is obtained.

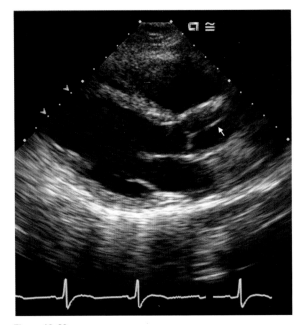

Figure 16–28.

The next best step for diagnostic evaluation is:

A. Perform transesophageal echocardiography
B. Move the transducer up an interspace
C. Use a higher-frequency transducer
D. Use fundamental instead of harmonic imaging
E. Obtain a contrast computed tomography study of the aorta

QUESTION 5

A 56-year-old man with a long history of hypertension presented to the Emergency Department with the sudden onset of severe tearing chest pain. His electrocardiogram showed only nonspecific ST changes. Urgent echocardiography at the bedside was performed, starting with subcostal images.

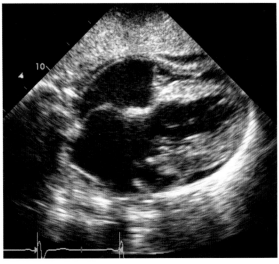

Figure 16–29.

Based on the clinical history and this image, the echocardiographic exam should next focus on:

A. Calculation of LV ejection fraction
B. Evaluation of regional ventricular systolic function
C. Imaging of the ascending aorta
D. Measurement of tricuspid regurgitant jet velocity
E. Respiratory variation in RV and LV diastolic filling

QUESTION 6

TEE imaging was requested to evaluate for endocarditis in a 32-year-old man with fevers and bacteremia.

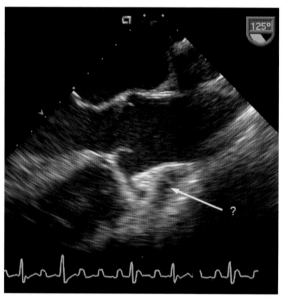

Figure 16–30.

This finding (arrow) is most consistent with:

A. Normal finding
B. Sinus of Valsalva aneurysm
C. Aortic annular abscess
D. Aortic pseudoaneurysm
E. Aortic dissection

QUESTION 7

This echocardiographic image was recorded in a 22-year-old man.

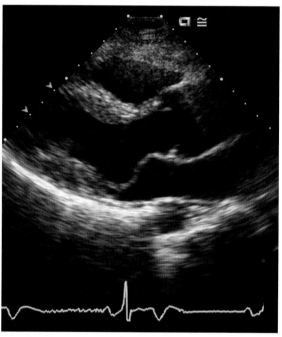

Figure 16–31.

The most likely diagnosis is:

A. Normal aorta
B. Sinus of Valsalva aneurysm
C. Aortic dissection
D. Marfan syndrome
E. Takayasu's arteritis
F. Bicuspid aortic valve

QUESTION 8

This 32-year-old man with no prior medical issues, other than a normally functioning bicuspid aortic valve, presents with the acute onset of severe chest pain. Which of the following diagnoses is most likely in the patient based on this image?

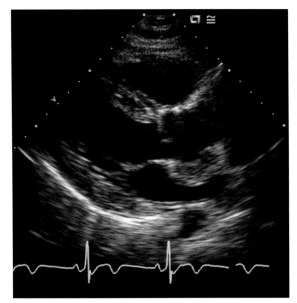

Figure 16–32.

A. Acute myocardial infarction
B. Aortic dissection
C. Pulmonary embolus
D. Paravalvular abscess
E. Aortic intramural hematoma

QUESTION 9

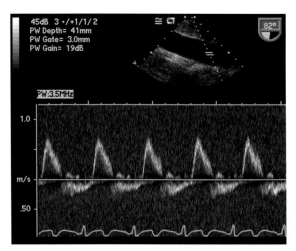

Figure 16–33.

This flow signal obtained on TEE is most consistent with the diagnosis of:

A. Aortic coarctation
B. Aortic regurgitation
C. Inferior vena cava obstruction
D. Branch pulmonary stenosis
E. Persistent left superior vena cava

ANSWERS

ANSWER 1

This suprasternal notch long-axis view of the aortic arch shows the:

1: B, Ascending aorta
2: A, Descending aorta
3: D, Left atrium
4: E, Right pulmonary artery

The LV is not well seen in this view. The right pulmonary artery is seen in cross section under the aortic arch, but the image plane does not include the left pulmonary artery. The azygous vein arises from the inferior vena cava, courses superiorly adjacent to the spine receiving the drainage of the intercostal veins, and then enters the superior vena cava above the right mainstem bronchus. When normal in size it is rarely seen by echocardiography and lies medial to the descending thoracic aorta.

ANSWER 2

Descending thoracic aorta

This is a low parasternal 4-chamber view with the transducer over the RV apex in this supine patient, showing a foreshortened view of the right and LVs, the right and left atria, and a bit of the aortic valve. Posterior to the left atrium, the tubular structure is the descending thoracic aorta, which is mildly dilated in this case. The identity of this structure can be confirmed by rotating the image plane 90 degrees to show the vessel in cross section. In addition, color and pulsed Doppler can be used to demonstrate the normal systolic flow pattern.

ANSWER 3: D

This apical 2-chamber view shows the descending thoracic aorta posterior to the left atrium. The descending aorta is dilated and there is a linear echo-density in the vessel lumen (*arrow in figure*), suggesting an aortic dissection. The pulmonary artery is not seen in this view. Thrombi are rarely seen in the pulmonary artery by echocardiography. Although specific, thrombus is not a sensitive finding for diagnosis of pulmonary embolism. A diagnosis of acute myocardial infarction depends on identification of a new regional wall motion abnormality of the LV, which was not present in this case. An aortic dissection might present with a mediastinal hematoma, which would be seen from the parasternal window. Costochondritis does not have any associated echocardiographic findings.

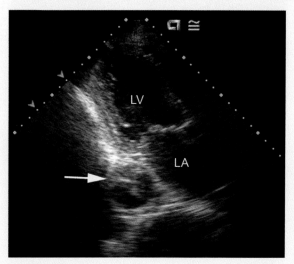

Figure 16–34.

ANSWER 4: B

The linear echo seen in the aorta most likely is a reverberation from the anterior aortic wall or a beam width artifact from the aortic closure line. Linear parallel reverberations artifacts also are seen posterior to the ascending aorta. Other findings that support an ultrasound artifact include the normal-size aorta, the normal aortic valve closure (not asymmetric as might be expected with a bicuspid valve), and the low pretest likelihood of aortic dissection in a young man with no risk factors for dissection (e.g., no evidence of Marfan syndrome, hypertension, or a bicuspid aortic valve). There also was no aortic regurgitation on color Doppler evaluation. A reverberation artifact can be avoided by using a different transducer position and moving up one interspace showed a normal aorta without luminal echodensities in this patient, and the reverberations posterior to the aorta also are no longer seen.

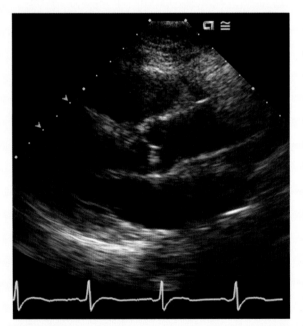

Figure 16–35.

A higher-frequency transducer would increase resolution in the near field but would not affect the reverberation artifact. Fundamental imaging also would not change this finding. If this echo finding was present in multiple views, or was associated with other abnormal findings, further evaluation with TEE or with computed tomographic imaging might be appropriate.

ANSWER 5: C

This patient's clinical history is strongly suggestive of acute aortic dissection and the presence of a small pericardial effusion is an ominous sign, suggesting partial rupture into the pericardium. The immediate next step should be evaluation of the ascending aorta, which in this patient showed a definite dissection flap (*arrow*) on a transthoracic echocardiographic parasternal long-axis view.

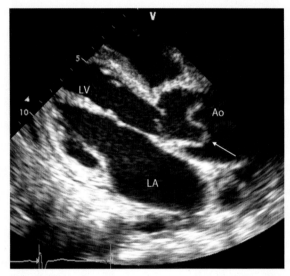

Figure 16–36.

When aortic dissection is suspected and transthoracic imaging is not diagnostic, further prompt evaluation by TEE or computed tomographic imaging is recommended because urgent surgical intervention can be lifesaving. In a clinically stable patient, evaluation of global and regional ventricular function is appropriate but unlikely to change therapy acutely in this patient with a nondiagnostic electrocardiogram (low likelihood of acute myocardial infarction) and no signs of acute heart failure. Pulmonary embolism may result in an acute elevation in pulmonary pressures but is unlikely to cause a pericardial effusion. Tamponade physiology, resulting in respiratory variation in RV and LV diastolic filling, can occur with aortic dissection but would be evident clinically as a low blood pressure or pulsus paradoxus, and treatment requires identification of the underlying cause—aortic dissection in this case.

ANSWER 6: A

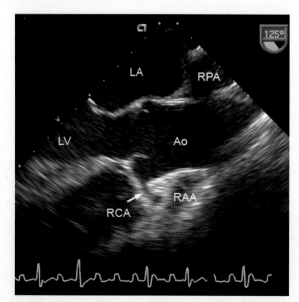

Figure 16–37.

This TEE long-axis view of the aorta shows a normal aortic valve with thin leaflets open in systole, the origin of the right coronary artery (RCA), and the tip of the right atrial appendage (RAA) immediately superior to the right coronary artery. The right pulmonary artery (RPA) is seen in circular cross section posterior to the aorta and superior to the LA. A sinus of Valsalva aneurysm communicates with one of the aortic sinuses and can be smooth walled (especially if congenital) or may have an irregular border if due to infection or with rupture of a congenital aneurysm. Aortic annular abscess occurs with endocarditis, most often with associated valvular vegetations, and may be echodense or may communicate with the aortic lumen. An aortic pseudoaneurysm due to a contained aortic rupture typically is larger than seen on this image and has a contour consistent with a high-pressure chamber. There are no linear echoes within the aortic lumen in this image, and the aortic size and contour appear normal.

ANSWER 7: D

This parasternal long-axis view shows a mildly dilated aorta (4.2 cm at the sinuses) with effacement of the sinotubular junction consistent with Marfan syndrome. This aorta is not normal for a 22-year-old man. In addition, the anterior mitral leaflet is long with systolic sagging toward the left atrium, as is typical with Marfan syndrome. A sinus of Valsalva aneurysm is characterized by asymmetric dilation of one of the sinuses, not symmetric as in this case. There is no intimal flap to suggest aortic dissection.

Takayasu's arteritis and other forms of aortitis, such as syphilis, are associated with increased thickness of the aortic wall due to the inflammatory process. With a bicuspid valve, aortic dilation may be present, but there often is some asymmetry or systolic doming of the aortic valve and effacement of the sinotubular junction is uncommon.

ANSWER 8: E

Bicuspid aortic valve disease is associated with dilation of the aortic sinuses and ascending aorta and with a higher risk of aortic dissection, which often occurs at a younger age (<45 years) than dissection related to hypertension or atherosclerosis. This parasternal long-axis view shows a markedly dilated ascending aorta (>5 cm) in this patient with bicuspid valve, but there is no luminal flap to suggest an aortic dissection. Instead there is a marked echodensity in the posterior aortic sinus that parallels the aortic wall, consistent with an aortic intramural hematoma. In terms of clinical management, aortic intramural hematoma and aortic dissection have similar adverse outcomes; because there is involvement of the ascending aorta, this patient underwent prompt aortic root replacement. An acute myocardial infarction would be evident as a regional wall motion abnormality and the patient does not have risk factors for early coronary artery disease. Pulmonary embolus is rarely seen on echocardiography (and the pulmonary artery is not seen on this view) so that alternate diagnostic approaches are recommended when pulmonary embolism is a concern. Indirect signs of pulmonary embolism on echocardiography include elevated pulmonary pressures and right-sided heart dysfunction, but these are not sensitive signs for making a diagnosis. The appearance of the posterior aortic root in this case might be mistaken for a paravalvular abscess; however, this diagnosis is unlikely because the patient does not have a consistent clinical history and there is no evidence for a valvular vegetation or valve dysfunction. At surgical inspection this was an intramural hematoma, not an abscess.

ANSWER 9: B

This pulsed Doppler was recorded from a TEE approach with the transducer turned posteriorly and the image plane rotated to 90 degrees to show the descending aortic in long axis. The flow signal shows antegrade flow in systole and with continuous (or holo-) diastolic flow reversal. This pattern is consistent with aortic valve regurgitation with retrograde flow back across the valve in diastole. Regurgitation is severe based on reversal in the distal descending aorta. A patent ductus would result in a similar flow pattern due to runoff from the aorta into the pulmonary artery in diastole. With aortic coarctation, antegrade velocity is increased and there is continuous *forward* flow in diastole. Branch pulmonary stenosis might be detected with the probe turned anteriorly, but it often is difficult to visualize branch pulmonary vessels on TEE and stenosis would be associated with high-velocity systolic flow. A persistent left superior vena cava would have a typical venous flow pattern with low-velocity antegrade systolic and diastolic flow. Inferior vena cava flow also would show a venous flow pattern; with obstruction, velocities would be higher and more continuous but both systolic and diastolic antegrade flow would be present.

The Adult with Congenital Heart Disease

BASIC PRINCIPLES

Identification of cardiac chambers and vessels

■ Identification of the chambers, great vessels, and their connections is the first step in echocardiographic evaluation of the patient with congenital heart disease (see Echo Exam).

Key points

❑ The RV and LV are distinguished based on the atrioventricular valve anatomy and position, the presence or absence of a moderator band, and the presence or absence of a muscular infundibular region. (Figure 17–1)

❑ The size and location of the ventricular chamber is not reliable for distinguishing the anatomic LV from RV.

❑ The RV tends to have a more triangular shape, whereas the LV is more ellipsoid, but shape can be unreliable when severe dilation is present.

❑ The aorta and pulmonary artery are identified by their distal anatomy; the pulmonary artery bifurcates into right and left pulmonary arteries, whereas the aorta supplies the head and neck arteries via the arch. (Figure 17–2)

❑ In addition to anatomic definitions, the ventricle that pumps oxygenated blood into the aorta is called the systemic ventricle and the ventricle that pumps systemic venous return into the pulmonary artery is called the pulmonic ventricle.

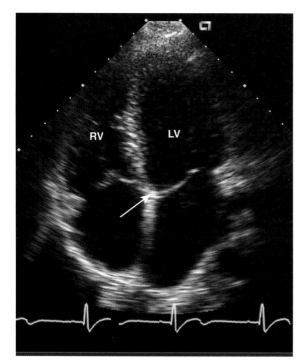

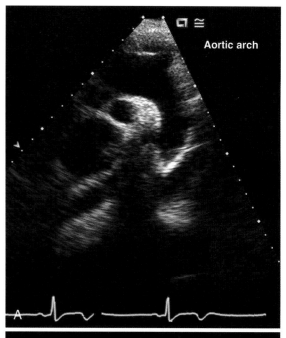

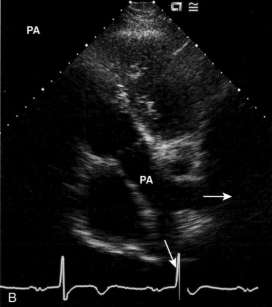

Figure 17–1. In this patient with congenital heart disease, the anatomic RV and LV are identified in the apical 4-chamber view based on morphologic features that include a more apical position of the tricuspid versus mitral annulus (*arrow*) and the moderator band and trabeculations in the RV. The atrioventricular valves are associated with the correct anatomic ventricle, even when atrial or great vessel connections are discordant. Mitral and tricuspid valve anatomy were confirmed in other views. This patient with a patent ductus arteriosus mild LV and LA enlargement but an otherwise unremarkable 4-chamber view.

Valve stenosis and regurgitation

■ Valve stenosis and regurgitation are evaluated using the same methods as for acquired valve disease.

Key points

❏ Congenital valve stenosis may be valvular, subvalvular, or supravalvular.
❏ Delineation of the level of obstruction using pulsed and color Doppler is necessary, in addition to CW Doppler measurements.

Intracardiac shunts

■ Intracardiac shunts are detected and quantitated using multiple Doppler modalities.

Key points

❏ Intracardiac shunts are detected based on the presence of a flow disturbance on the downstream side of the shunt with color or pulsed Doppler.

Figure 17–2. The aortic arch (A), in a suprasternal notch view, is identified by the arch and head and neck vessels. The pulmonary artery (B), from a low parasternal view, is identified based on its bifurcation.

❏ The velocity and shape of the CW Doppler signal across an intracardiac shunt reflects the pressure difference across the shunt and is a key factor in determining shunt location.
❏ The pulmonic-to-systemic flow ratio is calculated based on transpulmonic stroke volume and transaortic stroke volume.

Complex disease

- Complex congenital heart disease should be evaluated at centers with established Adult Congenital Heart Disease programs.

Key points

- ❏ This chapter includes a basic approach for simple conditions or patients with a well-established diagnosis.
- ❏ More complex cases require additional data acquisition by sonographers and physicians with expertise in congenital heart disease.

STEP-BY-STEP APPROACH

Basic transthoracic echo exam

- A structured study sequence is needed to ensure that all the images and Doppler flows needed for diagnosis are recorded.
- Most adult echocardiography laboratories acquire images and Doppler data in a similar sequence as for a standard adult study.
- With complex disease, the sonographer and physician work together during image acquisition to ensure the needed data are obtained.

Step 1: Review the clinical history

- Review the details of any previous surgical or percutaneous procedures.
- Obtain reports (and images when possible) of any previous diagnostic tests.
- Determine the specific objectives of the current examination.

Key points

- ❏ Knowledge of previous procedures and diagnostic studies ensures the current exam provides additional information and focuses on the key clinical issues.
- ❏ Complete evaluation of the adult with congenital heart disease often requires multiple diagnostic modalities; the echocardiographic examination provides only part of the needed information.

Step 2: Acquire images and Doppler data from the parasternal window

Parasternal long-axis view

- ❏ The position and angle of the transducer needed to obtain a long-axis view help identify an abnormal cardiac position in the chest (dextroversion or dextrocardia).

- ❏ Great vessel morphology and location are evaluated in the long-axis view.
- ❏ The connections of the great vessels to the ventricles are determined.
- ❏ Doppler is used to evaluate for valve regurgitation, areas of stenosis, and intracardiac shunts.

Key points

- ❏ Medial and lateral angulation of the transducer shows the relationship of the great vessels to each other and to the ventricular chambers.
- ❏ The pulmonary artery normally is anterior and runs perpendicular to the aorta; an anteriorly located aorta that lies parallel with the pulmonary artery suggests transposition of the great vessels. (Figure 17–3)
- ❏ The transducer is moved up one or more interspaces to follow the great vessel(s) seen in the long-axis view, allowing differentiation of the aorta from the pulmonary artery.
- ❏ Ventricular and atrial septal defects can be identified with color Doppler while slowly scanning from lateral to medial in the long-axis image plane and from apex to base in the short axis plane.
- ❏ Standard measurements of great vessels and cardiac chambers are recorded in the long-axis view.
- ❏ The transducer location for image acquisition is recorded because this information cannot be determined from the images themselves.

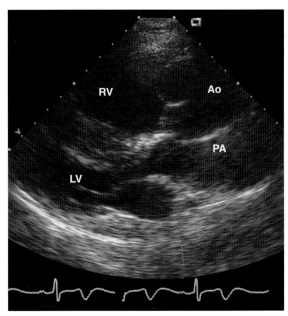

Figure 17–3. In a parasternal long-axis image of a patient with TGA, the anterior-posterior locations of the aorta (larger and anterior) and pulmonary artery (smaller and posterior) are opposite the normal position and the vessels lie parallel to each, rather than in the normal crisscross relationship.

- An enlarged coronary sinus suggests a persistent left superior vena cava (SVC). If needed, this can be confirmed with intravenous administration of saline contrast via the left upper extremity; after injection, contrast will appear in the coronary sinus before it drains into the RA. 2D imaging may confirm a persistent left SVC if a large vessel is seen branching off from the left subclavian vein.

Parasternal short axis view

- The short-axis view shows the relationship of the semilunar (aortic and pulmonic) valves.
- Basal ventricular size, systolic function, and septal motion are evaluated.
- Ventricular and atrial septal defects are demonstrated using color Doppler. (Figure 17–4)
- A cleft anterior mitral valve leaflet, commonly associated with primum atrial septal defects, may be seen from a parasternal short-axis view of the mitral valve.

Key points

- The normal relationship of the aortic and pulmonic valve planes is perpendicular to each other. When both are seen in short axis in the same image plane, transposition of the great vessels is present. (Figure 17–5)
- The anterior-posterior and medial-lateral locations of the aorta and pulmonary artery at the base are evaluated; the aortic root is anterior to the pulmonary artery when transposition is present.

- Atrial and ventricular septal defects typically are well seen in the short-axis view.
- The location of a ventricular septal defect relative to the aortic valve helps distinguish a membranous from subpulmonic (or supracristal) defect.
- Pulsed and CW Doppler interrogation of any abnormal color flow signal is helpful for diagnosis based on the time course and velocity of flow.

Parasternal right ventricular inflow and outflow views

- The RV inflow view is helpful for evaluation of the RA, pulmonary atrioventricular valve, and annulus. (Figure 17–6)
- CW Doppler measurement of atrioventricular valve regurgitant velocity allows measurement of RV (or pulmonary) systolic pressure.
- The RV outflow view allows visualization of RV outflow obstruction, at the subvalvular, pulmonic valve, or supravalvular level.
- Doppler evaluation allows localization of the level of RV outflow obstruction and calculation of the gradient between the ventricle and pulmonary artery.

Key points

- Standard RV inflow and outflow views may be difficult to obtain when transposition is present.
- Slow angulation from the long-axis view toward the RV inflow view, using color Doppler, may

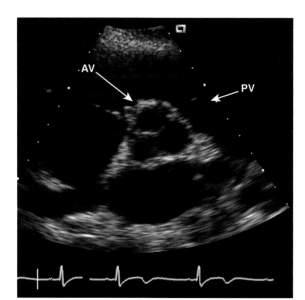

Figure 17–4. The normal aortic valve and pulmonic valve planes are perpendicular to each other so that the aortic valve (*AV*) is seen in short axis when the pulmonic valve (*PV*) is seen in long axis. Normally, the most anterior great vessel at the base of the heart is the pulmonary artery.

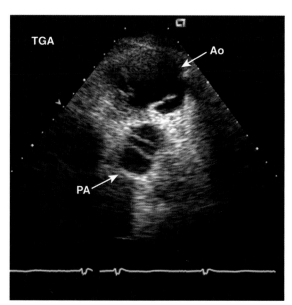

Figure 17–5. With TGA, the aorta is anterior to the pulmonary artery with a side-by-side (instead of crisscross) relationship of the great arteries. The semilunar valves are both in the same image plane so that the aortic and pulmonic valves are both seen in cross section in a short-axis view.

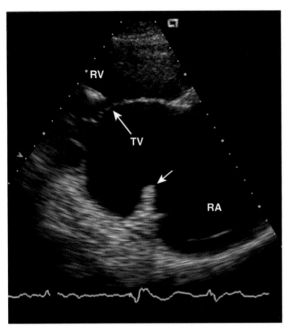

Figure 17–6. The RV inflow view in a patient with Ebstein's anomaly of the tricuspid valve shows the apical displacement of the septal leaflet from the annulus (*short arrow*), with the atrialized portion of the RV between the annulus and leaflet attachment level.

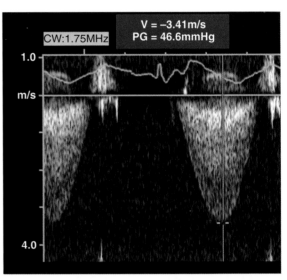

Figure 17–7. From a parasternal window, CW Doppler was used to record this high-velocity systolic ejection signal from the region of the pulmonic valve in a patient with pulmonic stenosis. This signal might be due to subpulmonic or valvular stenosis; two-dimensional imaging and color Doppler are helpful in localizing the level of obstruction.

be helpful for diagnosis of atrial and ventricular septal defect.

❑ When right (or pulmonic) ventricular outflow tract obstruction is present, ventricular systolic pressure does *not* equal pulmonary systolic pressure; instead, the transpulmonic gradient is subtracted from ventricular systolic pressure to determine pulmonary systolic pressure. (Figure 17–7)

❑ Evaluation of RV outflow obstruction requires color and pulsed Doppler to determine the anatomic location of the increase in velocity and CW Doppler to measure the peak velocity.

Step 3: Acquire images and Doppler data from the apical window

■ The morphology, size, and function of both ventricles are evaluated in the 4-chamber, 2-chamber, and long-axis views.

■ The atrioventricular valves are evaluated using two-dimensional imaging, color Doppler, and CW Doppler.

■ Anterior angulation from the 4-chamber view often allows imaging of the connection from each ventricle to the great vessels. (Figure 17–8)

■ Ventricular inflow and outflow signals are recorded using pulsed and CW Doppler.

Key points

❑ The normal transducer orientation is used to ensure correct identification of the location and anatomy of each ventricle.

❑ The apical view often allows recognition of the anatomic RV based on the shorter distance from the annulus to the apex, compared with the LV, as well as presence of the moderator band.

❑ The atrioventricular valves are evaluated using standard Doppler approaches.

❑ With anterior angulation to image the great vessels, the bifurcation of the pulmonary artery and the curve of the aortic arch may be visualized, helping with identification of the ventricular to great vessel connections.

❑ With posterior angulation, the size and location of the coronary sinus are evaluated.

❑ Atrial anatomy and size may be evaluated, although the distance of these chambers from the transducer may limit detailed evaluation, particularly in patients with an interatrial baffle repair.

❑ Evaluation of the interatrial septum may be limited by ultrasound dropout because the atrial septum is parallel to the ultrasound beam.

Step 4: Acquire images and Doppler data from the subcostal window

■ The subcostal 4-chamber view allows evaluation of the interatrial septum. (Figure 17–9)

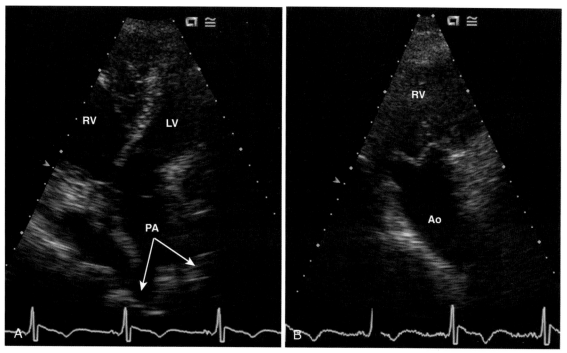

Figure 17–8. In this patient with TGA, from the apical 4-chamber view, the transducer is angulated anteriorly to show (A) the pulmonary artery (PA) with its bifurcation (arrows) and then (B) the ascending aorta (Ao), which has coronary ostia and an arch. This view is helpful for documenting which ventricle ejects into each great vessel. In this patient with transposition of the great vessels and an interatrial baffle repair, the RV ejects into the anteriorly located aorta and the LV ejects into the more posteriorly located pulmonary artery.

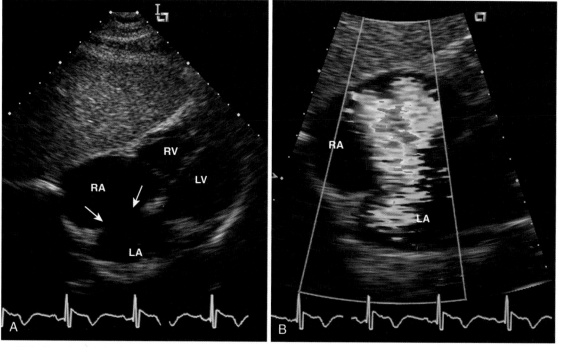

Figure 17–9. The subcostal view is ideal to evaluate for a secundum ASD. In this patient, the RA and RV are enlarged and there is an apparent defect in the center of the atrial septum (A). Because the ultrasound beam is perpendicular to the atrial septum from this window, this likely is a true defect and not echo dropout. Color flow imaging (B) confirms the large defect with left to right flow.

- RV size and systolic function often are best evaluated from the subcostal view.
- The entrance of the inferior vena cava provides clear identification of the RA chamber.

Key points

- ❑ The ultrasound beam is perpendicular to the interatrial septum from the subcostal view so that ultrasound dropout, simulating an atrial defect, is less likely. This view is optimal for two-dimensional and color Doppler detection of an atrial septal defect or patent foramen ovale.
- ❑ In adults, the free wall of the RV may not be well seen in apical views. The subcostal view provides a more standard image plane of the RV, with the ultrasound beam perpendicular to the RV free wall, and thus is more reliable for evaluation of RV size and function.
- ❑ The junction of the inferior vena cava and RA provides anatomic information on atrial situs, in addition to allowing estimation of RA pressure.

Step 5: Acquire images and Doppler data from the suprasternal notch window

- A standard transducer orientation allows identification of aortic arch position and anatomy.
- Aortic coarctation is evaluated (or excluded) based on CW Doppler descending aortic flow. (Figures 17–10 and 17–11)
- Images and pulsed Doppler flows in the superior vena cava are useful in many types of congenital heart disease.

Key points

- ❑ A right-sided aortic arch may be missed if the transducer or image orientation is reversed.
- ❑ Normal systolic and diastolic flow in the descending aorta excludes a diagnosis of aortic coarctation.

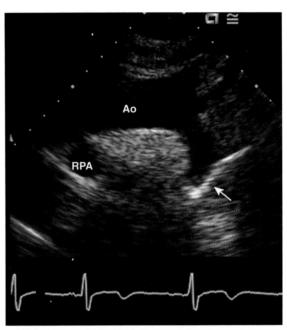

Figure 17–10. The suprasternal notch view is used to evaluate aortic coarctation. However, on two-dimensional imaging even a normal descending aorta appears to taper (*arrow*) because the curvature of the vessel results in an oblique plane through the vessel.

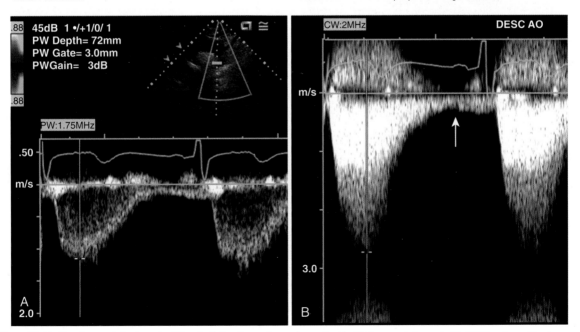

Figure 17–11. Flow is recorded using pulsed Doppler in the descending aorta proximal to (*A*) the coarctation and with CW Doppler as blood passes through the narrowed segment (*B*). When a severe coarctation is present, there is persistent antegrade flow in diastole (*arrow*) due to a higher diastolic pressure proximal, compared with distal, to the coarctation.

- The superior vena cava typically is to the right of the ascending aorta. Flow patterns are important when obstruction is present or when the superior vena caval flow has been redirected into the pulmonary artery.
- The right pulmonary artery is seen inferior to the arch. When ultrasound penetration is optimal, the LA and pulmonary veins also may be identified.
- The branch pulmonary arteries may be seen in the parasternal short-axis view in some patients.
- An aortic to pulmonary artery shunt may be evaluated from the suprasternal notch view in some cases (e.g., patent ductus arteriosis, aortic to pulmonary window).

Step 6: Pulmonary pressure estimation

- In the absence of pulmonic stenosis, RV (and pulmonary) systolic pressure is calculated by the standard approach based on tricuspid regurgitant jet velocity and estimated RA pressure. (Figure 17–12)
- With complex congenital heart disease, estimation of pulmonary pressures depends on the exact cardiac anatomy.

Key points

- When pulmonic stenosis is present, the transpulmonic systolic gradient is subtracted from the estimated RV systolic pressure.
- With a large unrestricted ventricular septal defect and Eisenmenger's physiology, pulmonary artery and aortic pressures are equalized, even if there is no tricuspid regurgitation.
- With tricuspid atresia and Fontan physiology (direct connection of systemic venous return to the pulmonary artery) pulmonary pressures are low with a venous type blood flow pattern.
- Pulmonary diastolic pressure can be estimated from the end-diastolic pulmonic regurgitant velocity, plus an estimate of RV diastolic pressure. (Figure 17–13)
- The velocity through a ventricular septal defect reflects the LV to RV systolic pressure difference.

Step 7: Review and report study results

- Most adult congenital disease studies are reported in the standard format with additional sections for the congenital findings.

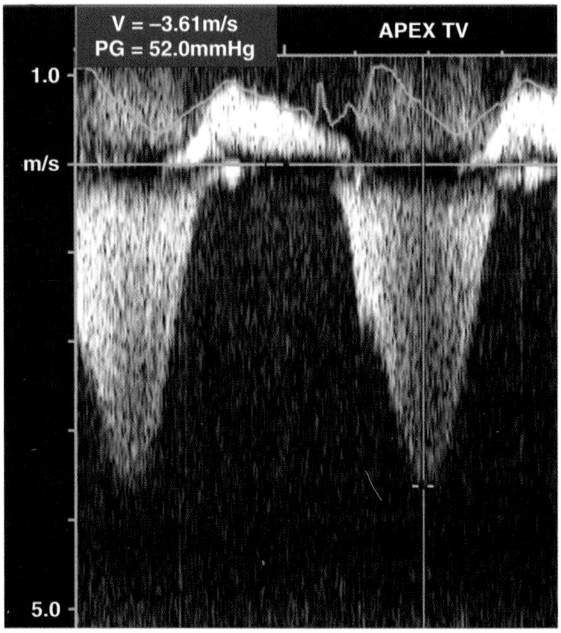

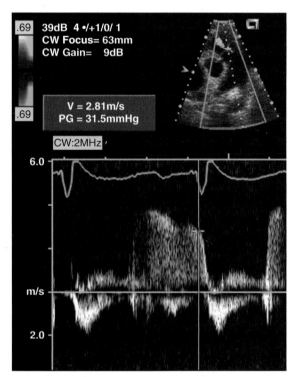

Figure 17–12. This tricuspid regurgitant jet shows a maximum velocity of 3.6 m/s, consistent with an RV to RA systolic pressure difference of 52 mm Hg, or an estimated RV systolic pressure of 62 mm Hg assuming an RA pressure of 10 mm Hg. However, this patient has pulmonic stenosis, so that the RV–to–pulmonary artery (*PA*) systolic gradient must be subtracted from the estimated RV pressure to estimate PA systolic pressure. This is the same patient as Figure 17–7, so estimated PA systolic pressure is 62 mm Hg – 47 mm Hg or 15 mm Hg.

Figure 17–13. The end-diastolic pulmonic regurgitant velocity reflects the diastolic PA–to–RV pressure gradient, 32 mm Hg in this case. Assuming an RV diastolic pressure of 10 mm Hg, estimated PA diastolic pressure is 32 mm Hg + 10 mm Hg = 42 mm Hg, consistent with severe pulmonary hypertension.

- The report describes the anatomy and physiology, with an indication of the level of certainty of each finding, depending on data quality.
- The echocardiographic findings are interpreted in view of the clinical history, previous surgical procedures, and current clinical indication.

Key points

- ❏ The findings in most patients with congenital disease can be described using a standard report format; however, with complex congenital heart disease, a more detailed narrative description is needed.
- ❏ The echocardiographic study should not be used to deduce the surgical history; instead, the surgical history should be reviewed to ensure the echocardiographic study provides a complete evaluation.
- ❏ The echocardiographic study should seek to answer the specific clinical question articulated by the referring physician.
- ❏ The current study should be compared with previous examinations (with side-by-side review of images when possible).

Step 8: Determine remaining anatomic/physiologic questions

- Initial evaluation of simple congenital heart disease and follow-up studies of more complex disease may require only transthoracic echocardiography.
- Additional diagnostic procedures often are needed for evaluation of complex congenital heart disease.

Key points

- ❏ Transthoracic echocardiography often cannot fully evaluate atrial-level anatomy and flow in patients with Fontan physiology or an interatrial baffle repair, due to the distance of the transducer from the structures of interest. (Figure 17–14)
- ❏ Extracardiac connections, such as arterial to pulmonary shunts, are difficult to assess by transthoracic echocardiography.
- ❏ Previous surgical procedures may result in shadowing or reverberations due to prosthetic valves, conduits, or patch material.
- ❏ Evaluation of branch pulmonary artery stenosis usually requires other diagnostic approaches.

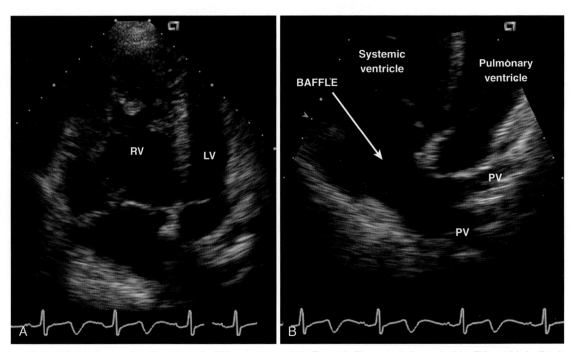

Figure 17–14. Apical 4-chamber view of a patient with TGA and an interatrial baffle repair. The systemic (anatomic right, *RV*) ventricle is dilated and hypertrophied as expected and the pulmonic (anatomic left, *LV*) ventricle is relatively normal size (*A*). The interatrial baffle is not well seen in the 4-chamber view, but the pulmonary venous channel is better seen by posterior angulation of the transducer with pulmonary veins (*PV*) draining into the baffle and then the systemic ventricle (*B*).

- Quantitation of RV volumes and systolic function is problematic with standard echocardiographic approaches.
- These areas of uncertainty or issues that cannot be addressed by echocardiography are identified at the end of the study with suggestions for appropriate additional diagnostic approaches.

Basic transesophageal approach

Step 1: Assess the risk of TEE and institute appropriate modifications in the study protocol

- The risk of conscious sedation is higher in some patients with congenital heart disease.
- Additional monitoring and sedation by an anesthesiologist may be needed in some cases.

Key points

- Risk of sedation is highest in patients with cyanosis, severe pulmonary hypertension, or Eisenmenger's physiology.
- Concurrent pulmonary or other medical conditions also may be present that increase procedural risk.
- Baseline oxygen saturation is assessed before beginning the procedure because patients may have significant chronic desaturation due to an intracardiac shunt.
- When risk is high or uncertain, a cardiac anesthesiologist should be asked to assist with the procedure.
- All health care providers involved in the study (e.g., physician, nurse, and sonographer) should understand and review any potential risks.

Step 2: Determine the objectives of the TEE study

- In consultation with the referring physician, the clinical data and transthoracic echocardiogram are reviewed to determine the specific areas of interest on the TEE study.
- A complete TEE study is performed whenever possible, putting priority on key elements if study length is constrained.

Key points

- TEE provides better visualization of posterior structures, such as the atrial septum, pulmonary veins, and interatrial baffle repairs. (Figure 17–15)
- TEE provides improved images when prosthetic material shadows posterior structures from the transthoracic approach.

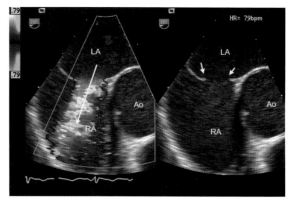

Figure 17–15. TEE provides superior images of the atrial septum. In this patient with a secundum ASD, the left to right flow across the defect is visualized with color Doppler (*left*) and the exact location and size (*arrows*) of the defect can be measured (*right*). Three-dimensional imaging also may be helpful to show the shape of the defect.

- Anterior and extracardiac structures, such as systemic venous return conduits, branch pulmonary stenosis, and arterial to pulmonic shunts, may be difficult to visualize on TEE. (Figure 17–16)
- Be sure all individuals involved in the TEE study understand the study objectives.

Step 3: TEE imaging sequence

- The standard imaging sequence, described in Chapter 3, is appropriate for adults with congenital heart disease.
- The examiner should ensure that all cardiac structures are evaluated by imaging and Doppler, preferably in at least two orthogonal views.

Key points

- Start with the standard TEE 4-chamber, 2-chamber, long-axis rotational series of images to provide an overview of cardiac anatomy.
- Follow a checklist to ensure all structures are evaluated:
  - Systemic and pulmonic ventricles (including anatomic identify, location, great vessel connections, and systolic function)
  - Aorta and pulmonary artery (including size, location, and connections to the ventricles)
  - Aortic and pulmonic valves (including anatomy and Doppler flows)
  - Systemic and pulmonic atrioventricular valves (anatomy and function)
  - Left and right atria (or interatrial baffle, Fontan conduit, etc.)
  - Atrial and ventricular septums
  - Location and flow patterns in all four pulmonary veins
  - Superior and inferior vena cava

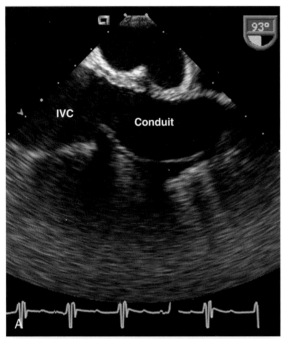

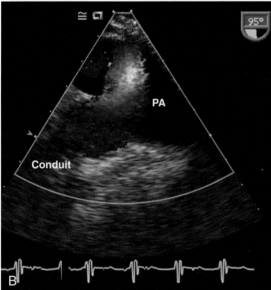

Figure 17–16. This patient has tricuspid atresia and a Fontan conduit from the inferior vena cava (*IVC*) to the pulmonary artery. The conduit is seen on TEE in a vertical image plane by turning the probe toward the patient's right side. The junction of the IVC and the conduit (*A*) is seen and then the probe is slowly withdrawn in the esophagus, keeping the conduit centered in the image plane (*B*) to show the flow from the conduit into the pulmonary artery.

- Coronary sinus
- Descending aorta
- ❏ Transgastric views may provide alternate views of the ventricles, atrioventricular valves, an aortic and pulmonic valves.
- ❏ Before completing the study, ask the nurse and sonographer if any imaging views or Doppler flows have been missed and if they have any other suggestions.

SPECIAL CONSIDERATIONS IN COMMONLY SEEN CONDITIONS

Atrial septal defect

- RV volume overload due to an atrial septal defect (ASD) results in the characteristic findings of RV enlargement and paradoxical septal motion.
- ASD are classified as:
  - Secundum (center of atrial septum)
  - Primum (adjacent to the atrioventricular valves)
  - Sinus venosus (near junction of superior or inferior vena cava)
- Anomalous pulmonary venous drainage into the RA or cavae also results in right-sided volume overload. (Figure 17–17)
- Both the anatomic size of an ASD (measured directly) and the physiologic effects (based on the amount of flow across the defect) are useful measures of disease severity.

Key points

- ❏ A secundum or primum ASD may be visualized on transthoracic imaging in parasternal short-axis, apical 4-chamber, and subcostal 4-chamber views. (see Figures 17–9 and 17–15)
- ❏ Color Doppler evidence of transatrial flow avoids mistaking echo dropout from an ASD, but care is needed to distinguish normal superior and inferior vena caval inflow from flow across the atrial septum.
- ❏ A primum ASD may be accompanied by a cleft anterior mitral leaflet. (Figure 17–18)
- ❏ An endocardial cushion defect is the association of a primum ASD with an adjacent ventricular septal defect, often with associated abnormalities of the atrioventricular valves.
- ❏ A sinus venosus ASD may be difficult to visualize on transthoracic imaging and often is suspected based on unexplained right-sided enlargement; on TEE imaging in the bicaval view with the probe rotated slightly rightward, the defect is seen at the junction of the superior vena cava with the RA. Anomalous pulmonary venous return may also be seen.
- ❏ The presence of RV dilation mandates a careful search for an ASD or anomalous pulmonary venous return using two-dimensional imaging, color Doppler, and an intravenous saline contrast study.
- ❏ When visualized, the diameter of the ASD should be directly measured from two images.
- ❏ Shunt flow, defined as the ratio of pulmonary blood flow (Qp) to systemic blood flow (Qs), is determined by calculating stroke volume in the pulmonary artery and aorta, with a ratio of more than 1.5:1 considered significant.

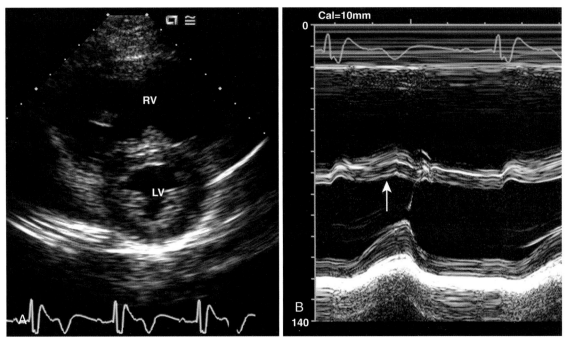

Figure 17–17. With right-sided volume overload (but normal pulmonary pressures) due an ASD, there is significant right-sided heart enlargement on two-dimensional imaging with a normal septal curvature at end-systole (*A*), and there is paradoxical septal motion seen on M-mode with anterior motion of the septum during systole and rapid posterior motion during diastole due to the increased right-sided diastolic filling volume.

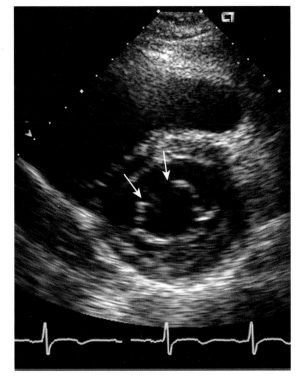

Figure 17–18. A cleft anterior mitral valve seen in a parasternal short-axis image with differing maximal excursion of the medial and lateral aspects of the cleft leaflet (*arrows*).

❑ Transesophageal imaging is more sensitive than transthoracic imaging for detection of a sinus venosus ASD or anomalous pulmonary venous return.

Ventricular septal defect

■ Ventricular septal defects (VSDs) are classified as:
  • Membranous (from just beneath the aortic valve to under the septal tricuspid leaflet)
  • Supracristal (from just beneath the aortic valve to under the pulmonic valve)
  • Inlet (between the mitral and tricuspid valves)
  • Muscular (anywhere in the muscular part of the ventricular septum)
■ Large uncorrected VSDs result in severe pulmonary hypertension early in life with equalization of pulmonary and systolic pressures and bidirectional shunting (Eisenmenger's physiology).
■ Small VSDs are associated with a high-pressure difference (and high velocity) between the LV and RV in systole.

Key points

❑ The anatomic site of a VSD is detected using the combination of 2D imaging and color Doppler to demonstrate systolic turbulence on the right side of the ventricular septum. (Figures 17–19 and 17–20)

❏ The VSD is confirmed using CW Doppler to demonstrate the high-velocity systolic ejection type Doppler curve. (Figure 17–21)

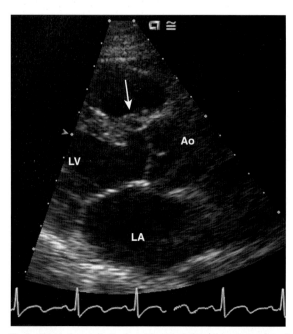

Figure 17–19. In a patient referred for a systolic murmur, the region of the membranous septum (*arrow*) appears abnormal in the standard parasternal long-axis view.

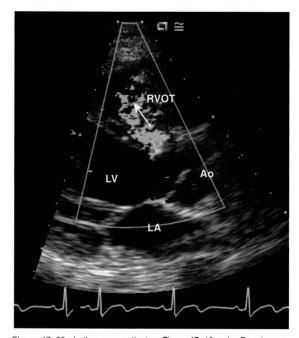

Figure 17–20. In the same patient as Figure 17–19, color Doppler confirms right to left flow consistent with a membranous VSD.

❏ The peak velocity of the VSD jet is related to the left to RV systolic pressure difference as stated in the Bernoulli equation: $\Delta P = 4V^2$

❏ A low velocity diastolic signal also may be seen corresponding to the diastolic pressure difference between the LV and RV.

❏ With Eisenmenger's physiology, a large VSD is seen on 2D imaging with bidirectional flow on color and spectral Doppler. Right and LV size and wall thickness are similar and the velocities in the mitral and tricuspid regurgitant jets are equal. (Figure 17–22)

Patent ductus arteriosus

■ Most patent ductus arteriosus (PDAs) are diagnosed and treated early in life, with only rare cases diagnosed in adults.

■ Continuous systolic and diastolic flow into the main pulmonary artery is the key findings in adults with a PDA.

Key points

❏ Color Doppler of the main pulmonary artery shows the diastolic flow from the PDA originating near the pulmonary artery bifurcation. (Figure 17–23)

❏ Pulsed Doppler evidence of continuous flow in the pulmonary artery is diagnostic; this flow differs from pulmonic regurgitation by being distal to the pulmonic valve, and the diastolic components extend into systole. (Figure 17–24)

❏ Diastolic flow reversal also may be seen in the descending thoracic aorta and should not be mistaken for aortic regurgitation.

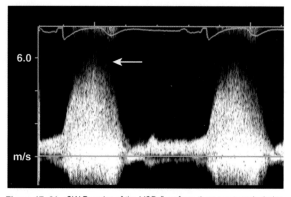

Figure 17–21. CW Doppler of the VSD flow from the parasternal window in the same patient as Figure 17–20 shows a very high velocity signal consistent with a small defect and a large systolic pressure gradient between the LV and RV in systole. There also is low velocity left to right flow in diastole.

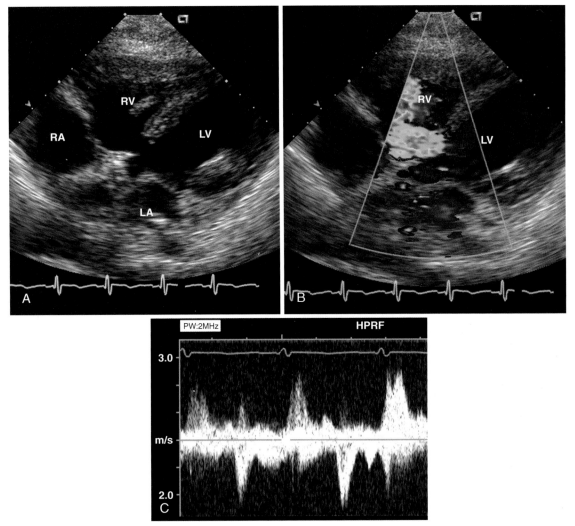

Figure 17–22. With a large VSD, as seen in this low parasternal 4-chamber view in a patient with trisomy 21, Eisenmenger physiology is present with equalization of RV and LV pressures, significant systemic oxygen desaturation, and cyanosis. Color flow shows both right to left (*B*) and left to right flow, and spectral Doppler showing relatively low-velocity bidirectional flow (*C*).

Aortic coarctation

- An aortic coarctation results in an increased systolic velocity and persistent diastolic antegrade flow in the descending thoracic aorta. (Figure 17–25)
- Descending aortic flow is recorded with CW Doppler from the suprasternal notch view.

Key points

- ❏ Doppler may underestimate the severity of coarctation due to nonparallel intercept angle between the eccentric jet and ultrasound beam.
- ❏ When the proximal velocity is also increased, the proximal velocity should be included in the pressure gradient calculation:

$$\Delta P = 4 \left(V_{max}^{2} - V_{prox}^{2} \right)$$

(see Figure 17–11).

- ❏ Imaging of the coarctation is rarely possible by transthoracic imaging in adults; TEE may be helpful in selected cases.
- ❏ Further evaluation of aortic coarctation with computed tomographic imaging or cardiac catheterization typically is needed.

Ebstein's anomaly

- Ebstein's anomaly is characterized by apical displacement of one or more tricuspid valve leaflets (Figure 17–26, and see Figure 17–6).
- Imaging the tricuspid annulus and leaflets in parasternal RV inflow and apical 4-chamber views usually is diagnostic.
- The segment of the RV between the annulus and displaced leaflet is "atrialized"; that is, ventricular

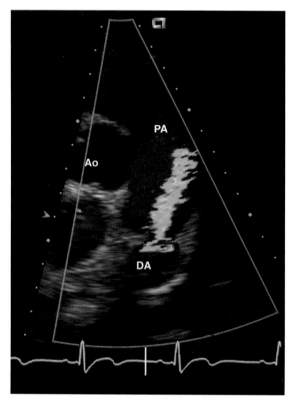

Figure 17–23. Patent ductus arteriosus seen in a parasternal short-axis image of the pulmonary artery. A color jet of diastolic flow is seen entering the pulmonary artery near its bifurcation, with the flow originating from the descending aorta (*DA*) just posterior to the pulmonary artery.

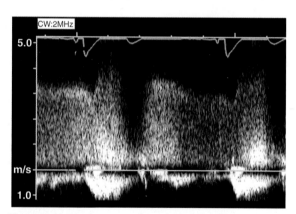

Figure 17–24. With a patent ductus arteriosus, CW Doppler shows continuous flow from the aorta into the pulmonary artery with the shape and velocity reflecting the pressure difference between the two vessels. For example, the increased systolic velocity corresponds to the increase in systemic blood pressure during systole.

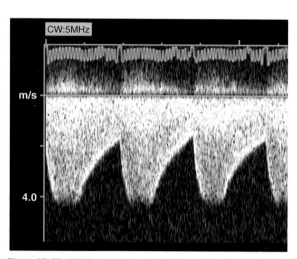

Figure 17–25. CW Doppler flow in the descending aorta in a patient with a severe aortic coarctation. The antegrade velocity more than 4 m/s is consistent with a pressure gradient of at least 64 mm Hg (possibly higher if the intercept angle is not parallel to blood flow), and persistent antegrade flow in diastole confirms severe obstruction.

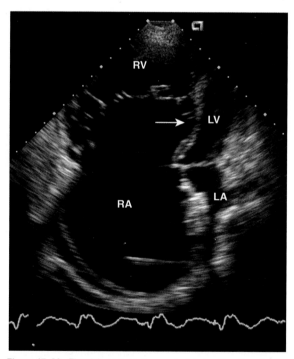

Figure 17–26. Ebstein's anomaly in an apical 4-chamber view showing severe apical displacement of the septal tricuspid valve leaflet (*arrow*).

myocardium is physiologically part of the atrial chamber.

Key points

❏ Ebstein's anomaly may be isolated or associated with an ASD and is common (about 15%-

40%) in patients with congenitally corrected transposition of the great vessels (see later section).

❏ Ebstein's anomaly is often associated with ventricular pre-excitation due to an accessory atrioventricular pathway (e.g., Wolf-Parkinson-White syndrome).

❏ In the apical 4-chamber view, a distance greater than 10 mm between the mitral and tricuspid leaflet insertions is diagnostic of Ebstein's anomaly.

❏ Ebstein's anomaly typically results in moderate or severe tricuspid regurgitation.

Complex congenital heart disease

Tetralogy of Fallot

- Tetralogy of Fallot (TOF) is characterized by:
  - A membranous (anteriorly misaligned) ventricular septal defect
  - An aorta that straddles the ventricular septum *and*
  - RV outflow obstruction *resulting in*
  - RV hypertrophy
- Most adults with TOF have undergone previous surgical repair with ventricular septal defect closure and relief of RV outflow obstruction. (Figure 17–27)
- The most common long-term issue after TOF repair is severe pulmonic regurgitation with progressive RV enlargement and eventual dysfunction.
- Patients with TOF usually have mild dilation of the aortic sinuses.

Key points

❏ RV outflow obstruction may be subvalvular, valvular, or supravalvular or may occur at more than one site, including branch pulmonary artery stenoses.

❏ Occasionally an adult patient with an untreated TOF will be diagnosed by echocardiography because the RV outflow obstruction prevents pulmonary hypertension.

❏ Severe pulmonic regurgitation typically is low velocity with a to-and-fro flow pattern by pulsed, CW, and color Doppler that may be overlooked due to the absence of turbulence. (Figure 17–28)

❏ Additional evaluation with cardiac magnetic resonance (CMR) imaging often is needed for quantitation of RV size and function.

Congenitally corrected transposition of the great arteries (L-TGA)

- The pathway of blood flow with L-TGA is:
  - Systemic venous return to the RA, then into the LV and out the pulmonary artery, *and*
  - Pulmonary venous return to the LA, then into the RV and out the aorta
- Some patients with L-TGA remain undiagnosed until adulthood because the flow of oxygenated and unoxygenated blood is physiologic, even

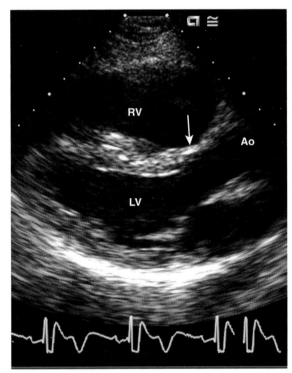

Figure 17–27. Parasternal long-axis view in a typical patient with repaired TOF. The RV outflow tract is enlarged; the basal septum is intact but has increased echogenicity (*arrow*) suggestive of VSD patch repair; and the aorta is mildly enlarged and slightly overrides the septum.

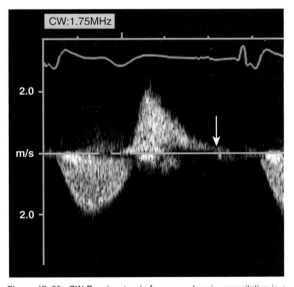

Figure 17–28. CW Doppler signal of severe pulmonic regurgitation in a patient with repaired TOF and persistent pulmonic regurgitation after surgical pulmonic valvotomy. The retrograde flow in diastole has a signal density similar to antegrade flow, consistent with similar volume flow rates. The diastolic deceleration slope is steep and reaches the baseline before the end of diastole (*arrow*), consistent with equalization of diastolic pulmonary artery and RV pressures.

though the anatomic RV serves as the systemic ventricle.

- Defects commonly associated with L-TGA include a ventricular septal defect, pulmonic stenosis, and Ebstein's anomaly of the systemic (tricuspid) atrioventricular valve, and complete heart block.

Key points

❑ L-TGA also is called "ventricular inversion" because the pattern of blood flow is normal other than the reversed positions of the ventricles (and the associated atrioventricular valves).

❑ Typically, the aortic annulus is anterior and to the left (the "L" in L-TGA) of the pulmonic valve.

❑ L-TGA is evident on echocardiography based on the systemic ventricle having the anatomic features of an RV (moderator band, apical annulus, and tricuspid valve). (Figure 17–29).

❑ The atrioventricular valves are associated with each ventricle so the systemic atrioventricular valve is the tricuspid valve and the pulmonary atrioventricular valve is the mitral valve.

❑ Long-term systolic dysfunction of the systemic ventricle may complicate L-TGA.

❑ Dextroversion (apex pointed toward the right) or mesocardia often is present with L-TGA, which limits acoustic access due to the retrosternal cardiac position.

Complete transposition of the great arteries (D-TGA)

- Complete transposition requires intervention at birth to provide mixing between the separated pulmonic and systemic blood flow circuits.

- D-TGA then is treated by redirection of blood flow in childhood with:
  - An interatrial baffle repair that redirects systemic and pulmonary venous inflow to restore a normal pattern of circulation, but with the anatomic RV serving as the systemic ventricle (Mustard or Senning repair) *or*
  - More recently, an arterial switch procedure with the aorta and pulmonary artery transected and reconnected to the correct ventricles

- The aorta is anterior and the great vessels are parallel to each other when D-TGA is present (see Figures 17–3 and 17–4).

- With an interatrial baffle repair, a major long-term issue is systolic dysfunction of the systemic (anatomic right) ventricle.

- With an arterial switch repair, a few patients develop systemic semilunar valve regurgitation, particularly of the neo-aortic valve with dilation of the proximal "aortic" root. (Figure 17–30)

Key points

❑ With an interatrial baffle repair, the circulatory pattern of oxygenated and unoxygenated blood

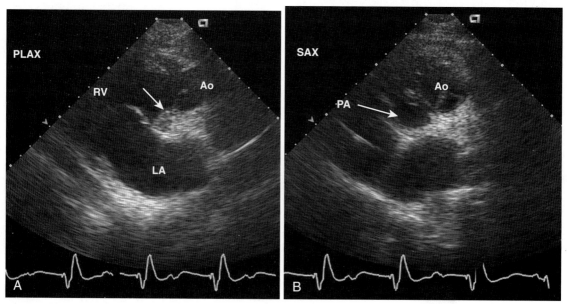

Figure 17–29. (A) Parasternal long-axis view in a patient with congenitally corrected L-TGA (ventricular inversion) shows the muscular ridge (*arrow*) between the systemic atrioventricular valve and aorta. This muscular band in the RV outflow tract identifies the anatomic RV (and tricuspid valve), which receives blood from the pulmonary veins and LA and ejects into the aorta. (B) in the short axis view (SAX), the position of the aorta (Ao) anterior to the pulmonary artery (PA) and the side-by-side relationship of the great arteries is evident.

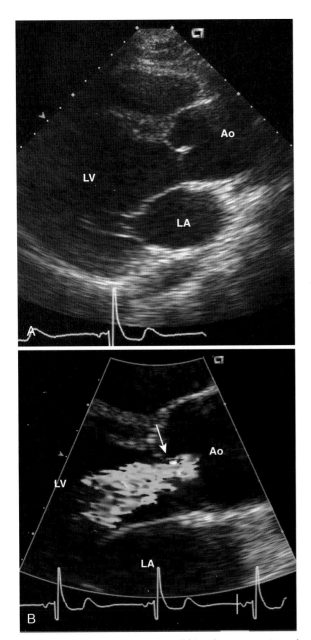

Figure 17–30. This 19-year-old man with TGA underwent a great vessel switch repair as an infant. The ventricular to great vessel relationships now are relatively normal as seen in this long-axis view. However, the sinuses of the transposed pulmonic valve (neo-aorta) are dilated to 4.6 cm (A) and central "aortic" regurgitation is present (B), with a vena contracta width of 0.5 cm.

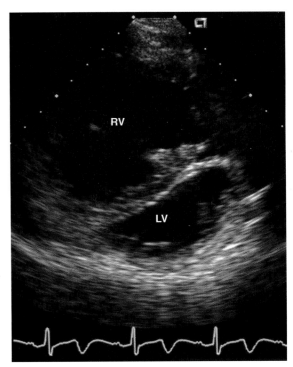

Figure 17–31. Short-axis view of the ventricles in a patient with TGA and an interatrial baffle repair. The RV is located anteriorly but serves as the systemic ventricle and is appropriately dilated and hypertrophied. The smaller, posteriorly located LV is the low-pressure pulmonic ventricle with systolic curvature of the septum reflecting the physiologic functions of each ventricle.

- ☐ Atrial baffle leaks and stenosis are difficult to evaluate by transthoracic imaging, typically requiring TEE or other imaging approaches.
- ☐ A lower Nyquist limit (i.e., signal aliasing at a lower velocity) and use of variance mode on the color display enhance detection of baffle leaks.
- ☐ With an arterial switch procedure, the neoaorta —the systemic semilunar valve and sinuses— was the anatomic pulmonic valve. The coronary arteries also were transposed to the neoaorta.
- ☐ Branch pulmonic stenosis can occur after an arterial switch repair related to moving the pulmonary artery anteriorly during the repair procedure.

Fontan physiology with tricuspid atresia

- ■ Fontan physiology refers to a direct valveless surgical connection from the systemic venous return to the pulmonary artery, without an intervening RV.
- ■ A Fontan repair is used for patients with only a single functional ventricle, including those with tricuspid atresia. (Figure 17–32)
- ■ Flow in a Fontan conduit is driven by the pressure gradient from the systemic venous return to the

is normal but the systemic ventricle is the anatomic RV and the pulmonic ventricle is the anatomic LV. (Figure 17–31)

- ☐ The atrioventricular valves are associated with each ventricle so the systemic atrioventricular valve is the tricuspid valve and the pulmonic atrioventricular valve is the mitral valve.

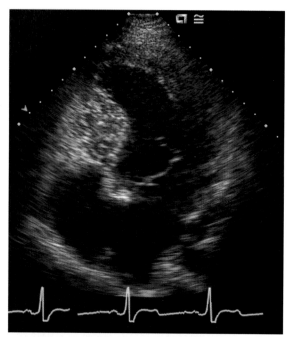

Figure 17–32. Apical view in a patient with tricuspid and pulmonic atresia shows only one ventricle and atrioventricular valve. The tricuspid valve is absent, with the small residual RV chamber (not visible in this view) communicating with the LV via a VSD. The right and left atria are connected by a large ASD. Pulmonary blood flow in this patient is provided by a right subclavian artery to pulmonary artery shunt.

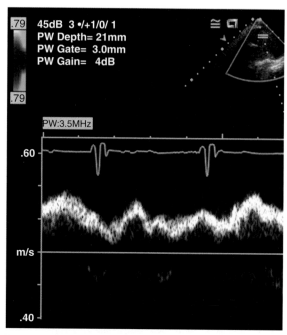

Figure 17–33. Flow in a Fontan conduit is similar to systemic venous flow, with low velocity forward flow in systole and diastole.

pulmonary artery, with a flow pattern similar to a normal systemic venous inflow. (Figure 17–33)

Key points

❏ There are many variations of the Fontan procedure:
  • Early Fontan repairs connected the RA to the pulmonary artery. These patients often have a severely enlarged RA with significant arrhythmias and may have obstruction of the pulmonary veins posterior to the dilated atrium.
  • More recent repairs include a direct connection of the superior vena cava to the right pulmonary artery with the inferior vena cava connected to the pulmonary artery by a conduit. This repair leaves the small residual RA (with the coronary sinus) in communication with the LA via an ASD.

❏ Transthoracic and transesophageal echocardiographic evaluation of a Fontan conduit is challenging and depends on the exact surgical repair and location of the conduit. (see Figure 17–16)

❏ Valved conduits connecting the RV to the pulmonary artery are used for other types of complex congenital heart disease. These patients do not have Fontan physiology because the RV provides pulsatile systolic pulmonary blood flow.

THE ECHO EXAM

Adult Congenital Heart Disease
Categories of Congenital Heart Disease

CONGENITAL STENOTIC LESIONS

Subvalvular
Valvular
Supravalvular
Peripheral great vessels (aortic coarctation)

CONGENITAL REGURGITANT LESIONS

Myxomatous valve disease
Ebstein's anomaly

ABNORMAL INTRACARDIAC COMMUNICATIONS

Atrial septal defect (ASD)
Ventricular septal defect (VSD)
Patent ductus arteriosus (PDA)

ABNORMAL CHAMBER AND GREAT VESSEL CONNECTIONS

Transposition of the great arteries (D-TGA)
Congenitally corrected transposition (L-TGA)
Tetralogy of Fallot (TOF)
Tricuspid atresia
Truncus arteriosus

Approach to the Echocardiographic Examination in Adults with Congenital Heart Disease

BEFORE THE EXAMINATION

Review the clinical history
Obtain details of any prior surgical procedures
Review results of prior diagnostic tests
Formulate specific questions

SEQUENCE OF EXAMINATION

Identify cardiac chambers, great vessels, and their connections
Identify associated defects, and evaluate the physiology of each lesion
Regurgitation and/or stenosis (quantitate as per Chapters 11 and 12)
Shunts (calculate $Q_p:Q_s$)
Pulmonary hypertension (calculate pulmonary pressure)
Ventricular dysfunction (measure ejection fraction if anatomy allows)

AFTER THE EXAMINATION

Integrate echo and Doppler findings with clinical data
Summarize findings
Identify which clinical questions remain unanswered, suggest appropriate subsequent diagnostic tests

Clues to the Identification of Cardiac Structures in Adults with Congenital Heart Disease

Structure	Anatomic Feature	Echo Approach
Right atrium	Inferior vena cava enters RA	Start with subcostal approach to identify RA
Right ventricle	Prominent trabeculation Moderator band Infundibulum Tricuspid valve Apical location of annulus	Apical 4-chamber view to compare annular insertions of AV valves, parasternal for valve anatomy and infundibulum
Pulmonary artery	Bifurcates	Parasternal long-axis view or apical 4-chamber view angulated very anteriorly
Left atrium	Pulmonary veins usually enter LA	TEE imaging for pulmonary vein anatomy
Left ventricle	Mitral valve Basal location of annulus Fibrous continuity between anterior mitral leaflet and semilunar valve	Apical 4-chamber view and parasternal long- and short-axis views.
Aorta	Gives rise to aortic arch and arterial branches.	Start with parasternal long-axis view and move transducer superiorly to follow vessel to its branches.

AV, atrioventricular; LA, left atrium; RA, right atrium; TEE, transesophageal echocardiography.

EXAMPLES

1. A 24-year-old with a history of a cardiac murmur has an echocardiogram that shows:

RV outflow velocity	1.6 m/s
Pulmonary artery velocity	3.1 m/s
Tricuspid regurgitant jet	3.4 m/s
Estimated right atrial pressure	5 mm Hg (small IVC with normal respiratory variation)

Because the RV outflow velocity is elevated, the maximum pulmonic valve gradient should be calculated using the proximal velocity in the Bernoulli equation:

$$\Delta P = 4 \left(V^2_{jet} - V^2_{prox} \right)$$

$$\Delta P = 4[(3.1)^2 - (1.6)^2] = 4[9.6 - 2.6] = 28 \text{ mm Hg}$$

If the proximal velocity is not included, the gradient would be overestimated at 38 mm Hg.

Estimated pulmonary systolic pressure is calculated by subtracting the pulmonic valve gradient from the estimated right ventricular pressure because pulmonic stenosis is present:

$$PAP = (\Delta P_{RV-RA} + P_{RA}) - \Delta P_{RV-PA}$$

$$PAP = (4V^2_{TR} + P_{RA}) - \Delta P_{RV-PA} = [4(3.4)^2 + 5)] - 28 = 23 \text{ mm Hg}$$

Thus, pulmonary artery systolic pressure is normal even though the tricuspid regurgitant jet indicates an RV systolic pressure of 51 mm Hg.

2. A 26-year-old woman undergoes echocardiography for symptoms of decreased exercise tolerance. She is found to have an enlarged RA and RV with paradoxic septal motion and the following Doppler data:

RV outflow velocity	
Velocity-time integral (VTI_{RVOT})	32 cm
Diameter	2.6 cm
Left ventricular outflow	
Velocity	1.1 m/s
Velocity-time integral (VTI_{LVOT})	16 cm
Diameter	2.4 cm

The right heart enlargement suggests an atrial septal defect may be present. The shunt ratio is calculated from the ratio of pulmonary flow (Q_p), measured in the RV outflow tract (RVOT), and systemic flow (Q_s), measured in the LV outflow tract (LVOT). At each site, cross-sectional area is calculated as the area of a circle:

$$CSA_{RVOT} = \pi(D/2)^2 = 3.14(2.6/2)^2 = 5.3 \text{ cm}^2$$

$$CSA_{LVOT} = \pi(D/2)^2 = 3.14(2.4/2)^2 = 4.5 \text{ cm}^2$$

Flow (stroke volume) at each site then is calculated:

$$Q_p = CSA_{RVOT} \times VTI_{RVOT} = 5.3 \text{ cm}^2 \times 32 \text{ cm} = 170 \text{ cm}^3$$

$$Q_s = CSA_{LVOT} \times VTI_{LVOT} = 4.5 \text{ cm}^2 \times 16 \text{ cm} = 72 \text{ cm}^3$$

so that

$$Qp:Qs = 170/72 = 2.4 \text{ to } 1$$

These calculations are consistent with a significant shunt that most likely will require closure to prevent progressive right heart dysfunction.

IVC, inferior vena cava.

SELF-ASSESSMENT QUESTIONS

QUESTION 1

A 23-year-old asymptomatic woman is referred for echocardiography to evaluate a murmur.

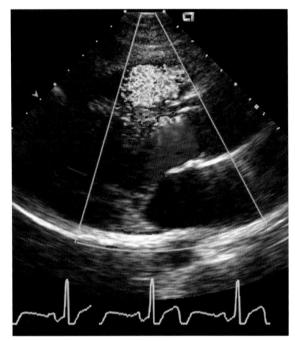

Figure 17–34.

The most likely diagnosis is:

A. Aortic coarctation
B. Bicuspid aortic valve
C. Ventricular septal defect
D. Ebstein's anomaly
E. Pulmonic stenosis

QUESTION 2

In the patient in Question 1, the maximum velocity in the CW Doppler signal is expected to be closest to which of the following?

A. 1 m/s
B. 2 m/s
C. 3 m/s
D. 4 m/s
E. 5 m/s

QUESTION 3

In evaluating a patient with complex congenital heart disease, you obtain the following image.

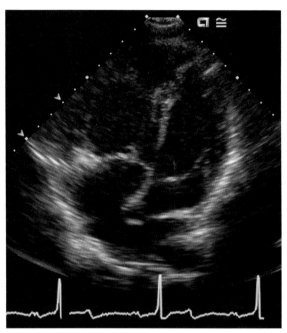

Figure 17–35.

Which feature in this image is most helpful in identification of the anatomic RV?

A. Triangular shape
B. Size relative to the other ventricle
C. Rightward and anterior location in chest
D. Wall thickness
E. Distance from apex to annulus

QUESTION 4

A 27-year-old woman undergoes echocardiography for a murmur during pregnancy and is found to have an ASD. The following measurements are made:

PULMONARY ARTERY	
Velocity	1.8 m/s
Velocity-time integral (VTI$_{RVOT}$)	36 cm
Diameter	2.6 cm
LV OUTFLOW	
Velocity	1.1 m/s
Velocity-time integral (VTI$_{LVOT}$)	25 cm
Diameter	2.2 cm
MITRAL VALVE	
Velocity-time integral (VTI$_{MV}$)	11 cm
Annulus diameter	3.3 cm

Calculate the pulmonic to systemic shunt ratio: _____

QUESTION 5

A 23-year-old woman with a history of surgery for repair of aortic coarctation in childhood is referred for echocardiography. Which of the following is most likely to be found in this patient?

A. Cleft mitral valve
B. Bicuspid aortic valve
C. Ventricular septal defect
D. Ebstein's anomaly
E. Pulmonic stenosis

QUESTION 6

A patient with an uncorrected Tetralogy of Fallot presents for echocardiographic evaluation. His blood pressure is 115/75 mm Hg, pulse is 76 bpm, and estimated RA pressure is 8 mm Hg. The following maximum systolic velocities are recorded with CW Doppler:

Aortic valve	1.3 m/s
Mitral valve	5.0 m/s
Pulmonic valve	3.6 m/s
Tricuspid valve	4.2 m/s

Calculate:

LV systolic pressure _____mm Hg
RV systolic pressure _____mm Hg
Pulmonary artery (PA) systolic pressure ___mm Hg
Velocity in the ventricular septal defect _____m/s

QUESTION 7

A 23-year-old patient with trisomy 21 is referred for echocardiography. On exam the blood pressure is 100/76 mm Hg, pulse is 88 bpm, and respiratory rate is 18/min. His hands show clubbing and cyanosis and the room air oxygen saturation is 79%. This echocardiographic image is obtained:

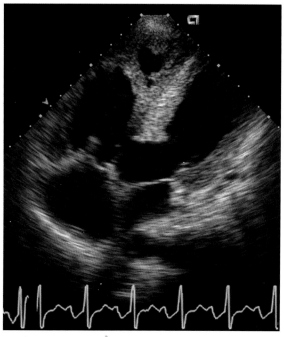

Figure 17–36.

The mitral regurgitant jet velocity is 4.7 m/s, the antegrade aortic velocity is 1.3 m/s, and the pulmonary artery systolic flow velocity is 0.9 m/s. Estimated RA pressure is 5 mm Hg based on normal size and respiratory variation in the inferior vena cava. There is only trace tricuspid regurgitation, and a CW Doppler tricuspid velocity could not be recorded.

Based on these data, estimated pulmonary systolic pressure is:

A. Not possible to determine
B. 120 mm Hg
C. 100 mm Hg
D. 80 mm Hg
E. 60 mm Hg

QUESTION 8

On a transthoracic echocardiogram in a 34-year-old woman with a previous atrial septal occluder device placement for neurologic events, a saline contrast study still shows contrast in the left heart within 1 to 2 beats of appearance in the right heart. TEE is requested to evaluate the placement of the device.

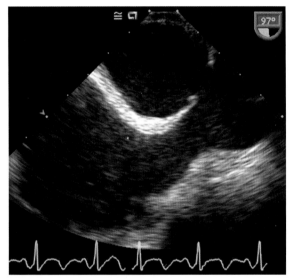

Figure 17–37.

Based on this image, which of the following is the most likely diagnosis?

A. Correct device placement with transpulmonary passage of contrast
B. Secundum ASD with an undersized occluder device
C. Anomalous pulmonary venous return
D. Sinus venous ASD
E. Normal device placement with expected LA spontaneous microbubbles

QUESTION 9

A 32-year-old man with no history of cardiac dysfunction is referred for echocardiography to evaluate a supraventricular arrhythmia. In the parasternal views an enlarged coronary sinus is noted. The most likely diagnosis is:

A. Coronary arterial-venous fistula
B. Persistent left superior vena cava
C. Secundum ASD
D. Ebstein's anomaly
E. Fontan physiology

QUESTION 10

Echocardiography is requested in a 24-year-old woman with complex congenital heart disease with palliative surgery in childhood. Her aortic and mitral valves show normal function with no significant regurgitation, but this Doppler flow tracing is recorded.

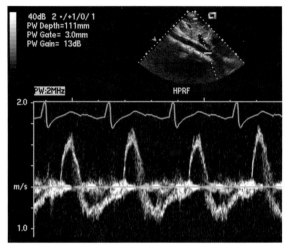

Figure 17–38.

This finding is most likely due to:

A. Severe tricuspid regurgitation
B. Anomalous pulmonary venous return
C. Aorto-pulmonary window
D. Aortic coarctation
E. Branch pulmonary stenosis

QUESTION 11

This echocardiographic image was obtained in a patient with congenital heart disease with a prior surgical repair.

The most likely diagnosis in this patient is:

A. Atrial septal defect
B. Cor triatriatum
C. Ebstein's anomaly
D. Tetralogy of Fallot
E. Transposition of the great arteries.

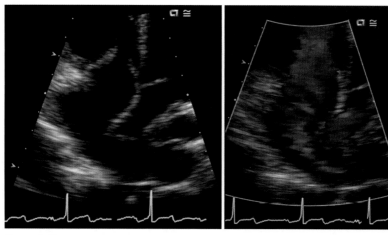

Figure 17–39.

QUESTION 12

This flow signal was obtained from the suprasternal notch window in a patient with operated congenital heart disease.

This flow signal most likely is due to a:

A. Blalock-Taussig shunt
B. Fontan conduit
C. Patent ductus arteriosus
D. Subclavian artery stenosis
E. Superior vena cava obstruction

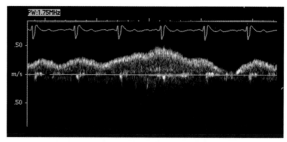

Figure 17–40.

ANSWERS

ANSWER 1: C

In this parasternal long-axis view, turbulent flow is seen in systole (mitral valve closed, aortic valve open) in the RV outflow tract. This is most likely due to a membranous ventricular septal defect. Aortic coarctation would result in high-velocity flow and turbulence in the descending thoracic aorta, which is not seen on this image. A bicuspid valve would be associated with an asymmetric aortic valve, systolic doming of the leaflets, and (possibly) an increased flow velocity in the ascending aorta. Ebstein's anomaly is associated with tricuspid regurgitation with a flow jet in the RA. Pulmonic stenosis would result in turbulent flow distal to the pulmonic valve, not in the RV outflow tract.

ANSWER 2: E

This patient has an asymptomatic small ventricular septal defect. The restrictive size of the defect is similar to a stenotic valve so that the velocity in the defect reflects the pressure difference between the systolic LV pressure (about 120 mm Hg with a normal systolic blood pressure) and RV systolic pressure (about 20 mm Hg in the absence of pulmonary hypertension). Thus, based on the Bernoulli $4V^2$ equation, the 100 mm Hg pressure difference between the LV and RV is equivalent to a velocity of 5 m/s.

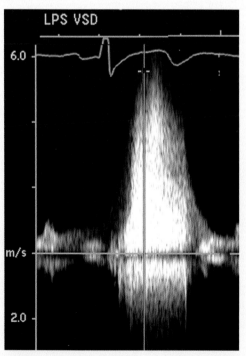

Pulmonary (and RV) systolic pressure should be normal in this patient with only a small volume of flow across the defect. Eisenmenger physiology, or equalization of systemic and pulmonary pressures, only occurs with larger VSDs that results in equalization of left and RV systolic pressures due to unrestricted flow between the ventricles in systole. Eisenmenger physiology typically occurs early in life and is associated with significant clinical symptoms and physical examination findings; echocardiography would not show turbulence in the RV outflow tract because the flow velocity across the defect is low in this situation.

ANSWER 3: E

This is an apical 4-chamber view in a patient with an interatrial baffle repair for transposition of the great vessels. The transducer is in the normal orientation at the apex, with the anatomic RV on the left and the anatomic LV on the right of the image. The RV is the systemic ventricle, with the interatrial baffle directing pulmonary venous return to the RV, which then ejects into the aorta. The atrioventricular valves go with the corresponding ventricles so that the anatomic RV has a tricuspid valve. The tricuspid valve annulus usually is slightly more apical than the mitral valve annulus (as seen on this image), so this is a reliable feature for identifying the RV. Occasionally, the tricuspid and mitral valve annulus are at the same level so that other features must be used for anatomic identification of the ventricular chambers. The presence of a moderator band is reliable for identification of the RV, but the degree of trabeculation is not reliable. The normal triangular shape, smaller size, and thinner walls of the RV are all altered when the anatomic RV serves as the systemic ventricle. With systemic pressures, the RV appropriately enlarges, hypertrophies, and changes shape, similar to an anatomic LV. The location of the RV and LV in the chest is abnormal in some patients with complex congenital heart disease and is not a reliable indicator of anatomy.

Figure 17–41.

ANSWER 4

Qp:Qs	2:1

The shunt ratio is calculated from the ratio of pulmonary flow (Q_p), measured in the RV outflow tract, and systemic flow (Q_s), measured in the LV outflow tract. At each site, cross-sectional area is calculated as the area of a circle:

$$CSA_{RVOT} = \pi(D/2)^2 = 3.14(2.6/2)^2 = 5.3 \text{ cm}^2$$

$$CSA_{LVOT} = \pi(D/2)^2 = 3.14(2.2/2)^2 = 3.8 \text{ cm}^2$$

Flow at each site then is calculated:

$$Q_p = CSA_{RVOT} \times VTI_{RVOT} = 5.3 \text{ cm}^2 \times 36 \text{ cm}$$
$$= 191 \text{ cm}^3 \text{ or mL}$$

$$Q_s = CSA_{LVOT} \times VTI_{LVOT} = 3.8 \text{ cm}^2 \times 25 \text{ cm}$$
$$= 95 \text{ cm}^3 \text{ or mL}$$

so that

$$Q_p : Q_s = 191/95 = 2:1$$

These calculations are consistent with a large shunt that likely is associated with right-sided heart enlargement and will require further evaluation and consideration of closure after pregnancy.

The transmitral volume flow rate should equal transaortic flow, in the absence of aortic or mitral regurgitation, and might provide an alternate site for calculation of systemic blood flow.

$$Q_{MV} = CSA_{MV} \times VTI_{MV} = 8.5 \text{ cm}^2 \times 11 \text{ cm}$$
$$= 94 \text{ cm}^3 \text{ or mL}$$

In this case, there is only a slight (1 mL) difference between transaortic and transmitral flow rates, which is within measurement error. Transmitral flow is rarely used for shunt ratio calculations because reproducible measurement of mitral annulus diameter is problematic.

ANSWER 5: B

In patients with an aortic coarctation, about 50% have a bicuspid aortic valve. Conversely, in patients with a bicuspid aortic valve, about 10% have an aortic coarctation, so that the presence of either of these conditions mandates a search for the other. A cleft mitral valve is most often associated with a primum atrial septal defect or an atrioventricular canal defect with a ventricular and atrial septal defect.

Ventricular septal defects are seen in several congenital conditions, such as tetralogy of Fallot and congenitally corrected transposition of the great arteries, or as an isolated anomaly, but are not associated with aortic coarctation. Ebstein's anomaly and pulmonic stenosis often accompany congenitally corrected transposition of the great vessels. Ebstein's anomaly of the tricuspid valve is associated with secundum atrial septal defect, arrhythmias due to pre-excitation and a bypass tract, and transposition of the great vessels.

ANSWER 6

LV systolic pressure	115 mm Hg
RV systolic pressure	79 mm Hg
PA systolic pressure	27 mm Hg
VSD velocity	3 m/s

LV systolic pressure is the same as systolic blood pressure (115 mm Hg) because there is no significant transaortic systolic gradient.

RV systolic pressure is calculated by adding the RV-to-RA systolic pressure difference to estimated RA pressure:

$$\text{RV pressure} = \Delta P_{RV-RA} + P_{RA} = 4V^2_{TR} + P_{RA}$$
$$= [4(4.2)^2 + 8)] = 79 \text{ mm Hg}$$

Pulmonary systolic pressure is calculated by subtracting the pulmonic valve gradient (from the estimated RV systolic pressure) because pulmonic stenosis is present:

$$\Delta P_{RV-PA} = 4V^2_{PA} = 52 \text{ mm Hg}$$

$$\text{PA pressure} = \text{RV pressure} - \Delta P_{RV-PA}$$
$$= \text{RV pressure} - 4V^2_{PA}$$
$$= 79 - 52 = 27 \text{ mm Hg.}$$

The velocity in the VSD reflects the systolic LV to RV pressure gradient.

Since

$$\text{LV pressure} - \text{RV pressure} = 115 - 79 = 36 \text{ mm Hg}$$

and

$$\Delta P_{VSD} = 4(V_{VSD})^2$$

then,

$$V_{VSD} = \sqrt{\Delta P_{VSD}/4} = \sqrt{(36/4)} = 3.0 \text{ m/s}$$

ANSWER 7: C

This apical 4-chamber view shows a large VSD, which has resulted in equalization of RV and LV systolic pressures as evidence by the similar size, shape, and wall thickness of the LV and RV (note the moderator band). If the patient had RV outflow obstruction (e.g., TOF), pulmonary pressures would be lower than ventricular pressure, but in that case there would be a systolic murmur on physical examination. Thus, this patient has Eisenmenger's physiology with equalization of systemic and pulmonary pressures --the cuff blood pressure and pulmonary pressure are the same. Bidirectional shunting across the ventricular defect results in severe arterial oxygen desaturation and clinical cyanosis. There is no murmur because the flow across the VSD is low velocity and unrestricted. Laboratory data likely include polycythemia. Given that pulmonary and systemic pressures are equalized with Eisenmenger's physiology, the best estimate of pulmonary pressure in this patient is the same as the systolic blood pressure or 100 mm Hg. When an adequate tricuspid regurgitant jet is not available, the velocity in the pulmonic regurgitation jet and the time to peak velocity in antegrade pulmonary flow may provide clues that pulmonary hypertension is present. The mitral regurgitant jet reflects the difference between the LV systolic pressure (100 mm Hg) and the LA pressure (about 10 mm Hg) with this 90 mm Hg pressure difference consistent with a velocity of 4.7 m/s.

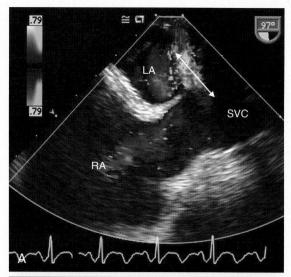

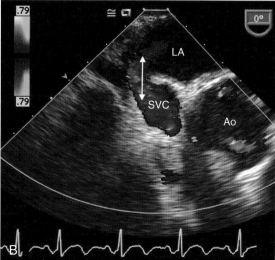

Figure 17–42.

ANSWER 8: D

This is the TEE bicaval view showing the RA, interatrial septum, and superior vena cava. The entrance of the inferior vena cava is also seen. The atrial septal occluder device is seen in the expected position and appears to completely cover the region of the fossa ovalis, where a secundum defect would be seen. However, adjacent to the superior aspect of the device, a discontinuity in the wall between the superior vena cava and LA is seen, suggestive of a sinus venous ASD. These defects also can occur near the inferior vena cava see Figure 17–42. Color Doppler confirmed bidirectional flow across this defect (A), and orthogonal views also demonstrated the defect (B).

By careful scanning between long- and short-axis views, the close relationship between the right superior pulmonary vein, sinus venosus defect, and superior vena cava was demonstrated. A saline contrast study was done once the defect was identified to confirm that this defect was the origin of the left-sided heart microbubbles. Transpulmonary passage of contrast would occur more than 3 beats after appearance in the right heart and could be confirmed by imaging a pulmonary vein during the contrast study. Anomalous pulmonary venous return without an associated sinus venosus septal defect does not result in right-to-left or bidirectional shunting (hence no contrast seen in the left heart). Although mechanical valves can cause left-sided heart microbubbles related to the impact of the valve occluders, spontaneous contrast has not been described with atrial septal occluder devices.

ANSWER 9: B

An enlarged coronary sinus most often is due to a persistent left superior vena cava. This is a variant seen in about 0.5% of normal individuals that results in an enlarged coronary sinus due to venous drainage via the coronary sinus into the RA. If needed, the diagnosis can be confirmed by saline contrast injected in a left arm vein appearing first in the coronary sinus, then in the RA; saline contrast injected in a right arm vein will appear in the RA but not the coronary sinus. A coronary arterial-venous fistula is a rare abnormality with drainage usually into a right-sided heart chamber; a dilated coronary sinus might occur but is unlikely. A secundum ASD results in RA and RV volume overload with chamber enlargement, but coronary sinus dimension is normal unless RA pressure is elevated. Ebstein's anomaly is associated with pre-excitation arrhythmias and is diagnosed based on apical displacement (>10 mm) of the tricuspid leaflet insertion, relative to the mitral annular plane. Fontan physiology describes the absence of a functional right heart with flow directly from the systemic venous return into the pulmonary artery, either via a conduit or an RA–to–pulmonary artery anastomosis. Although the coronary sinus may be dilated in this situation, the patient would have a history of cardiac surgery.

ANSWER 10: C

This is a Doppler recording of flow from the transthoracic subcostal view in the proximal abdominal aorta with normal antegrade systolic flow and abnormal holodiastolic flow reversal. Retrograde diastolic flow in the aorta may be due to any communication from the proximal aorta into a lower-pressure vessel or chamber; classically this finding is seen with severe aortic regurgitation. Other causes of aortic diastolic flow reversal include a patent ductus arteriosus and a systemic arterial to pulmonary arterial shunt such as a Blalock-Taussig shunt. This patient had pulmonary atresia and single-ventricle physiology with pulmonary blood flow supplied by a surgically created aortic-to-pulmonary window, which accounts for the flow pattern seen in the aorta. Severe tricuspid regurgitation causes systolic flow reversal in the inferior vena cava or hepatic veins. Anomalous pulmonary venous return may enter the inferior vena cava or RA junction and would show a typical low-velocity systolic and diastolic filling pattern. Aortic coarctation results in continued forward flow in the aorta in diastole, as well as an increased systolic velocity. Branch pulmonary stenosis results in a high systolic velocity and the pulmonary artery is not seen on this subcostal view.

ANSWER 11: E

This is an apical 4-chamber view, magnified to focus on the atrium and atrioventricular valves. The two-dimensional images show a linear echo across the atrial region with color Doppler showing laminar blood flow through this channel and then across an atrioventricular valve into a ventricle. These images are consistent with an interatrial baffle surgical repair (Mustard or Senning) for D-TGA. The baffle directs systemic venous return to the pulmonary artery via the anatomic LV and pulmonary venous return to the aorta via the anatomic RV. This corrects the pattern of blood flow to the pulmonary and systemic circuits but leaves the anatomic RV as the systemic ventricle. Adults with this surgical procedure are still seen in adult congenital centers, but the current approach to surgical repair for TGA is a great vessel switch procedure.

There is an apparent defect in the atrial septum because of the anatomy of the baffle repair, but there is no intracardiac shunt and no evidence for volume overload of the subpulmonic ventricle. Cor triatriatum is a partial membrane across the LA chamber, with normal ventricular and great vessel relationships. In Ebstein's anomaly, the anatomic tricuspid valve (the systemic atrioventricular valve in this case) is displaced apically, whereas this image shows the atrioventricular valve insertions at the same level. Tetralogy of Fallot includes a ventricular septal defect, an enlarged aorta, and RV outflow obstruction with RV hypertrophy, none of which are seen on these images.

ANSWER 12: B

This Doppler recording shows a continuous low-velocity (about 0.5 m/s) flow signal that peaks in late diastole to early systole but does not show an obvious relationship to the cardiac cycle. The flow signal seems to increase (beats 3 and 4) and decrease with timing, suggestive of respiratory variation. These findings are most consistent with a Fontan conduit with systemic venous return from the inferior vena cava directed into the right pulmonary artery (so the flow direction is toward the suprasternal notch). A Blalock-Taussig shunt is a connection from the systemic subclavian artery to pulmonary artery, so velocity would be higher (a higher-pressure drop from systemic to pulmonary artery) and flow would be directed away from the transducer. A patent ductus arteriosus results in continuous high-velocity diastolic and systolic flow into the pulmonary artery and diastolic flow reversal in the descending aorta. Subclavian artery stenosis causes a high-velocity systolic jet that may be mistaken for aortic stenosis if the location overlaps with the direction of the aortic flow signal. Superior vena cava obstruction results in a higher-velocity venous flow pattern directed away from the suprasternal notch transducer position.

MEDICAL LIBRARY
MORRISTON HOSPITAL

18 Intraoperative Transesophageal Echocardiography

STEP-BY-STEP APPROACH

Basic principles

- TEE is increasingly used to guide surgical and percutaneous cardiac procedures.
- TEE performance and interpretation occur simultaneously, with immediate communication of results to the physician performing the surgical or percutaneous procedure.
- More detailed information on intraoperative TEE is provided in the Otto Companion Series book Intraoperative Echocardiography: A Volume in Practical Echocardiography Series, edited by Don Oxorn, MD (Elsevier, 2011).

Key points

- ❏ Time constraints may require a focused examination.
- ❏ Altered loading conditions may affect evaluation of valve and ventricular function.
- ❏ Loading conditions should be matched on baseline and post-intervention studies.
- ❏ Urgent decision making based on TEE findings may be necessary.

- ❏ Limitations of the TEE data must be promptly recognized and communicated.
- ❏ Appropriate training and experience are needed for procedural TEE; at many institutions these TEE studies are performed and interpreted by qualified anesthesiologists.

Step 1: Review the pre-operative data

- For elective procedures, a complete diagnostic evaluation is performed prior to the planned intervention to ensure evaluation under normal loading conditions and to allow time for discussion and procedural planning.
- All pre-procedure images and diagnostic data should be reviewed, including coronary angiography, hemodynamics, cardiac MRI and CT imaging, as well as echocardiographic data.

Key points

- ❏ Intra-operative TEE provides:
  - confirmation of the diagnosis,
  - additional information on valve repairability,
  - a baseline study for comparison to post-procedure imaging,

- monitoring of LV function, and
- guidance for optimization of intravascular catheter and device placement.
- ❏ Unexpected findings on the baseline procedural TEE may require a change in the intervention, consultation with the referring cardiologist, or rescheduling of the procedure.
- ❏ In emergency situations, the baseline procedural TEE may be the primary diagnostic test; in this setting a complete study should be performed when allowed by time constraints.

Step 2: Consider effects of hemodynamic changes and surgical instrumentation

- Hemodynamic effects of sedation or anesthesia must be considered in the interpretation of procedural TEE imaging and Doppler data.
- Baseline and post-procedure data should be recorded at similar loading conditions, using volume infusion and pharmacologic agents, if needed, to match hemodynamic parameters.

Key points

- ❏ Assessment of hemodynamics and ventricular function is affected by:
  - positive pressure mechanical ventilation,
  - volume status,
  - myocardial "stunning" (when aortic cross-clamping is necessary),
  - effects of cardiopulmonary bypass, and
  - pharmacologic therapy.
- ❏ Basic hemodynamic parameters (heart rate and blood pressure) should be indicated on the recorded echocardiographic images to ensure matched loading conditions.
- ❏ When possible, cardiac output, filling pressures, and systemic vascular resistance also should be recorded with the TEE images.
- ❏ With cardiac surgery, TEE images will be affected by:
  - inversion of the LA appendage (looks like an LA mass) during mitral valve surgery,
  - reverberations and shadowing by intracardiac cannulas,
  - intracardiac air (Figure 18–1), and
  - electronic interference. (Figure 18–2)

Step 3: Baseline data acquisition

- A complete systemic TEE (see Chapter 3) is recommended when possible, but time constraints may require a limited study focused on the key diagnostic information.

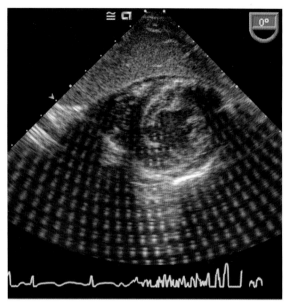

Figure 18–1. TEE in the operating room often is complicated by artifacts, such as the electronic interference pattern due to the use of electrocautery seen on this transgastric short-axis view. Diagnostic imaging should be performed when this artifact is absent as it may also affect the color Doppler signal.

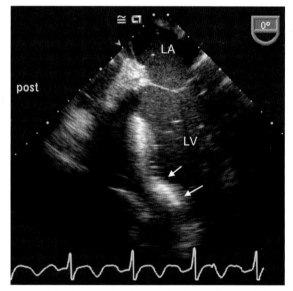

Figure 18–2. When weaning from cardiopulmonary bypass, TEE can assist in detection of intracardiac air. In this TEE 4-chamber view, isolated bubbles are seen in the LV chamber along with a denser area (arrows) due to an air collection in the apical aspect of the septum.

- Optimal diagnosis is ensured by use of a protocol with a consistent image sequence, and acquisition of images is obtained in standard TEE views.
- Images may be acquired either by:
  - obtaining all views from each transducer position (high esophageal, mid-esophageal, transgastric), first with imaging and then with Doppler, or

• evaluation of each anatomic structure by both imaging and Doppler in at least two orthogonal views—all four cardiac chambers, all four valves, both great arteries, systemic and pulmonary venous return, atrial appendage, and interatrial septum.

Key points

❑ As with any echocardiographic study, intraoperative TEE images should be obtained in standard long-axis, short-axis, 2-chamber, and 4-chamber image planes. (Figure 18–3 A, B, C)

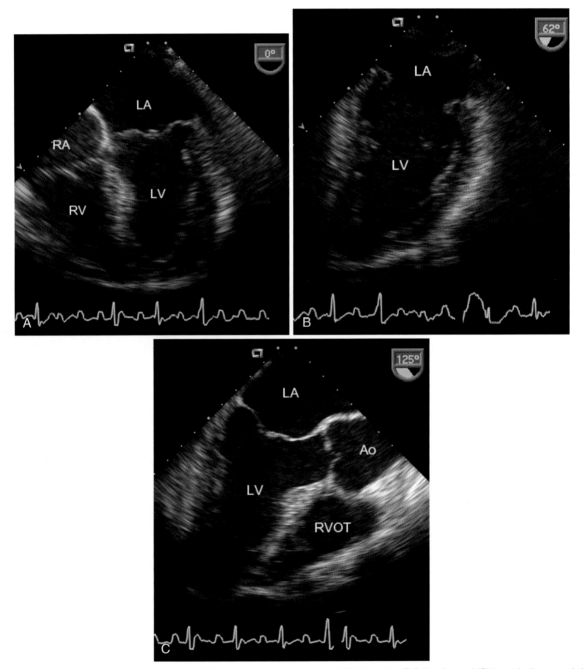

Figure 18–3. Whenever possible, the intraoperative TEE exam should start with standard (*A*) 4-chamber, (*B*) 2-chamber, and (*C*) long-axis views recorded at a depth to include the LV apex. Acquisition of these images takes only 1 to 2 minutes and allows evaluation of LV size, LV regional and global systolic function, RV size and systolic function, and allows a quick assessment of aortic, mitral, and tricuspid valve anatomy and motion.

- Color Doppler is helpful for evaluation of intra-cardiac flow patterns, particularly for evaluation of mitral regurgitation.
- Pulsed Doppler is useful for evaluation of pulmonary venous and transmitral flow patterns. The pulsed Doppler signal also may help in identification of anatomic structures when otherwise unclear.
- CW Doppler is helpful in selected cases but the possibility of a non-parallel intercept angle (and underestimation of velocity) must be considered due to the constraints on transducer positioning in the esophagus.
- Interference and technical artifacts that limit image quality may be reduced by re-positioning the transducer or pausing electronic devices while images are obtained.
- Standard instrument pre-sets, including transducer frequency, depth, gain, pre- and post-processing, and sector scan width may be adequate for some images, but adjustment often is needed during the examination.
- If the ECG signal is inadequate or subject to interference, cine loops can be acquired using a set time interval, instead of one- or two-beat clips, from the ECG.
- The structure of interest should be centered in the image, with depth and zoom adjusted to optimize the image.
- Color Doppler images should be recorded at a depth and sector width that just includes the area of interest (to optimize frame rate). (Figure 18–4 A, B, C)

Step 4: Post-procedure data acquisition

- After the procedure, TEE is repeated to assess the results of the intervention and to evaluate for potential complications and indicated text annotations on the acquired echo image.
- When possible, loading conditions on the post-operative TEE should be similar to the baseline study.

Key points

- The post-procedure TEE focuses on the views and Doppler flows needed to evaluate the effect of the procedure; obtaining data in similar views as the baseline study allows direct comparison of the images.
- With surgical procedures, the post-procedure TEE is performed after weaning from cardiopulmonary bypass and after restoration of hemodynamics similar to the baseline study.
- With percutaneous interventions, TEE data may be used continuously to guide the

procedure with repeat evaluations at each stage of the intervention.
- Instrument settings should be the same as on the baseline study to avoid differences due to technical factors, rather than to the procedure itself.

Step 5: Interpret and communicate findings

- Unlike a conventional diagnostic TEE, intraoperative and procedural TEE studies are interpreted and reported verbally simultaneously with image acquisition.
- In addition to the results themselves, the degree of certainty of each finding should be reported.

Key points

- TEE findings may prompt a change in surgical plans or additional procedures.
- If the findings are equivocal or images are low quality, this information should be communicated to avoid decision making based on inadequate data.
- Qualitative data often are adequate for decision making; when quantitative approaches are used, measurements and calculations that can be performed rapidly are preferred.
- TEE findings should be documented in the permanent medical record, as well as providing immediate results during the procedure.
- Intraoperative TEE images should be saved, as for any echocardiographic study, to allow comparison with future studies.

SPECIFIC CLINICAL APPLICATIONS

Monitoring left ventricular function

- Intraoperative TEE is useful for continuously monitoring LV function in high-risk patients undergoing noncardiac surgery and for evaluation of LV function after cardiac surgical procedures.
- Images of the LV allow monitoring of:
  - ventricular preload (LV volume),
  - global LV systolic function,
  - regional LV function, and
  - RV size and systolic function.

Key points

- In general, the size of the LV chamber reflects filling volume; monitoring allows optimization of preload.
- Small LV volumes with adequate filling pressures are seen with restrictive cardiomyopathy,

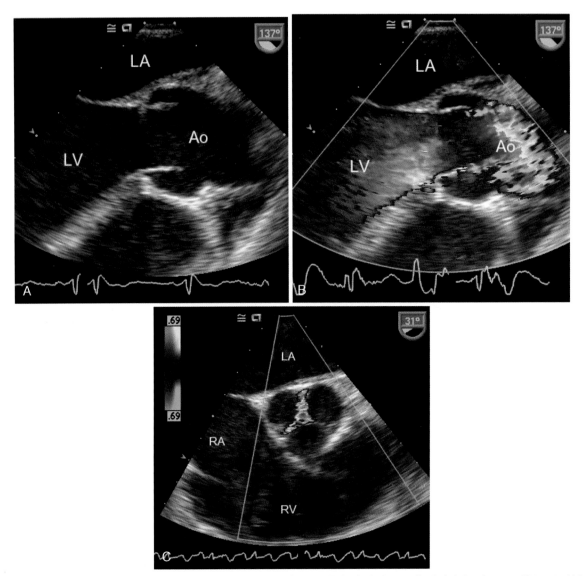

Figure 18–4. Color Doppler evaluation of aortic valve function is best performed with the depth decreased to include just the area of interest, which allows a higher frame rate. A, Both 2D valve images and color Doppler images in at least twp orthogonal views—(B) long axis and (C) short axis in this example—are recorded. This patient has only mild central aortic regurgitation seen in the short-axis view of the aortic valve.

pericardial constraint, severe RV dysfunction, or high contractility states.

❑ The transgastric short-axis view is often used for continuous monitoring of LV size and global and regional function, as it includes myocardial segments supplied by the three major coronary arteries. (Figure 18–5 and 18–6)

❑ TEE images of the LV apex are usually suboptimal, as the LV is typically foreshortened due to the constraints of transducer positioning in the esophagus.

❑ Changes in wall motion usually reflect ischemia; other causes include conduction defects, hypovolemia, and myocardial stunning after cardiopulmonary bypass.

❑ LV volumes and ejection fraction can be quantitated by tracing endocardial borders at end-diastole and end-systole in TEE 4-chamber and 2-chamber views, but the time needed for this approach limits utility for monitoring procedures.

❑ RV dysfunction may be due to ischemia, inadequate cardioplegia, or air embolism into the right coronary artery when separating from cardiopulmonary bypass.

Detection of aortic atheroma

■ Atheroma in the ascending aorta can be detected by TEE or epicardial scanning, which allows

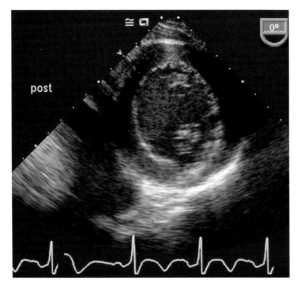

Figure 18–5. The transgastric short-axis view of the LV allows evaluation of overall LV size (reflecting preload or volume status), global ventricular systolic function, and regional dysfunction due to coronary disease.

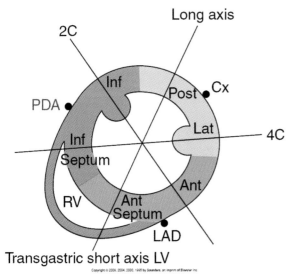

Transgastric short axis LV

Copyright © 2009, 2004, 2000, 1995 by Saunders, an imprint of Elsevier Inc.

Figure 18–6. The wall segments seen on the transgastric view, with the corresponding coronary artery supply, are shown on this schematic drawing. PDA, posterior descending coronary artery; LAD, left anterior descending coronary artery; Cx, circumflex coronary artery; Inf, inferior; Ant, anterior; Post, posterior; Lat, lateral.

placement of bypass grafts and aortotomy sites in areas of normal aortic tissue.

Key points

❐ The ascending aorta often is best visualized using a sterile epicardial transducer to ensure the absence of atheroma at the site of proximal coronary bypass graft anastomoses and at aortotomy sites.

❐ TEE imaging also may provide images of the ascending aorta, but atheroma lateral to the long-axis image plane may be missed.

Placement of coronary sinus catheter

■ With open surgical procedures, the coronary sinus catheter is placed under direct vision by the surgeon.
■ With minimally invasive surgical approaches, the coronary sinus catheter is placed percutaneously via the internal jugular vein using fluoroscopy and TEE to guide positioning of the catheter.

Key points

❐ Coronary sinus catheter placement for retrograde cardioplegia can be optimized using TEE guidance.
❐ Sometimes the valve of the coronary sinus impedes placement.
❐ Both placement in the coronary sinus and depth of insertion should be assessed by TEE.

Mitral valve repair

■ Baseline TEE allows precise delineation of mitral valve anatomy and the mechanism of regurgitation, which is helpful in planning the surgical repair.
■ Post-repair TEE allows evaluation of any residual mitral regurgitation and detection of complications.

Key points

❐ Mitral valve anatomy is best evaluated using rotational scanning from a mid-esophageal position. (Figure 18–7)
  • The central scallops of the anterior (A) and posterior (P) leaflets are seen in the 4-chamber and long-axis views.
  • The lateral (P1) and medial (P2) scallops of the posterior leaflets are seen in the bicommissural view at 60 to 90 degrees rotation.
  • Starting in the 4-chamber plane, the lateral scallops of the anterior (A1) and posterior (P1) leaflets can be seen by slightly withdrawing the probe, or tilting superiorly; medial segments (A3 and P3) are seen by advancing the probe or tilting posteriorly.
  • From the 2-chamber plane, all three scallops of the anterior leaflet are seen when the probe is turned toward the patient's right and all three scallops of the posterior leaflet are seen when the probe is turned leftward.
  • A transgastric short-axis view of the mitral valve, when possible, shows both leaflets.

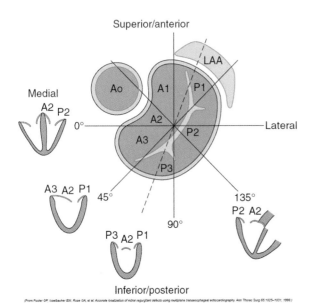

Superior/anterior

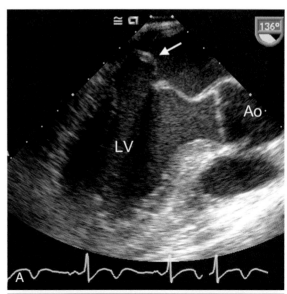

(From Foster GP, Isselbacher EM, Rose GA, et al: Accurate localization of mitral regurgitant defects using multiplane transesophageal echocardiography. Ann Thorac Surg 65:1025–1031, 1998.)

Figure 18–7. Reference view demonstrating the relationship of the TEE rotational imaging planes to the mitral valve with the probe positioned in the standard mid-esophageal position. A1, A2, A3, anterior mitral leaflet segments; P1, P2, P3, posterior mitral leaflet segments. *From Foster GP, Isselbacher EM, Rose GA, Torchiana DF, Akins CW, Picard MH: Accurate localization of mitral regurgitant defects using multiplane transesophageal echocardiography. Ann Thorac Surg. 65(4):1025–31, 1998.*

❏ 3D images of the mitral valve, showing the left atrial side of the valve, facilitate identification of prolapsing segments and flail chords and are recommended, when available.

❏ The direction of the mitral regurgitant jet is helpful in defining the mechanism of regurgitation. Severity of regurgitation is evaluated by (Figure 18–8 A, B):
  • vena contracta width,
  • CW Doppler signal intensity of regurgitant compared to antegrade flow,
  • pulmonary vein systolic flow reversal, and
  • proximal isovelocity surface area calculation of regurgitant orifice area (if needed).

❏ Post-repair, anatomic and functional results are evaluated using the same imaging views and Doppler measures as on the baseline study (Figure 18–9).
  • Loading conditions (esp. blood pressure) should be similar to the baseline study.
  • Use of the same imaging planes facilitates comparison of pre- and post-procedure data.
  • Doppler data are recorded with the same instrument settings to ensure detection of any residual regurgitation.

❏ The post-procedure TEE includes evaluation for the complications of mitral valve repair.
  • Persistent mitral regurgitation
  • Systolic anterior motion of the mitral leaflet
  • Functional mitral stenosis (Figure 18–10)
  • Ventricular systolic dysfunction

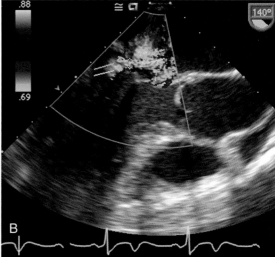

Figure 18–8. In this 56-year-old man undergoing surgical repair for mitral valve prolapse, (*A*) the baseline intraoperative TEE shows prolapse of the posterior mitral leaflet (*arrow*) in the long-axis view. Color Doppler imaging (*B*) confirms that posterior leaflet prolapse is the mechanism of regurgitation based on the presence of an anteriorly directed jet with a vena contracta width of 6 mm. Although this vena contracta width suggests only moderate regurgitation in this anesthetized patient, pre-operative quantitation was consistent with severe regurgitation in conjunction with elevated pulmonary pressures and clinical symptoms of exertional dyspnea.

Valve replacement

Step 1: Evaluate the patient and plan the surgical approach before the patient is in the operating room

■ In patients undergoing aortic or mitral valve replacement, anatomic and functional assessment should be completed before the patient is in the operating room.

■ Evaluation of the severity of valve stenosis by TEE is problematic for several reasons, so

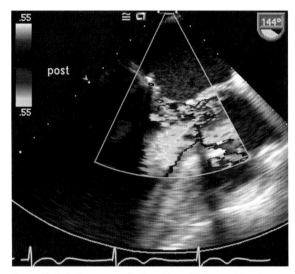

Figure 18-9. In the same patient as Figure 18-8, repeat imaging was performed after mitral valve repair with placement of an annuloplasty ring. Evaluation of mitral regurgitation was performed when blood pressure and heart rate were similar to the baseline study and using similar color Doppler instrumentation parameters. There was only trace detectable regurgitation.

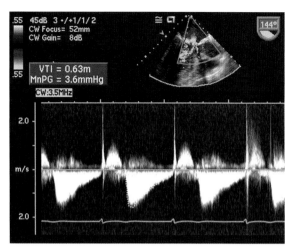

Figure 18-10. In the same patient as Figure 18-9, the antegrade trans-mitral flow was recorded with CW Doppler to ensure the absence of obstruction to LV inflow. CW Doppler also can be helpful for detection of residual mitral regurgitation, when present.

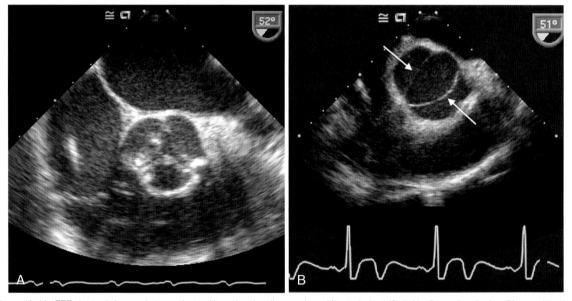

Figure 18-11. TEE short-axis images in two patients with aortic valve disease show: (*A*) a typical calcified tri-leaflet aortic valve in a 76-year-old patient with severe aortic stenosis showing marked restriction of systolic leaflet opening and (*B*) a bicuspid valve (*arrows*) in a 28-year-old man with no prior cardiac history who presented with acute aortic dissection.

intraoperative TEE decisions regarding stenosis severity should be avoided.
- Intraoperative severity of mitral regurgitation may transiently decrease relative to pre-operative severity due to the acute afterload reducing effects of general anesthesia.
- In patients with significant mitral regurgitation after attempted mitral valve repair, a second cardiopulmonary bypass pump run for valve replacement may be needed.

Key points

- ❏ A parallel alignment between the ultrasound beam and aortic velocity is rarely possible on TEE, resulting in underestimation of stenosis severity.
- ❏ Direct imaging and planimetry of aortic valve area is limited by reverberations and shadowing due to valve calcification; however, TEE aortic valve imaging is helpful for: (Figure 18–11)

- detection of a bicuspid aortic valve,
- assessment of the degree of valve calcification, and
- evaluation of aortic sinus and ascending aortic dilation.

❑ Mitral stenosis can be evaluated using the Doppler pressure half-time method because the TEE probe position allows a parallel alignment with antegrade transmitral flow.

❑ Planimetry of mitral valve area is sometimes possible on a transgastric short-axis view but may be inaccurate if the image plane is oblique or not at the leaflet tips; 3D imaging from a high TEE probe position allows better evaluation of mitral valve anatomy and is recommended, when available.

Step 2: Perform the baseline and intra-procedural TEE

- The baseline intraoperative TEE serves as a comparison to imaging after valve replacement.
- In addition to open surgical procedures, valve disease may be treated by transcatheter approaches with sequential TEE monitoring at each step of the procedure.

Key points

❑ Baseline images of LV global and regional function are recorded in standard views for comparison to post-procedure images.

❑ Valve anatomy and function are evaluated using standard imaging views and Doppler approaches, for comparison to post-procedure data.

❑ Transcatheter aortic valve implantation typically is monitored by TEE for:
- correct placement of the valve at the time of implantation, (Figure 18–12)
- evaluation of regurgitation (often paravalvular) after implantation, and
- evaluation of leaflet motion of the implanted valve.

❑ Mitral stenosis often is treated by percutaneous balloon valvotomy rather than by surgical valve replacement. (Figure 18–13)
- Transmitral mean gradient and pressure half-time valve area are monitored after each balloon dilation, along with invasive pressure measurements.
- Doppler evaluation for mitral regurgitation using standard approaches is repeated after each balloon dilation; an increase in regurgitant severity precludes further dilation attempts.

Step 3: Evaluate prosthetic valve function

- The post-procedure TEE allows detection of prosthetic valve dysfunction and assessment of LV systolic function.

- Knowledge of the structure and function of each prosthetic valve type is needed for correct interpretation of post-procedure data.

Key points

❑ A small amount of valve regurgitation is seen with a normally functioning prosthetic valve.

❑ Central regurgitation is common with a bioprosthetic valve; eccentric jets, with a variable pattern of regurgitation depending on valve type, are typical with mechanical valves.

❑ A small amount of paravalvular regurgitation may be seen but a large paravalvular leak may require immediate correction.

❑ Rarely, retained mitral leaflet tissue impairs normal motion of a mechanical mitral occluder.
   ❑ Recording images of leaflet/occluder motion and transvalvular Doppler flows in the OR provides a useful comparison for subsequent studies. (Figure 18–14 A, B, C, D)

Endocarditis

- Intraoperative TEE is essential in assessment of the degree of valve destruction and paravalvular involvement due to endocarditis.
- Post-procedure evaluation in the OR allows assessment of valve function after repair or replacement and provides a baseline for subsequent imaging studies.

Key points

❑ The baseline intraoperative TEE focuses on (Figure 18–15 A, B):
- presence and location of vegetations,
- mechanism of valve dysfunction,
- severity of regurgitation,
- paravalvular abscess, and
- detection of other complications (e.g., fistulas, pseudo-aneurysm).

❑ Extensive valve and paravalvular destruction in endocarditis often requires a complex surgical repair; knowledge of the surgical details is needed for correct interpretation of the post-procedure images.

Aortic dissection

- TEE is essential for accurate diagnosis of the presence and extent of aortic dissection; in urgent cases, diagnostic imaging may be performed in the operating room. (Figure 18–16 A, B)
- TEE distinguishes involvement of the ascending aorta (type A dissection) from a more distal (type B) dissection.
- Evaluation of aortic regurgitation is a key element of the examination because dilation of the sinuses

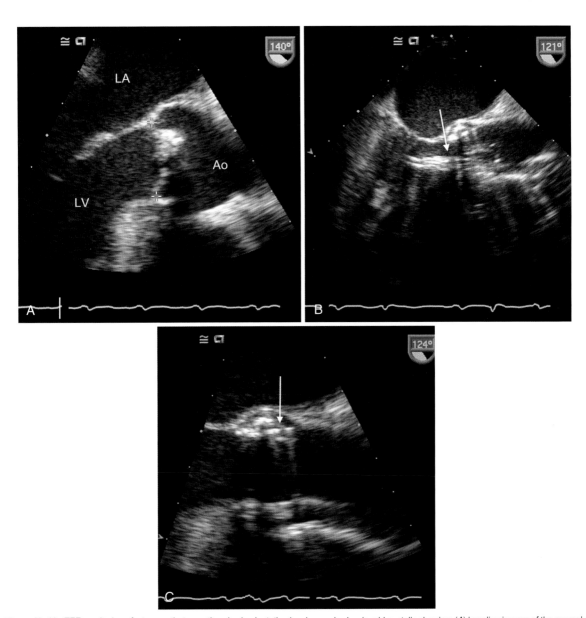

Figure 18–12. TEE monitoring of a transcatheter aortic valve implantation in a long-axis view in mid-systolic showing: (A) baseline images of the severely stenotic calcified valve, (B) the guiding catheter and unexpanded prosthetic valve (*arrow*) positioned across the valve, and (C) the stents of the prosthetic valve (*arrow*) now in the aortic position with relief of outflow obstruction.

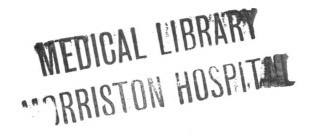
MEDICAL LIBRARY
MORRISTON HOSPITAL

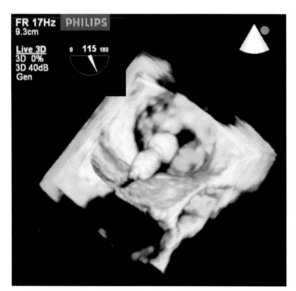

Figure 18–13. TEE 3D realtime imaging during percutaneous balloon mitral valvotomy shows the balloon catheter being positioned in the stenotic mitral orifice. *Images courtesy of Ed Gill, MD.*

or extension of the dissection into the valve can result in valve dysfunction.

Key points

❑ A complete examination of the aorta includes:
- Mid-esophageal views of the aortic sinuses and ascending aorta,
- Imaging of the descending thoracic aorta in a slow pull-back from the diaphragmatic level to the arch,
- High TEE views of the aortic arch, and
- Imaging of the os of the left subclavian artery (which delineates type A and type B dissections).

❑ In each view, long- and short-axis images are obtained (when possible).

❑ Color Doppler imaging improves identification of dissection flaps and provides visualization of flow in the true and false lumens.

❑ Aortic diameter is measured for each aortic segment at end-diastole at the white-black interface between the aortic lumen and vessel wall.

❑ The aortic valve is examined in standard long- and short-axis views, with color Doppler to detect and quantitate aortic regurgitant severity. (Figure 18–17 A, B)

❑ Pulsed Doppler evaluation of descending aortic flow is helpful in evaluation of aortic valve regurgitation.

❑ The coronary arteries are visualized, if possible, because the dissection flap may extend into the (most often, right) coronary ostium.

❑ Other indirect signs of aortic dissection include:
- Pericardial effusion (from extension into the pericardium, signaling impending aortic rupture), and
- LV regional wall motion abnormalities due to dissection extending into the coronary artery.

❑ After surgical repair, a persistent distal dissection flap is common.

Hypertrophic cardiomyopathy

■ Hypertrophic cardiomyopathy may be treated surgically by basal septal hypertrophy resection (myectomy) or may be treated percutaneously with catheter-based ablation of basal septal hypertrophy.

■ Echocardiography provides evaluation of the pattern of hypertrophy, baseline and post-procedure hemodynamics, and detection of procedural complications.

Key points

❑ Imaging allows assessment of the pattern and severity of septal hypertrophy, which is useful in procedural planning.

❑ Color Doppler localizes the level of outflow obstruction based on the location of the flow acceleration proximal to the aortic valve plane.

❑ CW Doppler alignment with the outflow tract velocity may be difficult by TEE; sterile epicardial scanning in the OR (transthoracic scanning for percutaneous procedures) is helpful if these data are needed for clinical decision making.

❑ After surgical resection, and at each stage of a percutaneous procedure, imaging and Doppler assessment of anatomic and hemodynamic results are documented.

❑ Systolic anterior motion of the mitral valve leaflet and accompanying mitral regurgitation may resolve after relief of outflow obstruction.

❑ Post-procedure imaging allows detection of complications, such as a ventricular septal defect, which is a rare complication of surgical myotomy-myectomy.

Ventricular assist devices

■ LV assist devices (LVADs) are increasingly used during complex cardiac procedures and long-term in patients with severe LV dysfunction.

■ The echocardiographer should be familiar with the specific type of LVAD being used; continual design advances require regular updates on implantation approaches and expected flow patterns. (Figure 18–18 A, B)

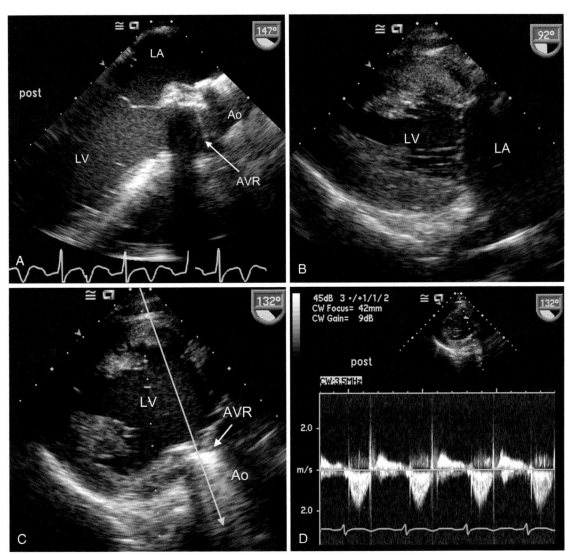

Figure 18–14. After placement of a mechanical aortic valve prosthesis, the long-axis view (A) shows the position of the valve with some post-operative thickening on the left atrial side of the valve, which is common. However, valve function is difficult to evaluate from this window because the LV outflow tract is shadowed by the prosthesis, limiting detection of aortic regurgitation, and it is not possible to align a CW Doppler beam parallel to LV outflow across the valve. B, From the transgastric 2-chamber view of the LV, the transducer is turned medially to (C) visualize the aortic valve replacement (AVR). With the Doppler beam aligned as shown in C, the CW Doppler signal of transvalvular flow (D) shows a normal velocity of 1.8 m/s and no aortic regurgitation. Although antegrade velocity may be underestimated due to a nonparallel intercept angle, these data are helpful in some clinical situations.

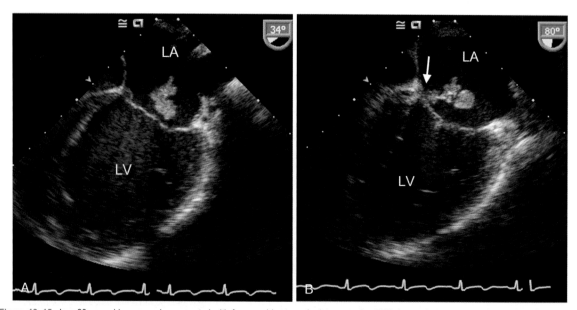

Figure 18–15. In a 28-year-old woman who presented with fever and bacteremia, intraoperative TEE demonstrates a vegetation on the left atrial side of the valve in systole in the 4-chamber view (*A*), but the attachment site of the vegetation and the mechanism of regurgitation are not well defined. Rotating the image plane toward the 2-chamber plane (*B*) now demonstrates the attachment of the 2 cm vegetation on the P2 scallop of the posterior leaflet. Color Doppler demonstrated a leaflet perforation adjacent to the vegetation. This information assisted in a successful mitral valve repair (not replacement) in this young woman.

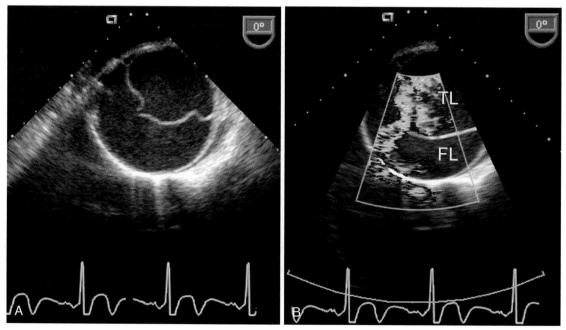

Figure 18–16. Intraoperative TEE imaging quickly demonstrates the presence of a dissection flap in the descending thoracic aorta (*A*) with color Doppler (*B*) showing a fenestration with flow from the true lumen (TL) into the false lumen (FL).

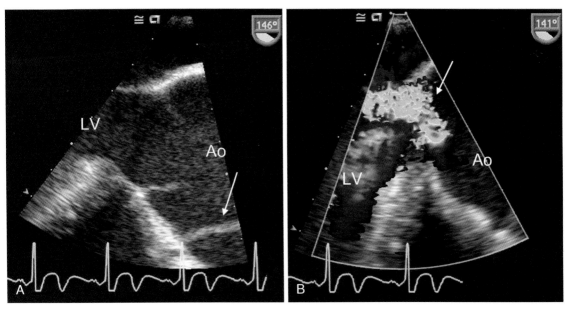

Figure 18–17. In the same patient as Figure 18–17, the ascending aorta is markedly dilated with a dissection flap (*arrow*), distinct from the open aortic valve leaflets in this image. Color Doppler (*B*) shows severe aortic regurgitation due to the combination of aortic dilation, dissection, and a bicuspid aortic valve.

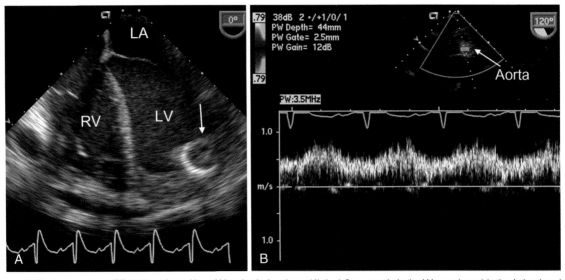

Figure 18–18. Intraoperative TEE in this patient with an LV assist device shows (*A*) the inflow cannula in the LV apex (*arrow*) in the 4-chamber view. In a high TEE long-axis view of the ascending aorta, a color Doppler signal is seen with pulsed Doppler confirming continuous flow from the LV assist device outflow cannula. Note that the aortic valve does not open in systole when an LV assist device is present.

Key points

❑ TEE evaluation is helpful during implantation of an LVAD for:
- Placement of inflow and outflow cannula,
- Ventricular volumes and systolic function,
- LVAD inflow and outflow velocities and flow patterns, and
- De-airing of the pump before activation.

❑ Typically, the LVAD inflow cannula is in the LV apex with the outflow cannula in the proximal ascending aorta.

❑ The aortic valve usually remains closed throughout the cardiac cycle because cardiac output now is directed through the LVAD; significant aortic regurgitation is a contraindication to LVAD placement.

❑ The LV is small (decompressed) when LVAD function is normal. LV contraction reflects the underlying disease process, with improvement due to disease resolution, not the LVAD.

❑ LVAD flow may be pulsatile or continuous (also called axial); each has a specific expected flow pattern.

❑ Complications of an LVAD that may be detected by echocardiography include:
- Intracardiac thrombus formation,
- Obstruction of inflow or outflow cannula due to positioning or thrombus,
- Regurgitation of LVAD valves (in some devices),
- Inadequate flow volumes, and
- Pericardial hematoma around the inflow cannula.

Heart transplantation

■ After orthotopic heart transplantation, intraoperative TEE allows evaluation of the anastomoses to the aorta, pulmonary artery, pulmonary veins, and vena cavae.

■ Intraoperative TEE provides a baseline assessment of LV and RV systolic function in the transplanted heart.

Key points

❑ Evaluation of LV and RV function in the OR is helpful in managing acute hemodynamics as the patient is stabilized after heart transplantation (Figure 18–19).

❑ Tricuspid regurgitation may be present early after transplantation if RV systolic dysfunction is present.

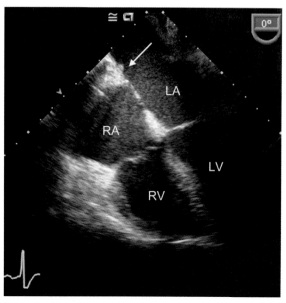

Figure 18–19. Intraoperative TEE was performed at baseline and after cardiac transplantation. This 4-chamber view shows the atrial anastomosis site (*arrow*). Other views were obtained to evaluate LV and RV systolic function and to measure antegrade aortic flow velocity.

Congenital heart disease

■ In patients undergoing surgery for congenital heart disease, it is essential that intraoperative TEE be performed by a skilled echocardiographer who is knowledgeable about congenital heart disease anatomy, physiology, and surgical approaches.

Key points

❑ Except for simple corrective procedures, such as closure of an isolated atrial septal defect, intraoperative TEE for congenital heart disease should be performed by echocardiographers with additional training in congenital heart disease.

❑ Additional information on intraoperative TEE for congenital heart disease is available in the Otto Companion Series book Echocardiography in Pediatric and Adult Congenital Heart Disease: A Volume in Practical Echocardiography Series edited by Karen Stout and Mark Lewin (Elsevier, 2011).

THE ECHO EXAM

Intraoperative Transesophageal Echocardiography

BASIC PRINCIPLES OF INTRAOPERATIVE TEE

- Establish diagnosis pre-operatively when possible
- The goals of the baseline TEE are to:
  - confirm the diagnosis,
  - provide additional information on repairability,
  - serve as comparison to post-procedure study,
  - assess LV and RV function, and
  - check for other abnormalities.
- Perform a complete study unless there are clinical or time constraints
- Record post-procedure images at similar loading conditions to baseline
- Communicate and discuss findings at time of study
- Report TEE findings in medical record and store TEE images

Recommended Image Acquisition for Intraoperative TEE

Window	Image Plane	Rotation angle (approx.)	Structure Visualized
Mid-esophagus	4-chamber	0°	LV, RV, LA, RA, mitral valve, TV, pulmonary veins
	Bicommissural	45–60°	LV, LA, mitral valve
	2-chamber	60-90°	LV, LA, LAA, mitral valve
	Long axis	120-140°	LV, LA , mitral valve, AV, Ao.
	Long axis, decreased depth	120-140°	AV and sinuses, mitral valve
	Long axis, higher in esophagus	120-140°	Asc. Ao
	Short-axis asc. ao.	0-30°	Asc. Ao, PA
	Short-axis aortic valve	30-60°	AV
	RV inflow-outflow	60-90°	RA, TV, RVOT, PV
	Bicaval view	80-110°	SVC, RA, IVC, atrial septum
Transgastric	Short-axis LV	0-20°	LV, RV
	Short-axis mitral valve	0-20°	Mitral valve
	2-chamber view	80-100°	LV, mitral valve, LA
	Long axis	80-100°	LV, mitral valve, AV
	RV inflow	80-100°	RA, TV, RV
Deep transgastric	4-chamber (with aorta)	0-20° with anteflexion	LV, LA, Ao, RV
Descending aorta	Short axis	0°	Desc Ao
	Long axis	90-110°	Desc Ao
Aortic arch	Long axis	0°	Arch, L brachio. vein
	Short axis	90°	Arch, PA

Modified from Shanewise JS, Cheung AT, Aronson S, et al: ASE/SCA guidelines for performing a comprehensive intraoperative multiplane transesophageal echocardiography examination: recommendations of the American Society of Echocardiography Council for Intraoperative Echocardiography and the Society of Cardiovascular Anesthesiologists Task Force for Certification in Perioperative Transesophageal Echocardiography. Anesth Analg 89:870–884, 1999.

Asc Ao, ascending aorta; Ao, aorta; arch, aortic arch; PA, pulmonary artery; PV, pulmonic valve; RA, right atrium; LA, left atrium; RV, right ventricle; LV, left ventricle; brachio., brachiocephalic; L, left; IVC, inferior vena cava; SVC, superior vena cava; LAA, left atrial appendage; TV, tricuspid valve.

SELF-ASSESSMENT QUESTIONS

QUESTION 1

A 54-year-old male presented to the emergency room 3 days ago with dyspnea and fatigue. Echocardiography demonstrated regional wall motion abnormalities in the inferior wall and RV free wall. In addition, color Doppler demonstrated a ventricular septal defect. On coronary angiography, there was severe three-vessel coronary disease with subtotal occlusion of the right coronary artery. He underwent coronary bypass grafting and repair of the ventricular septal defect and initially improved. Now he has a falling blood pressure and worsening hypoxia, and a repeat TEE was requested.

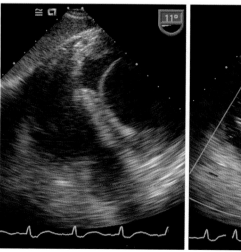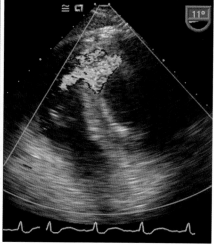

Figure 18–20.

These images are most consistent with:

A.   Papillary muscle rupture
B.   VSD patch dehiscence
C.   Mitral valve leaflet perforation
D.   Pericardial tamponade

QUESTION 2

A patient is sent for urgent aortic valve replacement and aortic root repair following diagnosis of an acute type A aortic dissection. The cardiothoracic surgeon requests guidance in placing cannula to retrograde deliver cardioplegia solution. You visualize and guide toward the:

A.   Coronary sinus
B.   Descending abdominal aorta
C.   Right coronary artery
D.   Left brachiocephalic vein

QUESTION 3

A 48-year-old with bioprosthetic aortic valve endocarditis is referred for repeat aortic valve replacement. Based on the pre-operative transthoracic images, there is significant aortic regurgitation. An intraoperative image is provided.

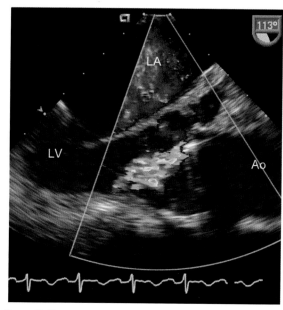

Figure 18–21.

Based on this image, you discuss with the surgeon the possibility of:

A. Mitral leaflet perforation
B. Aortic aneurysm
C. Pseudo-aneurysm
D. Vegetation

QUESTION 4

A 58-year-old presents to the emergency department with acute, severe chest and upper back pain and was diagnosed with an acute type A aortic dissection. A transthoracic image obtained in the emergency department and an intraoperative TEE recorded at the end of the surgical procedure are shown.

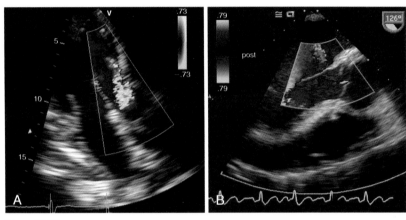

Figure 18–22.

The patient has undergone aortic root replacement with:

A. Resuspension of the aortic valve
B. Mechanical aortic valve replacement
C. Bioprosthetic aortic valve replacement
D. Transcatheter aortic valve implantation

QUESTION 5

A patient with heart failure underwent cardiac surgery with placement of a device. This systolic image was obtained at the end of the procedure.

The most likely device used in this patient was:

A. Prosthetic aortic valve
B. Biventricular pacing leads
C. Mitral annuloplasty ring
D. LV assist device
E. Intraaortic balloon pump

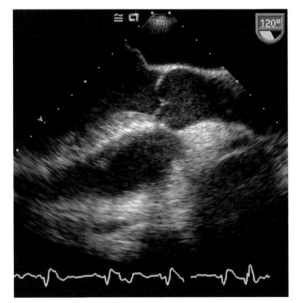

Figure 18–23.

QUESTION 6

In a 26-year-old woman undergoing surgical repair of a congenital intracardiac shunt, this transgastric image was obtained.

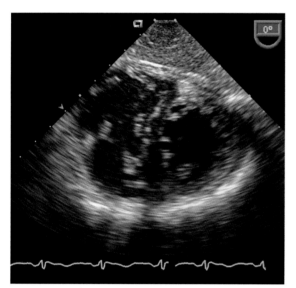

Figure 18–24.

The most likely diagnosis is:

A.   Atrial septal defect
B.   Ventricular septal defect
C.   Patent ductus arteriosus
D.   Fontan physiology
E.   Coronary arterio-venous fistula

QUESTION 7

During weaning from cardiopulmonary bypass in a patient undergoing coronary artery bypass grafting surgery, the following image was obtained:

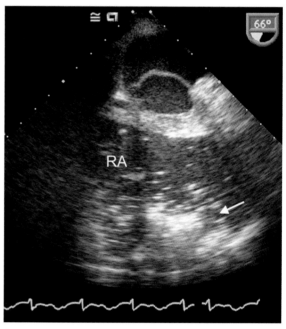

Figure 18–25.

The structure indicated by the arrow most likely is:

A.   Air
B.   Artifact
C.   Cannula
D.   Tumor
E.   Thrombus

QUESTION 8

On the TEE image, the structure between the arrows is the:

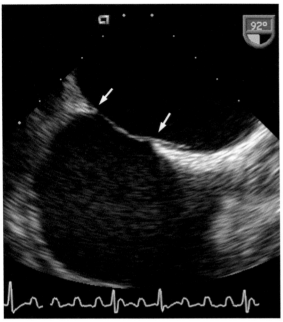

Figure 18–26.

A. Cor triatriatum
B. Crista terminalis
C. Eustachian valve
D. Fossa ovalis
E. Primum atrial septum

QUESTION 9

In this TEE image, the arrow points at:

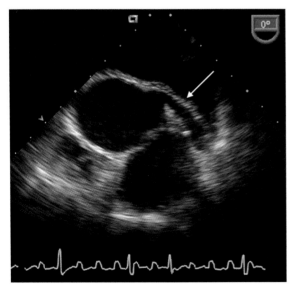

Figure 18–27.

A. LA appendage
B. Coronary sinus
C. Left main coronary artery
D. Right coronary artery
E. RA appendage

QUESTION 10

This Doppler tracing recording during an intraoperative TEE study shows blood flow velocities in the:

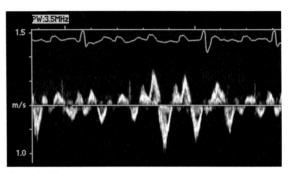

Figure 18–28.

A. Coronary sinus
B. Left atrial appendage
C. Superior vena cava
D. Coronary artery
E. Pulmonary vein

ANSWERS

ANSWER 1: B

This patient has had a complicated post-myocardial infarction course with multivessel coronary artery disease. The infarct-related vessel is the right coronary artery, which has led to regional wall motion abnormalities in the inferior wall, RV, and septum. Complications of the infarction include the ischemic VSD, which was patch repaired, in addition to coronary bypass grafting intraoperatively. The follow-up TEE images show persistent intracardiac shunting across the VSD, through the patch via color Doppler. Patch repair for ischemic VSDs is often less successful because the patch is sewn into friable, acutely injured tissue that can rupture easily. This patient subsequently underwent successful percutaneous closure of the ventricular septal defect.

Papillary muscle rupture is another potential complication of infarction. The posteromedial papillary muscle has a single coronary artery distribution, and ischemia and infarction of the muscle can lead to necrosis and rupture. The necrotic region shown in this case is in the septum, not the papillary muscle. Complications of papillary muscle rupture are severe mitral regurgitation. Mitral valve leaflet perforation is a complication of infective endocarditis and is seen as an abnormal regurgitant flow distant from expected commissural closure lines. Iatrogenic leaflet perforation is occasionally seen intraoperatively if the surgeon inadvertently nicks or injures a valve. If seen, the echocardiographer or anesthesiologist should draw attention to the surgeon so that additional repair may be performed, if needed. Pericardial tamponade is fluid in the pericardial space. Intraoperatively, the pericardium is open, and tamponade is not a concern. Post-operatively, echocardiography is useful to identify hematoma and focal tamponade.

ANSWER 2: A

Administration of retrograde cardioplegia solution is aided by TEE visualization of the coronary sinus for cannulation. The coronary sinus is best seen in the distal esophagus from the 4-chamber view, just as the transducer is at the gastroesophageal junction, and is seen as a vessel vertically crossing the middle of the scanning sector (Figure 18–29).

For minimally invasive surgery, smaller, steerable catheters have been developed to increase the success of coronary sinus cannulation, but still often require the aid of echocardiographic guidance in optimizing placement. Flow in the descending abdominal aorta is directed away from the heart and would not provide a conduit for retrograde cardioplegia. Selective cannulation of the right coronary artery would not

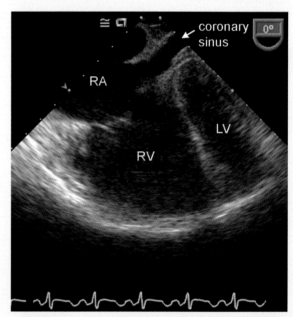

Figure 18–29.

provide enough myocardial distribution for the cardioplegia solution.

ANSWER 3: C

This TEE image shows the posterior aspect of the aorta with an echo-free space between the aorta and left atrium with to-and-fro flow (indicated by the double-headed arrow) between this space and the LV. These findings are consistent with a pseudo-aneurysm of the aortic-mitral intervalvular fibrosa, due to annular abscess with rupture into the LV. This explains the eccentric regurgitant jet that originates from the posterior aspect of the aortic valve annulus. Infection may extend into the adjacent mitral valve, but this image shows no evidence of a mitral valve vegetation, leaflet destruction, or perforation. Abnormal mitral regurgitation would be easily identified by TEE imaging and was not seen in this patient. The ascending aorta is normal in diameter with no evidence of an aortic aneurysm. The aortic valve replacement (AVR) casts a dense shadow anteriorly, obscuring the prosthetic valve leaflets and LV outflow tract (Figure 18–30).

ANSWER 4: A

The intraoperative image shows a normal-appearing aortic valve with thin leaflets and without supporting struts or a sewing ring to suggest either a mechanical or stented bioprosthetic valve. It is possible that a

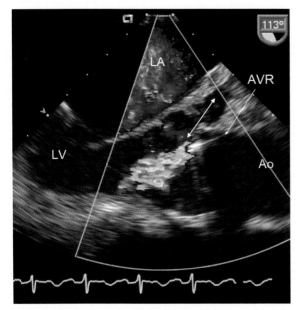

Figure 18-30.

stentless valved conduit may have been used in this case but it is more likely that the native valve has been re-suspended in the aortic graft. Transcatheter aortic valve implantation is used primarily for aortic stenosis, not regurgitation, and would show increased echogenicity in the peri-aortic region.

With aortic dissection, aortic regurgitation may be due to an intrinsic anatomic abnormality of the valve, such as a bicuspid aortic valve, or may be due to extension of the dissection into the base of the aortic valve. In this case, aortic regurgitation was due to prolapse of the dissected segment through a normal tri-leaflet aortic valve. The prolapsing tissue impeded leaflet coaptation, resulting in severe aortic regurgitation. Replacement of the ascending aorta with elimination of the dissection flap restored normal aortic leaflet closure. Thus, the aortic valve was re-suspended and had only mild regurgitation post-operatively.

ANSWER 5: D

This long-axis view in systole (the discontinuity in the ECG tracing indicates the timing of the still frame image) shows a closed aortic valve, as is typical with an LV assist device. The LV assist device pumps blood from an inflow cannula in the LV apex into an outflow cannula in the ascending aorta, thus bypassing the aortic valve, which remains closed during the cardiac cycle. Biventricular pacing leads are used to treat heart failure when there is a wide QRS indicating ventricular dyssynchrony, but the aortic valve would open normally. Neither a prosthetic aortic valve nor a mitral annuloplasty ring is seen on this

image. An intraaortic balloon pump would not be seen in this view, but aortic valve opening would be normal; the balloon pump inflates in the descending thoracic aorta during diastole to improve diastolic coronary perfusion pressure, with deflation in systole to reduce LV afterload.

ANSWER 6: A

This transgastric short-axis view of the LV and RV shows severe RV dilation with a normal systolic curvature of the septum, consistent with right heart volume overload. Of the lesions listed here, only an atrial septal defect with left to right shunting is associated with right heart volume overload. A ventricular septal defect is usually small in adults without associated chamber enlargement. A large ventricular septal defect would have resulted in Eisenmenger physiology by this age with equalization of right and LV systolic pressures; if this were present, the septum would be flattened in systole, as well as in diastole, due to pressure overload of the right heart. A patent ductus arteriosus leads to left heart chamber enlargement as the increased volume shunts from the descending aorta into the pulmonary bed and then left heart, without right heart volume overload. In Fontan physiology, the systemic venous return is directed to the pulmonary circuit without an intervening RV. A coronary arterio-venous fistula is rare and rarely results in right heart enlargement.

ANSWER 7: A

This view of the RA shows microbubbles in the right heart consistent with intracardiac air. The dense mass of echoes indicated by the arrow is consistent with an air collection at the superior aspect of the RA, near the RA appendage. Tumor or thrombus is unlikely given the clinical setting and the density of the echo signal. The appearance is not suggestive of an artifact. A cannula would show parallel smooth lines; the presence and position of a cannula could be confirmed by direct inspection in the operating room. TEE imaging is helpful in ensuring that all intracardiac air is eliminated before coming off bypass.

ANSWER 8: D

This is a bicaval view of the interatrial septum showing the thin fossa ovalis. The overlap at the superior (right side of figure) end of the fossa is typical and is the location where a patent foramen ovale is most often seen. Cor triatriatum is a congenital abnormality with a membrane across the LA chamber. The crista terminalis is a normal ridge of tissue between the smooth and trabeculated sections of the RA. A Eustachian valve occurs at the junction of the inferior vena cava with the RA, which is not seen in this view. The

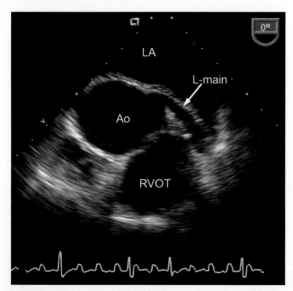

Figure 18–31.

the left main coronary artery arising from the left coronary cusp (Figure 18–31). The LA appendage is just lateral to the coronary artery. The coronary sinus would be seen in a 4-chamber view with posterior angulation or in a low TEE view of the RA and RV. The RA appendage is anterior to the aorta; in fact, a bit of the RA appendage is seen in this image anterior to the aorta and medial to the RV outflow tract (RVOT).

ANSWER 10: B

This Doppler tracing of flow from the LA appendage into the LA demonstrates regular low-velocity pulsatile flow consistent with atrial fibrillation (left side of tracing) or flutter (right side of tracing). Flow in the coronary sinus is challenging to record but would show a venous flow pattern. Flow in the superior vena cava and in the pulmonary vein would show a typical systemic venous flow pattern with systolic and diastolic filling velocities, and a small reversal of flow after atrial contraction. Coronary artery flow occurs predominantly in diastole.

primum atrial septum is the thicker segment adjacent to the atrioventricular valves.

ANSWER 9: C

This oblique short-axis view at the level of the aortic sinuses, just superior to the aortic valve leaflets, shows

INDEX

A

Abdominal aorta, proximal, 345-346, 345f, 347f
Abscess, paravalvular, 93, 300, 305-306, 306f
Accuracy, of echocardiography, 81-82, 82f
Acoustic impedance, 1, 2t
Acoustic shadowing, 16, 16f, 18-19, 337f, 340
Acute coronary syndrome (ACS), 147-149
Acute pericarditis, 147
Adult Congenital Heart Disease programs, 368
Advanced echocardiographic modalities, 65-80
 examination, 76t
 handheld echocardiography, 75
 intracardiac echocardiography (ICE), 72-74,
  73f
 intravascular echocardiography (IVUS), 74-75,
  74f
 myocardial mechanics, 70-72
 stress echocardiography, 65-69
 three-dimensional echocardiography, 69
Agitated saline contrast studies, 72, 72f
Air, intracardiac, 397f
Alfieri mitral valve repair technique, 280
Aliasing velocity, 239, 240f
American College of Cardiology/American
  Heart Association, 266, 319
Amplitude, 1, 2t
Anatomy, echographic terminology for, 21t
Aneurysms. *See also* Pseudoaneurysms
 aortic-mitral intervalvular fibrosa, 306, 307f
 atrial septal, 330, 331f, 338
 sinus of Valsalva, 364
Angina, 89
 unstable, 147
Angiosarcoma, 327
Ankylosing spondylitis, 350
Annuloplasty rings, mitral, 281, 281f
Aorta. *See also* Ascending aorta; Descending
  aorta; Descending thoracic aorta
 anatomy of, 21t
 atheroma, 332, 346f, 353
 identification, 366, 367f
 measurement, 25t, 218
 mid-ascending, 343f-344f
 pseudoaneurysm, 352-353, 353f
 transesophageal echocardiography of,
  347-350, 348f-350f
 transthoracic echocardiography of, 342-350,
  343f-347f
 upper limits of normal dimensions in, 348t
Aortic arch, 55, 345f-346f, 346
 color Doppler image, 16, 16f, 18-19
 suprasternal notch views, 33, 34f, 346, 346f,
  358, 358f, 362
Aortic coarctation, 372f, 379, 380f
Aortic dilation, 344f
 chronic, 350
Aortic dissection, 91
 ascending aorta in, 348f
 as chest pain cause, 147
 complications, 351-352
 descending thoracic aorta in, 349f

Aortic dissection *(Continued)*
 dissection flap identification, 350-351, 351f
 intraoperative transesophageal
  echocardiographic imaging, 404-406,
  408f
 with pericardial effusion, 359, 359f, 363
 type A, 413, 413f, 416-417
 type A differentiated from type B, 404, 408f
Aortic flow, antegrade, 246
Aortic jet velocity, 215-216, 216f-217f
 in atrial fibrillation, 220f
Aortic-mitral intervalvular fibrosa
 aneurysm, 306, 307f
 pseudoaneurysm, 412-413, 416, 417f
Aortic regurgitation, 50, 243-246
 antegrade aortic flow and stenosis evaluation,
  246
 aortic dissection-related, 352, 352f
 aortic root disease-related, 349
 chronic ventricular pressure evaluation, 246
 color Doppler imaging, 343
 continuous wave Doppler imaging, 11f, 245,
  245f, 262-263, 262f, 267
 descending aortic holodiastolic flow reversal
  in, 33
 determination of etiology, 243
 eccentric jet, 305f
 endocarditis-related, 303f, 308f
 evaluation, 218, 219f
 examination, 256t-257t
 flow, 245f
 holodiastolic flow reversal in, 345, 347f
 intraoperative transesophageal
  echocardiographic imaging, 400f
 with left ventricular dilation, 246, 246f
 regurgitant severity evaluation, 52f, 243
 regurgitant volume calculation, 241f
 retrograde flow, 361, 361f, 364-365
 severity evaluation, 242-245
 severity quantification, 257f
 stroke volume calculation, 263, 267
 volume overload evaluation, 246
Aortic root, 26
 anterior-posterior motion, 104-105, 105f
 components, 342
 dilation, 91
 parasternal window views, 343, 343f
 transesophageal echocardiographic imaging,
  51f, 347-348
Aortic sinus, calculation of dimensions, 348t
Aortic stenosis, 215-219
 with aortic regurgitation, 218, 246
 with chronic pressure overload, 218-219, 219f
 continuous wave Doppler imaging, 11f
 dobutamine stress echocardiography in,
  231-232, 231t, 236-237
 etiology determination, 215
 examination, 227t-228t
 M-mode tracing, 234, 238
 severity evaluation, 215-217, 231-232, 231t,
  235-237, 235f-236f
 transesophageal echocardiographic short axis
  view, 403f
Aortic valve(s). *See also* Bicuspid aortic valves;
  Bioprosthetic aortic valves
 anatomy and function, 21t, 348-349
 area calculation (AVA), 217, 218f

Aortic valve(s) *(Continued)*
 bicuspid, 404
 calcified, 215, 230, 235, 340
 cusps, 38, 38f, 41
 endocarditis of, 307f
 imaging artifacts, 8f
 sclerosis of, 180, 180f
 transesophageal echocardiographic evaluation,
  50-52, 51f
 two-dimensional guided M-mode imaging, 25f
 vegetations on, 300
 zoom mode imaging, 26, 26f
Aortic valve leaflets
 fluttering of, 25f
 trileaflet, 231, 236
 trileaflet, calcified, 403f
 trileaflet, parasternal short axis view, 28f
Aortic valve replacement. *See also* Bioprosthetic
  aortic valves; Prosthetic aortic valves
 intraoperative transesophageal
  echocardiography in, 402
 postoperative thickening, 407f
 with transcatheter implantation, 404, 405f,
  416-417
Apical "ballooning", 178
Apical biplane method
 for ejection fraction calculation, 168, 169f
 for left ventricular volume calculation, 101f
Apical four-chamber view, in dilated
  cardiomyopathy, 325f
Apical hypokinesis, 148f
Apical shadowing, 73f
Apical window views, 29-32
 in congenital heart disease in adults, 370, 371f
 four-chamber views, 29-31, 29f-31f
 long axis views, 29, 30f
 two-chamber views, 29-31, 30f
Arrhythmias
 dobutamine-related, 145
 myocardial infarction-related, 149
Arrhythmogenic right ventricular dysplasia
  (ARVD), 178
Artifacts
 in ascending aorta, 348
 common causes, 5
 Doppler, 11-12, 12t
 in intraoperative transesophageal
  echocardiography, 397f
 minimization, 11f
 mirror image, 12
 reflection, 5
 refraction, 5
 reverberation, 6f, 323, 359, 359f, 363
 shadow, 5, 11-12
 in tricuspid regurgitant jet velocity, 11f
 in two-dimensional imaging, 16, 19
Ascending aorta, 26f, 52f, 92, 94
 in aortic stenosis, 218
 atheroma, 400-401
 Dacron tube replacement, 353f
 dilated, 351f
 proximal, parasternal long axis view, 343f
 relationship to superior vena cava, 373
 transesophageal echocardiographic imaging,
  347f-348f
Atheroma, aortic, 332, 353, 354f
Atrial appendage flow, 48f

Page numbers followed by "f" indicate figures,
and "t" indicate tables.

419

MEDICAL LIBRARY
MORRISTON HOSPITAL